HANDBOOK OF
DIAGNOSTIC TESTS

SECOND EDITION

HANDBOOK OF
DIAGNOSTIC TESTS

SECOND EDITION

Springhouse Corporation
Springhouse, Pennsylvania

STAFF

Vice President
Matthew Cahill

Editorial Director
Darlene Cooke

Clinical Director
Judith Schilling McCann, RN, MSN

Art Director
John Hubbard

Managing Editor
H. Nancy Holmes

Clinical Project Manager
Carla M. Roy, RN, BSN, CCRN

Clinical Editors
Joanne M. Bartelmo, RN, MSN, CCRN;
Jill Curry, RN, BSN, CCRN; Collette Bishop
Hendler, RN, CCRN; Lori Musolf Neri, RN,
MSN, CCRN; Tracy L. Yeomans, RN, BSN, CCRN

Editors
Marcia Andrews, Peter H. Johnson, Vijay
S. Kothare, Doris Weinstock

Copy Editors
Brenna H. Mayer (manager), Karen C.
Comerford, Mary T. Durkin, Gretchen Fee,
Barbara Hodgson, Barbara Long, Pamela
Wingrod

Designers
Arlene Putterman (associate art director),
Linda Franklin (project manager), Joseph
John Clark, Donna S. Morris, Jeff Sklarow

Cover Illustrator
Joseph D. Fiedler

Manufacturing
Deborah Meiris (director), Patricia K.
Dorshaw (manager), Otto Mezei (book
production manager)

Typography
Diane Paluba (manager), Joyce Rossi
Biletz, Valerie Molettiere

Editorial Assistants
Beverly Lane, Marcia Mills, Liz Schaeffer

Indexer
Sara Spofford, RN

 A member of the Reed Elsevier plc group

Library of Congress Cataloging-in-Publication Data

Handbook of diagnostic tests — 2nd ed.
  p. cm.
  Rev ed of: Professional handbook of diagnostic tests. ©1995.
  Includes bibliographical references and index.
  1. Diagnosis — Handbooks, manuals, etc. I. Springhouse Corporation. II. Professional handbook of diagnostic tests.
  [DNLM: 1. Laboratory Techniques and Procedures handbooks. 2. Laboratory Techniques and Procedures nurses' instruction. 3. Diagnostic Imaging handbooks. 4. Diagnostic Imaging nurses' instruction. QY 39 H2368 1999]
RC71.P76 1999
616.07'54—dc21
DNLM/DLC   98-51301
ISBN 0-87434-982-6 (alk. paper)   CIP

CONTENTS

ix   *Contributors and Consultants*
xi   *Foreword*

Part One   **KEY DIAGNOSTIC FINDINGS IN MAJOR DISORDERS**   **1**

Part Two   **DIAGNOSTIC TESTS**   **83**

Chapter 1   **HEMATOLOGY AND COAGULATION TESTS**   **84**

   85   Red blood cells
   92   Hemoglobin
  102   White blood cells
  107   Platelet activity
  113   Coagulation

Chapter 2   **BLOOD CHEMISTRY TESTS**   **127**

  129   Arterial blood gases
  132   Electrolytes
  141   Cardiac enzymes and proteins
  145   Hepatic enzymes and proteins
  153   Pancreatic enzymes
  155   Special enzymes
  166   Lipids and lipoproteins
  173   Proteins and protein metabolites
  182   Pigments
  184   Carbohydrates

Chapter 3   **HORMONE TESTS**   **195**

  196   Pituitary hormones
  214   Thyroid and parathyroid hormones
  224   Adrenal and renal hormones
  232   Pancreatic and gastric hormones
  236   Gonadal hormones
  240   Placental hormones

Chapter 4   **VITAMIN AND TRACE ELEMENT TESTS**   **243**

  244   Vitamins
  250   Trace elements

CHAPTER 5 IMMUNOLOGIC TESTS 253

255 Immunohematology
264 General cellular function
269 General humoral function
277 Autoantibodies
290 Viruses
301 Bacteria and fungi
310 Miscellaneous tests

Chapter 6 URINE TESTS 319

321 Urinalysis
329 Enzymes
334 Hormones
341 Metabolites
351 Proteins and protein metabolites
361 Pigments
369 Sugars, ketones, and mucopolysaccharides
374 Vitamins
376 Minerals

Chapter 7 ADDITIONAL SPECIMEN TESTS 383

384 Respiratory system
387 Gastrointestinal system
402 Reproductive system
421 Miscellaneous tests

Chapter 8 CULTURES 437

438 General cultures
453 Genital cultures

Chapter 9 BIOPSY 459

460 Respiratory system
463 Gastrointestinal system
467 Reproductive system
472 Skeletal system
479 Other organ-specific biopsies

Chapter 10 ENDOSCOPY 489

490 Respiratory system
496 Gastrointestinal system
505 Reproductive system
508 Skeletal system

Chapter 11   ULTRASONOGRAPHY   513

514   Cardiovascular system
524   Gastrointestinal system
531   Miscellaneous tests

Chapter 12   RADIOGRAPHY   537

539   Neurologic system
545   Eye
548   Respiratory system
558   Cardiovascular system
562   Gastrointestinal system
583   Genitourinary system
604   Reproductive system
607   Skeletal system
611   Miscellaneous tests

Chapter 13   COMPUTED TOMOGRAPHY AND MAGNETIC RESONANCE IMAGING   615

616   Neurologic system
621   Gastrointestinal system
625   Musculoskeletal system
631   Miscellaneous tests

Chapter 14   NUCLEAR MEDICINE SCANS   639

640   Thyroid
643   Respiratory system
646   Cardiovascular system
651   Miscellaneous tests

Chapter 15   MONITORING AND CATHETERIZATION   665

666   Fetal monitoring
671   Neurologic monitoring
679   Cardiac monitoring and catheterization

Chapter 16   SPECIAL FUNCTION TESTS   709

710   Eyes and vision
716   Ears and hearing
723   Gastrointestinal function
726   Renal function
733   Miscellaneous tests

APPENDICES AND INDEX   745

746   *Appendix A: Normal laboratory test values*
748   *Appendix B: Normal and abnormal serum drug levels*
751   *Appendix C: Illustrated guide to home testing*
764   *Index*

CONTRIBUTORS AND CONSULTANTS

Deborah Becker, RN, MSN, CCRN, CRNP
Lecturer
University of Pennsylvania School of
   Nursing
Philadelphia

Susan J. Brown-Wagner, RN, MSN, CRNP,
  AOCN
Director, Oncology Service Line
Scottsdale (Ariz.) Healthcare

Lawrence Carey, BS, PharmD
Clinical Pharmacist Coordinator
Jefferson Home Infusion Service
Philadelphia

Joan T. Converse, MA, CLS(NCA), MT(ASCP)
MLT Program Director, Clinical
   Biochemistry Education
Mayo Medical Center
Rochester, Minn.

Kathleen Ellstrom, RN, PhD(C), CS
Pulmonary Clinical Nurse Specialist
University of California, Los Angeles

Harriet W. Ferguson, RN,C, MSN, EdD
Associate Professor, Department of
   Nursing
Temple University
Philadelphia

Ellie Z. Franges, RN, MSN, CCRN, CNRN
Director, Neuroscience Services
Sacred Heart Hospital
Allentown, Pa.

Geriann B. Gallagher, ND, APRN
Gerontological Nurse Practitioner
Advanced Practice Nursing Associates
Middletown, Conn.

Peggi Guenter, RN, PhD, CNSN
Editor-in-Chief, *Nutrition in Clinical*
   Practice
American Society for Parenteral and
   Enteral Nutrition
Silver Spring, Md.

Michél E. Lloyd, MT(ASCP), SBB
Technical Coordinator, Blood Bank
St. Luke's Hospital
Bethlehem, Pa.

Dawna Martich, RN, MSN
Clinical Manager
University Family Practice Associates, Inc.
Moon Township, Pa.

Kambiz Motamedi, MD
Resident in Diagnostic Radiology
Albert Einstein Medical Center
Philadelphia

Lori Musolf Neri, RN, MSN, CCRN
Clinical Instructor, University of
   Pennsylvania and Villanova (Pa.)
   University
Philadelphia
Staff Nurse, North Penn Hospital
Lansdale, Pa.

Gladys Purvis, RN, MSN, CCRN
Clinical Leader, Coronary Care Unit
Abington (Pa.) Memorial Hospital

Dorothy L. Rhoads, RN,C, MSN, CRNP
Ob/Gyn Nurse Practitioner
G.C.S.F. Ob/Gyn Associates
Willow Grove, Pa.

Teresa A. Richardson, BS, MT
Medical Technologist
St. Luke's Hospital
Quakertown, Pa.

Mary Jean Rutherford, MEd, MT(ASCP), SC
Program Director, Clinical Laboratory
   Science Programs
Arkansas State University
State University

Sylvia N. Schneider, RN, BSN
Staff Nurse
Graduate Hospital
Philadelphia

Karen E. Tumelty, RN, BSN
Nurse Clinician
Cooper Institute for Reproductive
   Hormonal Disorders, Inc.
Marlton, N.J.

FOREWORD

Medical knowledge at the end of the twentieth century continues to grow at an exponential rate. Keeping up with this growth is a daunting challenge for the busy clinician. The new edition of the *Handbook of Diagnostic Tests* provides an efficient way for all health care professionals to review the latest advances in medical diagnosis and treatment.

In clinical medicine, choosing the appropriate diagnostic tests and interpreting the results knowledgeably is often the difference between success and failure, especially when treating seriously ill patients. The *Handbook of Diagnostic Tests,* Second Edition, provides the latest information about commonly used tests in a format that is clear, concise, and easy to access.

Many of the newer diagnostic tests have had a dramatic effect on patient care. Changes in the diagnostic approach to patients suspected of having acute appendicitis provide a good example of how improvements in technology and increasing skill in interpreting imaging studies have changed patient care. Before abdominal and pelvic ultrasound examinations and computed tomography (CT) scanning were generally available, surgeons operating on a presumed diagnosis of appendicitis had an 80% diagnostic accuracy. Twenty percent of surgeries for possible appendicitis revealed no abnormalities, nor did they indicate that some other process (such as diverticulitis, pelvic inflammatory disease, mesenteric adenitis, and Crohn's disease) was responsible for the patient's symptoms. However, improving the preoperative diagnostic accuracy by waiting until symptoms become more definite risks a ruptured appendix. Today, the ready availability of abdominal ultrasound and CT scanning has greatly changed the management of these patients. When clinical findings are equivocal, an immediate ultrasound can be obtained. When the ultrasound suggests appendicitis, surgery is often done at an earlier stage in the disease than it might have otherwise. If the ultrasound examination is not diagnostic, a CT scan may clarify the diagnosis; sometimes it diagnoses appendicitis when the ultrasound is normal. With this approach, the diagnostic accuracy in patients with acute appendicitis is over 95% instead of 80%, meaning that thousands of patients every year can avoid unnecessary surgery and can sooner undergo safer and more appropriate therapy.

The *Handbook of Diagnostic Tests,* Second Edition, is a valuable guide to understanding how and when these newer diagnostic approaches are used and how to interpret the results. The book is divided into two sections. Part One presents the key diagnostic findings for more than 500 disorders arranged alphabetically. Besides providing a quick cross-reference linking specific disorders to tests, this section provides a sound foundation that the practitioner can use in developing a diagnostic and therapeutic strategy.

Part Two provides specific details about hundreds of diagnostic tests in a clear, consistent, and easy-to-use format. In addition to a general description of each test, its purpose, patient preparation and teaching, and any special equipment needed to obtain a specimen or perform the test, the format covers the steps of the procedure, patient care during it and afterward, precautions to ensure test quality and avoid patient complications, normal results, the clinical significance of abnormal results, and the factors that can interfere with test accuracy.

The book's content ranges over the entire scope of laboratory tests and diagnostic procedures that are important to clinicians. The first five chapters discuss tests done on blood samples, including blood chemistry, hematology, coagulation, and endocrine and immunologic assays. Chapters 6 through 8 cover urine, sputum, and bacteriologic testing. Chapter 9 discusses biopsies, and chapter 10 explains endoscopic procedures. The next three chapters convey the latest information on imaging modalities, including the use of ultrasound, plain X-rays, CT scanning, magnetic resonance imaging, and nuclear medicine scanning. Chapter 15 discusses clinical monitoring and catheterization studies, and the final chapter provides information about special function tests, including those for vision and hearing, gastric acidity, and renal function. What's more, tests within most chapters are logically organized by body system, making it easy to find relevant information.

New features in the second edition include a thorough review and updating of all tests and the addition of more than 35 tests, including new ones for cancer, Alzheimer's disease, deep-vein thrombosis, and osteoporosis, and a new type of mammography. Every test now includes a list of interfering factors, such as specific foods and drugs, that can skew test results. Also added are "clinical alert" icons that remind the practitioner of important clinical signs to watch for in certain procedures or point out when special testing procedures may be helpful. Three extremely useful new appendices include a quick-reference listing of normal laboratory values, normal and abnormal test levels for major therapeutic drugs, and a whole section of teaching aids for the most-used home self-tests.

The *Handbook of Diagnostic Tests,* Second Edition, is a comprehensive guide that provides essential information about hundreds of laboratory tests and diagnostic procedures. The information is current and presented with a practical, hands-on approach. I am sure it will prove to be a valuable reference source for all health care professionals, including nurses, medical technologists, radiographers, physician assistants, respiratory therapists, and students.

John Castagna, MD, FACS
General Surgeon, Torrance (Calif.) Memorial Hospital
Clinical Assistant Professor of Surgery,
University of California at Los Angeles
Specialist in advanced laparoscopic procedures

KEY DIAGNOSTIC FINDINGS IN MAJOR DISORDERS

Abbreviations used in Part One

The following list shows abbreviations that are used throughout Part One.

ABG	arterial blood gas
ALT	alanine aminotransferase
APTT	activated partial thromboplastin time
AST	aspartate aminotransferase
BUN	blood urea nitrogen
CBC	complete blood count
CK	creatine kinase
CSF	cerebrospinal fluid
CT	computed tomography
CXR	chest X-ray
DNA	deoxyribonucleic acid
ECG	electrocardiogram
EEG	electroencephalogram
ELISA	enzyme-liked immunosorbent assay
ESR	erythrocyte sedimentation rate
Hb	hemoglobin
hCG	human chorionic gonadotropin
HCT	hematocrit
Ig	immunoglobulin
KUB	kidney-ureter-bladder
LD	lactate dehydrogenase
MRI	magnetic resonance imaging
$Paco_2$	partial pressure of arterial carbon dioxide
Pao_2	partial pressure of arterial oxygen
PET	position emission tomography
PFT	pulmonary function test
PT	prothrombin time
PTT	partial thrombosplastin time
RBC	red blood cell
WBC	white blood cell

Abdominal aortic aneurysm

● CT scan, MRI, or ultrasonography reveals the size, shape, and location of the aneurysm.
● Anteroposterior and lateral X-rays of the abdomen may detect aortic calcification, which outlines the mass.
● Aortography shows the condition of vessels proximal and distal to the aneurysm and the extent of the aneurysm but may underestimate aneurysm diameter, because it visualizes only the blood flow channel and not the surrounding clot.

Abnormal premenopausal bleeding

● Serum hormone levels reflect adrenal, pituitary, or thyroid dysfunction.
● Urine 17-ketosteroids reveal adrenal hyperplasia, hypopituitarism, or polycystic ovarian disease.
● Pelvic ultrasonography rules out uterine masses.
● Hysteroscopy allows visualization of the endometrium.
● Endometrial biopsy rules out malignancy and should be performed in all patients who experience abnormal premenopausal bleeding.
● Pelvic examination and Papanicolaou smear rule out local or malignant causes.

Abruptio placentae

● History includes mild to moderate vaginal bleeding (usually during second half of pregnancy).
● Amniocentesis reveals "port wine" fluid.
● Coagulation tests reveal a rise in fibrin split product levels.
● CBC reveals decreased Hb level and platelet counts.
● Pelvic ultrasonography reveals abnormal echo patterns.

Acceleration-deceleration cervical injuries
- Full cervical spine CT scans or X-rays indicate absence of cervical fracture.
- If the X-rays are negative for obvious cervical fracture, examination emphasizes motor ability and sensation below the cervical spine to detect signs of nerve root compression.

Acquired immunodeficiency syndrome
- ELISA identifies the HIV-1 antibody.
- Western blot test may also reveal the HIV-1 antibody and should be performed after a positive ELISA to confirm the diagnosis (antibody may not be detected in late stages due to inability to mount an antibody response).
- CD4+ T-lymphocyte assay reveals a lymphocyte count < 200 cells/μl in an HIV-infected individual.

Actinomycosis
- Culture of tissue or exudate identifies *Actinomyces israelii*.
- Gram staining of excised tissue or exudates reveals branching gram-positive rods.
- CXR reveals lesions in unusual locations such as the shaft of a rib.

Acute leukemia
- Bone marrow aspiration indicates a proliferation of immature WBCs.
- Bone marrow biopsy reveals cancerous cells.
- CBC indicates pancytopenia with circulating blasts.

Acute poststreptococcal glomerulonephritis
- History includes recent streptococcal infection.
- Serum electrolyte studies show elevated calcium, chloride, phosphate, potassium, and sodium levels.

- BUN and serum creatinine levels are elevated.
- Urinalysis reveals RBCs, WBCs, mixed cell casts, and protein.
- Antistreptolysin-O test reveals elevated streptozyme titers, indicating a recent streptococcal infection (in 80% of patients).
- Anti-Dnase B titers are elevated, indicating a recent streptococcal infection.
- Serum complement assay levels are low, indicating recent streptococcal infection.
- Throat culture may show group A beta-hemolytic streptococci.
- KUB X-rays show bilateral kidney enlargement.
- Renal biopsy reveals histologic changes indicating glomerulonephritis.

Acute pyelonephritis
- Urinalysis reveals sediment containing leukocytes singly, in clumps, and in casts and, possibly, a few RBCs as well as low specific gravity and osmolality and a slight alkaline urine pH.
- Urine culture reveals more than 100,000 organisms/μl of urine.
- KUB X-rays may reveal calculi, tumors, or cysts in the kidneys and the urinary tract.
- Excretory urography may show asymmetrical kidneys.

Acute renal failure
- History includes renal disease.
- BUN and serum creatinine levels are elevated.
- ABG analysis indicates a blood pH < 7.35 and an HCO_3^- level < 22 mEq/L.

Acute respiratory failure in chronic obstructive pulmonary disease
- ABG measurements show progressive deterioration when compared with normal values for patient; increased

HCO_3^- level may indicate metabolic alkalosis or metabolic compensation for chronic respiratory acidosis.
● CXR reveals pulmonary pathology such as emphysema, atelectasis, lesions, pneumothorax, infiltrates, or effusions.
● Hb and HCT levels are decreased.
● Serum electrolyte studies reveal hypokalemia.
● WBC count is elevated if bacterial infection is present.
● ECG indicates arrhythmias that suggest cor pulmonale and myocardial hypoxia.

Acute tubular necrosis
● Urinalysis reveals urinary sediment containing RBCs and casts, specific gravity of 1.010 or less, and osmolality < 400 mOsm/kg.
● Urine sodium level is between 40 and 60 mEq/L.
● BUN and serum creatinine levels are elevated.
● Serum electrolyte studies reveal hyperkalemia.
● ABG analysis indicates blood pH < 7.25 and HCO_3^- level < 22 mEq/L.

Adenoid hyperplasia
● Nasopharyngoscopy or rhinoscopy reveals abnormal tissue mass.
● Lateral pharyngeal X-rays show oblation of the nasopharyngeal air column.

Adrenal hypofunction
● Plasma cortisol levels are decreased.
● Fasting blood glucose and serum sodium levels are decreased (in Addison's disease).
● Serum potassium and BUN levels are increased.
● CBC reveals increased HCT and elevated lymphocyte and eosinophil counts.
● X-rays reveal a small heart.
● Corticotropin level is increased.

● Rapid corticotropin test reveals low cortisol levels.
● Sweat test reveals elevated sodium level (> 46 mmol/L or mEq/L) and chloride level (> 43 mmol/L).
● Urine 17-hydroxycorticosteroid levels and urine 17-ketosteroid (17-KS) levels are decreased.

Adrenogenital syndrome
● Physical examination reveals pseudohermaphroditism in females or precocious puberty in patients of either sex.
● Urine 17-KS levels are elevated and can be suppressed by administering dexamethasone by mouth.
● Levels of urine hormone metabolites (particularly pregnanetriol) and plasma 17-hydroxyprogesterone are elevated.
● Urine 17-hydroxycorticosteroid levels are normal or decreased.
● Symptoms of adrenal hypofunction or adrenal crisis in the first week of life strongly suggest congenital adrenal hyperplasia; elevated serum calcium, chloride, and sodium levels (in the presence of excessive levels of urine 17-KS and pregnanetriol) and decreased urine aldosterone levels confirm it.

Age-related macular degeneration
● Indirect ophthalmoscopy reveals gross macular changes.
● I.V. fluorescein angiography reveals leaking vessels.
● Amsler's grid reveals visual field loss.

Albinism
● Family history suggests inheritance pattern.
● Inspection shows pale skin (in whites) and white-to-yellow hair.
● Microscopic examination of the skin and of hair follicles reveals the amount of pigment present.

- Pigmentation testing of plucked hair roots by incubating them in tyrosine distinguishes tyrosinase-positive albinism from tyrosinase-negative albinism; tyrosinase-positive hair roots will develop color.

Alcoholism

- History includes chronic and excessive ingestion of alcohol.
- Liver function studies reveal increased levels of serum cholesterol, LD, ALT, AST, and CK in patients with liver damage.
- Serum amylase and lipase levels are elevated (in pancreatitis).

Allergic rhinitis

- Personal or family history includes allergies.
- Sputum and nasal smears reveal a large numbers of eosinophils.
- Skin test for specific allergen is positive, supported by tested response to environmental stimuli.

Alport's syndrome

- Family history includes recurrent hematuria, deafness, and renal failure (especially in men).
- Urinalysis indicates presence of RBCs.
- Renal biopsy reveals histologic changes characteristic of Alport's syndrome.
- Blood tests reveal Ig and complement components.
- Eye examination may reveal cataracts and, less commonly, keratoconus, microspherophakia, myopia, nystagmus, and retinitis pigmentosa.

Alzheimer's disease

- History includes progressive personality, mental status, and neurologic changes.
- PET scan reveals alteration in the metabolic activity of the cerebral cortex.

- Elevated Tau proteins with low levels of soluble amyloid beta-protein precursor in CSF correlate with Alzheimer's disease.
- EEG and CT scan may help diagnose later stages of illness.
- Autopsy reveals neurofibrillary tangles, neuritic plaques, and granulovascular degeneration.

Amebiasis

- Culture of stool, sputum, or aspirates from abscesses, ulcers, or tissue reveal *Entamoeba histolytica* (cysts and trophozoites).
- CT scan may reveal abscess.

Amputation, traumatic

- History and examination reveal trauma to an extremity.
- CBC reveals decreased Hb and HCT, indicating hemorrhage.

Amyloidosis

- Histologic examination of tissue specimen (rectal mucosa, gingiva, skin, or nerve biopsy) or abdominal fat pad aspiration using a polarizing or electron microscope and appropriate tissue staining reveals amyloid deposits.
- Liver function studies are generally normal, except for slightly elevated serum alkaline phosphatase levels.
- ECG shows low voltage and conduction or rhythm abnormalities resembling those characteristic of myocardial infarction (with cardiac amyloidosis).
- Echocardiography (M-mode and two-dimensional) may detect myocardial infiltration.

Amyotrophic lateral sclerosis

- Upper and lower motor neuron degeneration occurs without sensory impairment.
- Electromyography may show abnormalities of electrical activity of involved muscles.

- Muscle biopsy may disclose atrophic fibers interspersed among normal fiber.
- Nerve conduction studies are usually normal.
- CSF analysis reveals increased protein content in one-third of patients.
- CT scan and EEG may help rule out other disorders.

Anal fissure

- Digital examination elicits pain and bleeding.
- Gentle traction on perianal skin allows for visualization of fistula.
- Anoscopy reveals longitudinal tear and confirms the diagnosis.
- Patient may complain of local itching, tenderness, or pain aggravated by bowel movements.

Anaphylaxis

- Patient's history, physical examination, and signs and symptoms establish the diagnosis. They may include a rapid onset of severe respiratory or cardiovascular symptoms after ingestion or injection of a drug, vaccine, diagnostic agent, food, or food additive or after an insect sting.

Ankylosing spondylitis

- Family history includes the disorder.
- X-rays reveal blurring of the bony margins of joints (in early stage), bilateral sacroiliac involvement, patchy sclerosis with superficial bony erosions, squaring of vertebral bodies, and "bamboo spine" (with complete ankylosis).
- Serum HLA-B27 is present in about 95% of patients with primary disease and 80% of patients with secondary disease.
- CBC reveals slightly elevated ESR and alkaline phosphatase and creatine phosphatase levels in active disease.
- Serum IgA levels may be elevated.

Anorectal abscess and fistula

Examination of rectum helps to distinguish type of abscess:

- Perianal abscess produces a red, tender, localized, oval swelling close to the anus, which may drain pus. Sitting or coughing increases pain.
- Ischiorectal abscess involves the entire perianal region on the affected side of the anus. Digital examination reveals a tender induration bulging into the anal canal, which may not produce drainage.
- Patient may report constipation, ribbon-formed stools, and pain with bowel movements.
- Submucous or high intramuscular abscess may produce a dull, aching pain in the rectum, tenderness and, occasionally, induration. Digital examination reveals a smooth swelling of the upper part of the anal canal or lower rectum.
- Pelvirectal abscess produces fever, malaise, and myalgia but no local anal or external rectal signs or pain. Digital examination reveals a tender mass high in the pelvis, perhaps extending into one of the ischiorectal fossae.
- Sigmoidoscopy, barium enema, and colonoscopy may be performed to rule out other conditions.

Anorectal stricture, stenosis, or contracture

- Visual inspection reveals narrowing of the anal canal.
- Digital examination reveals tenderness and tightness.

Anorexia nervosa

- History includes weight loss of 25% or greater with no organic basis, compulsive dieting and bulimic episodes or gorging and purging, and laxative or diuretic abuse.
- Emaciated appearance is accompanied by maintenance of physical vigor.

- CBC reveals decreased Hb levels, platelet levels, WBC count, and ESR.
- Bleeding time is prolonged (due to thrombocytopenia).
- Serum creatinine, BUN, uric acid, cholesterol, total protein, albumin, sodium, potassium, chloride, and calcium levels are decreased.
- Fasting blood glucose level is decreased.
- ECG reveals nonspecific ST interval, T-wave changes, prolonged PR interval, and ventricular arrhythmias.
- Additional diagnostic testing may be performed to rule out other disorders that may cause wasting.

Anthrax
- History includes exposure to wool, hides, or other animal products.
- Inspection reveals a large, pruritic, painless skin lesion.
- Tissue culture with Gram stain reveals large gram-positive rods.
- Drainage cultures reveal *Bacillus anthracis*.
- Indirect hemagglutination reveals a fourfold rise in titer.

Aortic insufficiency
- Cardiac catheterization shows reduced arterial diastolic pressure, aortic insufficiency, and valvular abnormalities.
- Echocardiography reveals left ventricular enlargement and changes in left ventricular function; it may show a dilated aortic root, a flail leaflet, thickening of the cusps, or valve prolapse.
- Doppler echocardiography readily detects mild degrees of aortic insufficiency that may be inaudible. It also shows a rapid, high-frequency, diastolic fluttering of the anterior mitral leaflet that results from aortic insufficiency.
- ECG may show left ventricular hypertrophy, ST-segment depression, and T-wave inversion.

- Radionuclide angiography helps to determine the degree of regurgitant blood flow and assess left ventricular function.

Aortic stenosis
- Cardiac catheterization reveals the pressure gradient across the aortic valve (indicating the severity of obstruction), increased left ventricular end-diastolic pressures (indicating left ventricular dysfunction), and the number of cusps.
- CXR shows valvular calcification, left ventricular enlargement, dilation of the ascending aorta, pulmonary venous congestion and, in later stages, left atrial, pulmonary artery, right atrial, and right ventricular enlargement.
- Echocardiography demonstrates a thickened aortic valve and left ventricular wall and possible coexistent mitral valve stenosis.
- Doppler echocardiography allows calculation of the aortic pressure gradient.
- ECG reveals left ventricular hypertrophy and ST-segment and T-wave abnormalities. As hypertrophy progresses in severe aortic stenosis, left atrial enlargement is noted. Up to 10% of patients have atrioventricular and intraventricular conduction defects.

Aplastic or hypoplastic anemia
- CBC reveals normochromic and normocytic RBCs with a total count of 1 million or less as well as decreased platelet, neutrophil, and WBC counts.
- Serum iron is elevated. (Hemosiderin is present and tissue iron storage is visible microscopically.)
- Bleeding time is prolonged.
- Bone marrow biopsy yields a "dry tap" or shows severely hypocellular or aplastic marrow, with a varying amount of fat, fibrous tissue, or gelatinous replacement; absence of tagged

iron and megakaryocytes; and depression of erythroid elements.

Appendicitis
• History includes right upper quadrant abdominal pain that eventually localizes in lower right quadrant, plus patient complaints of nausea and vomiting, anorexia, and obstipation.
• Temperature is elevated.
• WBC count is elevated, with increased numbers of immature cells.

Arm and leg fractures
• History includes trauma to extremity.
• Physical examination reveals pain and difficulty moving parts distal to the injury.
• Anteroposterior and lateral X-rays of extremity reveal fracture.

Arterial occlusive disease
• Arteriography demonstrates the type (thrombus or embolus), location, and degree of obstruction, and the collateral circulation.
• Doppler ultrasonography and plethysmography show decreased blood flow distal to the occlusion.
• Ophthalmodynamometry helps determine degree of obstruction in the internal carotid artery by comparing ophthalmic artery pressure to brachial artery pressure on the affected side. More than a 20% difference between pressures suggests insufficiency.

Asbestosis
• History includes occupational, family, or neighborhood exposure to asbestos fibers.
• CXR reveals fine, irregular, and linear diffuse infiltrates; extensive fibrosis results in "honeycomb" or "ground glass" appearance. X-rays also show pleural thickening and calcification, with bilateral oblation of costophrenic angles.

• PFTs reveal decreased vital capacity, forced vital capacity (FVC), and total lung capacity; decreased or normal forced expiratory volume in 1 second (FEV_1); a normal ratio of FEV_1 to FVC; and reduced diffusing capacity for carbon dioxide.
• ABG analysis may reveal decreased Pao_2 and $Paco_2$.

Ascariasis
• Stools contain ova or roundworm.
• Vomitus contains roundworm.
• CXR reveals infiltrates, patchy areas of pneumonitis, and widening of hilar shadows.

Aspergillosis
• History includes ocular trauma or surgery.
• CXR reveals crescent-shaped radiolucency surrounding a circular mass.
• Culture of exudate identifies *Aspergillus.*

Asphyxia
• History includes change in mental status and alteration of respiratory pattern.
• ABG analysis reveals $Pao_2 < 60$ mm Hg and $Paco_2 > 50$ mm Hg.
• CXR may reveal presence of foreign body, pulmonary edema, or atelectasis.
• Toxicology screening may reveal abnormal Hb or ingestion of drugs or chemicals.
• PFTs may indicate respiratory muscle weakness.

Asthma
• PFTs may reveal:
– forced expiratory flow < 75%
– forced expiratory volume in 1 second of 83% or below
– tidal volumes < 5 to 7 ml/ kg of body weight
– residual volume > 35% of total lung capacity.

- ABG analysis may demonstrate Pa_{O_2} < 75 mm Hg and Pa_{CO_2} > 45 mm Hg (indicating severe bronchial obstruction).
- CBC reveals eosinophil count > 7%.
- CXR shows hyperinflation.

Asystole

ECG reveals a waveform that is almost a flat line. Characteristic findings include the following:

- Atrial rhythm is usually indiscernible. No ventricular rhythm is present.
- Atrial rate is usually indiscernible. No ventricular rate is present.
- P wave may or may not be present.
- PR interval is not measurable.
- QRS complex is absent, or occasional escape beats are present.
- T wave is absent.
- QT interval is not measurable.

Ataxia-telangiectasia

- History and physical examination reveal the presence of ataxia, telangiectasia, and recurrent sinopulmonary infection.
- Serum analysis shows absent or deficient levels of IgA or IgE.
- Examination of thymic tissue reveals absence of Hassall's corpuscles.

Atelectasis

- Chest auscultation reveals decreased or absent breath sounds.
- CXR reveals characteristic horizontal lines in the lower lung zones (in widespread atelectasis) and dense shadows (with segmental or lobar collapse) with hyperinflation of neighboring lung.

Atopic dermatitis

- History includes clinical manifestations of allergy symptoms such as asthma, hay fever, or urticaria.
- CBC reveals elevated eosinophil count.

- Serum analysis shows elevated IgE levels.
- Tissue culture may be performed to rule out bacterial, viral, or fungal superinfections.

Atrial fibrillation

ECG reveals the following:

- Both atrial and ventricular rhythms are grossly irregular.
- The atrial rate, almost indiscernible, usually exceeds 400 beats/minute. The ventricular rate usually varies from 100 to 150 beats/minute, but can be < 100 beats/minute.
- P wave is absent. Erratic baseline f (fibrillatory) waves appear instead. These chaotic f waves represent atrial tetanization from rapid atrial depolarizations. When f waves are pronounced, the arrhythmia is called coarse atrial fibrillation. When they are not pronounced, the arrhythmia is called fine atrial fibrillation.
- PR interval is indiscernible.
- Duration and configuration of QRS complex are usually normal. If ventricular conduction is aberrant, the QRS complex may be wide and abnormally shaped.
- T wave is indiscernible.
- QT interval is not measurable.
- Atrial fib-flutter, a rhythm that frequently varies between a fibrillatory line and flutter waves, may appear.

Atrial flutter

ECG reveals the following:

- Atrial rhythm is regular. Ventricular rhythm depends on the atrioventricular (AV) conduction pattern; it's often regular, although cycles may alternate. An irregular pattern may herald atrial fibrillation or indicate a block.
- Atrial rate is 250 to 400 beats/minute. Ventricular rate depends on the degree of AV block; usually, it's 60 to 100 beats/minute, but it may accelerate to 125 to 150 beats/minute.

- P wave is saw-toothed, referred to as flutter or F waves.
- PR interval isn't measurable.
- Usually, duration of QRS complex is within normal limits; however, the complex may be widened if F waves are buried within.
- T wave isn't identifiable.
- QT interval isn't measurable because T wave can't be identified.
- The patient may develop an atrial rhythm that frequently varies between a fibrillatory line and F waves. This is called atrial fib-flutter; the ventricular response is irregular.

Atrial septal defect

- Echocardiography measures right ventricular enlargement, may locate the defect, and shows volume overload in the right heart.
- ECG reveals incomplete or complete right bundle-branch block in nearly all cases.
- Cardiac catheterization reveals a left-to-right shunt, determines the extent of shunting and pulmonary vascular disease, detects the size and location of pulmonary venous drainage, and the atrioventricular valves' competence.

Atrial tachycardia

ECG reveals the following:
- Both atrial and ventricular rhythms are regular.
- Atrial rate is characterized by three or more consecutive ectopic atrial beats occurring at a rate between 160 and 250 beats/minute; the rate rarely exceeds 250 beats/minute. The ventricular rate depends on the atrioventricular conduction ratio.
- Usually positive, the P wave may be aberrant, invisible, or hidden in the previous T wave. If visible, it precedes each QRS complex.
- PR interval may be unmeasurable if the P wave can't be distinguished from the preceding T wave.

- Duration and configuration of QRS complex are usually normal.
- T wave usually can't be distinguished.
- QT interval is usually within normal limits, but may be shorter because of the rapid rate.

Atrioventricular (AV) block, third-degree

ECG reveals the following:
- Both atrial and ventricular rhythms are regular.
- Atrial rate, which is usually within normal limits, exceeds the ventricular rate. The slow ventricular rate ranges from 40 to 60 beats/minute, but this rate is determined by the block's location and the origin of the subsidiary impulse.
- P wave has normal size and configuration.
- PR interval is not measurable because the atria and ventricles beat independently (AV dissociation).
- Configuration of the QRS complex depends on where the ventricular beat originates. A high AV junctional pacemaker produces a narrow QRS complex; a pacemaker in the bundle of His produces a wide QRS complex; a ventricular pacemaker produces a wide, bizarre QRS complex.
- T wave has normal size and configuration.
- QT interval may or may not be within normal limits.

B-cell deficiency

- History includes recurrent infections.
- Family history includes infection as cause of death.
- IgM, IgA, and IgG levels are decreased (after age 6 months).
- Tissue biopsy may show B cells but no plasma cells (B cells mature to form plasma cells as part of a normal immune response) in acquired hypogammaglobulinemia.

Basal cell carcinoma
- Inspection reveals skin lesions.
- Tissue biopsy reveals basal cell carcinoma.

Bell's palsy
- Inspection reveals facial paresthesia with an inability to raise the eyebrow, close the eyelid, smile, show the teeth, or puff the cheek.
- EEG distinguishes temporary conduction defect from pathologic interruption of nerve fibers (after 10 days).

Benign prostatic hyperplasia
- History includes problems with urination.
- Rectal examination reveals enlarged prostate gland.
- Prostate biopsy reveals histologic changes characteristic of benign prostatic hyperplasia.
- Excretory urography may indicate urinary tract obstruction, hydronephrosis, calculi, or tumors, and filling and emptying defects in the bladder.
- Elevated BUN and creatinine levels suggest impaired renal function.
- Urinalysis and urine culture show hematuria, pyuria, and, when bacterial count exceeds 100,000/μl, infection.
- Cystourethroscopy indicates prostate enlargement (usually performed immediately before surgery to help determine the best operative procedure).

Berylliosis
- History includes occupational, family, or neighborhood exposure to beryllium dust, fumes, or mists.
- In acute berylliosis, CXR reveals acute miliary process or patchy acinous filling, and diffuse infiltrates with prominent peribronchial markings.
- In chronic berylliosis, CXR reveals reticulonodular infiltrates, hilar adenopathy, and large coalescent infiltrates in both lungs.
- PFTs reveal decreased lung capacity.

Bladder cancer
- Cystoscopy with biopsy reveals the presence of malignant cells and may reveal that the bladder is fixed to the pelvic wall or prostate.
- Arylsulfatase A levels are elevated.
- Retrograde cystography evaluates bladder structure and integrity and confirms the diagnosis.
- Excretory urography reveals an early-stage or infiltrating tumor, ureteral obstruction, or a rigid deformity of the bladder wall. This test may also delineate functional problems in the upper urinary tract and help assess the degree of hydronephrosis.
- Urinalysis indicates presence of blood and malignant cytology.
- Ultrasonography may detect metastases in tissue beyond the bladder and can distinguish a bladder cyst from a bladder tumor.
- Pelvic arteriography reveals tumor invasion of the bladder wall.
- CT scan reveals the thickness of the involved bladder wall and detects enlarged retroperitoneal lymph nodes.

Blastomycosis
- Culture of skin lesions, pus, sputum, or pulmonary secretions reveals *Blastomyces dermatitidis*.

Blepharitis
- History includes irritated eyes and rubbing of the eyes.
- Tissue culture of ulcerated lid margin reveals *Staphylococcus aureus* (with ulcerative blepharitis).
- Inspection detects presence of nits (with pediculosis).

Blood transfusion reaction
- Crossmatching reveals conflicting blood types.
- Urinalysis reveals hemoglobinuria.
- Antibody screening reveals anti-A or anti-B antibodies in the blood.

● Serum haptoglobin level falls below pretransfusion level after 24 hours.
● Blood cultures may indicate bacterial contamination.

Blunt and penetrating abdominal injuries

● History includes trauma to abdomen or chest area.
● CXR or abdominal X-ray indicates presence of free air.
● Peritoneal lavage reveals blood, urine, bile, stool, or pus.
● Serum amylase level > 239 U/L indicates pancreatic injury.
● Hb and HCT levels show a serial decrease.
● Excretory urography and retrograde cystography indicate renal and urinary tract damage.
● CT scan indicates abdominal organ rupture.
● Exploratory laparotomy reveals specific injuries when other clinical evidence is incomplete.

Blunt chest injuries

● History includes trauma to chest area.
● With hemothorax, percussion reveals dullness.
● With tension pneumothorax, percussion reveals tympany.
● CXR may indicate rib and sternal injuries, pneumothorax, flail chest, pulmonary contusion, lacerated or ruptured aorta, diaphragmatic rupture, lung compression, or hemothorax.
● CT scan reveals aortic laceration or rupture, or diaphragmatic rupture.
● CK-MB level shows mild elevation.

Bone tumor, primary malignant

● Physical examination detects palpable mass over bony area.
● Biopsy reveals malignant cells.
● Bone X-ray and radioisotope bone scan reveal tumor location and size.

● CT scan reveals tumor location and size
● MRI reveals tumor.
● Serum alkaline phosphatase level is elevated (in patients with sarcomas).

Botulism

● Offending toxin is detected in the patient's serum, stool, gastric content, or the suspected food.
● Electromyography shows diminished muscle action potential after a single supramaximal nerve stimulus.

Brain abscess

● History includes congenital heart disease or infection, especially of the middle ear, mastoid, nasal sinuses, heart, or lungs.
● CT scan or MRI reveals site of abscess.
● Arteriography highlights the abscess with a halo.
● Culture of drainage reveals causative organism, such as *Staphylococcus aureus, Streptococcus viridans,* or *Streptococcus hemolyticus.*

Breast cancer

● Breast examination is abnormal.
● Mammography, ultrasonography, or thermography indicates presence of mass.
● Surgical biopsy reveals malignant cells.
● Carcinoembryonic antigen levels are > 20 ng/ml
● Serum or urine of woman who isn't pregnant contains hCG.

Bronchiectasis

● History includes recurrent bronchial infections, pneumonia, and hemoptysis.
● CXR show pleural thickening, areas of atelectasis, and scattered cystic changes.

Bronchitis, chronic

- CXRs may show hyperinflation and increased bronchovascular markings.
- PFTs demonstrate increased residual volume, decreased vital capacity and forced expiratory flow, and normal static compliance and diffusing capacity.
- ABG analysis reveals decreased PaO_2 and normal or increased $PaCO_2$.
- Sputum culture reveals the presence of microorganisms and neutrophils.
- ECG may detect atrial arrhythmias; peaked P waves in leads II, III, and aV_F; and, occasionally, right ventricular hypertrophy.
- Bronchography reveals location and extent of disease.

Brucellosis

- History includes contact with animals.
- Agglutinin titers within 3 weeks of illness are elevated.
- Multiple blood cultures, bone marrow culture, and biopsy of infected tissue indicate presence of *Brucella* bacteria.

Buerger's disease

- History includes intermittent claudication of the palm of the hand and the instep.
- Doppler ultrasonography reveals diminished circulation in the peripheral vessels.
- Plethysmography reveals decreased circulation in the peripheral vessels.

Burns

- History includes exposure to heat, electricity, or chemicals.
- Examination reveals depth of skin and tissue damage and area affected.
- Urinalysis may reveal myoglobinuria and hemoglobinuria.
- ABG analysis reveals reduced respiratory function.

- Fiber-optic bronchoscopy may reveal epithelial damage to the trachea and bronchi.
- Serum protein studies show increased albumin levels.
- BUN level is increased due to increased protein catabolism.
- Fibrin split products are increased.
- Serum magnesium levels are suppressed.
- Osmotic fragility is high (increased tendency to hemolysis).
- Changes are noted in serum electrolyte levels, including elevated potassium and decreased sodium levels.
- WBC count reveals leukocytosis.

Calcium imbalance

- In hypocalcemia:
  - serum calcium level is < 4.5 mEq/L.
- In hypercalcemia:
  - serum calcium level is > 5.5 mEq/L
  - urinalysis reveals increased calcium precipitation.

  Note: Because approximately one-half of serum calcium is bound to albumin, changes in serum protein must be considered when interpreting serum calcium levels.

Cancer of the vulva

- Papanicolaou test reveals abnormal cells.
- Tissue biopsy reveals malignant cells.
- Vulva staining (with toluidine blue dye) indicates diseased tissues.

Candidiasis

- Culture of skin, vaginal scrapings, pus, sputum, blood, or tissue reveals *Candida albicans*.

Cardiac tamponade

- CXR reveals slightly widened mediastinum and cardiomegaly.
- Echocardiography reveals pericardial effusion with signs of right ventricular and atrial compression.

• Pulmonary artery monitoring reveals increased right atrial pressure, right ventricular diastolic pressure, and central venous pressure.

Cardiogenic shock

• Auscultation detects gallop rhythm, faint heart sounds, and a holosystolic murmur (with ruptured ventricular septum or papillary muscles).
• Pulmonary artery pressure monitoring reveals the following:
– increased pulmonary artery pressure
– increased pulmonary artery wedge pressure
– increased systemic vascular resistance
– increased peripheral vascular resistance
– decreased cardiac output.
• Invasive arterial pressure monitoring reveals hypotension.
• CK levels are increased.
• ABG analysis may show metabolic acidosis and hypoxia.
• ECG shows acute myocardial infarction, ischemia, or ventricular aneurysm.

Carpal tunnel syndrome

• Physical examination reveals decreased sensation to light touch or pinpricks in the affected fingers.
• Tinel's sign is positive.
• Wrist-flexion test reveals positive Phalen's sign.
• Compression test provokes pain and paresthesia along the distribution of the median nerve.
• Electromyography detects a median nerve motor conduction delay of more than 5 milliseconds.

Cataract

• Eye examination reveals the white area behind the pupil (unnoticeable until the cataract is advanced).

• Ophthalmoscopy or slit-lamp examination reveals a dark area in the normally homogeneous red reflex.

Celiac disease

• Tissue biopsy of the small bowel reveals a mosaic pattern of alternating flat and bumpy areas on the bowel surface (due to an almost total absence of villi) and an irregular, blunt, and disorganized network of blood vessels (usually prominent in the jejunum).
• Stool samples (after 72-hour collection) reveal excess fat.
• Human leukocyte antigen (HLA) test reveals presence of HLA-B8 antigen.
• D-xylose absorption test reveals depressed blood and urine D-xylose levels.
• Upper GI series followed by a small-bowel series demonstrates protracted barium passage: Barium shows up in a segmented, coarse, scattered, and clumped pattern; the jejunum shows generalized dilation.
• Glucose tolerance test indicates poor glucose absorption.
• Low serum carotene levels, indicating malabsorption
• CBC indicates decreased Hb and HCT levels as well as decreased WBC and platelet counts.
• Decreased serum albumin, sodium, potassium, cholesterol, and phospholipid levels
• PT may be shortened.

Cerebral aneurysm

• History includes headache and change in mental status (usually with rupture or leakage).
• Angiography shows location and size of unruptured aneurysm.
• CT scan reveals location of clot, hydrocephalus, areas of infarction, and extent of blood spillage within the cisterns around the brain.

Cerebral contusion
- History includes head trauma.
- CT scan reveals ischemic tissue and hematoma.
- Skull X-ray indicates fracture is absent.

Cerebral palsy
Infant displays the following characteristics:
- difficulty sucking or keeping food in his mouth
- infrequent voluntary movement
- arm or leg tremors with movement
- crossing legs when lifted from behind rather than pulling them up or "bicycling"
- legs difficult to separate to change diapers
- persistent use of one hand, or ability to use hands well but not legs.

Cerebrovascular accident
- Patient reports sudden onset of motor or sensory impairment.
- CT scan detects structural abnormalities, edema, and lesions, such as nonhemorrhagic infarction and aneurysms.
- Cerebral angiography reveals disruption or displacement of the cerebral circulation by occlusion or hemorrhage.
- Ultrasonography of carotid and cerebral arteries may reveal occlusion.
- Digital abstraction angiography evaluates the patency of the cerebral vessels and identifies their position in the head and neck. It also detects and evaluates lesions and vascular abnormalities.
- PET scan provides data on cerebral metabolism and cerebral blood flow changes, especially in ischemic stroke.
- Single-photon emission tomography identifies cerebral blood flow and helps diagnose cerebral infarction.
- EEG may detect reduced electrical activity in an area of cortical infarction.

- Transcranial Doppler studies examine the size of intracranial vessels and the direction of blood flow.
- MRI allows evaluation of the lesion's location and size.

Cervical cancer
- Papanicolaou (Pap) test reveals abnormal cells.
- Cone biopsy of cervical tissue reveals malignant cells.
- Colposcopy determines the source of the abnormal cells seen on the Pap test.

Cesarean birth
The following test findings indicate the need for cesarean birth:
- X-ray pelvimetry may reveal cephalopelvic disproportion and malpresentation.
- Ultrasonography may reveal pelvic masses that interfere with vaginal delivery and fetal position.
- Amniocentesis may reveal Rh isoimmunization, fetal distress, or fetal genetic abnormalities.
- Auscultation of fetal heart rate (fetoscope, Doppler unit, or electronic fetal monitor) may reveal acute fetal distress.

Chalazion
- Visual examination and palpation of the eyelid reveal a small bump or nodule.
- Tissue biopsy rules out meibomian gland cancer.

Chancroid
- History includes sexual contact with a partner with chancroid.
- Tissue culture of ulcer exudate, bubo aspirate, or blood reveals *Haemophilus ducreyi*.

Chlamydial infections
- History includes sexual contact with a partner with chlamydial infection.

• Culture of site indicates *Chlamydia trachomatis* (findings may reveal urethritis, cervicitis, salpingitis, endometritis, or proctitis).
• Culture of blood, pus, or CSF reveals *C. trachomatis* (findings may reveal epididymitis, prostatitis, or lymphogranuloma venereum).

Chloride imbalance

• In hypochloremia, serum chloride level is < 98 mEq/L.
• In hyperchloremia, serum chloride level is > 108 mEq/L.

Cholelithiasis and related disorders

• Ultrasonography of the gallbladder indicates presence of stones.
• Percutaneous transhepatic cholangiography reveals gallbladder disease.
• Endoscopic retrograde cholangiopancreatography visualizes the biliary tree.
• Hida scan of the gallbladder reveals obstruction of the cystic duct.
• Oral cholecystography shows stones in the gallbladder and biliary duct obstruction.
• Technetium-labeled iminodiacetic acid scan of the gallbladder indicates cystic duct obstruction and acute or chronic cholecystitis if the gallbladder can't be seen.
• Blood studies may reveal elevated serum alkaline phosphatase, LD, AST, and total bilirubin levels and icteric index.
• WBC count is slightly elevated during a cholecystitis attack.

Cholera

• Patient reports voluminous, gray-tinged diarrhea.
• Stool or vomitus culture reveals presence of *Vibrio cholerae*.
• Agglutination and other clear reactions to group- and type-specific antisera provide definitive diagnosis.

• Dark-field microscopic examination of fresh stool shows rapidly moving bacilli.
• Immunofluorescence allows for rapid diagnosis.

Choriocarcinoma

• Radioimmunoassay of hCG levels, performed frequently, provides early and accurate diagnosis; levels that are extremely elevated for early pregnancy indicate gestational trophoblastic disease.
• Histologic examination of possible hydatid vessels confirms the diagnosis.
• Ultrasonography performed after the third month shows grapelike clusters rather than a fetus.
• Amniography reveals the absence of a fetus (performed only when the diagnosis is in question).
• Doppler ultrasonography demonstrates the absence of fetal heart tones.
• Hb, HCT, and RBC count are abnormal.
• Fibrinogen levels are abnormal.
• PT and PTT are abnormal.
• WBC count and ESR are increased.
• CXR, CT scan, and MRI may identify choriocarcinoma metastasis.
• Lumbar puncture may detect early cerebral metastasis if hCG is in CSF.

Chronic fatigue and immune dysfunction syndrome

• History includes persistent or relapsing debilitating fatigue or tendency to tire easily.
• Average level of activity is < 50% of normal for 6 months or more.
• Fatigue doesn't resolve with bed rest.
• Diagnostic tests rule out other illnesses, such as Epstein-Barr virus, leukemia, and lymphoma.

Chronic glomerulonephritis

• Urinalysis reveals proteinuria, hematuria, cylindruria, and RBC casts.
• BUN level is elevated.

- Serum creatinine level is elevated.
- Kidney X-rays or ultrasonography reveals small kidneys.
- Renal biopsy indicates presence of underlying disease.

Chronic granulomatous disease

- History inlcudes osteomyelitis, pneumonia, liver abscess, or chronic lymphadenopathy in a young child.
- Nitroblue tetrazolium (NBT) test reveals impaired NBT reduction, indicating abnormal neutrophil metabolism.
- Neutrophil function test measures the rate of intracellular killing by neutrophils; in chronic granulomatous disease, killing is delayed or absent.

Chronic lymphocytic leukemia

- CBC reveals numerous abnormal lymphocytes.
- WBC count is mildly but persistently elevated in early stages.
- Granulocytopenia is present.
- Bone marrow aspiration and biopsy reveal lymphocytic invasion.

Chronic mucocutaneous candidiasis

- Inspection reveals large, circular lesions.
- Culture of affected area indicates presence of *Candida.*

Chronic renal failure

- History includes chronic progressive debilitation.
- BUN level is elevated.
- Serum creatinine level is elevated.
- Serum potassium level may be elevated.
- ABG analysis reveals blood pH < 7.35 and HCO_3^- level < 22 mEq/L.
- Urinalysis may show proteinuria, glycosuria, erythrocytes, leukocytes, and casts.
- Kidney biopsy identifies underlying pathology.

Cirrhosis and fibrosis

- Liver biopsy reveals destruction and fibrosis of hepatic tissue.
- Abdominal X-rays show liver size and cysts or gas within the biliary tract or liver, liver calcification, and massive ascites.
- CT and liver scans determine the liver size, identify liver masses, and reveal hepatic blood flow and obstruction.
- Esophagogastroduodenoscopy reveals bleeding esophageal varices, stomach irritation or ulceration, or duodenal bleeding and irritation.
- ALT, AST, total serum bilirubin, and indirect bilirubin levels are elevated.
- Serum albumin and protein levels are decreased.
- PT is prolonged.
- HCT, Hb, and serum electrolyte levels are decreased.

Coal worker's pneumoconiosis

- History includes exposure to coal dust.
- In simple coal worker's pneumoconiosis (CWP), CXR reveals small opacities (< 10 mm in diameter) prominent in the upper lung fields.
- In complicated CWP, CXR reveals one or more large opacities (1 to 5 cm in diameter), possibly exhibiting cavitation.
- PFTs reveal decreased lung capacity.

Coarctation of the aorta

- Physical examination reveals resting systolic hypertension, absent or diminished femoral pulses, and wide pulse pressure.
- CXR reveals notching of the undersurfaces of the ribs due to collateral circulation.
- Echocardiography reveals left ventricular muscle thickening, coexisting aortic valve abnormalities, and the coarctation site.

- Aortography locates the site and extent of coarctation.
- ECG may reveal left ventricular hypertrophy.

Coccidioidomycosis

- Skin test indicates a positive reaction for coccidioidin.
- Immunodiffusion of sputum and pus from lesions and tissue biopsy reveal presence of *Coccidioides immitis* spores.
- Complement fixation reveals presence of IgG antibodies.
- Serum Ig levels help establish diagnosis.

Colorado tick fever

- History includes recent exposure to ticks.
- Serum studies indicate presence of Colorado tick fever virus.
- Patient may have leukopenia.

Colorectal cancer

- Hemoccult test (guaiac) reveals blood in stools.
- Proctoscopy or sigmoidoscopy reveals presence of mass.
- Colonoscopy reveals lesion.
- Tissue biopsy reveals malignant cells.
- Barium X-ray reveals lesion.
- Carcinoembryonic antigen level is > 5 ng/ml.

Common variable immunodeficiency

- Circulating B-cell count is normal.
- Serum IgM, IgA, and IgG levels are decreased, suggesting diminished synthesis or secretion.
- Antigenic stimulation reveals an inability to produce specific antibodies.
- X-rays may reveal signs of chronic lung disease or sinusitis.

Complement deficiencies

- Total serum complement level is low.
- Specific assays may confirm deficiency of specific complement components.

Concussion

- History includes head trauma, with or without loss of consciousness.
- Patient demonstrates amnesia with regard to traumatic event.
- Patient reports headache.
- Neurologic examination results are normal for patient.
- Skull X-ray and CT scan may be negative.

Congenital hip dysplasia

- Ortolani's or Trendelenburg's sign is positive.
- Inspection reveals extra thigh fold on affected side, higher buttock fold on the affected side, restricted abduction of the affected hip.
- X-ray reveals the location of the femur head and a shallow acetabulum.

Conjunctivitis

- Inspection reveals inflammation of the conjunctiva.
- Stained smear of conjunctival scrapings reveal monocytes (viral conjunctivitis), polymorphonuclear cells (bacterial conjunctivitis), or eosinophils (allergic conjunctivitis).
- Conjunctival culture reveals causative organism.

Cor pulmonale

- Pulmonary artery pressure measurements reveal increased right ventricular and pulmonary artery pressures as well as elevated right ventricular systolic, pulmonary artery systolic, and pulmonary artery diastolic pressures.
- CXR reveals large central pulmonary arteries and rightward enlargement of cardiac silhouette.
- Echocardiography reveals right ventricular enlargement.

Corneal abrasion

- History includes eye trauma or prolonged wearing of contact lenses.
- Fluorescein stain of the cornea turns the injured area green during flashlight examination.
- Slit-lamp examination discloses the depth of the abrasion.

Corneal ulcers

- History includes eye trauma or use of contact lenses.
- Flashlight examination reveals irregular corneal surface.
- Fluorescein dye, instilled in the conjunctival sac, stains the outline of the ulcer.

Coronary artery disease

- History includes angina and risk factors for coronary artery disease.
- ECG reveals ischemia and, possibly, arrhythmias during an anginal attack. ECG returns to normal when pain ceases.
- Coronary angiography reveals coronary artery stenosis or obstruction, collateral circulation, and the arteries' condition beyond the narrowing.
- Myocardial perfusion imaging with thallium-201 during treadmill exercise detects ischemic areas.

Corrosive esophagitis and stricture

- History includes chemical ingestion.
- Oropharyngeal burns (indicated by white membranes and edema of the soft palate and uvula).
- Endoscopy (in the first 24 hours after ingestion) delineates the extent and location of the esophageal injury and assesses depth of the burn; 1 week after ingestion, this test helps assess stricture development.
- Barium swallow, performed 1 week after ingestion and every 3 weeks thereafter, as ordered, identifies segmental spasm or fistula.

Cri du chat syndrome

- History includes cat cry, facial disproportions, microencephaly, small birth size, and poor physical and mental development.
- Karyotype reveals deleted short arms of chromosome 5.

Crohn's disease

- History includes frequent stools and abdominal cramping.
- Barium enema reveals the string sign (segments of stricture separated by normal bowel).
- Sigmoidoscopy and colonoscopy reveal patchy areas of inflammation.
- Biopsy of bowel tissue reveals histologic changes indicative of Crohn's disease.

Cryptococcosis

- Inspection may reveal signs of meningeal irritation.
- Sputum, urine, prostatic secretion culture; bone marrow aspirate or biopsy; or pleural biopsy reveals *Cryptococcus neoformans.*
- Blood culture reveals *C. neoformans* (with severe infection).
- CXR reveals pulmonary lesion.
- Cryptococcal antigen and positive cryptococcal culture occurs in 90% of tests.

Cushing's syndrome

- Serum cortisol levels are consistently elevated.
- 24-hour urine sample demonstrates elevated free cortisol levels.
- Dexamethasone suppression test reveals a cortisol level of 5 g/dl or greater (failure to suppress).
- Urine 17-hydroxycorticosteroid levels are elevated.
- Urine 17-ketosteroid levels are elevated.
- Ultrasonography, CT scan, or angiography localize adrenal tumors.

- CT scan of the head identifies pituitary tumors.

Cutaneous larva migrans
- Patient displays characteristic migratory lesions.
- History includes contact with warm, moist soil within the past several months.

Cystic fibrosis
- Family history includes the disorder.
- Pulmonary disease or pancreatic insufficiency (absence of trypsin) is present.
- Sweat test reveals sodium level 79 to 148 mmol/L and chloride level 14 to 30 mmol/L or mEq/L.
- DNA testing may locate the Delta 508 deletion and help to confirm the diagnosis.
- PFTs evaluate lung function.
- Sputum culture allows the detection of concurrent infectious disease.
- ABG analysis helps determine pulmonary status.
- CXR helps diagnose respiratory obstruction and monitor its progress.

Cystinuria
- Family history includes renal disease or kidney stones.
- Chemical analysis of calculi shows cystine crystals, with a variable amount of calcium.
- Clearance of cystine, lysine, arginine, and ornithine is elevated.
- Urinalysis with amino acid chromatography indicates aminoaciduria, as evidenced by the presence of cystine, lysine, arginine, and ornithine.
- Urine pH is usually < 5.
- Microscopic examination of urine shows hexagonal, flat cystine crystals.
- Cyanide-nitroprusside test is positive.
- Excretory urography or KUB X-rays reveal size and location of calculi.

Cytomegalovirus infection
- Culture of urine, saliva, throat, or blood or biopsy specimens reveal virus.
- Indirect immunofluorescent test reveals IgM antibody.

Dacryocystitis
- History includes constant tearing.
- Culture of discharge from tear sac reveals *Staphylococcus aureus* and, occasionally, beta-hemolytic streptococci in acute dacryocystitis; culture reveals *Streptococcus pneumoniae* or *Candida albicans* in the chronic form.
- Dacryocystography locates the atresia.

Decompression sickness
- History includes rapid decompression.
- Physical examination reveals incapacitating joint and muscle pain, and neurologic and respiratory disturbance.

Dermatitis
- Family history includes allergy and chronic inflammation.
- Patient demonstrates characteristic distribution of skin lesions.
- Serum IgE levels are elevated.

Dermatophytosis
- Inspection reveals skin lesions.
- Microscopic examination or culture of lesion scrapings reveals infective organism.
- Wood's light examination may reveal types of tinea capitis.

Diabetes insipidus
- History includes head trauma or neurologic surgery.
- Urinalysis reveals almost colorless urine of low osmolality (< 300 mOsmol/kg) and low specific gravity (< 1.005).

Diabetes mellitus
- In nonpregnant adults, findings include:
- symptoms of uncontrolled diabetes and a random blood glucose level ≥ 200 mg/dl
- fasting plasma glucose level ≥ 126 mg/dl on at least two occasions
- in a patient with normal fasting glucose, a blood glucose level > 200 mg/dl during the 2nd hour of a glucose tolerance test and on at least one other occasion during the glucose tolerance test.
- Ophthalmologic examination may show diabetic retinopathy.
- Urinalysis reveals presence of acetone.

DiGeorge's syndrome
- History includes facial anomalies in infant.
- T-lymphocyte assay shows decreased or absent T cells.
- B-lymphocyte assay shows elevated B cells.
- CT scan or MRI shows thymus is absent.
- Serum calcium levels are < 8 mg/dl.

Dilated cardiomyopathy
- CXR reveals cardiomegaly, usually affecting all heart chambers.
- CXR may show pulmonary congestion, pleural or pericardial effusion, or pulmonary venous hypertension.
- ECG may reveal ST-segment and T-wave changes.
- Echocardiography reveals left ventricular thrombi, global hypokinesia, and degree of left ventricular dilation.

Diphtheria
- Inspection reveals characteristic thick, patchy grayish green membrane over the mucous membranes of the pharynx, larynx, tonsils, soft palate, and nose.

- Throat culture or culture of other suspect lesions reveals *Corynebacterium diphtheriae*.

Dislocated or fractured jaw
- History includes trauma to jaw or face.
- Maxillary or mandibular mobility is abnormal.
- X-ray of the jaw shows fracture.

Dislocations and subluxations
- Inspection confirms joint deformity.
- X-ray is negative for fracture but may reveal dislocation or subluxation.
- Arthroscopy reveals dislocation or subluxation.

Disseminated intravascular coagulation
- Patient displays abnormal bleeding in the absence of a known hematologic disorder.
- Platelet count is < 100,000/μl.
- Fibrinogen is < 175 mg/dl.
- PT is > 15 seconds.
- Partial PTT is > 60 seconds.
- Fibrin split products reveal fibrin degradation products > 100 μg/ml.
- D-dimer test (a specific fibrinogen test for disseminated intravascular coagulation) is positive.
- Fibrin degradation products are increased, > 45 μg/dl.

Diverticular disease
- Upper GI series reveals barium-filled pouches in the esophagus and upper bowel.
- Barium enema reveals barium-filled pouches in the lower bowel; barium outlines diverticula filled with stool.

Down syndrome
- History includes hypotonia at birth.
- Karyotype reveals chromosome abnormality.
- Prenatal ultrasonography may suggest Down syndrome if a duodenal ob-

struction or an atrioventricular canal defect is present.
● Maternal serum alpha-fetoprotein levels are reduced.
● Amniocentesis reveals the translocated chromosome.

Dysfunctional uterine bleeding
● History includes excessive vaginal bleeding.
● Organic, systemic, psychogenic, and endocrine causes of bleeding are ruled out.
● Dilatation and curettage and biopsy reveal endometrial hyperplasia.

Dysmenorrhea
● History includes abdominal pain related to menstruation.
● Pelvic examination may reveal the physical cause.
● Laparoscopy may reveal an underlying cause such as endometriosis or uterine leiomyoma.
● Dilatation and curettage may reveal an underlying cause such as cervical stenosis or pelvic inflammatory disease.

Dyspareunia
● History includes discomfort during sexual intercourse.
● Pelvic examination may reveal a physical disorder as underlying cause of discomfort.

Ectopic pregnancy
● Serum pregnancy test shows presence of hCG.
● Real-time ultrasonography (performed if serum pregnancy test is positive) reveals no intrauterine pregnancy.
● Culdocentesis (performed if ultrasonography detects the absence of a gestational sac in the uterus) reveals free blood in the peritoneum.
● Laparoscopy (performed if culdocentesis is positive) reveals pregnancy outside the uterus.

Electric shock
● History includes electrical contact, voltage, and length of contact.
● Physical examination reveals electrical burn.
● ECG reveals ventricular fibrillation or other arrhythmias that progress to fibrillation or myocardial infarction.
● Urine myoglobin test is positive.

Emphysema
● Examination reveals barrel chest, pursed-lip breathing, and use of accessory muscles of respiration; palpation may reveal decreased tactile fremitus and decreased chest expansion; percussion may reveal hyperresonance; auscultation may reveal decreased breath sounds, crackles and wheezing on inspiration, prolonged expiratory phase with grunting respirations, and distant heart sounds.
● In advanced disease, CXR may show a flattened diaphragm, reduced vascular markings at the lung periphery, overaeration of the lungs, a vertical heart, enlarged anteroposterior chest diameter, and large retrosternal air space.
● PFTs indicate increased residual volume and total lung capacity, reduced diffusing capacity, and increased inspiratory flow.
● ABG analysis usually shows reduced Pao_2 and normal $Paco_2$ until late in the disease when $Paco_2$ increases.
● ECG may reveal tall, symmetrical P waves in leads II, III, and aV_F; a vertical QRS axis; and signs of right ventricular hypertrophy late in the disease.
● RBC count usually demonstrates an increased Hb level late in the disease, when the patient has persistent severe hypoxia.

Encephalitis
● Lumbar puncture reveals elevated CSF pressure and clear CSF, with

slightly elevated WBC and protein levels.

- CSF or blood culture reveals virus.
- Serologic studies (in herpes encephalitis) may show rising titers of complement-fixing antibodies.
- EEG reveals abnormalities such as generalized slowing of waveforms.

Endocarditis

- Auscultation reveals a loud, regurgitant murmur.
- Blood cultures (three or more during a 24- to 48-hour period) reveal infecting organism.
- WBC count is elevated.
- ESR is elevated.
- Serum creatinine level is elevated.
- Echocardiography or transesophageal echocardiography reveals valvular damage and endocardial vegetation.

Endometriosis

- Pelvic examination reveals multiple tender nodules on uterosacral ligaments or in the rectovaginal septum, which enlarge and become more tender during menses.
- Palpation may uncover ovarian enlargement in patients with endometrial cysts on the ovaries or thickened, nodular adnexa (as in pelvic inflammatory disease).
- Laparoscopy shows small, blue powder burns on the peritoneum or the serosa of any pelvic or abdominal structure.
- Barium enema rules out malignant or inflammatory bowel disease.

Enterobiasis

- Collecting a sample from the perianal area with a cellophane tape swab leads to identification of the *Enterobius* ova.
- History includes pruritus ani as well as recent contact with infected person or infected articles.

Enterocolitis

- Stool Gram stain reveals numerous gram-positive cocci and polymorphonuclear leukocytes with few gram-negative rods.
- Stool culture identifies *Staphylococcus aureus* as the causative organism.
- Blood studies reveal leukocytosis, moderately increased BUN level, and decreased serum albumin level.

Epicondylitis

- History includes traumatic injury or strain associated with athletic activity.
- Examination reveals pain with wrist extension and supination with lateral involvement, or with flexion and pronation with epicondyle involvement.
- X-rays are normal at first, but later bony fragments, osteophyte sclerosis, or calcium deposits appear.
- Arthrography is normal with some minor irregularities on the tendon undersurface.
- Arthrocentesis identifies causative organism if joint infection is suspected.

Epidermolysis bullosa

- Skin biopsy of a freshly induced blister reveals type of epidermolysis bullosa.
- Fetoscopy and biopsy provide prenatal diagnosis of the severe scarring forms (at 20 weeks' gestation).

Epididymitis

- History includes unilateral, dull aching pain radiating to the spermatic cord, lower abdomen, and flank.
- Physical examination shows characteristic waddle, as an attempt to protect the groin and scrotum when walking.
- WBC count in urine is increased.
- Urine culture and sensitivity tests reveal causative organism.
- Elevated serum WBC count indicates infection.

Epiglottitis

- Throat examination reveals a large, edematous, bright red epiglottis.
- Direct laryngoscopy reveals swollen, beefy-red epiglottis (not done if significant obstruction is suspected or immediate intubation is not possible).
- Lateral neck X-rays show an enlarged epiglottis and distended hypopharynx.

Epilepsy

- CT scan provides brain density readings indicating abnormalities in internal structures.
- EEG may show paroxysmal abnormalities and helps classify the disorder.
- MRI helps identify the cause of the seizure by providing clear images of the brain in regions where bone normally hampers visualization.

Epistaxis

- History includes trauma to the nose, chemical irritation, sinus infection, or coagulopathy.
- Inspection with a bright light and nasal speculum locates the site of bleeding.

Erectile dysfunction

- Detailed sexual history reveals persistent or recurrent partial or complete failure to attain or maintain erection until completion of sexual activity or a persistent or recurrent lack of a subjective sense of sexual excitement and pleasure during sexual activity.
- Urologic screening rules out urogenital problems.
- Neurologic evaluation rules out neurologic dysfunction.
- Drug history rules out medication use as a causative factor.

Erysipeloid

- History includes occupational exposure to *Erysipelothrix insidiosa* and skin injury.
- Examination reveals purple erythema of the skin, persisting over several days.
- Full-thickness skin biopsy taken from the edge of the lesion results in isolation of *E. insidiosa*.

Erythroblastosis fetalis

- Maternal history reveals risk factors for incompatibility of fetal and maternal blood, such as erythroblastotic stillbirths, abortions, previously affected children, previous anti-Rh titers, and blood transfusions.
- Maternal blood typing indicates mother is Rh-negative (titers determine changes in the degree of maternal immunization).
- Amniocentesis reveals an increase in bilirubin levels (indicating possible hemolysis) and elevations in anti-Rh titers.
- Radiologic studies may show edema and, in hydrops fetalis, the halo sign (edematous, elevated, subcutaneous fat layers) and the Buddha position (fetus's legs are crossed).
- Direct Coombs' test of umbilical cord blood confirms maternal-newborn Rh incompatibility.
- An umbilical cord Hb count < 10 g signals severe disease.
- Stained RBC examination reveals many nucleated peripheral RBCs.

Esophageal cancer

- X-rays of the esophagus, with barium swallow and motility studies, reveal structural and filling defects and reduced peristalsis.
- CXR or esophagography reveals pneumonitis.

- Esophagoscopy, punch-and-brush biopsies, and exfoliative cytologic tests confirm esophageal tumors.
- Bronchoscopy may reveal tumor growth in the tracheobronchial tree.
- Endoscopic ultrasonography (combined with endoscopy and ultrasonography) identifies depth of tumor penetration.
- Mediastinoscopy reveals lesion and extent of disease.
- Esophageal biopsy reveals malignant cells.

Esophageal diverticula
- Barium swallow reveals characteristic out-pouching in esophagus.
- Esophagoscopy rules out other lesions as cause.

Exophthalmos
- Physical examination reveals forward displacement of the eyeballs.
- Exophthalmometer readings reveal the degree of anterior projection and asymmetry between the eyes to be > 12 mm.
- X-rays show orbital fracture or bony erosion by an orbital tumor.
- CT scan identifies lesions in optic nerve, orbit, or ocular muscle within the orbit.

Extraocular motor nerve palsies
- Neuro-ophthalmologic examination reveals third nerve palsy (ptosis, exotropia, pupil dilation, and unresponsiveness to light, inability to move and accommodate), fourth nerve palsy (diplopia and inability to rotate eye downward and upward), or sixth nerve palsy (one eye turning, with the other eye unable to abduct beyond midline).
- Skull X-rays rule out intracranial tumor.
- CT scan and MRI rule out tumor.

- Cerebral angiography rules out vascular abnormalities.
- Blood studies rule out diabetes.
- Culture and sensitivity tests reveal infective organism (for sixth nerve palsy resulting from infection).

Extrapulmonary tuberculosis
- Acid-fast smear reveals *Mycobacterium tuberculosis*.
- Tuberculin skin test is positive.
- CXR reveals primary pulmonary nodular infiltrates and cavitations (often, however, CXR is negative in extrapulmonary tuberculosis).
- Fluid specimen culture (urine, synovial fluid) reveals *M. tuberculosis*.

Fallopian tube cancer
- History includes unexplained postmenopausal bleeding.
- Papanicolaou test reveals abnormal cells.
- Ultrasonography defines tumor mass.
- Barium enema rules out intestinal obstruction.
- Laparotomy and biopsy reveal malignant cells.

Fanconi's syndrome
- 24-hour urine testing reveals excessive excretion of glucose, phosphate, amino acids, HCO_3^-, and potassium.
- Phosphorus and nitrogen levels are elevated (with increased renal dysfunction).
- Serum alkaline phosphatase levels are elevated (with rickets).
- Serum potassium level is decreased.
- Serum HCO_3^- level is < 22 mEq/L.

Fatty liver
- Examination reveals large, tender liver.
- Liver function studies reveal low albumin, elevated globulin, elevated total

bilirubin, low aminotransferase and, commonly, elevated cholesterol levels.
- PT is prolonged.
- Liver biopsy reveals excessive fat.

Femoral and popliteal aneurysms
- Palpation reveals a pulsating mass above or below the inguinal ligament (in femoral aneurysm) or in the popliteal space (in popliteal aneurysm).
- Arteriography or ultrasonography reveals location and size of aneurysm.

Folic acid deficiency anemia
- Serum folate level is decreased.
- Reticulocyte count is decreased.
- Schilling test is positive.
- Serum blood studies show macrocytosis, increased mean corpuscular volume, and abnormal platelets.

Folliculitis, furunculosis, and carbunculosis
- Examination reveals pustule, painful nodule, or abscess on areas with hair growth.
- Wound culture identifies *Staphylococcus aureus*.
- CBC may reveal leukocytosis.
- In carbunculosis, history includes preexistent furunculosis.

Galactorrhea
- History includes milk secretion more than 21 days after weaning.
- Breast palpation results in expression of secretions.
- Microscopic examination reveals fat droplets in fluid.
- Prolactin levels are > 200 ng/ml.
- CT scan rules out pituitary tumor.
- Mammography rules out tumor.

Galactosemia
- Deficiency of the enzyme galactose-1-phosphate uridyl transferase in RBCs indicates classic galactosemia; decreased galactokinase level in RBCs indicates galactokinase deficiency.
- Serum and urine galactose levels are increased.
- Ophthalmoscopy reveals punctate lesions in the fetal lens nucleus.
- Liver biopsy reveals acinar formation.
- Liver enzyme levels (AST and ALT) are elevated.
- Urinalysis reveals presence of albumin.
- Amniocentesis provides prenatal diagnosis (recommended for heterozygous and homozygous parents).

Gallbladder and bile duct carcinoma
- Liver function test may show elevated urobilirubin levels and may show elevated levels of bile and bilirubin.
- Serum bilirubin levels are elevated (5 to 390 mg/dl).
- Patient may be jaundiced.
- PT is prolonged.
- Serum alkaline phosphatase levels are consistently elevated.
- Liver-spleen scan identifies abnormality.
- Cholecystography shows stones or calcifications.
- MRI may show areas of tumor growth.
- Cholangiography outlines common bile duct obstruction.
- Ultrasonography of the gallbladder shows a mass.
- Endoscopic retrograde cholangiopancreatography identifies tumor site.
- Biopsy reveals malignant cells.

Gas gangrene
- History includes recent surgery or a deep puncture wound with rapid onset of pain and crepitation around the wound.
- Anaerobic cultures of wound drainage reveal *Clostridium perfringens*.

- Gram stain of wound drainage reveals large, gram-positive, rod-shaped bacteria.
- X-rays reveal gas in tissues.
- Blood studies reveal leukocytosis and, later, hemolysis.

Gastric carcinoma
- Barium X-rays with fluoroscopy reveal tumor or filling defect in the outline of the stomach, loss of flexibility and distensibility, and abnormal gastric mucosa with or without ulceration.
- Gastroscopy with fiber-optic endoscope visualizes mucosal lesions and allows gastroscopic biopsy (biopsy reveals malignant cells).
- Photography with fiber-optic endoscope provides a permanent record of gastric lesions that may help determine disease progression and effect of treatment.
- CT scans, CXR, liver and bone scans, and liver biopsy may rule out specific organ metastasis.

Gastritis
- History includes gastric discomfort or bleeding.
- Gastroscopy demonstrates inflammation of mucosa and confirms diagnosis.
- Stools or vomitus may contain occult blood.
- Hb and HCT levels are decreased if bleeding has occurred.

Gastroenteritis
- History includes acute onset of diarrhea accompanied by abdominal pain and discomfort.
- Stool or blood culture reveals causative bacteria, parasites, or amoebae.
- Barium enema reveals inflammation.

Gastroesophageal reflux
- Barium swallow with fluoroscopy may be normal except in patients with advanced disease; in children, barium esophagography under fluoroscope reveals reflux.
- Esophageal acidity test reveals pH of 1.5 to 2.0.
- Acid perfusion test elicits pain or burning.
- Gastroesophageal reflux scanning detects radioactivity in the esophagus.
- Endoscopy and biopsy identify pathologic mucosal changes.

Gaucher's disease
- Bone marrow aspiration reveals Gaucher's cells.
- Direct assay of glucocerebrosidase activity, which can be performed on venous blood, shows absent or deficient activity.
- Liver biopsy reveals increased glucosylceramide accumulation.
- Serum acid phosphatase levels are increased.
- Platelet count and serum iron level are decreased.

Genital herpes
- History includes oral, vaginal, or anal sexual contact with an infected person or other direct contact with lesions.
- Examination reveals vesicles on the genitalia, mouth, or anus.
- Tissue culture and histologic biopsy of vesicular fluid reveals herpes simplex virus type 2.

Genital warts
- Dark-field examination of scrapings from wart cells shows marked vascularization of epidermal cells, which helps to differentiate genital warts from condylomata lata.
- Applying 5% acetic acid (white vinegar) to the warts turns them white, indicating papillomas.

Giardiasis

- History includes such risk factors as recent travel to an endemic area, participation in sexual activity involving oral-anal contact, ingestion of suspect water, or institutionalization.
- Stool specimen shows cysts.
- Duodenal aspirate or biopsy shows trophozoites.
- Small-bowel biopsy shows parasitic infection.

Glaucoma

- History includes gradual loss of peripheral vision.
- Tonometry (using an applanation, Schiøtz, or pneumatic tonometer) reveals increased intraocular pressure.
- Gonioscopy determines the angle of the anterior chamber of the eye, differentiating between chronic open-angle glaucoma and acute angle-closure glaucoma.
- Ophthalmoscopy reveals cupping and atrophy of the optic disk.
- Slit-lamp examination visualizes anterior structures of the eye, demonstrating effects of glaucoma.
- Perimetry or visual field tests evaluate the extent of visual field loss of open-angle deterioration.
- Fundus photography reveals changes in the optic disk.

Glycogen storage diseases

- Type Ia:
- Liver biopsy reveals normal glycogen synthetase and phosphorylase enzyme activities but reduced or absent glucose-6-phosphatase activity.
- Liver biopsy reveals normal glycogen structure, but elevated amounts.
- Serum glucose levels are low.
- Plasma studies reveal high levels of free fatty acids, triglycerides, cholesterol, and uric acid.
- Injection of glucagon or epinephrine increases pyruvic and lactic acid levels but doesn't increase blood glucose levels.
- Glucose tolerance test curve reveals depletional hypoglycemia and reduced insulin output.
- Type II (Pompe's):
- Muscle biopsy reveals increased concentration of glycogen with normal structure and decreased alpha-1,4-glucosidase level.
- ECG (in infants) shows large QRS complexes in all leads, inverted T waves, and a shortened PR interval.
- Electromyography (in adults) demonstrates muscle fiber irritability and myotonic discharges.
- Amniocentesis reveals a deficiency in alpha-1,4-glucosidase level.
- Placenta or umbilical cord examination shows an alpha-1,4-glucosidase deficiency.
- Liver biopsy shows deficient debranching activity and increased glycogen concentration.
- Type III (Cori's):
- Laboratory tests (in children only) may reveal elevated AST or ALT levels and an increase in erythrocyte glycogen.
- Type IV (Andersen's):
- Liver biopsy demonstrates deficient branching enzyme activity and that the glycogen molecule has longer outer branches.
- Type V (McArdle's):
- Serum studies indicate no increase in venous levels of lactate in sample drawn from extremity after ischemic exercise.
- Muscle biopsy reveals a lack of phosphorylase activity and an increased glycogen content.
- Type VI (Hers'):
- Liver biopsy shows decreased phosphorylase beta activity and increased glycogen concentration.
- Type VII:
- Serum studies indicate no increase in venous levels of lactate in sample

drawn from extremity after ischemic exercise.
– Muscle biopsy shows deficient phosphofructokinase and a marked rise in glycogen concentration.
– Blood studies reveal low erythrocyte phosphofructokinase activity and reduced half-life of RBCs.
– Muscle biopsy shows deficient phosphofructokinase with a marked rise in glycogen concentration with normal structure.
• Type VIII:
– Liver biopsy shows deficient phosphorylase beta activity and increased liver glycogen levels.
– Blood studies show deficient phosphorylase beta kinase in leukocytes.

Goiter, simple

• History includes residence in an area known for nutritionally related risk factors (such as iodine-depleted soil or malnutrition) or ingestion of goitrogenic medications or foods.
• Serum thyroid-stimulating hormone or triiodothyronine concentration is high or normal.
• Serum thyroxine concentrations are low to normal.
• Uptake of ^{131}I is normal or increased.
• Protein-bound iodine is low to normal.
• Urinary excretion of iodine is low.

Gonorrhea

• History includes sexual contact with a partner with gonorrhea.
• Culture from site of infection (urethra, cervix, rectum, pharynx) reveals *Neisseria gonorrhoeae.*
• Culture of joint fluid and skin lesions reveals gram-negative diplococci (gonococcal arthritis).
• Culture of conjunctival scrapings confirms gonococcal conjunctivitis.
• Complement fixation and immunofluorescent assays of serum reveal antibody titers four times the normal rate.

Goodpasture's syndrome

• Immunofluorescence of alveolar basement membrane shows linear deposition of Ig as well as C_3 and fibrinogen.
• Immunofluorescence of glomerular basement membrane (GBM) shows linear deposition of Ig combined with detection of circulating anti-GBM antibody.
• Lung biopsy shows interstitial and intra-alveolar hemorrhage with hemosiderin-laden macrophages.
• CXR reveals pulmonary infiltrates in a diffuse, nodular pattern.
• Renal biopsy reveals focal necrotic lesions and cellular crescents.
• Serum creatinine and BUN levels typically increase two to three times normal.
• Urinalysis may reveal RBCs and cellular casts, granular casts, and proteinuria.

Gout

• Microscopic analysis of synovial fluid obtained by needle aspiration reveals needlelike intracellular crystals of sodium urate; presence of monosodium urate monohydrate crystals confirms diagnosis.
• Serum uric acid levels are normal, but may be increased; the higher the level, the more likely a gout attack.
• Urine uric acid levels are increased (in approximately 20% of patients).
• X-rays reveal damage to the articular cartilage and subchondral bone (in chronic gout).

Granulocytopenia

• Patient demonstrates marked neutropenia.
• WBC count is markedly decreased.
• CBC reveals few observable granulocytes.
• Bone marrow aspiration reveals a scarcity of granulocytic precursor cells beyond the most immature forms.

Guillain-Barré syndrome
- History includes minor febrile illness 1 to 4 weeks before current symptoms.
- Examination reveals progressive muscle weakness.
- CSF analysis reveals normal WBC count, rising protein levels (peaks in 4 to 6 weeks), and increasing pressure.
- Electromyography reveals repeated firing of the same motor unit instead of widespread sectional stimulation.
- Electrophysiologic studies may reveal marked slowing of nerve conduction velocities.

Haemophilus influenzae infection
- Blood culture reveals *H. influenzae* infection.
- CBC reveals polymorphonuclear leukocytosis and, in young children with severe infection, leukopenia.

Hearing loss
- Audiometry identifies and quantifies hearing loss.
- The Weber, the Rinne, and Schwabach tests differentiate between conductive and sensorineural hearing loss.
- Auditory brain stem response and behavioral tests may help to identify neonatal or infant hearing loss.
- CT scan evaluates vestibular and auditory pathways.
- Pure tone audiometry identifies the presence and degree of hearing loss.
- MRI detects acoustic tumors and lesions.

Heart failure
- Auscultation reveals dyspnea or crackles.
- CXR reveals increased pulmonary vascular markings, interstitial edema, or pleural effusion and cardiomegaly.
- Pulmonary artery monitoring reveals elevated pulmonary artery and capillary wedge pressures and elevated left ventricular end-diastolic pressure in left-sided heart failure, and elevated right atrial pressure or central venous pressure in right-sided heart failure.

Hemochromatosis
- Serum or plasma iron concentration is elevated.
- Transferrin levels are increased to 70% to 100% saturation.
- 24-hour urine collection shows excretion of iron after administration of deferoxamine, an iron-chelating agent.
- Liver biopsy may also confirm diagnosis.

Hemophilia
- History suggests disorder runs in family.
- History includes prolonged bleeding after surgery or trauma or of episodes of spontaneous bleeding into muscles or joints.
- Hemophilia A:
  – Factor VIII assay is 0% to 55% of normal.
  – APTT is prolonged.
  – Platelet count and function, bleeding time, and PT are normal.
- Hemophilia B:
  – Factor IX assay is deficient.
  – APTT is prolonged.
- Hemophilia C:
  – Assay testing reveals deficient factor XI. but normal factors VIII and IX levels (rules out hemophilias A and B).
  – PTT is prolonged.
- CT scan rules out intracranial bleeding.
- Arthroscopy rules out joint bleeding.
- Endoscopy rules out GI bleeding.

Hemorrhoids
- History includes intermittent rectal bleeding after defecation.
- Examination reveals hemorrhoids protruding from rectum.
- Proctoscopy reveals internal hemorrhoids.

- Anoscopy and flexible sigmoidoscopy identify internal hemorrhoids and rule out polyps or fistulae.

Hemothorax

- History includes recent trauma to chest area.
- Chest percussion reveals dullness.
- Chest auscultation reveals decreased to absent breath sounds on the affected side.
- Thoracentesis reveals blood or serosanguineous fluid.
- CXR reveals pleural fluid with or without mediastinal shift.
- ABG studies show respiratory failure.
- Hb levels may be decreased depending on the degree of blood loss.

Hepatic encephalopathy

- History includes liver disease, with symptoms beginning with slight personality changes progressing to mental confusion and coma.
- Serum ammonia levels are > 33 µmol/L.
- EEG shows slowing waves as the disease progresses.

Hepatitis, viral

- Hepatitis profile identifies serum antigens and antibodies (serum markers) specific to the causative virus, establishing the type of hepatitis (types A, B, C, D, and E).
- PT is prolonged (more than 3 seconds longer than normal indicates liver damage).
- AST and ALT levels are elevated.
- Serum alkaline phosphatase levels are elevated.
- Serum and urine bilirubin levels are elevated (with jaundice).
- Serum albumin is decreased and serum globulin is increased.
- Liver biopsy and liver scan show patchy necrosis.

Hereditary hemorrhagic telangiectasia

- History includes an established family pattern of bleeding disorders.
- Examination reveals localized aggregations of dilated capillaries on the skin of the face, ears, scalp, hands, arms, and feet, and under the nails; characteristic telangiectases are raised or flat, nonpulsatile, violet in color, blanche under pressure, and bleed easily.
- Bone marrow aspiration shows depleted iron stores, which confirms secondary iron deficiency anemia.
- Platelet count may be abnormal.

Herniated disk

- History includes unilateral low back pain radiating to the buttocks, legs, and feet, often associated with a previous traumatic injury or back strain.
- X-rays show degenerative changes and rule out other abnormalities.
- MRI also rules out spinal compression.
- LeSegue's test causes resistance and pain, as well as loss of ankle or knee-jerk reflex.
- Myelography pinpoints the level of herniation and reveals spinal canal compression by herniated disk material.
- CT scan identifies soft tissue and bone abnormalities.
- Electromyelography confirms nerve involvement.
- Neuromuscular tests identify motor and sensory loss and leg muscle weakness.

Herpangina

- Examination reveals vesicular lesions on the mucous membranes of the soft palate, tonsillar pillars, and throat.
- Cultures of mouth washings or stool reveal the coxsackieviruses.
- Antibody titers are elevated.

Herpes simplex
● Examination reveals edema with small vesicles on an erythematous base that rupture, leaving a painful ulcer followed by yellow crusting.
● Isolation of virus from local lesions and biopsy reveal *Herpesvirus hominis*.

Herpes zoster
● Examination reveals small, red, nodular skin lesions that spread unilaterally around the thorax or vertically over the arms or legs and vesicles filled with clear fluid or pus.
● Examination of vesicular fluid and infected tissue reveals eosinophilic intranuclear inclusions and varicella virus.
● Lumbar puncture shows increased CSF pressure; CSF analysis shows increased protein levels and possibly, pleocytosis (with central nervous system involvement).

Hiatal hernia
● CXR reveals air shadow behind the heart (with large hernia).
● Barium swallow with fluoroscopy reveals outpouching at lower end of the esophagus and identifies diaphragmatic abnormalities.
● Serum Hb and HCT levels may be decreased (with paraesophageal hernia).
● Endoscopy and biopsy rule out varices and other small gastroesophageal lesions.
● Esophageal motility studies reveal esophageal motor or lower esophageal pressure abnormalities.
● pH studies reveal reflux of gastric contents.
● Acid perfusion test reveals heartburn resulting from esophageal reflux.

Hirschsprung's disease
● Rectal biopsy reveals absence of ganglion cells.

● Barium enema studies reveal a narrowed segment of distal colon with a sawtooth appearance and a funnel-shaped segment above it; barium is retained longer than the usual 12 to 24 hours.
● Rectal manometry detects failure of the internal anal sphincter to relax and contract.
● Upright films of the abdomen show marked colonic distention.

Histoplasmosis
● History includes an immunocompromised condition or exposure to contaminated soil in an endemic area.
● Tissue biopsy and sputum culture reveal *Histoplasma capsulatum* (in acute primary and chronic pulmonary histoplasmosis).
● Histoplasmosis skin test is positive.
● Complement fixation test results and agglutination titers are increased.

Hodgkin's disease
● Lymph node biopsy reveals Reed-Sternberg's abnormal histiocyte proliferation and nodular fibrosis and necrosis.
● CT scan shows lymph node abnormality.
● Lymphangiography shows lymph node abnormality.
● Bone marrow, liver, mediastinal, and spleen biopsies; abdominal CT scan; and lung and bone scans identify organ involvement.
● Blood studies show normochromic anemia (in 50% of patients) and elevated, normal, or reduced WBC count and differential showing any combination of neutrophilia, lymphocytopenia, monocytosis, and eosinophilia.
● Serum alkaline phosphatase levels are increased.

Hookworm disease
● Stool specimen reveals hookworm ova.

- Blood studies show decreased Hb (in severe cases) and markedly increased WBC count with eosinophil count elevation.

Huntington's disease
- History includes family inheritance pattern along with progressive chorea and dementia, with usual onset between ages 35 and 40.
- PET scan identifies disease.
- DNA analysis identifies marker for gene linked to the disease.
- Evoked potential studies reveal bilateral abnormal P100 latencies.
- Pneumoencephalography reveals the characteristic butterfly dilation of the brain's lateral ventricles.
- CT scan reveals brain atrophy.

Hydatidiform mole
- History includes vaginal bleeding, ranging from brownish red spotting to bright red hemorrhage.
- Examination reveals an abnormally enlarged uterus; pelvic examination reveals grapelike vesicles.
- Histologic identification of hydatid vesicles after passage helps confirm diagnosis.
- Ultrasonography shows grapelike structures rather than a fetus; use of a Doppler ultrasonic flowmeter demonstrates the absence of fetal heart tones.
- Amniography reveals the absence of a fetus.
- WBC count and ESR are increased.
- Hb, HCT levels, RBC count, PT, PTT, fibrinogen levels, and hepatic and renal function studies are abnormal.
- Serum hCG levels are elevated 100 days or more after the last menstrual period.
- Serum human placental lactogen levels are subnormal.

Hydrocephalus
- Examination reveals an abnormally large head size for age.

- Skull X-rays reveal thinning of the skull with separation of sutures and widening of the fontanels.
- Ventriculography reveals enlargement of the brain's ventricles.
- Angiography, CT scan, or MRI of the brain reveals areas of altered density and rules out intracranial lesions.

Hydronephrosis
- KUB X-rays reveal bilateral kidney enlargement.
- Renal ultrasonography reveals large, echo-free, central mass that compromises the renal cortex.
- Excretory urography reveals abnormal kidneys.
- Urine studies reveal the inability to concentrate urine, a decreased glomerular filtration rate and, possibly, pyuria (if infection is present).

Hyperaldosteronism
- Serum potassium levels are persistently low (in the absence of edema, diuretic use, GI loss, or abnormal sodium intake).
- Low plasma renin level after volume depletion by diuretic administration and upright posture and a high plasma aldosterone level after volume expansion by salt loading confirms primary hyperaldosteronism in a hypertensive patient without edema.
- Serum HCO_3^- level is elevated with ensuing alkalosis resulting from the loss of hydrogen and potassium in the distal tubules.
- Serum and urine aldosterone levels are increased.
- Plasma volume levels are increased.
- Adrenal angiography or CT scan reveals adrenal tumor.
- Suppression testing reveals decreased plasma aldosterone and urine metabolites (secondary hyperaldosteronism) or normal plasma aldosterone and urine metabolites (primary hyperaldosteronism).

- ECG reveals ST-segment depression and the presence of U waves, indicating hypokalemia.
- CXR shows left ventricular hypertrophy from chronic hypertension.
- CT scan, ultrasonography, or MRI identifies tumor location.

Hyperbilirubinemia

- Patient is jaundiced.
- Serum bilirubin levels are > 10 mg/dl.

Hyperemesis gravidarum

- History includes uncontrolled nausea and vomiting that persists beyond the first trimester of pregnancy.
- Examination reveals substantial weight loss.
- Serum sodium, chloride, potassium, and protein levels are decreased.
- BUN level is elevated.
- Urinalysis reveals ketonuria and proteinuria.

Hyperlipoproteinemia

- Type I (Fredrickson's hyperlipoproteinemia, fat-induced hyperlipemia, idiopathic familial):
– Chylomicrons (very-low-density lipoproteins [VLDL], low-density lipoproteins [LDL], high-density lipoproteins [HDL]) are present in plasma 14 hours or more after last meal.
– Serum chylomicron and triglyceride levels show high elevation; serum cholesterol levels are slightly elevated.
– Serum lipoprotein lipase levels are decreased.
– Leukocytosis is present.
- Type II (familial hyperbetalipoproteinemia, essential familial hypercholesterolemia):
– Plasma concentrations of LDL are increased.
– Serum LDL and cholesterol levels are elevated.
– Increased LDL levels are detected by amniocentesis.

- Type III (familial broad-beta disease, xanthoma tuberosum):
– Serum beta-lipoprotein levels are abnormal.
– Cholesterol and triglyceride levels are elevated.
– Glucose levels are slightly elevated.
- Type IV (endogenous hypertriglyceridemia, hyperbetalipoproteinemia):
– Plasma VLDL levels are elevated.
– Plasma triglyceride levels are moderately increased.
– Serum cholesterol levels are normal or slightly elevated.
– Glucose tolerance is mildly abnormal.
– History includes early coronary artery disease.
- Type V (mixed hypertriglyceridemia, mixed hyperlipidemia):
– Chylomicrons are present in plasma.
– Plasma VLDL levels are elevated.
– Serum cholesterol and triglyceride levels are elevated.

Hyperparathyroidism

- Serum parathyroid hormone levels are increased.
- Serum calcium levels are increased.
- Urine cyclic adenosine monophosphate test reveals failure to respond to parathyroid hormone.
- X-rays show diffuse demineralization of bones, bone cysts, outer cortical bone absorption, and subperiosteal erosion of the radial aspect of the middle fingers.
- X-ray spectrophotometry demonstrates increased bone turnover.
- Radioimmunoassay shows increased concentration of parathyroid hormone with accompanying hypercalcemia.
- Serum phosphorus levels are increased.
- Serum and urine chloride, uric acid, creatinine, and alkaline phosphatase levels are increased; basal acid secretion is present.

• Serum immunoreactive gastrin levels are increased.

Hyperpituitarism
• Growth hormone (GH) immunoassay shows increased plasma GH levels.
• Glucose suppression test shows failure to suppress GH level to below accepted norm of 5 mg.
• Skull X-rays, CT scan, arteriography, and pneumoencephalography reveal the presence and extent of a pituitary lesion.
• Bone X-rays reveal a thickening of the cranium (especially of frontal, occipital, and parietal bones) and of the long bones, as well as osteoarthritis in the spine.

Hypersplenism
• I.V. infusion of chromium-labeled RBCs or platelets reveals high spleen-liver ratio of radioactivity, indicating splenic destruction or sequestration.
• CBC shows decreased Hb levels, WBC count, and platelet count, and elevated reticulocyte count.
• Examination reveals splenomegaly.

Hypertension
• Serial blood pressure measurements on a sphygmomanometer are more than 140/90 mm Hg.
• Urinalysis reveals presence of protein, RBCs, WBCs, or glucose.
• Excretory urography may reveal renal atrophy.
• BUN and serum creatinine levels are normal or elevated, suggesting renal disease.

Hyperthyroidism
• Radioimmunoassay shows increased serum thyroxine and triiodothyronine levels.
• Thyroid scan reveals increased uptake of ^{131}I.
• Thyroid-releasing hormone (TRH) stimulation test reveals failure of the thyroid-stimulating hormone level to rise within 30 minutes after administration of TRH.
• Autoantibody tests reveal presence of thyroid-stimulating Ig.

Hypervitaminoses A and D
• History includes accidental or misguided use of supplemental vitamin preparations.
• Serum vitamin A level is > 90 μg/dl (hypervitaminosis A).
• Serum vitamin D level is > 100 ng/ml (hypervitaminosis D).
• Serum carotene level is > 250 μg/dl (hypercarotenemia).
• X-rays show calcification of tendons, ligaments, and subperiosteal tissues (hypervitaminosis D).

Hypoglycemia
• Blood glucose studies reveal abnormally low levels (< 45 mg/dl).
• c-peptide assay identifies fasting hypoglycemia.

Hypogonadism
• Serum and urine gonadotropin levels are increased in primary, or hypergonadotropic, hypogonadism and decreased in secondary, or hypogonadotropic, hypogonadism.
• Chromosomal analysis identifies the cause.
• Testicular biopsy and semen analysis reveal impaired spermatogenesis and low testosterone levels.
• X-rays and bone scans show delayed closure of epiphyses and immature bone age.

Hypoparathyroidism
• Radioimmunoassay shows decreased serum parathyroid hormone levels.
• Urine and serum calcium levels are decreased.
• Serum phosphorus levels are increased.
• Urine creatinine levels are decreased.

- X-rays show increased bone density and malformation.
- Cyclic adenosine monophosphate test demonstrates a ten- to twentyfold increase (26 to 74 nmol/dl).
- ECG shows increased QT and ST intervals due to hypercalcemia.

Hypopituitarism

- Radioimmunoassay shows decreased plasma levels of some or all pituitary hormones.
- Serum thyroxine levels are decreased (with thyroid dysfunction).
- Arginine test reveals failure of human growth hormone (hGH) levels to rise after arginine infusion (with pituitary dysfunction).
- Insulin tolerance test reveals failure of stimulation or a blunted response of hGH levels (with hypothalamic-pituitary-adrenal axis dysfunction).
- Urine 17-ketosteroid levels are decreased (with hypoadrenalism).
- Levels of serum pituitary hormones (follicle-stimulating hormone, luteinizing hormone, and thyroid-stimulating hormone) are decreased.
- CT scan, pneumoencephalography, or cerebral angiography confirms the presence of tumors inside or outside the sella turcica.

Hypothermic injuries

- History includes severe and prolonged exposure to cold.
- Core body temperature is < 95° F (35° C)
- Physical examination shows burning, tingling, numbness, swelling, pain, and mottled blue-gray skin in exposed areas.

Hypothyroidism in adults

- Radioimmunoassay shows low serum levels of thyroid hormones.
- Serum thyroid-stimulating hormone level may be increased (due to thyroid insufficiency) or decreased (due to hypothalamic or pituitary insufficiency).
- Radioactive iodine uptake test reveals below normal percentages of iodine uptake.
- Radionuclide thyroid imaging reveals "cold spots."
- Thyroid ultrasonography identifies cysts or tumors.
- Serum antithyroid antibodies are elevated (in autoimmune thyroiditis).

Hypothyroidism in children

- Elevated serum thyroid-stimulating hormone levels are associated with low triiodothyronine and thyroxine levels.
- Thyroid scan (^{131}I uptake test) shows decreased uptake levels and confirms the absence of thyroid tissue in athyroid children.
- Gonadotropin levels are increased and compatible with sexual precocity in older children.
- Hip, knee, and thigh X-rays reveal absence of the femoral or tibial epiphyseal line and delayed skeletal development that is markedly inappropriate for the child's chronological age.

Hypovolemic shock

- History includes recent loss of blood volume.
- Blood pressure auscultation reveals mean arterial pressure under 60 mm Hg in adults and a narrowing pulse pressure.
- Blood studies show low Hb and HCT levels, low RBC count, and low platelet levels.
- Serum potassium, sodium, LD, creatinine, and BUN levels are elevated.
- Urine specific gravity is > 1.020.
- Urine osmolality is elevated.
- Urine creatinine levels are decreased.
- ABG measurements show decreased pH, decreased PaO_2, and increased $PaCO_2$ levels.

Idiopathic hypertrophic subaortic stenosis

• Echocardiography shows increased thickness of the intraventricular septum and abnormal motion of the anterior mitral leaflet during systole, occluding left ventricular outflow in obstructive disease.
• Cardiac catheterization reveals elevated left ventricular end-diastolic pressure and, possibly, mitral insufficiency.
• ECG usually demonstrates left ventricular hypertrophy, T-wave inversion, left anterior hemiblock, Q waves in precordial and inferior leads, ventricular arrhythmias and, possibly, atrial fibrillation.
• Phonocardiography confirms an early systolic murmur.

Idiopathic thrombocytopenic purpura

• Platelet count is markedly decreased.
• Bleeding time is prolonged.
• Bone marrow studies show an abundance of megakaryocytes (platelet precursors) and a shortened circulating platelet survival time.

IgA deficiency

• Serum IgA levels are < 15% of total Ig or < 60 mg/dl.
• IgA is usually absent from secretions.

Impetigo

• Inspection reveals characteristic lesions.
• Microscopic visualization, Gram stain, or culture of exudate identifies *Staphylococcus aureus* as causative organism.
• WBC count may be elevated.

Inactive colon

• History includes dry, hard, infrequent stools.

• Digital rectal examination reveals stools in the lower portion of the rectum and a palpable colon.
• Proctoscopy reveals unusually small colon lumen, prominent veins, and an abnormal amount of mucus.
• Upper GI series and barium enema rule out tumor.
• Fecal occult blood test is negative.

Inclusion conjunctivitis

• History includes sexual contact with a partner infected with *Chlamydia trachomatis.*
• Examination reveals swollen, reddened lower eyelids, excessive tearing, and a moderately purulent discharge.
• Conjunctival scraping reveals cytoplasmic inclusion bodies in conjunctival epithelial cells and many polymorphonuclear leukocytes; culture for bacteria is negative.

Infantile autism

• History includes symptom development before age 30 months.
• Denver Developmental Screening Test shows delayed development, especially of social and language skills.
• IQ testing indicates retardation.
• Evaluation reveals impairment in social interaction skills, verbal and nonverbal communication, and imaginative activity and a markedly restricted range of activities and interests.

Infectious mononucleosis

• WBC count is elevated during 2nd and 3rd week of illness, with lymphocytes and monocytes making up 50% to 70% of WBCs (10% of lymphocytes are abnormal).
• Heterophil agglutination tests indicate the presence of heterophil antibodies; testing at 3- to 4-week intervals reveals a rise to four times normal levels.

- Indirect immunofluorescence shows antibodies to Epstein-Barr virus and cellular antigens.
- Liver function studies are abnormal.

Infectious myringitis

- Otoscopic examination shows small, reddened, inflamed blebs in the ear canal, on the tympanic membrane, and in the middle ear (with bacterial invasion).
- Culture of exudate identifies infective organism.

Infertility, female

- History includes inability to achieve pregnancy after having regular intercourse, without contraception, for at least 1 year.
- Progesterone blood levels reveal a luteal phase deficiency.
- Follicle-stimulating hormone levels are decreased.
- Hysterosalpingography reveals tubal obstruction or uterine abnormalities.
- Endoscopy shows tubal obstruction or uterine abnormalities.
- Laparoscopy visualizes abdominal and pelvic areas and may reveal peritubular adhesions or ureterotubal obstruction.
- Postcoital (Sims-Huhner) test shows inadequate motile sperm cells in cervical fluid after intercourse.
- Immunologic or antibody testing detects spermicidal antibodies in the sera of the female.

Infertility, male

- History includes abnormal sexual development, delayed puberty, or infertility in previous relationships.
- Medical history also includes prolonged fever, mumps, impaired nutritional status, previous surgery, or trauma to genitalia.
- Semen analysis reveals subnormal sperm counts, decreased sperm motility, abnormal morphology, or absence of viable spermatozoa.
- Urine 17-ketosteroid levels are decreased.
- Serum testosterone levels are decreased.

Influenza

- Nose and throat culture identifies the causative virus.
- Cold agglutinin titers are elevated.
- Serum antibody titers are increased.
- WBC count is decreased and lymphocytes are increased (uncomplicated cases).

Inguinal hernia

- History includes sharp or "catching" pain when lifting or straining, with excessive coughing, or following a recent pregnancy.
- Examination reveals a swelling or lump in the inguinal area.
- Palpation of the inguinal area, while the patient is performing Valsalva's maneuver, reveals pressure against the fingertip (indirect hernia) or pressure against the side of the finger (direct hernia).
- Abdominal X-ray rules out obstruction.
- WBC count may be elevated.

Insect bites and stings

- Tick:
- History reveals exposure in woods and fields and complaints of itching.
- After several days, tick paralysis (acute flaccid paralysis, starting as paresthesia and pain in legs and resulting in respiratory failure from bulbar paralysis) occurs.
- Bee, wasp, or yellow jacket:
- History reveals painful sting.
- Examination reveals protruding stinger (bees), edema, urticaria, or pruritus.
- Systemic reaction (anaphylaxis), indicating hypersensitivity, usually ap-

pears within 20 minutes and may include weakness, chest tightness, dizziness, nausea, vomiting, abdominal cramps, and throat constriction.

• Brown recluse (violin) spider:
– History reveals exposure to dark areas (outdoor privy, barn, woodshed) in south-central United States with reaction within 2 to 8 hours of the bite.
– Examination reveals localized vasoconstriction with ischemic necrosis at bite site and small, reddened puncture wound forming a bleb and becoming ischemic, proceeding to a dark, hard center in 3 to 4 days and an ulcer within 2 to 3 weeks.
– Pain is minimal initially, but increases over time.
– Commonly, fever, chills, malaise, weakness, nausea, vomiting, edema, seizures, joint pains, petechiae, cyanosis, and phlebitis develop.
– Rarely, thrombocytopenia and hemolytic anemia develop and lead to death within 24 to 48 hours (usually in a child or patient with previous history of cardiac disease).

• Scorpion:
– In nonlethal types, history reveals symptoms lasting from 24 to 78 hours and including local swelling and tenderness, sharp burning sensation, skin discoloration, paresthesia, lymphangitis with regional gland swelling, and anaphylaxis (rare).
– In lethal types, history reveals symptoms including immediate sharp pain, hyperesthesia, drowsiness, itching (nose, throat, mouth), impaired speech, and generalized muscle spasms (including jaw muscle spasms, laryngospasm, incontinence, seizures, nausea, and vomiting).

• Black widow spider:
– History reveals exposure to dark areas (outdoor privy, barn, woodshed) in southern United States between April and November and report of pinprick

sensation followed by dull, numbing pain.
– Examination reveals edema and tiny red bite marks, rigidity of stomach muscles, and severe abdominal pain (10 to 40 minutes after bite).
– Muscle spasms develop in extremities.
– Ascending paralysis occurs, causing difficulty in swallowing and labored, grunting respirations.
– Other symptoms include extreme restlessness, vertigo, sweating, chills, pallor, seizures (especially in children), hyperactive reflexes, hypertension, tachycardia, thready pulse, circulatory collapse, nausea, vomiting, headache, ptosis, eyelid edema, urticaria, pruritus, and fever.

Intestinal obstruction

• History includes progressive, colicky abdominal pain and distention.
• Abdominal X-ray reveals the presence and location of intestinal gas or fluid.
• In X-ray, small-bowel obstruction appears as a typical "stepladder" pattern of alternating gas and fluid levels.
• In X-ray, large-bowel obstruction reveals a distended, air-filled colon or a closed loop of sigmoid with extreme distention.
• Serum sodium, chloride, and potassium levels may decrease because of vomiting.
• WBC count may be normal or slightly elevated if necrosis, peritonitis, or strangulation occurs.
• Serum amylase level may increase.
• Sigmoidoscopy, colonoscopy, or barium enema may help identify the cause of obstruction.

Intussusception

• Barium enema reveals characteristic coiled spring sign and delineates the extent of intussusception.

- Upright abdominal X-rays may show a soft-tissue mass and signs of complete or partial obstruction, with dilated loops of bowel.
- Elevated WBC count may indicate obstruction, strangulation, or bowel infarction.

Iodine deficiency

- Serum thyroxine levels are low, with high ^{131}I uptake.
- 24-hour urine collection reveals low iodine levels.
- Serum thyroid-stimulating hormone levels are high.
- Radioiodine uptake test traces ^{131}I in the thyroid 24 hours after administration.

Iron deficiency anemia

- Bone marrow studies reveal depleted or absent iron stores and normoblastic hyperplasia.
- Hb level is decreased.
- HCT level is decreased.
- Serum iron levels are low, with high iron binding capacity.
- Serum ferritin levels are low.
- RBC count is low, with microcytic and hypochromic cells.
- GI studies rule out or confirm the bleeding.

Irritable bowel syndrome

- History includes diarrhea alternating with constipation and bowel upset related to diet or psychological stress.
- Sigmoidoscopy may reveal spastic contraction.
- Barium enema may reveal colonic spasm and tubular appearance of descending colon.
- Colonoscopy, rectal examination, or rectal biopsy may rule out other disorders.
- Fecal tests for occult blood, parasites, and pathogenic bacteria are negative.

Junctional tachycardia

ECG findings include the following:
- Atrial and ventricular rhythms are usually regular. The atrial rhythm may be difficult to determine if the P wave is absent or hidden in the QRS complex or preceding T wave.
- Atrial and ventricular rates exceed 100 beats/minute (usually between 100 and 200 beats/minute). The atrial rate may be difficult to determine if the P wave is absent or hidden in the QRS complex, or precedes the T wave.
- P wave is usually inverted. It may occur before or after the QRS complex, be hidden in the QRS complex, or be absent.
- If the P wave precedes the QRS complex, the PR interval is shortened (< 0.12 second). Otherwise, the PR interval can't be measured.
- Duration of QRS complex is within normal limits. The configuration is usually normal.
- T-wave configuration is usually normal, but may be abnormal if the P wave is hidden in the T wave. Fast rate may make the T wave indiscernible.
- QT interval is usually within normal limits.

Juvenile angiofibroma

- Nasopharyngeal mirror or nasal speculum reveals a blue mass in the nose or nasopharynx.
- Nasal X-rays reveal a bowing of the posterior wall of the maxillary sinus.
- Angiography reveals the size and location of the tumor and also shows the source of vascularization.

Keratitis

- History includes recent infection of the upper respiratory tract accompanied by cold sores.
- Slit-lamp examination reveals one or more small branchlike (dendritic) lesions (caused by herpes simplex virus).

- Touching the cornea with cotton reveals reduced corneal sensation.

Kidney cancer
- Renal ultrasonography and CT scan identify renal tumor.
- Excretory urography, nephrotomography, and KUB X-ray identify renal tumor.
- Liver function studies show increased alkaline phosphatase, bilirubin, and transaminase levels.
- PT is prolonged.
- Blood studies show anemia, polycythemia, hypercalcemia, and increased ESR.
- Urinalysis reveals hematuria.
- Antegrade urography and cytologic studies reveal malignancy.
- Renal biopsy reveals malignant cells.
- Radionuclide renal imaging reveals malignant tumor.

Klinefelter syndrome
- Karyotype obtained by culturing lymphocytes from the patient's peripheral blood shows chromosome abnormality.
- Testosterone level is depressed after puberty.
- Urine 17-ketosteroid levels are decreased.
- Follicle-stimulating hormone levels are increased.

Kyphosis
- History includes severe pain.
- Examination reveals curvature of the thoracic spine and bone destruction.
- X-rays reveal vertebral wedging, Schmorl's nodes, irregular plates, and possibly mild scoliosis of 10 to 20 degrees.

Labyrinthitis
- History includes nausea and vomiting, hearing loss, and severe vertigo from any movement of the head.

- Examination reveals spontaneous nystagmus with jerking movements of the eyes toward the unaffected ear.
- Culture of drainage identifies infective organism.
- Audiometry reveals sensorineural hearing loss.
- CT scan rules out brain lesion.

Laryngeal cancer
- History includes hoarseness that lasts longer than 2 weeks.
- Laryngoscopy reveals lesion.
- Laryngeal tomography, CT scan, or laryngography defines the borders of a lesion.
- Laryngeal biopsy reveals malignant cells.
- CXR identifies metastasis.

Laryngitis
- History includes hoarseness, ranging from mild to complete loss of voice.
- Indirect laryngoscopy reveals red, inflamed and, occasionally, hemorrhagic vocal cords, with rounded rather than sharp edges, and exudate; bilateral swelling may be present, which restricts movement but doesn't cause paralysis.

Lassa fever
- History includes recent travel to an endemic area.
- Throat washings, pleural fluid, or blood cultures reveal Lassa virus.
- Antibody titer reveals Lassa immunoglobulins.

Legg-Calvé-Perthes disease
- Examination reveals restricted abduction and rotation of the hip.
- Hip X-rays (taken every 3 to 4 months) reveal flattening of the femoral head or deformity, new bone formation, and eventually regeneration of the joint.
- Bone scan reveals involvement of anterolateral portion of the femoral head.

- Aspiration and culture of synovial fluid rule out joint sepsis.

Legionnaires' disease

- Cultures of respiratory tract secretions and tissue culture identify *Legionella pneumophila.*
- Direct immunofluorescence testing reveals *L. pneumophila.*
- Indirect fluorescent serum antibody testing shows convalescent serum with a fourfold or greater rise in antibody titer for *L. pneumophila.*
- CXR reveals patchy, localized infiltration, which progresses to multilobar consolidation, pleural effusions and, in fulminant disease, opacification of the entire lung.
- Blood studies show leukocytosis, increased ESR, and increases in alkaline phosphatase, ALT, and AST levels.
- ABG measurements show decreased PaO_2 and, initially, decreased $PaCO_2$.
- Bronchial washings, blood and pleural fluid cultures, and transtracheal aspirate studies rule out pulmonary infections.

Leishmaniasis

- Scrapings from edges of lesion identify species of *Leishmania.*
- *Leishmania* skin test is positive.

Leprosy

- Examination reveals skin lesions and muscular and neurologic deficits.
- Biopsy of skin lesions, peripheral nerves, or smear of skin or ulcerated mucous membranes allows identification of *Mycobacterium leprae.*

Lichen planus

- Examination reveals generalized eruptions of flat, glistening purple papules marked with white lines or spots appearing linearly or coalescing into plaques.
- Skin biopsy reveals lichen planus.

Listeriosis

- Cultures of blood, CSF, cervical or vaginal lesion drainage, or lochia from a mother with an infected fetus reveal *Listeria monocytogenes.*
- CBC reveals monocytosis.

Liver abscess

- Liver scan reveals filling defects at the area of the abscess longer than ¾″ (1.9 cm).
- Hepatic ultrasonography reveals defects caused by abscess.
- CT scan reveals a low-density, homogenous area with well-defined borders.
- CXR reveals the diaphragm on the affected side to be raised and fixed.
- Blood tests show elevated levels of AST, ALT, alkaline phosphatase, and bilirubin.
- Serum albumin is decreased.
- WBC count is elevated.
- Blood cultures and percutaneous liver aspiration identify causative organism.
- Stool cultures and serologic and hemagglutination tests isolate *Entamoeba histolytica* (in amoebic abscesses).

Liver cancer

- Needle biopsy or open biopsy reveals malignant cells.
- Alpha-fetoprotein levels are elevated in 70% of patients with hepatocellular carcinoma.
- Liver scan shows filling defects.
- Liver function tests are abnormal.
- CXR rule out metastasis to lungs.
- Arteriography may define large tumors.
- Serum electrolyte measurements show increased levels of sodium.
- Serum glucose levels are decreased.
- Cholesterol levels are decreased.

Lower urinary tract infection

- Microscopic urinalysis reveals RBC and WBC counts > 10/high-power field.
- Clean-catch urinalysis reveals bacterial count of more than 100,000/ml.
- Voiding cystoureterography or excretory urography shows congenital anomalies predisposing the patient to urinary tract infections.

Lung abscess

- Auscultation of the chest may reveal crackles and decreased breath sounds.
- CXR shows a localized infiltrate with one or more clear spaces, usually containing air or fluid.
- Percutaneous aspiration of an abscess or bronchoscopy may be used to obtain cultures to identify the causative organism.
- Blood and sputum cultures and Gram stain identify causative organism.
- WBC count is elevated.

Lung cancer

- CXR reveals lesion or mass.
- Sputum cytology reveals malignant cells.
- Bronchoscopy reveals site of mass.
- Biopsy reveals malignant cells.
- Tissue biopsy reveals evidence of metastasis.

Lupus erythematosus

- Examination reveals classic butterfly rash occurring over the nose and cheeks.
- Antinuclear antibody, anti-DNA, and lupus erythematosus cell tests are positive.
- Urine studies may show RBCs, WBCs, urine casts, sediment, and protein loss.
- CXR reveals pleurisy or lupus pneumonitis.
- Blood studies may show decreased serum complement (C_3 and C_4) levels,

indicating active disease; ESR is usually elevated; leukopenia, mild thrombocytopenia, and anemia also may be evident.
- ECG may show a conduction defect (with cardiac involvement or pericarditis).
- Renal biopsy identifies progression and extent of renal involvement.

Lyme disease

- History includes recent travel to endemic areas or exposure to ticks.
- Examination reveals the classic skin lesion called erythema chronicum migrans, beginning as a red macule or papule at the tick bite site growing in size to as large as 2″ (5 cm), described as hot and pruritic, with bright red outer rims and white centers.
- Mild anemia and elevated ESR, leukocyte count, serum IgM level, and AST level support the diagnosis.
- Antibody titers, ELISA, or blood culture may reveal *Borrelia burgdorferi;* lumbar puncture with CSF analysis allows for identification of antibodies to *B. burgdorferi* (if Lyme disease involves the central nervous system).

Lymphocytopenia

- Lymphocyte count is markedly decreased.
- Bone marrow aspiration and lymph node biopsies identify the cause.

Magnesium imbalance

- Hypomagnesemia:
– Serum magnesium levels are < 1.5 mEq/L.
– Serum potassium and calcium levels are decreased.
– ECG shows tachyarrhythmias, slightly prolonged PR interval, prolonged QT interval, slightly prolonged QRS complex, ST-segment depression, prominent U waves, and broad flattened T waves.

- Hypermagnesemia:
– Serum magnesium levels are
> 2.5 mEq/L.
– Serum potassium and calcium levels
are elevated.
– ECG shows prolonged PR interval,
prolonged QRS complex, and elevated
T wave.

Malaria
- History includes travel to an endemic
area, recent blood transfusion, or I.V.
drug use.
- Blood smears reveal parasites in
RBCs.
- Indirect immunofluorescent serum
antibody tests reveal malaria (2 weeks
after onset).
- CBC shows decreased Hb level and a
normal or decreased WBC count.
- Urinalysis reveals protein and WBCs
in urine sediment.
- Serum blood studies show a reduced
platelet count, prolonged PT, prolonged
PTT, and decreased plasma fibrinogen
levels (in falciparum malaria).

Malignant brain tumor
- Skull X-ray, brain scan, CT scan, or
MRI reveals lesion.
- Biopsy of lesion reveals malignant
cells.
- Lumbar puncture shows increased
protein levels and decreased glucose
levels in CSF; increased CSF pressure,
indicating increased intracranial pressure; and, occasionally, tumor cells in
CSF.

Malignant lymphoma
- Examination reveals enlarged lymph
nodes.
- Biopsy of lymph nodes, tonsils, bone
marrow, liver, bowel, or skin reveals
malignant cells.
- CXR; lymphangiography; liver,
bone, and spleen scans; CT scan of the
abdomen; and excretory urography
show disease progression.

- Serum uric acid level is normal or elevated.
- Serum calcium level may be elevated, indicating bone lesions.

Malignant melanoma
- Examination reveals skin lesion or
nevus with recent changes in appearance.
- Excisional biopsy and full-depth
punch biopsy reveal malignant cells.
- Urine test reveals melanin.

Mallory-Weiss syndrome
- History includes recent bout of
forceful vomiting followed by vomiting blood or passing blood rectally (after a few hours to several days).
- Endoscopy identifies esophageal
tear.
- Angiography reveals bleeding site.
- Serum HCT level are decreased.
(Measurements help to quantify blood
loss.)

Marfan syndrome
- History includes disease in close rel-
atives.
- Examination reveals skeletal defor-
mities and ectopia lentis.
- X-rays reveal skeletal abnormalities.
- Echocardiography detects aortic root
dilation.

Mastitis and breast
engorgement
- History includes breast discomfort or
other symptoms of inflammation in a
lactating woman.
- Examination reveals redness, swelling, warmth, hardness, tenderness,
cracks or fissures of the nipple, and enlarged lymph nodes.
- Cultures of expressed milk identify
infective organism (generalized mastitis).
- Cultures of breast skin identify infective organism (localized mastitis).

Mastoiditis

- X-rays of the mastoid area reveal hazy mastoid air cells, and the bony walls between the cells appear decalcified.
- Otoscopy reveals a dull, thickened, and edematous tympanic membrane, if the membrane isn't concealed by obstruction.
- Culture and sensitivity tests identify causative organism.
- Audiometry shows a conductive hearing loss.

Medullary cystic disease

- Family history includes medullary cystic disease.
- Arteriography and excretory urography demonstrate small kidneys.
- Kidney biopsy shows structural abnormalities.
- Blood studies show profound anemia.
- Serum alkaline phosphatase level is elevated (in young patients).

Medullary sponge kidney

- Excretory urography reveals a characteristic flowerlike appearance of the pyramidal cavities when they fill with contrast material.
- Urinalysis is normal, but may show increased WBC count and casts (with infection) or an increased RBC count (with hematuria).

Ménière's disease

- History includes vertigo, tinnitus, and hearing loss or distortion.
- Audiometric studies indicate a sensorineural hearing loss and loss of discrimination and recruitment.
- MRI rules out brain lesions or tumors.
- Auditory brain stem response test rules out cochlear or retrocochlear lesion as the cause of hearing loss.

Meningitis

- Lumbar puncture reveals cloudy CSF, elevated CSF pressure, high protein level, and depressed glucose concentration.
- CSF culture and sensitivity tests reveal gram-positive or gram-negative organisms.
- CXR shows pneumonitis or lung abscess, tubercular lesions, or granulomas (secondary to fungal infection).
- Sinus and skull X-rays may help identify cranial osteomyelitis, paranasal sinusitis, or skull fracture.
- WBC count shows leukocytosis.
- CT scan rules out cerebral hematoma, hemorrhage, or tumor.
- Brudzinski's and Kernig's signs are positive.

Meningococcal infection

- Blood, CSF, or lesion culture reveals *Neisseria meningitidis*.
- Platelet and clotting levels are decreased (with skin or adrenal hemorrhages).

Menopause

- History includes menstrual cycle irregularities.
- Papanicolaou test results show changes indicating the influence of estrogen deficiency on vaginal mucosa.
- Radioimmunoassay blood studies show decreased estrogen levels, plasma estradiol level of 0 to 30 pg/ml, and estrone level of 14 to 103 pg/ml.
- Pelvic examination, endometrial biopsy, and dilatation and curettage rule out suspected organic disease.
- Serum follicle-stimulating hormone level is 30 to 100 mIU/ml.
- Plasma luteinizing hormone level is 20 to 100 IU/L.

Metabolic acidosis

- ABG analysis reveals:
– pH < 7.35 (in severe acidosis, pH may fall to 7.10)

– $Paco_2$ normal or < 34 mm Hg
– HCO_3^- level may be < 22 mEq/L.
● Anion gap is > 14 mEq/L.
● Serum potassium levels are usually elevated.
● Blood glucose and serum ketone body levels are elevated (in diabetes mellitus).
● Plasma lactic acid levels are elevated (in lactic acidosis).

Metabolic alkalosis

● ABG analysis reveals:
– pH > 7.45.
– HCO_3^- level > 29 mEq/L
– $Paco_2$ may be > 45 mm Hg (indicating respiratory compensation).
● Serum electrolyte levels usually show decreased potassium, calcium, and chloride levels.
● ECG shows a low T wave merging with a P wave and atrial or sinus tachycardia.

Mitral insufficiency

● Cardiac catheterization may indicate signs of mitral insufficiency, including increased left ventricular end-diastolic volume and pressure, increased atrial and pulmonary artery wedge pressures, and decreased cardiac output.
● CXR may demonstrate left atrial and ventricular enlargement, pulmonary venous congestion, and calcification of the mitral leaflets.
● Echocardiography may reveal abnormal motion of the valve leaflets, left atrial enlargement, and a hyperdynamic left ventricle.
● ECG may show left atrial and ventricular hypertrophy, sinus tachycardia, or atrial fibrillation.

Mitral stenosis

● Cardiac catheterization shows a diastolic pressure gradient across the mitral valve and elevated left atrial and pulmonary artery pressures, as well as an elevated pulmonary artery wedge pres-

sure. Catheterization may also reveal elevated right ventricular pressure, decreased cardiac output, and abnormal contraction of the left ventricle. Note that this test may not be indicated in patients who have isolated mitral stenosis with mild symptoms.
● CXR shows left atrial and left ventricular enlargement (in severe mitral stenosis), straightening of the left border of the cardiac silhouette, enlarged pulmonary arteries, dilation of the pulmonary veins of the upper lobes of the lungs, and mitral valve calcification.
● Echocardiography may disclose thickened mitral valve leaflets and left atrial enlargement.
● ECG can reveal atrial fibrillation, right ventricular hypertrophy, left atrial enlargement (in sinus rhythm), and right axis deviation.

Motion sickness

● History includes nausea, vomiting, dizziness, headache, fatigue, diaphoresis, or difficulty breathing related to a sensation of motion.
● If problem is persistent and affects the person's lifestyle, audiometry and vestibular tests may rule out vertigo.

Multiple endocrine neoplasia

● Family history reveals inheritance pattern, confirmed by genetic testing.
● Evaluation of signs and symptoms suggests multiple endocrine neoplasia.
● Diagnostic tests reveal hyperplasia, adenoma, or carcinoma in two or more endocrine glands, confirmed by biopsy.

Multiple myeloma

● CBC shows moderate to severe anemia; differential may show 40% to 50% lymphocytes but seldom more than 3% plasma cells.
● Rouleaux formation is seen on differential smear results.

- Analysis of urine proteins reveals Bence-Jones protein, proteinuria, and hypercalciuria.
- Serum calcium levels are elevated.
- Serum electrophoresis shows an elevated globulin spike, which is electrophoretically and immunologically abnormal.
- Excretion tests show phenolsulfonphthalein level > 25% in 15 minutes, > 80% in 2 hours.
- Bone marrow aspiration detects myelomatous cells.
- KUB X-rays reveal bilateral renal enlargement.
- X-rays reveal multiple, sharply circumscribed osteolytic lesions, especially on the skull, pelvis, and spine.

Multiple sclerosis

- History includes multiple neurologic attacks with characteristic remissions and exacerbations.
- EEG results are abnormal.
- CSF analysis reveals elevated gamma globulin fraction of IgG (with normal serum gamma globulin levels).
- MRI reveals multifocal white matter lesions resulting from demyelination.
- Evoked potential studies show slowed conduction of nerve impulses (in 80% of patients).
- CT scan may show lesions within the brain's white matter.

Mumps

- History includes inadequate immunization and exposure to person infected with mumps.
- Examination reveals swelling and tenderness of the parotid glands and one or more of the other salivary glands.
- Antibody titer increases fourfold 3 weeks after acute phase of illness.
- Serum amylase level may be elevated.

Muscular dystrophy

- History includes progressive muscle weakness and evidence of genetic transmission.
- Muscle biopsy reveals fat and connective tissue deposits, degeneration and necrosis of muscle fibers and, in Duchenne's and Becker's dystrophies, a deficiency of the muscle protein dystrophin.
- Electromyography shows short, weak bursts of electrical activity in affected muscles.
- Genetic testing identifies the gene defect (in some patients).
- Urine creatinine, serum CK, LD, ALT, and AST levels are elevated.

Myasthenia gravis

- History includes progressive muscle weakness and muscle fatigability that improves with rest.
- Tensilon test is positive, showing improved muscle function after an I.V. injection of edrophonium or neostigmine.
- Serum acetylcholine receptor antibodies test is positive in symptomatic adults.
- Electromyography reveals motor unit potentials that are initially normal but progressively diminish in amplitude with continuing contractions.
- CXR or CT scan may show a thymoma.

Mycosis fungoides

- History includes multiple, varied, and progressively severe skin lesions.
- Biopsy of lesions reveals lymphoma cells.
- Fingerstick smear reveals Sézary cells (abnormal circulating lymphocytes), found in the erythrodermic variants of mycosis fungoides (Sézary syndrome).

Myelitis and acute transverse myelitis

- WBC count is normal or slightly elevated.
- CSF analysis may show normal or increased lymphocyte and protein levels and allows for isolation of the causative agent.
- Throat washings may reveal the causative virus (in poliomyelitis).
- CT scan or MRI may rule out spinal tumor.
- Examination may reveal focal neck and back pain with development of paresthesia and sensory loss.

Myocardial infarction

- History includes substernal chest pain, with radiation.
- Serial 12-lead ECG may be normal or inconclusive during the first hours after a myocardial infarction (MI); may reveal serial ST-segment depression (in subendocardial MI) and ST-segment elevation and Q waves (in transmural MI).
- Cardiac enzyme tests reveal elevated CK levels, with CK-MB isoenzyme > 5% of total CK over a 72-hour period.
- Echocardiography shows ventricular wall dyskinesia (with a transmural MI).
- Radioisotope scans using I.V. technetium 99m pertechnetate show "hot spots," indicating damaged muscle.
- Myocardial perfusion imaging with thallium-210 reveals a "cold spot" in most patients during the first few hours after a transmural MI.

Myocarditis

- History includes recent febrile upper respiratory tract infection, viral pharyngitis, or tonsillitis.
- Cardiac examination reveals supraventricular and ventricular arrhythmias, S_3 and S_4 gallops, a faint S_1, possibly a murmur of mitral insufficiency,

and a pericardial friction rub (in patients with pericarditis).
- Endomyocardial biopsy reveals histologic changes consistent with myocarditis.
- Cardiac enzyme levels, including CK, CK-MB, serum AST, and LD, are elevated.
- WBC count and ESR are elevated.
- Antibody titers such as antistreptolysin-O are elevated.
- ECG shows diffuse ST-segment and T-wave abnormalities, conduction defects, and other ventricular and supraventricular arrhythmias.
- Cultures of stool, throat, pharyngeal washings, or other body fluids identify the causative bacteria or virus.

Nasal papillomas

- Examination reveals inverted papillomas as large, bulky, highly vascular, and edematous; color varies from dark red to gray; consistency, from firm to friable.
- Examination may also reveal exophytic papillomas that are raised, firm, and rubbery; color varies from pink to gray; papillomas are securely attached by a broad or pedunculated base to the mucous membrane.
- Biopsy reveals histologic findings characteristic of papillomas.

Nasal polyps

- X-rays of sinuses and nasal passages reveal soft tissue shadows over the affected areas.
- Examination with a nasal speculum reveals nasal obstruction and a dry, red surface with clear or gray growths; large growths may resemble tumors.

Near-drowning

- History includes recent water submersion.
- Auscultation of the lungs reveals rhonchi and crackles.

- ABG analysis reveals:
- – pH < 7.35
- – PaO$_2$ < 75 mm Hg
- – HCO$_3^-$ level < 22 mEq/L.
- ECG may show supraventricular tachycardia, premature ventricular contractions, and nonspecific ST-segment and T-wave abnormalities.

Necrotizing enterocolitis
- Anteroposterior and lateral abdominal X-rays reveal nonspecific intestinal dilation and, in later stages, gas or air in the intestinal wall.
- Platelet count is decreased.
- Serum sodium levels are < 135 mEq/L.
- Serum bilirubin levels (indirect, direct, and total) may be elevated.
- Blood and stool cultures are positive for *Escherichia coli, Clostridia, Salmonella, Pseudomonas,* or *Klebsiella.*
- Hb level is decreased.
- PT and PTT are prolonged.
- Fibrin degradation products are increased.
- Guaiac test detects occult blood in stool.

Nephrotic syndrome
- Urinalysis shows marked proteinuria and reveals increased number of hyaline, granular, and waxy, fatty casts and oval fat bodies.
- Renal biopsy provides histologic identification of the lesion.
- Triiodothyronine resin uptake percentage is high with a low or normal free thyroxine level.
- Serum protein electrophoresis reveals decreased albumin and gamma globulin levels and markedly increased alpha$_2$ and beta globulin levels.
- Serum triglyceride, phospholipid, and cholesterol levels are elevated.

Neurofibromatosis
- Examination reveals café-au-lait spots and multiple pedunculated nodules (neurofibromas) of varying sizes on the nerve trunks of the extremities and on the nerves of the head, neck, and body.
- X-rays and CT scan reveal widening internal auditory meatus and intervertebral foramen.
- Myelography reveals spinal cord tumors.
- Lumbar puncture with CSF analysis reveals elevated protein concentration.

Neurogenic arthropathy
- History includes painless joint deformity.
- X-rays reveal soft-tissue swelling or effusion (early stage), articular fracture, subluxation, erosion of articular cartilage, periosteal new bone formation, and excessive growth of marginal new bodies or resorption.
- Vertebral examination reveals narrowing of vertebral disk spaces, deterioration of vertebrae, and osteophyte formation.
- Synovial biopsy reveals bony fragments and bits of calcified cartilage.

Neurogenic bladder
- History includes neurologic disease or spinal cord injury.
- CSF analysis shows increased protein level indicating cord tumor; increased gamma globulin level may indicate multiple sclerosis.
- X-rays of the skull and vertebral column show fracture, dislocation, congenital anomalies, or metastasis.
- Myelography shows spinal cord compression.
- Electromyelography confirms presence of peripheral neuropathy.
- Cystometry reveals abnormal micturition and vesical function.
- External sphincter electromyography reveals detrusor-external sphincter dyssynergia.
- Voiding cystourethrography reveals neurogenic bladder.

- Whitaker test reveals bladder abnormality.

Nezelof syndrome
- History includes failure to thrive, poor eating habits, weight loss, and recurrent infections in children.
- Family history may reveal genetic transmission.
- T-lymphocyte assay reveals defective T cells that are moderately to markedly decreased in number.

Nocardiosis
- History reveals progressive pneumonia despite antibiotic therapy.
- Culture of sputum or discharge identifies *Nocardia.*
- Biopsy of lung or other tissue identifies *Nocardia.*
- CXR shows fluffy or interstitial infiltrates, nodules, or abscesses.

Nonspecific genitourinary infections
- History includes sexual contact with a partner with a nonspecific genitourinary infection.
- Cultures of prostatic, cervical, or urethral secretions reveal excessive polymorphonuclear leukocytes but few, if any, specific organisms.

Nonviral hepatitis
- History includes exposure to hepatotoxic chemicals or drugs.
- Serum ALT levels are > 56 U/L.
- Serum AST levels are > 40 U/L.
- Serum total and direct bilirubin levels are elevated (with cholestasis).
- Serum alkaline phosphatase levels are elevated.
- Differential WBC count reveals elevated eosinophils.

Nystagmus
- Inspection reveals involuntary eye movement.

- Positional testing causes nystagmus to occur.
- Electronystagmography reveals nystagmus.
- Vestibular acuity tests may rule out a vestibular lesion as the cause.
- X-rays may rule out structural defects.

Obesity
- Observation and comparison of height and weight to a standardized table reveals weight exceeding ideal body weight by 20% or more. In morbid obesity, body weight > 200% of standard range.
- Measurement of the thickness of subcutaneous fat folds with calipers reveals excess body fat.

Optic atrophy
- Slit-lamp examination reveals a pupil that reacts sluggishly to direct light stimulation.
- Ophthalmoscopy shows pallor of the nerve head from loss of microvascular circulation in the disk and deposit of fibrous or glial tissue.
- Visual field testing reveals a scotoma and, possibly, major visual field impairment.

Orbital cellulitis
- Examination reveals eyelid edema and purulent discharge.
- Culture of eye discharge identifies *Streptococcus, Staphylococcus,* or *Pneumococcus* as the causative organism.

Ornithosis
- History includes recent exposure to birds.
- *Chlamydia psittaci* is recovered from mice, eggs, or tissue culture inoculated with the patient's blood or sputum.
- Comparison of acute and convalescent sera shows a fourfold rise in antibody titers during convalescent phase.

- CXR reveals patchy lobar infiltrate.

Osgood-Schlatter disease
- Examination reveals pain during internal rotation of the tibia while extending the knee from 90 degrees flexion, which subsides immediately with external rotation of the tibia.
- X-rays may reveal epiphyseal separation and soft tissue swelling (up to 6 months after onset) and eventual bone fragmentation.

Osteoarthritis
- History includes deep, aching joint pain, particularly after exercise or weight bearing, usually relieved by rest; and morning stiffness that lasts < 30 minutes.
- Examination may reveal nodes in the distal and proximal joints that become red, swollen, and tender.
- X-rays reveal narrowing of the joint space or margin, cystlike bony deposits in joint space and margins, sclerosis of the subchondral space, joint deformity due to degeneration or articular damage, bony growths at weight-bearing areas, and fusion of joints.

Osteogenesis imperfecta
- Examination reveals blue sclera and deafness.
- X-rays reveal multiple old fractures and skeletal deformities.
- Skull X-ray shows wide sutures with small, irregularly shaped islands of bone (wormian bones).

Osteomyelitis
- History includes sudden pain in the affected bone accompanied by tenderness, heat, swelling, and restricted movement.
- Blood cultures identify *Staphylococcus aureus, Streptococcus pyogenes, Pneumococcus, Pseudomonas aeruginosa, Escherichia coli,* or *Proteus vulgaris* as the causative organism.

- Bone scan shows infection site in early stages of illness.
- X-ray reveals abnormal areas of calcification (may not be evident until 2 to 3 weeks).
- ESR is elevated (> 20 mm/hour).
- WBC count reveals leukocytosis.

Osteoporosis
- X-rays may reveal typical degeneration in the lower thoracic and lumbar vertebrae; vertebral bodies may appear flattened and more dense than normal.
- Photon absorptiometry reveals deterioration of bone mass.
- Bone biopsy reveals thin, porous, but otherwise normal-looking bone.
- Bone densitometry reveals decreased bone density.

Otitis externa
- Examination reveals pain on palpation of the tragus or auricle.
- Otoscopy reveals a swollen external ear canal (sometimes to the point of complete closure), periauricular lymphadenopathy (tender nodes in front of the tragus, behind the ear, or in the upper neck) and, occasionally, regional cellulitis.
- In fungal otitis externa, examination reveals thick, red epithelium after removal of growth.
- Microscopic examination or culture and sensitivity tests identify *Aspergillus niger* or *Candida albicans* as the causative organism for fungal otitis externa; *Pseudomonas, Proteus vulgaris, Streptococcus*, or *Staphylococcus aureus* as the causative organism for bacterial otitis externa.
- In chronic otitis externa, examination of the ear canal reveals a thick red epithelium.

Otitis media
- In acute suppurative otitis media:

– Otoscopy reveals obscured or distorted bony landmarks of the tympanic membrane.
– Pneumatoscopy may show decreased tympanic membrane mobility.
– Examination shows that pulling on the auricle does not exacerbate the pain.
• In acute secretory otitis media:
– Otoscopy demonstrates tympanic membrane retraction, causing the bony landmarks to appear more prominent, with clear or amber fluid detected behind the tympanic membrane, possibly with a meniscus and bubbles.
– If hemorrhage into the middle ear has occurred, the tympanic membrane appears blue-black.
• In chronic otitis media:
– History discloses recurrent or unresolved otitis media; otoscopy shows thickening, and sometimes scarring, and decreased mobility of the tympanic membrane.
– Pneumatoscopy reveals decreased or absent tympanic membrane movement.
• History of recent air travel or scuba diving suggests barotitis media.

Otosclerosis
• Rinne test reveals bone conduction lasting longer than air conduction (normally, the reverse is true); as otosclerosis progresses, bone conduction deteriorates.
• Audiometric testing reveals hearing loss ranging from 60 dB in early stages to total loss as the disease advances.
• Weber's test reveals sound lateralizing to the more affected ear.

Ovarian cancer
• Examination reveals abdominal mass.
• CT scan shows the abdominal tumor.
• Pelvic ultrasonography reveals mass.
• Exploratory laparotomy with biopsy reveals malignant cells.

• Transvaginal ultrasonography shows ovarian enlargement and growth.
• Transvaginal Doppler color flow imaging reveals ovarian growth.
• Carcinoembryonic antigen levels are > 20 ng/ml.
• Serum hCG levels are elevated in a nonpregnant woman.
• Barium enema reveals obstruction and size of tumor.

Ovarian cysts
• Pelvic ultrasonography reveals ovarian mass.
• Laparoscopy reveals a bubble on the surface of the ovary, which may be clear, serous, or mucus-filled.
• hCG titers are highly elevated (with theca-lutein cysts).
• Progesterone levels are elevated.

Paget's disease
• X-rays reveal increased bone expansion and density (before overt symptoms appear).
• Bone scan reveals radioisotope concentrates in areas of active lesions (early pagetic lesions).
• Bone biopsy reveals characteristic mosaic pattern.
• Serum alkaline phosphatase level is highly elevated.
• Urine hydroxyproline levels are increased (> 45 mg/24 hours).

Pancreatic cancer
• Ultrasonography, CT scan, or MRI reveals mass size and locations.
• Laparotomy and biopsy reveal malignant cells.
• Barium swallow shows neoplasm or changes in the duodenum or stomach indicating carcinoma of the head of the pancreas.
• Endoscopic retrograde cholangiopancreatography shows mass and abnormalities of the pancreatic ducts.

- Cholangiography shows obstructed bile ducts caused by carcinoma of the pancreas.
- Secretin test reveals an abnormal volume of secretions, HCO_3^-, or enzymes.
- Serum alkaline phosphatase and serum bilirubin levels are markedly elevated with biliary obstruction.
- Plasma insulin immunoassay reveals measurable serum insulin (with islet cell tumors).
- Stool guaiac testing shows presence of occult blood, suggesting ulceration in GI tract or ampulla of Vater.

Parainfluenza

- History includes symptoms of respiratory illness.
- Serum antibody titers differentiate parainfluenza from other respiratory illnesses.
- Blood culture reveals virus (rarely done).

Parkinson's disease

- History and examination reveal muscle rigidity, akinesia, and pill-roll tremors increasing during stress or anxiety.
- Urinalysis reveals decreased dopamine levels.
- Evoked potential studies reveal bilateral abnormal P100 latencies.

Pediculosis

- In pediculosis capitis, examination reveals oval, grayish nits that can't be shaken loose.
- In pediculosis corporis, examination reveals characteristic skin lesions and nits found on clothing.
- In pediculosis pubis, examination reveals nits attached to pubic hairs, which feel coarse and grainy to the touch.

Pelvic inflammatory disease

- History includes recent sexual intercourse, intrauterine device insertion, childbirth, or abortion.
- Cultures and Gram stain of secretions from the endocervix or cul-de-sac identify *Neisseria gonorrhoeae* or *Chlamydia trachomatis* as the infective organism.
- Ultrasonography reveals an adnexal or uterine mass.
- Laparoscopy reveals infection or abscess.

Penetrating chest wounds

- Examination reveals chest wound and a sucking sound during breathing.
- Hb and HCT levels are markedly decreased, indicating severe blood loss.
- CXR reveals pneumothorax and possible lung laceration.

Penile cancer

- Tissue biopsy reveals malignant cells.
- Examination reveals small circumscribed lesion, pimple, or sore on the penis, which may be accompanied by pain, hemorrhage, dysuria, purulent discharge, and urinary meatal obstruction (in late stages).

Peptic ulcers

- History includes heartburn, midepigastric pain, or gastric bleeding.
- Endoscopy reveals ulcer.
- Upper GI X-rays show abnormalities in the mucosa.
- Gastric secretory studies show hyperchlorhydria.
- Biopsy rules out malignancy.
- Stool guaiac testing reveals presence of occult blood.

Perforated eardrum

- History includes trauma to the ear accompanied by severe earache and bleeding from the ear.

- Direct visual inspection of the tympanic membrane with an otoscope confirms perforation; flaccid, thin areas indicate previous perforation.
- Audiometric testing reveals hearing loss.

Pericarditis

- Chest auscultation reveals pericardial friction rub.
- Pericardial fluid culture identifies infecting organism (in bacterial or fungal pericarditis).
- ECG reveals ST-segment elevation in the standard limb leads and most precordial leads without the significant changes in QRS morphology that occur with myocardial infarction.
- ECG may also reveal atrial ectopic rhythms and diminished QRS voltage (with pericardial effusion).
- Echocardiography reveals an echo-free space between the ventricular wall and the pericardium (with pericardial effusion).

Peritonitis

- Examination reveals severe abdominal pain with direct or rebound tenderness.
- Abdominal X-rays reveal edematous and gaseous distention of the small and large bowel, or air in the abdominal cavity (with perforation of a visceral organ).
- Paracentesis reveals bacteria in fluid, exudate, pus, blood, or urine.
- CXR may show elevation of the diaphragm.
- Elevated WBC count indicates leukocytosis.

Pernicious anemia

- Hb level is markedly decreased.
- RBC count is decreased.
- Mean corpuscular volume is increased (> 120 μm^3).
- Serum vitamin B_{12} assay reveals levels < 190 ng/L.

- Schilling test reveals $< 3\%$ excretion of radioactive B_{12} in urine in 24 hours.
- Bone marrow aspiration reveals erythroid hyperplasia with increased numbers of megaloblasts but few normally developing RBCs.
- Gastric analysis reveals absence of free hydrochloric acid after histamine or pentagastrin injection.

Pharyngitis

- Examination reveals generalized redness and inflammation of the posterior wall of the pharynx and red, edematous mucous membranes studded with white or yellow follicles.
- Exudate is usually confined to the lymphoid areas of the throat, sparing the tonsillar pillars.
- Throat culture identifies the infective organism, most often *Streptococcus*.

Phenylketonuria

- Family history indicates presence of autosomal recessive gene.
- Guthrie screening test reveals elevated serum phenylalanine levels.
- Drops of 10% ferric chloride solution added to a wet diaper turns a deep, bluish-green color, indicating phenylpyruvic acid in the urine.
- Serum tyrosine level is < 33.2 $\mu mol/L$ in infants age 1 week or less.
- Urine testing reveals presence of phenylpyruvic acid.

Pheochromocytoma

- History includes acute episodes of hypertension, headache, sweating, and tachycardia, particularly in a patient with hyperglycemia, glycosuria, and hypermetabolism.
- 24-hour urine test reveals increased excretion of total free catecholamine and its metabolites, vanillylmandelic acid, and metanephrine.
- Total plasma catecholamines may show levels 10 to 50 times higher than normal.

- Angiography reveals an adrenal medullary tumor.
- Excretory urography with nephrotomography, adrenal venography, or CT scan helps localize a tumor.

Phosphorus imbalance

- Hypophosphatemia:
– Serum phosphorus level is < 1.7 mEq/L or 2.5 mg/dl.
– Urine phosphorus level is > 1.3 g/24 hours.
- Hyperphosphatemia:
– Serum phosphorus level is > 2.6 mEq/L or 4.5 mg/dl.
– Serum calcium level is < 9 mg/dl.
– Urine phosphorus level is < 0.9 g/24 hours.

Photosensitivity reactions

- History includes recent exposure to light or certain chemicals.
- Examination reveals erythema, edema, desquamation, and hyperpigmentation (characteristic skin eruptions).
- Photopatch test for ultraviolet A and B may identify the causative light wavelength.

Pilonidal disease

- Examination reveals a series of openings along the midline of the intergluteal fold with thin, brown, foul-smelling drainage or a protruding tuft of hair; pressure on the sinus tract produces purulent drainage.
- Culture of discharge from the infected sinus reveals staphylococci or skin bacteria (usually not bowel bacteria).

Pituitary tumors

- Skull X-rays with tomography reveal enlargement of the sella turcica or erosion of its floor and enlargement of the paranasal sinuses and mandible, thickened cranial bones, and separated teeth (if growth hormone predominates).
- Carotid angiography reveals displacement of the anterior cerebral and internal carotid arteries (with enlarging tumor mass).
- Intracranial CT scan may confirm the existence of the adenoma and accurately depict its size.
- Orbital radiography shows superior orbital fissure enlargement.
- MRI of the brain differentiates healthy, benign, and malignant tissues and blood vessels.
- Tangent screen examination reveals bitemporal hemianopia.
- Urine free cortisol levels are > 108 μg/24 hours.
- Human growth hormone levels are > 5 ng/ml in men, > 10 ng/ml in women.
- Urine 17-hydroxycorticosteroid levels are > 10 mg/24 hours in men, > 6 mg/24 hours in women, and > 5 mg/24 hours in children.

Pityriasis rosea

- Examination reveals slightly raised oval lesion, approximately 2 to 6 cm in diameter, changing to yellow-tan or erythematous patches with scaly edges approximately 0.5 to 1 cm in diameter on the trunk and extremities.

Placenta previa

- History includes painless bleeding during third trimester of pregnancy.
- Pelvic ultrasonography reveals abnormal echo patterns.
- Pelvic examination (performed only immediately before delivery) reveals only cervix and minimal descent of fetal presenting part.

Plague

- History includes exposure to rodents (bubonic plague).
- Culture of skin lesion reveals *Yersinia pestis.*
- WBC count is elevated; WBC differential reveals increased polymorphonuclear leukocytes.

- CXR reveals fulminating pneumonia (with pneumonic plague).

Platelet function disorders
- History includes excessive bleeding or bruising.
- Bleeding time is prolonged.
- PT and PTT are normal.
- Platelet count is normal.
- Platelet function tests measure platelet release reaction and aggregation to identify defective mechanism.

Pleural effusion and empyema
- CXR reveals radiopaque fluid in dependent regions.
- Lung auscultation reveals decreased breath sounds.
- Percussion detects dullness over the effused area, which doesn't change with respiration.
- Pleural fluid analysis reveals:
– transudative effusions with decreased specific gravity
– empyema with acute inflammatory WBCs and microorganisms
– empyema or rheumatoid arthritis with extremely decreased pleural fluid glucose levels.

Pleurisy
- Auscultation of the chest reveals characteristic pleural friction rub — a coarse, creaky sound heard during late inspiration and early expiration, directly over the area of pleural inflammation.
- Palpation may reveal coarse vibration.

Pneumocystis carinii pneumonia
- History includes an immunocompromising condition (such as human immunodeficiency virus infection, leukemia, and lymphoma) or procedure (such as organ transplantation).
- Histologic studies of sputum specimen confirm presence of *P. carinii.*

- CXR shows slowly progressing, fluffy infiltrates and occasional nodular lesions or a spontaneous pneumothorax.
- Gallium scan of the chest shows increased uptake over the lungs even if the CXR appears relatively normal.

Pneumonia
- Percussion reveals dullness; auscultation discloses crackles, wheezing, or rhonchi over the affected lung area as well as decreased breath sounds and decreased vocal fremitus.
- CXR discloses infiltrates, confirming the diagnosis.
- Gram stain and culture of sputum show acute inflammatory cells.
- WBC count indicates leukocytosis in bacterial pneumonia and a normal or low count in viral or mycoplasmal pneumonia.
- Blood cultures reflect bacteremia and help determine the causative organism.

Pneumothorax
- History includes sudden, sharp pain and shortness of breath.
- CXR reveals air in the pleural space and, possibly, mediastinal shift.
- Examination reveals overexpansion and rigidity of the affected chest side; in tension pneumothorax, examination may reveal neck vein distention.
- Palpation of chest reveals crackling beneath the skin and decreased vocal fremitus.
- Chest auscultation reveals decreased or absent breath sounds on the affected side.
- ABG measurements reveal pH < 7.35, Pao_2 < 80 mm Hg, and $Paco_2$ > 45 mm Hg.

Poisoning
- History includes ingestion, inhalation, injection of, or skin contact with a poisonous substance.

- Toxicologic studies (including drug screens) reveal poison in the mouth, vomitus, urine, stool, or blood or on the victim's hands or clothing.
- CXR (with inhalation poisoning) reveals pulmonary infiltrates or edema, or aspiration pneumonia (with petroleum distillate inhalation).

Poliomyelitis

- Throat culture or stool examination reveals poliovirus.
- Convalescent serum antibody titers rise fourfold from acute titers.
- CSF pressure and protein levels may be slightly increased.
- WBC count may be elevated initially, mostly due to polymorphonuclear leukocytes, which constitute 50% to 90% of the total count; thereafter, the number of cells is diminished with mononuclear leukocytes accounting for most of them.

Polycystic kidney disease

- Family history includes polycystic kidney disease.
- Physical examination reveals large bilateral, irregular masses in the flanks.
- Excretory or retrograde urography reveals enlarged kidneys, with elongation of pelvis, flattening of the calyces, and indentations caused by cysts.
- Excretory urography of the newborn shows poor excretion of contrast agent.
- Ultrasonography, CT scan, and radioisotope scans of the kidney show kidney enlargement and presence of cysts. CT scan also demonstrates multiple areas of cystic damage.

Polycythemia, secondary

- RBC mass is increased.
- Hb, HCT, mean corpuscular volume, and mean corpuscular Hb levels are increased.
- Urine erythropoietin and blood histamine levels are elevated.

- Arterial oxygen saturation may be decreased.
- Bone marrow biopsies reveal hyperplasia confined to the erythroid series.

Polycythemia, spurious

- Hb and HCT levels and RBC count are elevated.
- RBC mass is normal.
- WBC count is normal.

Polycythemia vera

- Laboratory studies confirm polycythemia vera by showing increased RBC mass and normal arterial oxygen saturation in association with splenomegaly or two of the following:
  – elevated platelet count
  – elevated WBC count
  – elevated leukocyte alkaline phosphatase level
  – elevated serum B_{12} elevation or unbound B_{12}-binding capacity.
- Bone marrow biopsy reveals panmyelosis.
- Serum and urine uric acid levels are increased.

Polymyositis and dermatomyositis

- Muscle biopsy reveals necrosis, degeneration, regeneration, and interstitial chronic lymphocytic infiltration.
- Muscle enzyme levels (CK, aldolase, AST) are elevated and not attributable to hemolysis of RBCs or hepatic or other diseases.
- Urine creatine level is markedly increased.
- Electromyography reveals polyphasic short-duration potentials, fibrillation, and bizarre high-frequency repetitive changes.
- Antinuclear antibodies are positive.

Porphyrias

- Screening tests reveal porphyrins or their precursors (such as aminolevulin-

ic acid and porphobilinogen) in urine, stool, blood, or skin biopsy.
• Urinary lead level is > 400 mg/24-hour collection.

Potassium imbalance

• Hypokalemia:
– Serum potassium levels are < 3.5 mEq/L.
– ECG shows flattened T waves, elevated U waves, and depressed ST segment.
• Hyperkalemia:
– Serum potassium levels are > 5 mEq/L.
– ECG shows tall, tented T waves; widened QRS complex; prolonged PR interval; flattened or absent P waves; and depressed ST segment.

Precocious puberty in females

• X-rays of hands, wrists, knees, and hips reveal advanced bone age and possible premature epiphyseal closure.
• Androstenedione level is > 3 ng/ml.
• Radioimmunoassay for estrogen levels and follicle-stimulating hormone levels are abnormally high for age.
• Vaginal smear for estrogen secretion reveals abnormally high levels.
• Urinary test for gonadotropic activity and excretion of 17-ketosteroids show abnormally high levels.

Precocious puberty in males

• Detailed patient history reveals recent growth pattern, behavior changes, family history of precocious puberty, or hormonal ingestion.
• In true precocious puberty:
– Serum levels of luteinizing and follicle-stimulating hormones and corticotropin are elevated.
– Plasma tests for testosterone demonstrate elevated levels (equal to those of an adult male).
– Evaluation of ejaculate indicates true precocity by revealing presence of live spermatozoa.

– Skull and hand X-rays reveal advanced bone age.
• In pseudoprecocious puberty:
– Chromosome analysis may demonstrate an abnormal pattern of autosomes and sex chromosomes.
– Steroid excretion levels, such as testosterone and 24-hour 17-ketosteroid levels, are elevated.

Pregnancy

• Serum hCG level is elevated.
• Urine hCG level is elevated.
• Pelvic examination reveals changes to uterus consistent with pregnancy.
• Ultrasonography reveals presence of fetus in the uterus.

Pregnancy-induced hypertension

• Mild preeclampsia:
– Systolic blood pressure is 140 mm Hg or shows a rise of 30 mm Hg or more above the patient's normal systolic pressure (measured on two occasions, 6 hours apart).
– Diastolic blood pressure is 90 mm Hg or shows a rise of 15 mm Hg or more above the patient's normal diastolic pressure (measured on two occasions, 6 hours apart).
– Proteinuria (urine protein level is > 500 mg/24 hours).
• Severe preeclampsia:
– Blood pressure measurements are 160/110 mm Hg or higher (measured on two occasions, 6 hours apart) on bed rest.
– Proteinuria is increased (urine protein level ≥ 5 g/24 hours).
– Patient has oliguria (urine output ≤ 400 ml/24 hours).
– Deep tendon reflexes are hyperactive.
• Eclampsia:
– History and examination reveal signs of severe preeclampsia and seizure activity.
– Ophthalmoscopic examination may reveal vascular spasm, papilledema,

retinal edema or detachment, and arteriovenous nicking or hemorrhage.

Premature labor

● Physical examination reveals rhythmic uterine contractions, cervical dilation and effacement, possible rupture of membranes, expulsion of cervical mucus plug, and bloody discharge occurring before expected date of delivery.
● Vaginal examination reveals progressive cervical effacement and dilation.
● Pelvic ultrasonography identifies fetus' position in the mother's pelvis.

Premature rupture of the membranes

● History includes passage of amniotic fluid before the expected date of delivery.
● Examination reveals amniotic fluid in the vagina.
● Nitrazine paper test of fluid from posterior fornix turns deep blue.
● Fluid from posterior fornix smeared on slide and allowed to dry takes on a fernlike pattern.

Premenstrual syndrome

● History includes menstruation-related symptoms, including mild to severe personality changes, nervousness, irritability, fatigue, lethargy, depression, breast tenderness or bloating, joint pain, headache, diarrhea, and exacerbations of skin, respiratory, or neurologic problems recorded for 2 to 3 months.
● Serum estrogen and progesterone levels are normal (ruling out hormonal imbalance).

Pressure ulcers

● History includes immobility, malnutrition, or skin irritation.
● Inspection reveals skin breakdown.
● Wound culture and sensitivity identify the infecting organisms.

Proctitis

● In acute proctitis, sigmoidoscopy reveals edematous, bright-red or pink rectal mucosa that's thick, shiny, friable, and possibly ulcerated.
● In chronic proctitis, sigmoidoscopy reveals thickened mucosa, loss of vascular pattern, and stricture of the rectal lumen.
● Biopsy reveals absence of malignant cells.

Progressive systemic sclerosis

● History includes Raynaud's phenomenon.
● Antinuclear antibody test is positive, revealing low titer and speckled pattern.
● Hand X-rays reveal terminal phalangeal tuft resorption, subcutaneous calcification, and joint space narrowing and erosion.
● CXR shows bilateral basilar pulmonary fibrosis.
● Rheumatoid factor is positive in approximately one third of patients.
● ESR is elevated.
● Urinalysis reveals proteinuria, microscopic hematuria, and casts (with renal involvement).

Prostatic cancer

● Digital rectal examination reveals small, hard nodule in prostate area.
● Serum prostate-specific antigen levels are elevated.
● Serum prostatic acid phosphatase is > 3.7 ng/ml (> 3.7 ng/ml in 17% of men with prostatic adenocarcinoma).
● Serum alkaline phosphatase level is elevated.
● Biopsy reveals malignant cells.

Prostatitis

● Examination reveals tender, indurated, swollen, and warm prostate.
● Urine samples, taken at start of voiding, midstream, after doctor massages the prostate, and final specimen, reveal

a significant increase in colony count of the prostatic specimens.

Protein-calorie malnutrition
• History includes poor diet lacking in protein.
• Examination reveals a small, gaunt, and emaciated appearance with no adipose tissue; dry and "baggy" skin; general weakness; sparse hair and dull brown or reddish yellow eyes; and slow pulse rate and respirations.
• Anthropometry reveals height and weight < 80% of standard for the patient's age and sex, and below standard arm circumference and triceps skinfolds.
• Serum albumin and pre-albumin levels are markedly decreased.

Pruritus ani
• History includes perianal itching, irritation, or superficial burning.
• Rectal examination identifies no fissures or fistulas.
• Biopsy rules out carcinoma.

Pseudomembranous enterocolitis
• History includes sudden onset of copious, watery or bloody diarrhea; abdominal pain; and fever.
• Rectal biopsy reveals characteristic histologic changes, such as plaquelike lesions on the colonic mucosal surface consisting of fibrinopurulent exudate and necrotic epithelial debris.
• Stool cultures identify *Clostridium difficile*.

Pseudomonas *infections*
• Culture of blood, spinal fluid, urine, exudate, or sputum identifies the *Pseudomonas* organism.
• Gram stain reveals gram-negative bacillus.

Psoriasis
• Examination reveals dry, cracked, encrusted lesions (erythematous plaques) accompanied by itching on the scalp, chest, elbows, knees, back, or buttocks.
• Skin biopsy reveals psoriasis.
• Serum uric acid level is elevated, without indications of gout.

Psoriatic arthritis
• Examination reveals psoriatic lesions.
• X-rays reveal erosion of terminal phalangeal tufts, "whittling" of the distal end of the terminal phalanges, "pencil-in-cup'" deformity of the distal interphalangeal joints, sacroiliitis, and atypical spondylitis with syndesmophyte formation, resulting in hyperostosis and vertebral ossification.
• Rheumatoid screening test is nonreactive.
• ESR is elevated.
• Serum uric acid levels are increased.

Ptosis
• Examination reveals drooping of the upper eyelid.
• Measurement of palpebral fissure widths, range of lid movement, and relation of lid margin to upper border of the cornea reveal the severity of illness.

Puerperal infection
• History includes fever within 48 hours after delivery or abortion.
• Culture of lochia, blood, incisional exudate (from cesarean incision or episiotomy), uterine tissue, or material collected from the vaginal cuff reveals *Streptococcus,* coagulase-negative staphylococci, *Clostridium perfringens, Bacteroides fragilis,* or *Escherichia coli* as the causative organism.
• Elevated WBC count shows leukocytosis and an increased sedimentation rate.

- Pelvic examination reveals induration without purulent discharge (parametritis).
- Culdoscopy shows adnexal induration and thickening.

Pulmonary edema

- Examination reveals respiratory distress.
- Chest auscultation reveals crackles in the lung fields.
- ABG analysis usually shows decreased PaO_2 (hypoxia) and variable $PaCO_2$. Profound respiratory alkalosis and acidosis may occur; metabolic acidosis occurs when cardiac output is low.
- CXR shows diffuse haziness of the lung fields and, often, cardiomegaly and pleural effusions.
- Pulmonary artery catheterization reveals elevated pulmonary wedge pressures.

Pulmonary embolism and infarction

- Lung scan reveals perfusion defects in areas beyond occluded vessels.
- Pulmonary angiography reveals emboli.
- CXR shows areas of atelectasis, elevated diaphragm and pleural effusion, prominent pulmonary artery and, occasionally, a wedge-shaped infiltrate suggesting pulmonary infarction.
- ECG may show right axis deviation; right bundle-branch block; tall, peaked P waves; ST-segment depression; T-wave inversion; and supraventricular tachycardia.
- Auscultation reveals right ventricular gallop, increased intensity of the pulmonic component of S_2, crackles, and pleural rub at the site of the embolism.
- ABG analysis may show decreased PaO_2 and $PaCO_2$ levels.

Pulmonary hypertension

- Pulmonary artery catheterization reveals elevated pulmonary systolic pressure and pulmonary artery wedge pressure.
- Pulmonary angiography reveals filling defects in pulmonary vasculature.
- PFTs may show decreased flow rates and increased residual volume (with underlying obstructive disease); total lung capacity may be decreased (with underlying restrictive disease).
- ABG analysis reveals decreased PaO_2.
- ECG shows right axis deviation and tall or peaked P waves in inferior leads (with right ventricular hypertrophy).

Pulmonic insufficiency

- Cardiac catheterization shows pulmonic insufficiency, increased right ventricular pressure, and associated cardiac defects.
- CXR shows enlargement of the right ventricle and pulmonary artery.
- Echocardiography shows right ventricular or right atrial enlargement.
- ECG may be normal in mild cases or show right ventricular or right atrial hypertrophy.

Pulmonic stenosis

- Cardiac catheterization reveals increased right ventricular pressure, decreased pulmonary artery pressure, and an abnormal valve orifice.
- CXR usually reveals a normal heart size and normal lung vascularity, although the pulmonary arteries may be evident. With severe obstruction and right-sided heart failure, CXR may reveal right atrial and ventricular enlargement.
- Echocardiography reveals the abnormality in the pulmonic valve.
- ECG results may be normal in mild cases, or they may indicate right axis deviation and right ventricular hypertrophy. High amplitude P waves in

leads II, III, aV_F, and V_1 indicate right atrial enlargement.

Rabies

- History reveals recent animal bite.
- Throat and saliva culture identifies virus.
- Serum fluorescent rabies antibody test is positive.
- WBC count is elevated, with increased polymorphonuclear and large mononuclear cells.
- Urine glucose, acetone, and protein levels are elevated.

Radiation exposure

- History includes exposure to radiation and nausea and vomiting.
- CBC reveals decreased Hb and HCT levels, and decreased WBC, platelet, and lymphocyte counts.
- Bone marrow studies reveal blood dyscrasias.
- X-rays may show bone necrosis.
- Geiger counter measurement reveals the amount of radiation in an open wound.

Rape-trauma syndrome

- History includes rape or attempted rape, accompanied by feelings of anxiety, grief, anger, fear, or revenge.
- Examination shows signs of physical trauma.
- X-rays reveal fractures.
- Vaginal specimen is positive for semen.
- Fingernail and pubic hair scrapings may help to identify alleged rapist.
- Semen analysis may help to identify alleged rapist.

Raynaud's disease

- History and examination reveal changes in skin color induced by cold or stress, bilateral involvement, minimal cutaneous gangrene or absence of gangrene, and clinical symptoms of 2 years' duration or more.
- Cold stimulation test demonstrates Raynaud's syndrome.
- Arteriography reveals no underlying secondary disease.

Rectal polyps

- Proctosigmoidoscopy or colonoscopy reveals type, size, and location of polyps.
- Biopsy reveals histologic changes consistent with polyps.
- Barium enema reveals polyps high in the colon.
- Stool guaiac testing reveals presence of occult blood.

Rectal prolapse

- In complete prolapse, visual examination reveals the full thickness of the bowel wall and, possibly, the sphincter muscle protruding and mucosa falling into bulky, concentric folds.
- In partial prolapse, visual examination reveals only partially protruding mucosa and a smaller mass of radial mucosal folds.

Reiter's syndrome

- History includes venereal or enteric infection.
- Human leukocyte antigen (HLA) testing reveals presence of HLA-B27.
- Analysis of urethral discharge and synovial fluid reveals numerous WBCs, mostly polymorphonuclear leukocytes.
- Synovial fluid analysis reveals increased complement and protein; fluid is grossly purulent.
- WBC count and ESR are elevated.

Relapsing fever

- History includes recurrent fever for 5 to 15 days.
- Blood smear shows spirochetes.
- WBC count is elevated, with increase in lymphocytes (although WBC count may be within normal limits).
- ESR is increased.

Renal calculi

- KUB X-rays reveal renal calculi.
- Excretory urography reveals size and location of calculi.
- Kidney ultrasonography reveals obstructive changes.
- Urine culture may reveal urinary tract infection.
- Urinalysis may be normal or may show increased specific gravity, acid or alkaline pH (depending on the type of stone), hematuria, crystals, casts, and pyuria (with or without WBCs).
- 24-hour urine collection shows presence of calcium oxalate, phosphorus, or uric acid.

Renal infarction

- Urinalysis reveals proteinuria and microscopic hematuria.
- Urine enzyme levels, especially LD and alkaline phosphatase, are elevated.
- Serum ALT, AST, and LD levels are elevated.
- Excretory urography shows diminished or absent excretion of contrast dye (with vascular occlusion or urethral obstruction).
- Isotopic renal scan demonstrates absent or reduced blood flow to the kidneys.
- Renal arteriography reveals infarction.

Renal tubular acidosis

- Urine studies reveal pH > 6, low titratable acids and ammonia content, increased HCO_3^- and potassium levels, and low specific gravity (< 1.005).
- Blood pH is < 7.35.
- Serum HCO_3^- level is < 22 mEq/L.
- Serum potassium and phosphorus levels are decreased.

Renal vein thrombosis

- Excretory urography reveals enlarged kidneys and diminished excretory function (in acute thrombosis);

urography contrast medium seems to "smudge" necrotic renal tissue.
- In chronic thrombosis, excretory urography may show ureteral indentations that result from collateral venous channels.
- Renal venography reveals filling defects.
- Renal biopsy reveals characteristic histologic changes.
- Urinalysis reveals gross or microscopic hematuria, proteinuria (> 2 g/day in chronic disease), casts, and oliguria.
- Blood studies show leukocytosis, hypoalbuminemia, hyperlipemia, and thrombocytopenia.

Renovascular hypertension

- Isotopic renal blood flow scan and rapid-sequence excretory urography demonstrate abnormal renal blood flow and discrepancies in kidney size and shape.
- Renal arteriography reveals the arterial stenosis or obstruction.
- Samples from both the right and left renal veins allow for comparison of plasma renin levels with those in the inferior vena cava; renin level is increased in the affected kidney.

Respiratory acidosis

- ABG measurements reveal:
- pH < 7.35
- $Paco_2$ > 45 mm Hg
- HCO_3^- level of 22 to 26 mEq/L in the acute stage and > 26 mEq/L in the chronic stage.

Respiratory alkalosis

- ABG measurements reveal:
- pH > 7.45
- $Paco_2$ < 35 mm Hg (in acute stage)
- HCO_3^- level normal in the acute stage and < 22 mEq/L in the chronic stage.

Respiratory distress syndrome, adult

- Initial ABG measurements reveal:
  – pH > 7.45
  – PaO_2 < 60 mm Hg
  – $PaCO_2$ < 35 mm Hg.
- ABG measurements following progression of illness reveal:
  – pH < 7.35
  – decreased PaO_2 (despite oxygen therapy)
  – $PaCO_2$ level > 45 mm Hg
  – HCO_3^- level < 22 mEq/L.
- Serial CXRs initially show bilateral infiltrates; later X-rays reveal ground glass appearance and eventually "whiteouts" of both lungs.

Respiratory distress syndrome, child

- CXR reveals fine reticulonodular pattern (may be normal for first 6 to 12 hours after birth).
- ABG measurements reveal pH < 7.35 and PaO_2 < 75 mm Hg.
- Chest auscultation reveals normal or diminished air entry and crackles (rare in early stages).
- Amniocentesis reveals lecithin-sphingomyelin ratio of < 2 (used to assess risk of respiratory distress syndrome).

Respiratory syncytial virus infection

- Cultures of nasal and pharyngeal secretions identify respiratory syncytial virus infection (not always reliable).
- Serum antibody titers elevated (maternal antibodies may impair results before age 6 months)
- CXR may reveal pneumonia.
- Indirect immunofluorescence and ELISA tests are positive.

Restrictive cardiomyopathy

- CXR reveals massive cardiomegaly, affecting all four chambers of the heart, pericardial effusion, and pulmonary congestion (advanced stage).
- Echocardiography detects increased left ventricular muscle mass and differences in end-diastolic pressures between the ventricles.
- Carotid palpation reveals blunt carotid upstroke with small volume.
- Cardiac catheterization demonstrates increased left ventricular end-diastolic pressure.
- ECG may show low-voltage complexes, hypertrophy, atrioventricular conduction defects, or arrhythmias.

Retinal detachment

- Ophthalmoscopy reveals the usually transparent retina to be gray and opaque.
- In severe detachment, ophthalmoscopy reveals folds in the retina and a ballooning out of the area.
- Indirect ophthalmoscopy reveals retinal tears.
- Ocular ultrasonography shows a dense sheetlike echo on a B-scan.

Retinitis pigmentosa

- Family history indicates a possible predisposition to retinitis pigmentosa.
- Electroretinography shows a retinal response time slower than normal or absent.
- Visual field testing (using a tangent screen) detects ring scotomata.
- Fluorescein angiography shows white dots (areas of dyspigmentation) in the epithelium.
- Ophthalmoscopy may initially show normal fundi but later reveals characteristic black pigmentary disturbance.

Reye's syndrome

- History includes recent viral disorder with varying degrees of encephalopathy and cerebral edema.
- ALT level is > 56 U/L.
- AST level is > 40 U/L.

- Liver biopsy reveals fatty droplets uniformly distributed throughout cells.
- PT and PTT are prolonged.
- CSF analysis reveals WBCs < 10/µl; in coma, CSF pressure is increased.
- Serum ammonia levels are elevated.
- Serum fatty acid and lactate levels are elevated.
- Serum glucose levels are normal or low.

Rheumatic fever and rheumatic heart disease

- History includes streptococcal infection.
- Examination reveals joint pain and swelling and one or more of the following symptoms: carditis, polyarthritis, chorea, erythema marginatum, or subcutaneous nodules.
- C-reactive protein is positive.
- Antistreptolysin-O titer is elevated (within 2 months of onset).
- Echocardiography and cardiac catheterization reveal valvular damage.
- Cardiac enzymes may be elevated (in severe carditis).

Rheumatoid arthritis

- Serum rheumatoid factor is > 80 IU/ml.
- X-rays reveal bone demineralization and soft-tissue swelling (in early stages), loss of cartilage and narrowing of joint spaces, and cartilage and bone destruction, erosion, subluxations, and deformities.
- Synovial fluid analysis reveals increased volume and turbidity but decreased viscosity and complement (C_3 and C_4) levels, and elevated WBC count.
- ESR is increased.
- CBC shows moderate decrease in RBC count, Hb, and HCT and slight leukocytosis.

Rheumatoid arthritis, juvenile

- History includes persistent joint stiffness and pain in the morning or after periods of inactivity.
- Antinuclear antibody test may be positive in patients who have pauciarticular juvenile rheumatoid arthritis (JRA) with chronic iridocyclitis.
- Rheumatoid factor is present in 15% of patients with JRA, as compared with 85% of patients with rheumatoid arthritis.
- Early changes seen on X-ray include soft-tissue swelling, effusion, and periostitis in affected joints.
- In later X-ray studies, osteoporosis and accelerated bone growth may appear, followed by subchondral erosions, joint space narrowing, bone destruction, and fusion.
- CBC usually shows decreased Hb levels, increased neutrophil count, increased platelet levels, and elevated ESR.
- Blood studies reveal elevated C-reactive protein, serum haptoglobin, Ig, and C_3 complement levels.
- Human leukocyte antigen (HLA) testing reveals presence of HLA-B27, forecasting later development of ankylosing spondylitis.

Rocky Mountain spotted fever

- History includes tick bite or travel to a tick-infested area.
- Complement fixation test shows a fourfold rise in convalescent antibodies compared to acute titers.
- Blood culture identifies *Rickettsia rickettsii*.
- Decreased platelet count indicates thrombocytopenia during 2nd week of illness.
- WBC count is elevated during 2nd week of illness.

Rosacea

- Examination reveals vascular and acneiform lesions without the comedones characteristically associated with acne vulgaris; in severe cases, rhinophyma is seen.

Roseola infantum
• History includes high fever (103° to 105° F [39.4° to 40.4° C]) followed by rash 48 hours after fever subsides
• Examination reveals maculopapular, nonpruritic rash that blanches on pressure.

Rubella
• History includes exposure to infected person.
• Examination reveals maculopapular rash, beginning on the face and spreading to the trunk and extremities.
• Examination also reveals lymphadenopathy.
• Cell cultures of throat, blood, urine, and CSF reveal rubella virus.
• Convalescent serum antibody titers rise fourfold from acute titers.

Rubeola
• History includes exposure to person infected with the measles virus (patient may be unaware of contact).
• Examination reveals the pathognomonic Koplik's spots.
• Cultures of blood, nasopharyngeal secretions, and urine identify measles virus (during the febrile period).
• Serum antibody titers appear within 3 days after onset of the rash and reach peak titers 2 to 4 weeks later.

Salmonellosis
• Culture of blood, stool, urine, bone marrow, pus, or vomitus identifies gram-negative bacilli of the genus *Salmonella*.
• Widal's test reveals a fourfold rise in titer.

Sarcoidosis
• Kveim-Siltzbach skin test confirms discrete epithelioid cell granuloma.

• CXR reveals bilateral hilar and right paratracheal adenopathy with or without diffuse interstitial infiltrates; occasionally, large nodular lesions appear in lung parenchyma.
• Lymph node, skin, or lung biopsy reveals noncaseating granulomas with negative cultures for mycobacteria and fungi.
• PFTs show decreased total lung capacity and compliance and decreased diffusing capacity.
• Tuberculin skin test, fungal serologies, and sputum cultures for mycobacteria and fungi and biopsy cultures are negative.

Scabies
• Visual examination of the contents of the scabietic burrow may reveal itch mite.
• Mineral oil placed over the burrow, followed by superficial scraping and examination of expressed material, reveals ova or mite feces.
• Pediculicide administration to affected area clears skin.

Scarlet fever
• History includes recent streptococcal pharyngitis.
• Examination reveals strawberry tongue and fine erythematous rash that blanches on pressure.
• Pharyngeal culture identifies group A beta-hemolytic streptococci.
• CBC reveals granulocytosis and, possibly, a reduced RBC count.

Schistosomiasis
• History includes travel to endemic areas.
• Urine, stool, or lesion biopsy reveals ova.
• WBC count reveals eosinophilia.

Scoliosis
• Examination reveals unequal shoulder height, elbow levels, and heights of

iliac crests and asymmetry of the paraspinal muscles.

- Scoliosometer (an apparatus for measuring curvature of the spinal column) reveals angle of trunk rotation to be abnormal.
- Anterior, posterior, and lateral spinal X-rays reveal degree of curvature and flexibility of the spine.

Septal perforation and deviation

- History and examination reveal whistle on inspiration, rhinitis, epistaxis, nasal crusting, and watery discharge.
- Inspection of the nasal mucosa with bright light and a nasal speculum reveals perforation or deviation.

Septic arthritis

- Synovial fluid Gram stain and culture or biopsy of synovial membrane reveals gram-positive cocci *(Staphylococcus aureus, Streptococcus pyogenes, Streptococcus pneumoniae,* or *Streptococcus viridans)*, gram-negative cocci *(Neisseria gonorrhoeae* or *Haemophilus influenzae)*, or gram-negative bacilli *(Escherichia coli, Salmonella,* or *Pseudomonas)* as the causative organism.
- Joint fluid analysis reveals gross pus or watery, cloudy fluid of decreased viscosity, with markedly elevated WBCs/μl, containing primarily neutrophils.
- Culture of skin exudate, sputum, urethral discharge, stool, urine, blood, or nasopharyngeal secretions is positive for causative organism.
- Skeletal X-rays show distention of joint capsules, followed by narrowing of joint space (indicating cartilage damage), and erosions of bone (joint destruction).
- WBC count may be elevated with many polymorphonuclear cells; ESR is increased.

Septic shock

- History includes infection accompanied by fever, confusion, nausea, vomiting, and hyperventilation.
- Blood cultures identify gram-negative bacteria *(Escherichia coli, Klebsiella, Enterobacter, Pseudomonas, Proteus,* or *Bacteroides)* or gram-positive bacteria *(Streptococcus pneumoniae, S. pyogenes,* or *Actinomyces)* as the causative organism.
- WBC count is elevated.
- Pulmonary artery catheterization reveals decreased central venous pressure, pulmonary artery pressures, wedge pressure, cardiac output (may be initially elevated), and systemic vascular resistance.
- ABG measurements reveal decreased $Paco_2$, low or normal HCO_3^- level, and pH > 7.45 (in early stages); as shock progresses, decreasing $Paco_2$, Pao_2, HCO_3^- level, and pH indicate the development of metabolic acidosis with hypoxemia.
- Serum BUN and creatinine levels increase; creatinine clearance decreases.
- Urine osmolality is < 400 mOsm; ratio of urine osmolality to plasma osmolality is < 1.5.
- ECG reveals ST-segment depression, inverted T waves, and arrhythmias.

Severe combined immunodeficiency disease

- History includes overwhelming infections during the first year of life.
- T-cell count and function are severely diminished.
- Lymph node biopsy reveals absence of lymphocytes.

Shigellosis

- Microscopic examination of a fresh stool may reveal mucus, RBCs, and polymorphonuclear leukocytes.
- Stool culture identifies *Shigella.*
- Hemagglutinating antibodies may be present, indicating severe infection.

Sickle cell anemia
- Family history includes homozygous inheritance.
- Stained blood smear reveals sickle cells.
- Hb electrophoresis reveals HbS.
- CBC may reveal decreased RBC count and elevated WBC and platelet counts.
- ESR is decreased.
- Serum iron levels are increased.

Sideroblastic anemias
- Bone marrow aspirate reveals ringed sideroblasts.
- Microscopic examination reveals RBCs that are hypochromic or normochromic and slightly macrocytic; red cell precursors may be megaloblastic, with anisocytosis and poikilocytosis.
- Hb levels are decreased.
- Serum iron and transferrin levels are increased.

Silicosis
- History includes occupational exposure to silica dust.
- Examination reveals decreased chest expansion, diminished intensity of breath sounds, areas of hyporesonance and hyperresonance, fine to medium crackles, and tachypnea (with chronic silicosis).
- CXR reveals the following:
– small, discrete, nodular lesions distributed throughout both lung fields but typically concentrated in the upper lung zones
– enlarged hilar lung nodes that exhibit "eggshell" calcification (in simple silicosis)
– one or more conglomerate masses of dense tissue (in complicated silicosis).
- PFTs reveal:
– reduced forced vital capacity (in complicated silicosis)
– reduced forced expiratory volume (in obstructed disease)
– reduced maximal voluntary ventilation (in restrictive and obstructive disease)
– reduced diffusing capacity for carbon monoxide when fibrosis destroys alveolar walls and oblates pulmonary capillaries, or when fibrosis thickens the alveolar capillary membrane.
- ABG measurements reveal:
– significantly decreased PaO_2 (in the late stages of chronic or complicated disease)
– decreased or normal $PaCO_2$ in early stages; may increase as restrictive pattern develops.

Sinus bradycardia
- ECG reveals:
– regular atrial and ventricular rhythm
– atrial and ventricular rates < 60 beats/minute
– P wave of normal size and configuration with a P wave preceding each QRS complex
– PR interval within normal limits and constant
– QRS complex of normal duration and configuration
– T wave of normal size and configuration
– QT interval within normal limits, but possibly prolonged.

Sinus tachycardia
- ECG reveals:
– regular atrial and ventricular rhythms
– atrial and ventricular rates > 100 beats/minute (usually between 100 and 160 beats/minute)
– P wave of normal size and configuration with a P wave preceding each QRS complex
– PR interval within normal limits and constant
– QRS complex of normal duration and configuration
– T wave of normal size and configuration

– QT interval within normal limits, but commonly shortened.

Sinusitis

- Nasal examination reveals inflammation and pus.
- Sinus X-rays reveal cloudiness in the affected sinus, air-fluid levels, or thickened mucosal lining.
- Transillumination allows inspection of the sinus cavities by passing a light through them; in sinusitis, purulent drainage prevents passage of light.

Sjögren's syndrome

- ESR is elevated.
- Hypergammaglobulinemia is present.
- Rheumatoid factor test is positive (75% to 90% of patients).
- Antinuclear antibody test is positive (50% to 80% of patients).
- Schirmer's tearing test is positive for tearing deficiency.
- Lower lip biopsy shows salivary gland infiltration by lymphocytes.
- History and examination reveal two of the following three conditions: xerophthalmia, xerostomia (with salivary gland biopsy showing lymphocytic infiltration), and associated autoimmune or lymphoproliferative disorder.

Skull fractures

- History includes recent head trauma.
- Skull X-ray shows fracture (minor vault fractures may not be visible).
- Neurologic examination evaluates cerebral function.
- Cerebral angiography reveals vascular disruption from internal pressure and injury.
- CT scan, echoencephalography, air encephalography, MRI, and radioactive scanning reveal cranial nerve injury or intracranial hemorrhage from ruptured blood vessels. These tests also help to localize subdural or intracerebral hematomas.

Snakebites, poisonous

- Examination reveals fang marks.
- Bleeding time and PTT are prolonged.
- Hb and HCT levels are decreased.
- Platelet count is sharply decreased.
- Urinalysis may reveal hematuria.
- CXR may show pulmonary edema or emboli.
- ECG may reveal tachycardia and ectopic beats.

Sodium imbalance

- Hyponatremia:
– Serum sodium level is < 135 mEq/L.
– Urine sodium level is > 100 mEq/24 hours.
– Serum osmolality is low.
- Hypernatremia:
– Serum sodium level is > 145 mEq/L.
– Urine sodium level is < 40 mEq/24 hours.
– Serum osmolality is high.

Spinal cord defects

- Examination reveals a protruding sac on the spine.
- Transillumination of sac reveals meningocele.
- Spinal X-ray shows bone defect (in spina bifida occulta).
- CT scan reveals hydrocephalus (in 90% of patients).

Spinal injuries without cord damage

- History includes trauma, metastatic disease, infection, or endocrine disorder.
- Physical examination reveals the location and level of injury.
- Spinal X-rays reveal fracture.
- Myelography reveals spinal mass.
- Lumbar puncture reveals increased CSF pressure, indicating spinal trauma or lesion.

Spinal neoplasms
• Lumbar puncture reveals clear yellow CSF with increased protein levels.
• X-rays show distortions of intervertebral foramina, changes in vertebrae or collapsed areas in the vertebral body, and localized enlargement of the spinal canal indicating an adjacent block.
• Myelography identifies the level of the lesion.
• CT scan and MRI show cord compression and tumor location.
• Radioisotope bone scan reveals evidence of metastatic invasion of the vertebrae by showing increased osteoblastic activity.
• Biopsy reveals malignant cells.

Sporotrichosis
• Examination reveals small, painless, movable subcutaneous nodules with discoloration and ulceration.
• Cultures of either sputum, pus, or bone drainage identify *Strongyloides schenckii*.

Sprains and strains
• History includes recent injury or chronic overuse of extremity.
• Examination reveals pain (local with a sprain, sharp and transient with a strain), swelling, and ecchymoses (rapid onset with a sprain; may take several days with a strain).
• X-ray of the extremity does not indicate fracture.

Squamous cell carcinoma
• Examination reveals ulcerated nodule with indurated base.
• Biopsy reveals squamous cell carcinoma.

Staphylococcal scalded skin syndrome
• Examination reveals three-stage progression of erythema, exfoliation, and desquamation.

• Skin lesions are positive for Group 2 *Staphylococcus aureus*.

Stomatitis and other oral infections
• Examination reveals inflammation of the oral mucosa or surrounding area.
• Smear of ulcer exudate reveals fusiform bacillus or spirochete as the causative organism (in Vincent's angina).

Strabismus
• Visual acuity test reveals the degree of visual defect.
• Hirschberg's method detects malalignment.
• Retinoscopy identifies refractive error.
• Maddox rods test identifies specific muscle involvement.
• Convergence test shows distance at which convergence is sustained.
• Duction test reveals limitation of eye movement.
• Cover-uncover test demonstrates eye deviation and the rate of recovery to original alignment.
• Alternate-cover test shows intermittent or latent deviation.

Strongyloidiasis
• History includes travel to endemic area.
• Stool specimen contains *Strongyloides stercoralis* larvae.
• Sputum specimen contains eosinophils and larvae.
• Hb level is decreased.
• WBC count with differential shows eosinophils at 450 to 700/µl.

Stye
• Visual examination reveals abscess of the lid glands.
• Abscess culture reveals a staphylococcal organism.

Sudden infant death syndrome

- Autopsy reveals:
– small or normal adrenal glands
– petechiae over the visceral surface of the pleura, within the thymus, and in the epicardium
– well-preserved lymphoid structures
– pathologic changes suggesting chronic hypoxemia
– edematous, congestive lungs fully expanded in the pleural cavities
– liquid blood in the heart (not clotted)
– curd from the stomach inside the trachea.

Syndrome of inappropriate antidiuretic hormone secretion

- History includes recent weight gain despite anorexia, nausea, and vomiting.
- Serum osmolality is < 280 mOsm/kg of water.
- Serum sodium level is < 123 mEq/L.
- Urine sodium level is > 20 mEq/L without diuretics.

Syphilis

- History includes sexual contact with partner with syphilis.
- Culture of lesion identifies *Treponema pallidum*.
- The fluorescent treponemal antibody-absorption test identifies antigens of *T. pallidum* in tissue, ocular fluid, CSF, tracheobronchial secretions, and exudates from lesions.
- Venereal Disease Research Laboratory (VDRL) slide test and rapid plasma reagin test are positive, detecting nonspecific antibodies.
- In neurosyphilis:
– CSF analysis reveals elevated total protein level.
– VDRL slide test is reactive.
– Cell count > 5 mononuclear cells/µl.

Taeniasis

- History includes travel to endemic areas; exposure to eating undercooked, infected beef, pork, or fish; or in dwarf tapeworm, exposure to an infected person.
- Laboratory observation reveals tapeworm ova or body segments in stool.
- Beef tapeworm reveals:
– crawling sensation in perianal area
– intestinal obstruction and appendicitis.
- Pork tapeworm reveals:
– seizures, headaches, personality changes (often overlooked in adults).
- In fish tapeworm:
– anemia (Hb as low as 6 to 8 g).
- Dwarf tapeworm reveals:
– no symptoms (mild infestation)
– anorexia, diarrhea, restlessness, dizziness, and apathy (severe infestation).

Tay-Sachs disease

- Family history includes Eastern European Jewish ancestry or history of the disease. Diagnostic screening may detect carriers of autosomal recessive gene.
- Serum analysis shows deficiency of hexosaminidase A.
- Ophthalmic examination reveals optic nerve atrophy and a distinctive cherry-red spot on the retina.

Tendinitis and bursitis

- History includes unusual strain or injury 2 to 3 days before onset of pain or heat-aggravated joint pain.
- Examination reveals localized pain and inflammation at joint.
- X-rays (in late stages) reveal bony fragments, osteophyte sclerosis, or calcium deposits.
- Arthrography is usually normal, with occasional small irregularities on the undersurface of the tendon.

Testicular cancer

- Physical examination reveals testicular mass.
- Transillumination confirms tumor.
- Biopsy reveals malignant cells.

• Excretory urography reveals ureteral deviation (indicates node involvement).
• Testosterone levels are > 1,200 ng/dl or < 300 ng/dl.
• Urine testing indicates presence of hCG.
• Serum alpha-fetoprotein and beta-hCG levels are increased.

Testicular torsion

• Physical examination reveals tense, tender swelling in the scrotum or inguinal canal and hyperemia of the overlying skin.
• Doppler ultrasonography reveals testicular torsion.

Tetanus

• History includes trauma and absence of tetanus immunization.
• Meningitis, rabies, phenothiazine or strychnine toxicity, or other conditions that mimic tetanus are ruled out.
• Cultures are positive for an anaerobic spore forming rod clostridium tetani.

Tetralogy of Fallot

• Echocardiography reveals septal overriding of the aorta, the ventricular septal defect (VSD), and pulmonary stenosis, and detects hypertrophy of walls of the right ventricle.
• Cardiac catheterization shows pulmonary stenosis, the VSD, and the overriding aorta and rules out other cyanotic heart defects.
• Auscultation reveals a loud systolic heart murmur, which may diminish or obscure the pulmonic component of S_2.
• Palpation may reveal a cardiac thrill at the left sternal border and an obvious right ventricular impulse.
• ECG shows right ventricular hypertrophy, right axis deviation and, possibly, right atrial hypertrophy.
• CXR reveals decreased pulmonary vascular marking (depending on the severity of pulmonary obstruction) and a boot-shaped cardiac silhouette.

Thalassemia

• Thalassemia major reveals:
– lowered RBC count and Hb level
– elevated reticulocyte level
– elevated bilirubin and urinary and fecal urobilinogen levels
– low serum folate level
– X-rays of the skull and long bones showing a thinning and widening of the marrow space
– Hb electrophoresis revealing a significant rise in HbF and a slight increase in HbA_2
– peripheral blood smear revealing extremely thin and fragile RBCs, pale nucleated RBCs, and marked anisocytosis.
• Thalassemia intermedia reveals:
– hypochromic and microcytic RBCs.
• Thalassemia minor reveals:
– hypochromic and microcytic RBCs
– Hb electrophoresis revealing a significant increase in HbA_2 and a moderate rise in HbF.

Thoracic aortic aneurysm

• CXR reveals widening of the aorta.
• CT scan or MRI reveals location and size of aneurysm.
• Aortography reveals the lumen of the aneurysm, its size and location and, in dissecting aneurysm, the false lumen.

Throat abscesses

• History includes staphylococcal or streptococcal infection.
• Retropharyngeal abscess is indicated by:
– history of nasopharyngitis or pharyngitis
– soft, red bulging of the posterior pharyngeal wall
– X-rays that reveal the larynx pushed forward and a widened space between the posterior pharyngeal wall and vertebrae

– pharyngeal culture that identifies infective organism.

● Examination reveals swelling of the soft palate on the abscessed side of the throat, with displacement of the uvula to the opposite side; red, edematous mucous membranes; and tonsil displacement toward the midline.

● Throat culture reveals streptococcal or staphylococcal infection.

Thrombocytopenia

● Platelet count is markedly decreased.
● Bleeding time is prolonged.
● PT and PTT are normal.
● Bone marrow studies reveal an increased number of megakaryocytes (platelet precursors) and shortened platelet survival.

Thrombophlebitis

● Homans' sign is positive.
● Doppler ultrasonography reveals reduced blood flow to a specific area and obstruction to venous flow.
● Plethysmography reveals decreased circulation distal to affected area.
● Phlebography reveals filling defects and diverted blood flow.

Thyroid cancer

● History includes exposure to radiation therapy or a family history of thyroid cancer.
● Examination reveals an enlarged, palpable node in the thyroid gland, neck, lymph nodes of the neck, or vocal cords.
● Thyroid scan reveals a "cold," nonfunctioning nodule.
● Thyroid biopsy reveals a well-encapsulated, solitary nodule of uniform but abnormal structure.
● Serum calcitonin assay reveals an elevated fasting calcitonin and an abnormal response to calcium stimulation (with medullary cancer).

Thyroiditis

● Autoimmune thyroiditis reveals:
– positive precipitin test
– high titers of thyroglobulin
– microsomal antibodies present in serum.
● Subacute granulomatous thyroiditis reveals:
– elevated ESR
– increased thyroid hormone levels
– decreased thyroidal radioiodine uptake.

Tic disorders

● History identifies stressors that may be related to symptoms.
● Examination reveals recurrent, involuntary movements involving the facial muscles, coughing, sniffling, or jerking head movements.
● Psychogenic tics are ruled out.

Tinea versicolor

● Wood's light examination reveals lesions.
● Microscopic examination of skin scrapings shows hyphae and clusters of yeast.

Tonsillitis

● Examination reveals generalized inflammation of the pharyngeal wall and swollen tonsils that project from between the pillars of the fauces and exude white or yellow follicles, with inflamed uvula.
● Purulent drainage appears when pressure is applied to the tonsillar pillars.
● Throat culture identifies infective organism, commonly beta-hemolytic streptococci.

Torticollis

● History includes painless neck deformity.
● Examination reveals enlargement of the sternocleidomastoid muscle.

- Cervical spine X-rays are negative for bone or joint disease but may reveal an associated disorder such as tuberculosis, scar tissue formation, or arthritis (in acquired torticollis).

Toxic epidermal necrolysis

- Examination reveals scalded skin with no history of burn.
- Nikolsky's sign (skin sloughs off with slight friction) appears in erythematous areas.
- Culture and Gram stain identify infective organism.
- WBC count reveals leukocytosis.

Toxic shock syndrome

- Culture of vaginal discharge or lesions identifies *Staphylococcus aureus.*
- CK level is elevated.
- BUN level is elevated.
- Serum creatinine level is elevated.
- AST level is > 56 U/L and ALT level is > 40 U/L.
- Platelet count is markedly decreased.

Toxocariasis

- History includes pica, eosinophilia, or recent exposure to a dog.
- Massive leukocytosis develops.
- Hypereosinophilia develops.
- Antibodies to *Toxocara canis* are present in serum.
- Liver biopsy contains *T. canis* larvae.

Toxoplasmosis

- History includes exposure to a cat or ingestion of uncooked meat.
- Blood, body fluid, or tissue tests positive for *Toxoplasma gondii* antibodies.
- *T. gondii* is identified in mice after their inoculation with specimens of patient's body fluids, blood, and tissue.

Tracheoesophageal fistula and esophageal atresia

- Examination reveals respiratory distress and drooling in a newborn.

- Catheter (#10 or #12 French) meets obstruction when passed through the nose at 4″ to 5″ (10 to 13 cm) distal from the nostrils.
- CXR demonstrates the position of the catheter and can show a dilated, air-filled upper esophageal pouch, pneumonia in the right upper lobe, or bilateral pneumonitis.
- Abdominal X-ray reveals gas in the bowel in a distal fistula (but none in a proximal fistula or atresia without fistula).
- Cinefluorography defines the upper pouch by allowing visualization on a fluoroscopic screen and differentiates between overflow aspiration from a blind end (atresia) and aspiration due to passage of liquids through a tracheoesophageal fistula.

Trachoma

- Examination reveals follicular conjunctivitis with corneal infiltration and upper lid or conjunctival scarring, with symptoms persisting for 3 weeks.
- Microscopic examination of a Giemsa-stained conjunctival scraping reveals cytoplasmic inclusion bodies, some polymorphonuclear reaction, plasma cells, Leber's cells (large macrophages containing phagocytosed debris), and follicle cells.

Transposition of the great arteries

- Echocardiography reveals the reversed position of the aorta and the pulmonary artery and records echoes from both semilunar valves simultaneously, due to the aortic valve displacement.
- Cardiac catheterization reveals decreased oxygen saturation in left ventricular blood and aortic blood; increased right atrial, right ventricular, and pulmonary artery oxygen satura-

tion; and right ventricular systolic pressure equal to systemic pressure.
- Dye injection during catheterization reveals the transposed vessels and the presence of any other cardiac defects.
- CXR shows right atrial and ventricular enlargement causing the heart to appear oblong (within days to weeks) and increased vascular markings, except when pulmonic stenosis exists.
- ECG reveals right axis deviation and right ventricular hypertrophy (may be normal in a neonate).
- ABG measurements reveal hypoxia and secondary metabolic acidosis.

Trichinosis
- History includes ingestion of raw or improperly cooked pork or pork products.
- Stools contain mature worms and larvae during the invasion stage.
- Skeletal muscle biopsy reveals encysted larvae 10 days after ingestion.
- Antibody titers are elevated during acute and convalescent stage.
- During acute stages, serum liver enzymes (AST, LD, and CK) are elevated.
- Eosinophil count is elevated.

Trichomoniasis
- History includes sexual contact with person with trichomoniasis.
- Microscopic examination of vaginal or seminal discharge identifies *Trichomonas vaginalis*.
- Culture of clear urine specimens may also reveal *T. vaginalis*.
- Examination reveals vaginal erythema; edema; frank excoriation; a frothy, malodorous, greenish yellow vaginal discharge; and, rarely, a thin, gray pseudomembrane over the vagina.
- Cervical examination shows punctate cervical hemorrhages, giving the cervix a strawberry appearance.

Trichuriasis
- History includes ingestion of food contaminated with nematoid ova.
- Stool specimen contains whipworm ova.

Tricuspid insufficiency
- Cardiac catheterization shows markedly decreased cardiac output; mean right atrial and right ventricular end-diastolic pressures may be elevated.
- CXR reveals right atrial and ventricular enlargement.
- Echocardiography shows right ventricular dilation and paradoxical septal motion. It may show prolapsing or flailing of the tricuspid valve leaflets. Doppler echocardiography provides estimates of pulmonary artery and right ventricular systolic pressure.
- ECG reveals right atrial hypertrophy and right or left ventricular hypertrophy. ECG also may reveal atrial fibrillation or incomplete right bundle-branch block.

Tricuspid stenosis
- Cardiac catheterization shows increased right atrial pressure and decreased cardiac output; it may also show an increased pressure gradient across the tricuspid valve.
- CXR reveals right atrial and superior vena cava enlargement.
- Echocardiography reveals a thick tricuspid valve with reduced mobility and right atrial enlargement.
- ECG shows right atrial hypertrophy and right ventricular hypertrophy. Atrial fibrillation may be present. Tall, peaked P waves are seen in lead II and prominent, upright P waves are seen in lead V_1, indicating right atrial enlargement.

Trigeminal neuralgia

- History includes pain in the superior mandibular or maxillary area, without sensory or motor impairment.
- Examination reveals splinting on the affected side of the face while talking.
- Skull X-rays, tomography, and CT scans rule out sinus or tooth infections and tumors.

Tuberculosis

- Stains and cultures of sputum, CSF, urine, and abscess drainage reveal heat-sensitive, nonmotile, aerobic, acid-fast bacilli.
- CXR shows nodular lesions, patchy infiltrates, cavity formation, scar tissue, and calcium deposits.
- Auscultation reveals crepitant crackles, bronchial breath sounds, wheezes, and whispered pectoriloquy.
- Chest percussion reveals a dullness over the affected area.
- Tuberculin skin test reveals that the patient has been infected with tuberculosis.

Tularemia

- History includes exposure to animals or ticks.
- Lymph nodes, sputum, or gastric washings identify *Francisella tularensis*.
- Agglutination test reveals a rise in antibody titers.
- Skin test (with a diluted specimen of *F. tularensis*) has a positive reaction (90% of patients).

Typhus, epidemic

- Weil-Felix reaction reveals a fourfold rise in agglutination titer 8 to 12 days after infection.
- Complement fixation for group-specific typhus antigens is positive 8 to 12 days after infection.

Ulcerative colitis

- History includes recurrent bloody diarrhea and GI disturbances.
- Sigmoidoscopy shows increased mucosal friability, decreased mucosal detail, and thick inflammatory exudate.
- Biopsy reveals histologic changes characteristic of ulcerative colitis.
- Colonoscopy identifies the extent of the disease.
- Barium enema identifies the extent of the disease and detects complications.
- ESR increases, correlating with severity of attack.
- Serum potassium and magnesium levels are decreased.
- CBC shows decreased Hb level and leukocytosis.
- Serum albumin level is decreased.
- PT is prolonged.

Undescended testes

- Examination of scrotum reveals unpalpable testes, either unilateral or bilateral.
- Buccal smear identifies genetic sex by showing a male sex chromatin pattern.
- Serum gonadotropin levels confirm the presence of testes.

Urticaria and angioedema

- History includes exposure to medications, food, and environmental influences.
- Skin testing reveals specific allergens.
- Serum C4 and C1 esterase inhibitor levels are decreased (confirming hereditary angioedema).
- CBC, urinalysis, ESR, and CXR rule out inflammatory infections.

Uterine cancer

- Endometrial, cervical, and endocervical biopsies reveal malignant cells.

- Schiller's test shows cancerous tissues resisting stain.
- Cervical biopsies and endocervical curettage identify degree of cervical involvement.
- Barium enema reveals bladder or rectal involvement.

Uterine leiomyomas

- History includes abnormal endometrial bleeding.
- Pelvic palpation reveals round or irregular mass.
- Ultrasonography shows a dense mass.
- Hysterosalpingography reveals asymmetric uterus.
- Laparoscopy reveals lumps on the uterus.
- CBC reveals decreased RBC count and Hb and HCT levels.

Uveitis

- Slit-lamp examination reveals a "flare and cell" pattern, which looks like light passing through smoke, and an increased number of cells over the inflamed area.
- Examination with a special lens, slit-lamp, and ophthalmoscope identifies active inflammatory fundus lesions involving the retina and choroid.
- Serologic tests indicate toxoplasmosis (in posterior uveitis).

Vaginal cancer

- Papanicolaou test reveals abnormal cells.
- Vaginal examination, aided by Lugol's solution, reveals lesion.
- Lesion biopsy reveals malignant cells.
- Gallium scan shows abnormal gallium activity.

Vaginismus

- History and examination rule out physical disorders causing muscle constriction.
- Pelvic examination reveals involuntary constriction of the musculature surrounding the outer portion of the vagina.
- Detailed sexual history reveals involuntary spastic contraction of the lower vaginal muscles, possibly coexisting with dyspareunia, preventing intercourse.

Varicella

- History includes exposure to person infected with chickenpox, although the patient may be unaware of contact.
- Examination reveals crops of small, erythematous macules on the trunk or scalp progressing to papules and then clear vesicles on a erythematous base; vesicles become cloudy and break, and then form a scab.
- Vesicular fluid tests positive for herpesvirus varicella-zoster.

Variola

- History includes exposure to infected person.
- Aspirate from vesicles and pustules reveals variola virus.
- Complement fixation detects antibodies to variola virus.
- Microscopic examination of smears from lesions shows variola virus.

Vascular retinopathies

- Central retinal artery occlusion:
– Ophthalmoscopy (direct or indirect) shows emptying of retinal arterioles.
– Slit-lamp examination reveals, within 2 hours of occlusion, clumps or segmentation in the artery. Later examination shows a milky white retina around the optic disk (resulting from swelling and necrosis of ganglion cells caused by reduced blood supply). Other find-

ings include a cherry-red spot in the macula (which subsides after several weeks).
– Ophthalmodynamometry measures approximate relative pressures in the central retinal arteries and indirectly assesses internal carotid artery blockage.
– Ultrasonography reveals blood vessel conditions in the neck.
– Digital subtraction angiography identifies carotid occlusion.
– MRI helps identify the reason for obstruction by revealing carotid or other obstruction.
– Contrast-enhanced computed tomography scan discloses the diseased carotid artery.
● Central retinal vein occlusion:
– Ophthalmoscopy (direct or indirect) reveals retinal hemorrhage, retinal vein engorgement, white patches among hemorrhages, and edema around the optic disk.
– Ultrasonography confirms or rules out occluded blood vessels.
● Diabetic retinopathy:
– Slit-lamp examination shows thickening of retinal capillary walls.
– Indirect ophthalmoscopy demonstrates retinal changes, such as microaneurysms (earliest change), retinal hemorrhages and edema, venous dilation and beading, exudates, vitreous hemorrhage, proliferation of fibrin into vitreous from retinal holes, growth of new blood vessels, and microinfarctions of nerve fiber layer.
– Fluorescein angiography shows leakage of fluorescein from dilated vessels and differentiates between microaneurysms and true hemorrhages.
● Hypertensive retinopathy:
– Ophthalmoscopy (direct or indirect) performed in early disease discloses hard and shiny deposits, tiny hemorrhages, narrowed arterioles, nicking of the veins where arteries cross them (re-

ferred to as arteriovenous nicking), and elevated arterial blood pressure. The same test in later disease shows cotton wool patches, exudates, retinal edema, papilledema caused by ischemia and capillary insufficiency, hemorrhages, and microaneurysms.
– History reveals hypertension and decreased vision.

Vasculitis
● Polyarteritis nodosa:
– History includes hypertension, abdominal pain, myalgia, headache, joint pain, and weakness.
– ESR is elevated.
– Leukocytosis, anemia, and thrombocytosis are present.
– C_3 complement is depressed.
– Rheumatoid factor is > 80 IU/ml.
– Circulating immune complexes are present.
– Tissue biopsy shows necrotizing vasculitis.
● Allergic angiitis and granulomatosis:
– History includes asthma.
– Eosinophilia is present.
– Tissue biopsy may show granulomatous inflammation with eosinophilic infiltration.
● Polyangiitis overlap syndrome:
– History includes allergy.
– Eosinophilia is present.
– Tissue biopsy that may show granulomatous inflammation with eosinophilic infiltration.
● Wegener's granulomatosis:
– Leukocytosis is present.
– Tissue biopsy reveals necrotizing vasculitis with granulomatous inflammation.
– ESR and IgA and IgG levels are elevated.
– Rheumatoid factor titer is low.
– Circulating immune complexes are present
● Temporal arteritis:
– Hb level is decreased.

– ESR is elevated.

– Tissue biopsy shows panarteritis with infiltration of mononuclear cells, giant cells within vessel wall, fragmentation of internal elastic lamina, and proliferation of intima.

• Takayasu's arteritis:

– Hb level is decreased.

– Leukocytosis is present.

– Lupus erythematosus cell preparation is positive and ESR is elevated.

– Arteriography shows calcification and obstruction of affected vessels.

– Tissue biopsy shows inflammation of adventitia and intima of vessels and thickening of vessel walls,

• Hypersensitivity vasculitis:

– History includes exposure to an antigen, such as a microorganism or a drug.

– Tissue biopsy may show leukocytoclastic angiitis (usually in postcapillary venules), with infiltration of polymorphonuclear leukocytes, fibrinoid necrosis, and extravasation of erythrocytes.

• Mucocutaneous lymph node syndrome:

– History and examination reveal fever, nonsuppurative cervical adenitis, edema, congested conjunctivae, desquamation of fingertips, and erythema of oral cavity, lips, and palms.

– Tissue biopsy may show intimal proliferation and infiltration of vessel walls with mononuclear cells.

Velopharyngeal insufficiency

• Examination reveals unintelligible speech.

• Fiber-optic nasopharyngoscopy permits monitoring of velopharyngeal patency during speech and may identify the insufficiency.

• Ultrasonography shows air-tissue overlap reflecting the degree of velopharyngeal sphincter incompetence; an opening of > 20 mm^2 results in unintelligible speech.

Ventricular aneurysm

• History includes persistent arrhythmias, onset of heart failure, or systemic embolization in a patient with left ventricular failure and a history of myocardial infarction.

• CXR reveals an abnormal bulge distorting the heart's contour (with large aneurysm).

• Left ventriculography reveals left ventricular enlargement, with an area of akinesia or dyskinesia and diminished cardiac function.

• Echocardiography reveals abnormal motion in the left ventricular wall.

Ventricular fibrillation

• ECG reveals the following:

– Atrial rhythm isn't measurable.

– Ventricular rhythm has no pattern or regularity.

– Atrial and ventricular rates aren't measurable.

– P wave isn't measurable.

– PR interval isn't measurable

– Duration of the QRS complex isn't measurable; configuration is wide and irregular.

– T wave isn't measurable.

Ventricular septal defect

• Echocardiography or MRI reveals a large defect and its location in the septum, estimates the size of a left-to-right shunt, suggests pulmonary hypertension, and identifies associated lesions and complications.

• Cardiac catheterization determines the size and exact location of the defect, calculates the degree of shunting, determines the extent of pulmonary hypertension, and detects associated defects.

• CXR is normal with small defects; in large defects, it shows cardiomegaly, left atrial and ventricular enlargement, and prominent pulmonary vascular markings.

• ECG is normal with small defects; in large defects, it shows left and right ventricular hypertrophy.

Ventricular tachycardia

• ECG reveals the following:
– Atrial rhythm isn't measurable. Ventricular rhythm is usually regular, but may be slightly irregular.
– Atrial rate can't be measured. Ventricular rate is usually rapid (140 to 220 beats/minute).
– P wave is usually absent. It may be obscured by and is dissociated from the QRS complex. Retrograde and upright P waves may be present.
– PR interval isn't measurable.
– QRS complex has a duration > 0.12 second, has a bizarre appearance, and usually has increased amplitude.
– T wave occurs in the opposite direction of the QRS complex.
– QT interval isn't measurable.

Vesicoureteral reflux

• History includes symptoms of urinary tract infection.
• Examination reveals hematuria or strong-smelling urine (in infants).
• Palpation may reveal a hard, thickened bladder (if posterior urethral valves are causing an obstruction in male infants).
• Cystoscopy reveals reflux.
• Urinalysis reveals bacterial count > 100,000/μl; specific gravity < 1.010, and increased pH.
• Excretory urography may show dilated lower ureter, ureter visible for its entire length, hydronephrosis, calyceal distortion, and renal scarring.
• Voiding cystourethrography identifies and determines the degree of reflux, shows when reflux occurs, and may also pinpoint the cause.
• Bladder catheterization identifies the amount of residual urine.

Vitamin A deficiency

• History includes inadequate dietary intake of foods high in vitamin A.
• Ocular examination reveals xerophthalmia, Bitot's spots, perforation, and scarring.
• Serum levels of vitamin A are < 20 μg/ dl.
• Carotene levels are < 40 μg/dl.

Vitamin B deficiencies

• History includes inadequate dietary intake of foods high in vitamin B.
• Serum cobalamin levels are < 150 pg/ml.
• Serum vitamin B_2 activity index is < 0.9.
• 24-hour urine test reveals:
– thiamine deficiency
– riboflavin deficiency
– niacin deficiency (levels < 0.05 mg/g)
– pyridoxine deficiency (if xanthurenic acid < 50 mg/day).

Vitamin C deficiency

• History includes inadequate intake of ascorbic acid
• Serum ascorbic acid levels are < 0.2 mg/dl and WBC ascorbic acid levels are < 30 mg/dl.

Vitamin D deficiency

• History includes inadequate dietary intake of preformed vitamin D.
• Serum vitamin D_3 levels are low or undetectable.
• Plasma calcium serum levels are < 7.5 mg/dl.
• Inorganic phosphorus serum levels are < 3 mg/dl.
• Serum citrate levels are < 2.5 mg/dl.
• Alkaline phosphatase levels are < 4 Bodansky units/dl.
• X-rays reveal characteristic bone deformities and abnormalities such as Looser's zones.

Vitamin E deficiency
- History includes diet high in polyunsaturated fatty acids fortified with iron but not vitamin E.
- Serum alpha-tocopherol levels are < 0.5 mg/dl in adults and < 0.2 mg/dl in infants.
- Serum CK levels are increased.
- Platelet levels are increased.

Vitamin K deficiency
- PT is 25% longer than the normal range of 10 to 20 seconds (in the absence of anticoagulant therapy or hepatic disease).
- Capillary fragility test is positive.

Vitiligo
- Examination reveals stark white skin patches.
- Wood's light examination in a darkened room detects vitiliginous patches; depigmented skin reflects the light, while pigmented skin absorbs it.

Vocal cord nodules and polyps
- History includes persistent hoarseness.
- Indirect laryngoscopy initially shows small red nodes; later, white solid nodes appear on one or both cords.
- Indirect laryngoscopy shows unilateral or, occasionally, bilateral, sessile or pedunculated polyps of varying size anywhere on the vocal cords.

Vocal cord paralysis
- History and examination reveal hoarseness or airway obstruction.
- Indirect laryngoscopy reveals one or both cords fixed in an adducted or partially abducted position.

Volvulus
- History includes sudden onset of severe abdominal pain.
- Examination reveals palpable abdominal mass.

- Abdominal X-rays reveal obstruction and abnormal air-fluid levels in the sigmoid and cecum (in midgut volvulus, abdominal X-rays may be normal).
- Barium enema reveals the following:
  – In cecal volvulus, barium fills the colon distal to the section of cecum.
  – In sigmoid volvulus in children, barium may twist to a point; in adults, barium may take on an "ace of spades" configuration.
- In midgut volvulus, upper GI series reveals obstruction and possibly a twisted contour in a narrow area near the duodenojejunal junction where barium will not pass.
- WBC count is elevated, indicating strangulation or bowel infarction.

Von Willebrand's disease
- History reveals family inheritance pattern.
- Bleeding time is prolonged.
- PTT is prolonged.
- Factor VIII-related antigens are decreased and factor VIII activity level is low.
- Clot retraction and platelet aggregation are normal.

Vulvovaginitis
- Examination reveals vaginal discharge and inflammation of the vulva.
- Culture of vaginal exudate identifies presence of Trichomonas vaginalis, Candida albicans, Gardnerella vaginitis, Neisseria gonorrhoeae, or Phthirus pubis.

Warts
- Visual examination reveals evidence of irregular growth on skin.
- Sigmoidoscopy may rule out internal involvement in recurrent anal warts.

Whooping cough
- Examination reveals forceful coughing that ends in a characteristic whoop.

- Nasopharyngeal swabs and sputum cultures identify *Bordetella pertussis* (in the early stages of illness).
- WBC count is markedly elevated, with 60% to 90% lymphocytes.

Wilms' tumor

- Examination reveals palpable abdominal mass in early childhood.
- Gallium scan reveals abnormal activity.
- Percutaneous renal biopsy reveals malignant cells.
- Excretory urography does not indicate neoplasm or extrarenal mass.

Wilson's disease

- Slit-lamp ophthalmic examination reveals Kayser-Fleischer rings (in advanced disease).
- Liver biopsy reveals excessive copper deposits and tissue changes indicative of chronic active hepatitis, fatty liver, or cirrhosis.
- Serum ceruloplasmin is < 22.9 mg/ dl.
- Serum copper is < 0.75 ng/ml.
- Urine copper is > 100 µg/24 hours (may be as high as 1,000 µg).

Wiskott-Aldrich syndrome

- History includes thrombocytopenia, bleeding disorders at birth, and recurrent infections.
- Platelet count is markedly decreased.
- IgE levels are normal or elevated, IgG and IgA levels are normal, and IgM levels are decreased.
- Isohemagglutinin levels are low or absent.
- Sputum and throat cultures commonly identify *Streptococcus pneumoniae,* meningococci, or *Haemophilus influenzae* as the causative organisms.

Wounds, open trauma

- History includes injury.
- Examination reveals open wound.

- X-rays show bone damage, extent of injury to the area and surrounding tissue, and retention of injuring object.
- Electromyography reveals isolated, irregular motor unit potentials with increased amplitude and duration indicating peripheral nerve injury.
- Nerve conduction studies reveal abnormal nerve conduction time indicating peripheral nerve injury.
- CBC reveals decreased Hb and HCT levels and increased WBC count.

X-linked infantile hypogammaglobulinemia

- Serum IgM, IgA, and IgG are decreased or absent (in patient at least 9 months old).
- Antigenic stimulation testing confirms an inability to produce specific antibodies, although cellular immunity remains intact.

Yellow fever

- Blood culture reveals presence of arbovirus.
- Urine albumin levels are increased (in 90% of patients).
- Antibody titer is elevated.

Zinc deficiency

- History includes excessive intake of foods containing iron, calcium, vitamin D, and the fiber and phytates in cereals.
- Serum zinc levels are < 121 µg/day.

PART TWO

DIAGNOSTIC TESTS

CHAPTER 1

Hematology and Coagulation Tests

RED BLOOD CELLS		85
85	Red blood cell count	88	Erythrocyte sedimentation rate
86	Hematocrit	89	Reticulocyte count
87	Red cell indices	90	Osmotic fragility

HEMOGLOBIN		92
92	Total hemoglobin	97	Heinz bodies
93	Fetal hemoglobin	98	Iron and total iron-binding
94	Hemoglobin electrophoresis		capacity
95	Sickle cell test	100	Ferritin
96	Unstable hemoglobin	101	Methemoglobin

WHITE BLOOD CELLS		102
102	White blood cell count	103	White blood cell differential

PLATELET ACTIVITY		107
107	Bleeding time	110	Capillary fragility
108	Platelet count	111	Platelet aggregation

COAGULATION		113
113	Activated partial thromboplastin time	118	Plasma thrombin time
114	Prothrombin time	119	Plasma fibrinogen
115	Activated clotting time	120	Fibrin split products
116	One-stage factor assay: Extrinsic coagulation system	121	Plasma plasminogen
		122	Protein C
117	One-stage factor assay: Intrinsic coagulation system	123	Euglobulin lysis time
		124	D-Dimer
		125	International normalized ratio

RED BLOOD CELLS

RED BLOOD CELL COUNT

The red blood cell (RBC) count, also called an erythrocyte count, is part of a complete blood count. It's used to detect the number of RBCs in a microliter (μl), or cubic millimeter (mm^3), of whole blood.

Purpose
- To provide data for calculating mean corpuscular volume and mean corpuscular hemoglobin, which reveal RBC size and hemoglobin content
- To support other hematologic tests for diagnosing anemia or polycythemia

Patient preparation
- Explain to the patient that this test is used to evaluate the number of RBCs and to detect possible blood disorders.
- Tell him that a blood sample will be taken. Explain who will perform the venipuncture and when.
- Reassure him that drawing a blood sample will take less than 3 minutes.
- Explain that he may feel slight discomfort from the tourniquet pressure and the needle puncture.
- If the patient is a child, explain to him (if he's old enough) and his parents that a small amount of blood will be taken from the finger or earlobe.
- Inform the patient that food or fluids need not be restricted before the test.

Procedure and posttest care
- For adults and older children, draw venous blood into a 7-ml *lavender-top* tube.

- For younger children, collect capillary blood in a microcollection device.
- If a hematoma develops at the venipuncture site, apply warm soaks.

Precautions
- Completely fill the collection tube.
- Invert the tube gently several times to mix the sample and the anticoagulant.
- Handle the sample gently to prevent hemolysis.

Reference values
Normal RBC values vary, depending on the type of sample and on the patient's age and sex, as follows:
- adult males: 4.5 to 5.5 million RBCs/ μl of venous blood
- adult females: 4 to 5 million RBCs/ μl of venous blood
- children ages 1 to 6: 3.9 to 5.3 million RBCs/μl of venous blood
- full-term infants: 4.1 to 6.1 million RBCs/μl of capillary blood at birth, decreasing to 3.8 to 5.6 million RBCs/μl at age 2 months, and increasing slowly thereafter.

Normal values may exceed these levels in patients living at high altitudes.

Abnormal findings
An elevated RBC count may indicate absolute or relative polycythemia. A depressed count may indicate anemia, fluid overload, or hemorrhage beyond 24 hours. Further tests, such as stained cell examination, hematocrit, hemoglobin, red cell indices, and white cell studies, are needed to confirm the diagnosis.

Interfering factors
- Failure to use the proper anticoagulant or to adequately mix the sample and the anticoagulant
- Hemoconcentration due to prolonged tourniquet constriction

- Hemodilution due to drawing the sample from the same arm used for I.V. infusion of fluids
- High white blood cell count (false-high test results in semiautomated and automated counters)
- Diseases that cause RBCs to agglutinate or form rouleaux (false decrease)
- Hemolysis due to rough handling of the sample or drawing the blood through a small-gauge needle for venipuncture
- Pregnancy

HEMATOCRIT

A hematocrit (HCT) test may be done separately or as part of a complete blood count. It measures percentage by volume of packed red blood cells (RBCs) in a whole blood sample; for example, an HCT of 40% indicates that a 100-ml sample of blood contains 40 ml of packed RBCs. Packing is achieved by centrifuging anticoagulated whole blood in a capillary tube so that red cells are tightly packed without hemolysis.

Purpose
- To aid diagnosis of polycythemia, anemia, or abnormal states of hydration
- To aid calculation of two red cell indices: mean corpuscular volume and mean corpuscular hemoglobin concentration

Patient preparation
- Explain to the patient that HCT is tested to detect anemia and other abnormal blood conditions.
- Tell him that a capillary blood sample will be taken. Explain who will perform the test and when.

- If the patient is a child, explain to him (if he's old enough) and his parents that a small amount of blood will be taken from the finger or earlobe.
- Inform the patient that food or fluids need not be restricted before the test.

Procedure and posttest care
- Perform a fingerstick, using a heparinized capillary tube with a red band on the anticoagulant end. Blood drawn from a capillary puncture has slightly lower HCT levels than blood drawn from a venipuncture.
- Fill the capillary tube from the red-banded end to about two-thirds capacity, and seal this end with clay.
- Alternatively, perform a venipuncture and fill a 7-ml *lavender-top* tube.
- If a hematoma develops at the venipuncture site, apply warm soaks.

Precautions
- Send the sample to the laboratory immediately.
- If you perform the test, place the tube in the centrifuge with the red end pointing outward.
- Fill the collection tube completely.
- Invert the tube gently several times to mix the sample.

Reference values
HCT is usually measured electronically. The results are 3% lower than manual measurements, which trap plasma in the column of packed RBCs.

Reference values vary, depending on the type of sample, the laboratory performing the test, and the patient's age and sex, as follows:
- neonates ages 0 to 2 weeks: 44% to 64%
- infants ages 2 weeks to 2 months: 39% to 59%
- infants ages 2 to 6 months: 35% to 49%
- infants ages 6 months to 1 year: 29% to 43%

- children ages 1 to 6: 30% to 40%
- children ages 6 to 16: 32% to 42%
- adult males: 42% to 52%
- adult females: 36% to 48%.

Abnormal findings

Low HCT suggests anemia, hemodilution, or massive blood loss. High HCT indicates polycythemia or hemoconcentration due to blood loss and dehydration.

Interfering factors

- Failure to fill the tube properly, to use the proper anticoagulant, or to adequately mix the sample and the anticoagulant
- Hemolysis due to rough handling of the sample or drawing the blood through a small-gauge needle for venipuncture
- Hemoconcentration due to tourniquet constriction for longer than 1 minute (increase, typically 2.5% to 5%)
- Drawing the blood from the same arm used for I.V. infusion
- Elevated blood glucose or sodium (possible increase due to erythrocyte swelling)
- Hemodilution or dehydration

RED CELL INDICES

Using the results of the red blood cell (RBC) count, hematocrit, and total hemoglobin tests, red cell indices (erythrocyte indices) provide important information about the size, hemoglobin concentration, and hemoglobin weight of an average RBC.

Purpose

- To aid diagnosis and classification of anemias

Patient preparation

- Explain to the patient that this test helps determine if he has anemia.
- Tell him that a blood sample will be taken. Explain who will perform the venipuncture and when.
- Reassure him that drawing a blood sample will take less than 3 minutes.
- Explain that he may feel slight discomfort from the tourniquet pressure and the needle puncture.

Procedure and posttest care

- Perform a venipuncture, and collect the sample in a 7-ml *lavender-top* tube.
- If a hematoma develops at the venipuncture site, apply warm soaks.

Precautions

- Completely fill the collection tube, and invert it gently several times to adequately mix the sample and the anticoagulant.
- Handle the sample gently to prevent hemolysis.

Reference values

The indices tested include mean corpuscular volume (MCV), mean corpuscular hemoglobin (MCH), and mean corpuscular hemoglobin concentration (MCHC).

MCV, the ratio of hematocrit (packed cell volume) to the RBC count, expresses the average size of the erythrocytes and indicates whether they are undersized (microcytic), oversized (macrocytic), or normal (normocytic). MCH, the hemoglobin-RBC ratio, gives the weight of hemoglobin in an average red cell. MCHC, the ratio of hemoglobin weight to hematocrit, defines the concentration of hemoglobin in 100 ml of packed RBCs. It helps to distinguish normally colored (normochromic) RBCs from paler (hypochromic) RBCs.

The range of normal red cell indices is as follows:

COMPARATIVE RED CELL INDICES IN ANEMIAS

	NORMAL VALUES (Normocytic, normochromic)	IRON DEFICIENCY ANEMIA (Microcytic, hypochromic)	PERNICIOUS ANEMIA (Macrocytic, normochromic)
MCV	82 to 98 μm^3	60 to 80 μm^3	95 to 150 μm^3
MCH	26 to 34 pg/cell	5 to 25 pg/cell	33 to 53 pg/cell
MCHC	31 to 37 g/dl	20 to 30 g/dl	33 to 38 g/dl

Key:
MCV = Mean corpuscular volume
MCH = Mean corpuscular hemoglobin
MCHC = Mean corpuscular hemoglobin concentration

- MCV: 82 to 98 μm^3
- MCH: 26 to 34 pg/cell
- MCHC: 31 to 37 g/dl.

Abnormal findings

Low MCV and MCHC indicate microcytic, hypochromic anemias caused by iron deficiency anemia, pyridoxine-responsive anemia, or thalassemia. A high MCV suggests macrocytic anemias caused by megaloblastic anemias, due to folic acid or vitamin B_{12} deficiency, inherited disorders of deoxyribonucleic acid synthesis, or reticulocytosis. Because MCV reflects the average volume of many cells, a value within the normal range can encompass RBCs of varying size, from microcytic to macrocytic. (See *Comparative red cell indices in anemias*.)

Interfering factors

- Failure to use the proper anticoagulant or to adequately mix the sample and the anticoagulant
- Hemolysis due to rough handling of the sample
- Hemoconcentration due to prolonged tourniquet constriction
- High white blood cell count (false-high RBC count in semiautomated and automated counters, invalidating MCV and MCHC results)
- Diseases that cause RBCs to agglutinate or form rouleaux (false-low RBC count)

ERYTHROCYTE SEDIMENTATION RATE

The erythrocyte sedimentation rate (ESR) measures the degree of erythrocyte settling in a blood sample during a specified time period. The ESR is a sensitive but nonspecific test that is frequently the earliest indicator of disease when other chemical or physical signs are normal. The ESR commonly increases significantly in widespread inflammatory disorders; elevations may be prolonged in localized inflammation and malignant disease.

Purpose

- To monitor inflammatory or malignant disease
- To aid detection and diagnosis of occult disease, such as tuberculosis, tis-

sue necrosis, or connective tissue disease

Patient preparation
• Explain to the patient that this test is used to evaluate the condition of red blood cells.
• Tell him that a blood sample will be taken. Explain who will perform the venipuncture and when.
• Reassure him that drawing a blood sample will take less than 3 minutes.
• Explain that he may feel slight discomfort from the tourniquet pressure and the needle puncture.
• Inform the patient that food or fluids need not be restricted before the test.

Procedure and posttest care
• Perform a venipuncture, and collect the sample in a 7-ml *lavender-top*, 4.5-ml *black-top*, or 4.5-ml *blue-top* tube. Check with the laboratory to determine its preference.
• If a hematoma develops at the venipuncture site, apply warm soaks.

Precautions
• Completely fill the collection tube, and invert it gently several times to thoroughly mix the sample and the anticoagulant.
• Because prolonged standing decreases the ESR, examine the sample for clots or clumps and send it to the laboratory immediately. It must be tested within 2 hours.
• Handle the sample gently to prevent hemolysis.

Reference values
The ESR normally ranges from 0 to 15 mm/hour in males, 0 to 20 mm/hour in females, and 0 to 10 mm/hour in children. Rates gradually increase with age.

Abnormal findings
The ESR rises in pregnancy, anemia, acute or chronic inflammation, tuberculosis, paraproteinemias (especially multiple myeloma and Waldenström's macroglobulinemia), rheumatic fever, rheumatoid arthritis, and some malignant diseases.

Polycythemia, sickle cell anemia, hyperviscosity, and low plasma fibrinogen or globulin levels tend to depress the ESR.

Interfering factors
• Failure to use the proper anticoagulant, to adequately mix the sample and the anticoagulant, or to send the sample to the laboratory immediately
• Hemolysis due to rough handling or excessive mixing of the sample
• Hemoconcentration due to prolonged tourniquet constriction
• Testing delayed more than 3 hours after sample collection (possible decrease)

RETICULOCYTE COUNT

Reticulocytes are nonnucleated, immature red blood cells (RBCs) that remain in the peripheral blood for 24 to 48 hours while maturing. They're generally larger than mature RBCs. In this test, reticulocytes in a whole blood sample are counted and expressed as a percentage of the total RBC count. Because the manual method of reticulocyte counting uses only a small sample, values may be imprecise and should be compared with RBC count or hematocrit.

Purpose
• To aid in distinguishing between hypoproliferative and hyperproliferative anemias

- To help assess blood loss, bone marrow response to anemia, and therapy for anemia

Patient preparation
- Explain to the patient that this test is used to detect anemia or to monitor its treatment.
- Tell him that a blood sample will be taken. Explain who will perform the venipuncture and when.
- Reassure him that drawing a blood sample will take less than 3 minutes.
- Explain that he may feel slight discomfort from the tourniquet pressure and the needle puncture.
- If the patient is an infant or child, explain to the parents that a small amount of blood will be taken from the finger or earlobe.
- Withhold antimalarials, antipyretics, azathioprine, chloramphenicol, corticotropin, dactinomycin, furazolidone (from infants), levodopa, methotrexate, phenacetin, and sulfonamides, as needed. If such medications must be continued, note this on the laboratory slip.
- Inform the patient that food or fluids need not be restricted before the test.

Procedure and posttest care
- Perform a venipuncture, and collect the sample in a 7-ml *lavender-top* tube.
- If a hematoma develops at the venipuncture site, apply warm soaks.
- Examine a stained smear of peripheral blood for the percentage of reticulocytes in relation to the number of RBCs present.
- Resume administration of medications withheld before the test.
- Monitor a patient with an abnormal reticulocyte count for trends or significant changes in repeated tests.

Precautions
- Completely fill the collection tube and invert it gently several times to mix the sample and the anticoagulant.
- Handle the sample gently to prevent hemolysis.

Reference values
Reticulocytes compose 0.5% to 2.5% of the total RBC count. In infants the normal reticulocyte count ranges from 2% to 5% at birth, decreasing to adult levels in 1 to 2 weeks.

Abnormal findings
A low reticulocyte count indicates hypoproliferative bone marrow (hypoplastic anemia) or ineffective erythropoiesis (pernicious anemia).

A high reticulocyte count indicates a bone marrow response to anemia caused by hemolysis or blood loss. The reticulocyte count may also increase after therapy for iron deficiency anemia or pernicious anemia.

Interfering factors
- Failure to use the proper anticoagulant or to adequately mix the sample and the anticoagulant
- Prolonged tourniquet constriction (false-low or false-high)
- Azathioprine, chloramphenicol, dactinomycin, and methotrexate (possible false-low)
- Corticotropin, antimalarials, antipyretics, furazolidone (in infants), levodopa (possible false-high)
- Sulfonamides (possible false-low or false-high)
- Recent blood transfusion (possible false-low due to hemodilution)

OSMOTIC FRAGILITY

Osmotic fragility measures red blood cell (RBC) resistance to hemolysis when exposed to a series of increasingly dilute saline solutions. The sooner hemolysis occurs, the greater the osmotic fragility of the cells.

Purpose
• To aid diagnosis of hereditary spherocytosis
• To supplement a stained cell examination to detect morphologic RBC abnormalities

Patient preparation
• Explain to the patient that this test is used to identify the cause of anemia.
• Tell him that a blood sample will be taken. Explain who will perform the venipuncture and when.
• Reassure him that drawing a blood sample will take less than 3 minutes.
• Explain that he may feel slight discomfort from the tourniquet pressure and the needle puncture.
• Inform him that food or fluids need not be restricted before the test.

Procedure and posttest care
• Perform a venipuncture, collecting the sample in a 7-ml *green-top* (heparinized) tube, or secure a special heparinized tube for collecting defibrinated blood.
• If a hematoma develops at the venipuncture site, apply warm soaks.

Precautions
• Because this test isn't routinely performed, notify the laboratory before drawing the sample.
• Completely fill the collection tube and invert it gently several times to mix the sample and anticoagulant thoroughly.
• Handle the sample gently to prevent accidental hemolysis.
• In some cases, RBCs don't hemolyze immediately; incubation in solution for 24 hours improves test sensitivity.

Reference values
Osmotic fragility values (percentage of RBCs hemolyzed) are determined by the tonicity of the saline. Reference values for the different tonicities are as follows:
• *0.5 g/dl sodium chloride (NaCl) solution (unincubated)*
– Males: 0.5% to 24.7% hemolysis
– Females: 0% to 23.1% hemolysis
• *0.6 g/dl NaCl solution (incubated)*
– Males: 18% to 55.2% hemolysis
– Females: 2.2% to 59.3% hemolysis
• *0.65 g/dl NaCl solution (incubated)*
– Males: 4% to 24.8% hemolysis
– Females: 0.5% to 28.9% hemolysis
• *0.75 g/dl NaCl solution (incubated)*
– Males: 0.5% to 8.5% hemolysis
– Females: 0.1% to 9.3% hemolysis

Abnormal findings
Low osmotic fragility (increased resistance to hemolysis) is characteristic of thalassemia, iron deficiency anemia, sickle cell anemia, and other red cell disorders in which codocytes (target cells) and leptocytes are found. Low osmotic fragility also occurs after splenectomy.

High osmotic fragility (increased tendency to hemolysis) occurs in hereditary spherocytosis, in spherocytosis associated with autoimmune hemolytic anemia, severe burns, or chemical poisoning, or in hemolytic disease of the newborn (erythroblastosis fetalis).

Interfering factors
• Failure to fill the tube completely, to use the proper anticoagulant, or to adequately mix the sample and the anticoagulant
• Hemolysis due to rough handling of the sample
• Presence of hemolytic organisms in the sample
• Severe anemia or other conditions with fewer RBCs available for testing
• Recent blood transfusion

HEMOGLOBIN

TOTAL HEMOGLOBIN

Total hemoglobin (Hb) is used to measure the amount of Hb found in a deciliter (dl, or 100 ml) of whole blood. It's usually part of a complete blood count. Hb concentration correlates closely with the red blood cell (RBC) count.

Purpose
• To measure the severity of anemia or polycythemia and to monitor response to therapy
• To obtain data for calculating mean corpuscular Hb and mean corpuscular Hb concentration

Patient preparation
• Explain to the patient that this test is used to detect anemia or polycythemia, or to assess his response to treatment.
• Tell him that a blood sample will be taken. Explain who will perform the venipuncture and when.
• Reassure him that drawing a blood sample will take less than 3 minutes.
• Explain that he may feel slight discomfort from the tourniquet pressure and the needle puncture.
• If the patient is an infant or child, explain to the parents that a small amount of blood will be taken from the finger or earlobe.
• Inform him that food or fluids need not be restricted before the test.

Procedure and posttest care
• For adults and older children, perform a venipuncture, and collect the sample in a 7-ml *lavender-top* tube.

• For younger children and infants, collect capillary blood in a pipette.
• If a hematoma develops at the venipuncture site, apply warm soaks.

Precautions
• Completely fill the collection tube and invert it gently several times to thoroughly mix the sample and the anticoagulant.
• Handle the sample gently to prevent hemolysis.

Reference values
Hb concentration varies, depending on the type of sample drawn (capillary blood samples for infants and venous blood samples for all others), and on the patient's age and sex, as follows:
• neonates ages 0 to 2 weeks: 14.5 to 24.5 g/dl
• infants ages 2 to 8 weeks: 12.5 to 20.5 g/dl
• infants ages 2 to 6 months: 10.7 to 17.3 g/dl
• infants ages 6 months to 1 year: 9.9 to 14.5 g/ dl
• children ages 1 to 6: 9.5 to 14.1 g/dl
• adult males: 14 to 17.4 g/dl
• adult females: 12 to 16 g/dl.

Abnormal findings
Low Hb concentration may indicate anemia, recent hemorrhage, or fluid retention, causing hemodilution.

Elevated Hb suggests hemoconcentration from polycythemia or dehydration.

Interfering factors
• Failure to use the proper anticoagulant or to adequately mix the sample and the anticoagulant
• Hemolysis due to rough handling of the sample
• Hemoconcentration due to prolonged tourniquet constriction

- Abnormal RBC size or drawing blood through a small-gauge needle
- Very high white blood cell counts, lipemia, or RBCs that are resistant to lysis (false-high)
- Dehydration (possible false-high)
- Hemodilution (possible false-low)

FETAL HEMOGLOBIN

Fetal hemoglobin (Hb), or Hb F, is a normal Hb produced in the red blood cells of a fetus and in smaller amounts in infants. It constitutes 50% to 90% of the Hb in a newborn; the remaining Hb consists of Hb A_1 and Hb A_2, the Hb in adults.

Under normal conditions, the body ceases to manufacture fetal Hb during the first years of life, and from that point on manufactures adult Hb. If this changeover doesn't occur and fetal Hb continues to constitute more than 5% of the Hb after age 6 months, an abnormality should be suspected, particularly thalassemia.

Purpose
- To diagnose thalassemia

Patient preparation
- Explain to the patient that this test is used to detect thalassemia disease.
- Tell him that a blood sample will be taken. Explain who will perform the venipuncture and when.
- Reassure him that drawing the sample will take less than 3 minutes.
- Explain that he may feel slight discomfort from the tourniquet pressure and the needle puncture.
- If the patient is a child, explain to his parents that a small amount of blood will be taken from the finger or earlobe.

- Inform the patient or his parents that food or fluids need not be restricted before the test.

Procedure and posttest care
- Perform a venipuncture and collect the sample of blood in a 15-ml *lavender-top* tube.
- For a young child, collect capillary blood in a microcollection device.
- If a hematoma develops at the venipuncture site, apply warm soaks.

Precautions
- Completely fill the collection tube, and invert it gently several times to mix the sample and the anticoagulant thoroughly.
- To avoid hemolysis, don't shake the tube vigorously.

Reference values
Normal values for fetal Hb range as follows:
- ages 0 to 30 days: 60% to 90%
- ages 1 to 23 months: 2%
- age 24 months to adult: 0% to 2%.

Abnormal findings
In beta-thalassemia major, fetal Hb may be 30% or more of the total Hb. Slight increases in fetal Hb concentration appear in a variety of unrelated hematologic disorders, such as aplastic anemia, homozygous sickle cell disease, and myeloproliferative disorders. Fetal Hb commonly increases to as much as 5% during normal pregnancy.

Interfering factors
- Hemolysis due to rough handling of the sample
- Delay in analyzing the specimen for more than 2 to 3 hours (possible false-high)

VARIATIONS OF HEMOGLOBIN TYPE AND DISTRIBUTION

HEMOGLOBIN	PERCENTAGE OF TOTAL HEMOGLOBIN	CLINICAL IMPLICATIONS
Hb A	95% to 100%	Normal
Hb A$_2$	4% to 5.8%	ß-thalassemia minor
	1.5% to 3%	Normal
	Under 1.5%	Hb H disease
Hb F	Under 2%	Normal
	2% to 5%	ß-thalassemia minor
	10% to 90%	ß-thalassemia major
	5% to 15%	ß-δ-thalassemia minor
	5% to 35%	Heterozygous hereditary persistence of fetal hemoglobin (HPFH)
	100%	Homozygous HPFH
	15%	Homozygous Hb S
Homozygous Hb S	70% to 98%	Sickle cell disease
Homozygous Hb C	90% to 98%	Hb C disease
Heterozygous Hb C	24% to 44%	Hb C trait

HEMOGLOBIN ELECTROPHORESIS

Hemoglobin (Hb) electrophoresis is probably the most useful laboratory method for separating and measuring normal and some abnormal Hb. Through electrophoresis, different types of Hb are separated to form a series of distinctly pigmented bands in a medium (cellulose acetate or starch gel). Results are then compared with those of a normal sample.

Hb A, A$_2$, S, C, and F are routinely checked, but the laboratory may change the medium or its pH to expand the range of this test.

Purpose
• To measure the amount of Hb A and to detect abnormal Hb
• To aid diagnosis of thalassemia
• To aid diagnosis of sickle cell disease or trait

Patient preparation
• Explain to the patient that this test is used to evaluate Hb.
• Tell him that a blood sample will be taken. Explain who will perform the venipuncture and when.
• Reassure him that drawing a blood sample will take less than 3 minutes.
• Explain that he may feel slight discomfort from the tourniquet pressure and the needle puncture.
• If the patient is an infant or child, explain to the parents that a small amount of blood will be taken from the finger or earlobe.
• Inform the patient that food or fluids need not be restricted before the test.

Procedure and posttest care
• Perform a venipuncture, and collect the sample in a 7-ml *lavender-top* tube.
• For very young children, collect capillary blood in a microcollection device.
• If a hematoma develops at the venipuncture site, apply warm soaks.

Precautions
• Completely fill the collection tube, and invert it gently several times to mix the sample and the anticoagulant. Do not shake the tube vigorously.
• Handle the sample gently to prevent hemolysis.

Reference values
In adults, Hb A accounts for 95% to 98% of all Hb; Hb A_2, 1.5% to 3%; and Hb F, less than 2%. In neonates, Hb F normally accounts for half the total. Hb S and Hb C are normally absent.

Abnormal findings
Hb electrophoresis allows identification of various types of Hb. Certain types may indicate a hemolytic disease. The chart on the opposite page shows some possible results and their associated conditions. (See *Variations of hemoglobin type and distribution*.)

Interfering factors
• Failure to fill the tube completely, to use the proper anticoagulant, or to adequately mix the sample and the anticoagulant
• Hemolysis due to rough handling of the sample
• Blood transfusion within the past 4 months

SICKLE CELL TEST

The sickle cell test, also known as the hemoglobin (Hb) S test, is used to detect sickle cells, which are severely deformed, rigid erythrocytes that may slow blood flow. Sickle cell trait (characterized by heterozygous Hb S) is found almost exclusively in people of African ancestry. It's present in nearly 8% of African Americans.

Although this test is useful as a rapid screening procedure, it may produce erroneous results. Hb electrophoresis should be performed to confirm the diagnosis if sickle cell disease is strongly suspected.

Purpose
• To identify sickle cell disease and sickle cell trait

Patient preparation
• Explain to the patient that this test is used to detect sickle cell disease.
• Tell him that a blood sample will be taken. Explain who will perform the venipuncture and when.
• Reassure him that drawing a blood sample will take less than 3 minutes.

• Explain that he may feel slight discomfort from the tourniquet pressure and the needle puncture.
• If the patient is an infant or child, explain to his parents that a small amount of blood will be taken from the finger or earlobe.
• Check the patient's history for a blood transfusion within the past 3 months.
• Inform him that food or fluids need not be restricted before the test.

Procedure and posttest care
• Perform a venipuncture, and collect the sample in a 7-ml *lavender-top* tube.
• For very young children, collect capillary blood in a microcollection device.
• If a hematoma develops at the venipuncture site, apply warm soaks.

Precautions
• Completely fill the collection tube and invert it gently several times to thoroughly mix the sample and the anticoagulant.
• Do not shake the tube vigorously.

Reference values
Results of this test are reported as positive or negative. A negative result suggests the absence of Hb S.

Abnormal findings
A positive result may indicate the presence of sickle cells, but Hb electrophoresis is needed to further diagnose the sickling tendency of cells. Rarely, in the absence of Hb S, other abnormal Hb may cause sickling.

Interfering factors
• Failure to fill the tube completely, to use the proper anticoagulant in the collection tube, or to adequately mix the sample and the anticoagulant
• Hemolysis due to rough handling of the sample

• Hb concentration < 10%, elevated Hb S levels in infants under age 6 months, or transfusion within 3 months of the test (possible false-negative)

UNSTABLE HEMOGLOBIN

Unstable hemoglobin (Hb) is a rare, congenital defect caused by amino acid substitutions in the structure of Hb. It's called "unstable" because of the ease with which the Hb decomposes. The presence of unstable Hb may lead to the formation of small masses called Heinz bodies, which accumulate on red blood cell membranes. Although Heinz bodies are usually removed by the spleen or liver, they may cause mild to severe hemolysis. Unstable Hb is best detected by precipitation tests (heat stability or isopropanol solubility).

Purpose
• To detect unstable Hb

Patient preparation
• Explain to the patient that this test is used to detect abnormal hemoglobin in the blood.
• Tell him that a blood sample will be taken. Explain who will perform the venipuncture and when.
• Reassure him that drawing a blood sample will take less than 3 minutes.
• Explain that he may feel slight discomfort from the tourniquet pressure and the needle puncture.
• As necessary, withhold antimalarials, furazolidone (from infants), nitrofurantoin, phenacetin, procarbazine, sulfonamides before the text because these drugs may induce hemolysis. If these medications must be continued, note this on the laboratory slip.

• Inform the patient that food or fluids need not be restricted before the test.

Procedure and posttest care
• Perform a venipuncture, and collect the sample in a 7-ml *lavender-top* tube.
• If a hematoma develops at the venipuncture site, apply warm soaks.
• Resume administration of medications withheld before the test.

Precautions
• Completely fill the collection tube, and invert it gently several times to mix the sample and the anticoagulant thoroughly.
• To avoid hemolysis, do not shake the tube vigorously.

Reference values
When no unstable Hb appears in the sample, the heat stability test result is negative; the isopropanol solubility test result is reported as stable.

Abnormal findings
A positive heat stability test result or unstable solubility test result, especially with hemolysis, strongly suggests the presence of unstable Hb.

Interfering factors
• Failure to fill the tube completely, to use the proper anticoagulant, or to adequately mix the sample and the anticoagulant
• Hemoconcentration due to prolonged tourniquet constriction
• Hemolysis due to rough handling of the sample
• Hemolysis due to antimalarials, furazolidone (in infants), nitrofurantoin, phenacetin, procarbazine, sulfonamides (possible false-positive or unstable results)
• High levels of Hb F (possible false-positive isopropanol)
• Recent blood transfusion

HEINZ BODIES

Heinz bodies are particles of decomposed hemoglobin that precipitate from the cytoplasm of red blood cells (RBCs) and accumulate on RBC membranes. Although Heinz bodies are removed from RBCs by the spleen, they're a major cause of hemolytic anemias.

Heinz bodies can be detected in a whole blood sample using phase microscopy or supravital stains; when they don't form spontaneously, various oxidant drugs may be added to the sample to induce their formation.

Purpose
• To help detect causes of hemolytic anemia

Patient preparation
• Explain to the patient that this test is used to determine the cause of anemia.
• Tell him that a blood sample will be taken. Explain who will perform the venipuncture and when.
• Reassure him that drawing a blood sample will take less than 3 minutes.
• Explain that he may feel slight discomfort from the tourniquet pressure and the needle puncture.
• Review the patient's drug history for medications that may affect test results. Withhold antimalarials, furazolidone, nitrofurantoin, phenacetin, procarbazine, and sulfonamides. If these medications must be continued, note this on the laboratory slip.
• Inform the patient that food or fluids need not be restricted before the test.

Procedure and posttest care
• Perform a venipuncture, collecting the sample in a 7-ml *lavender-top* tube.

● If a hematoma develops at the venipuncture site, apply warm soaks.
● Resume administration of medications withheld before the test.

Precautions
● Completely fill the sample collection tube and invert it gently several times to mix the sample and the anticoagulant; do not shake the tube vigorously.

Reference values
A negative test result indicates an absence of Heinz bodies.

Abnormal findings
The presence of Heinz bodies — a positive test result — may indicate an inherited RBC enzyme deficiency, the presence of unstable hemoglobin, thalassemia, or drug-induced RBC injury. Heinz bodies may also be present after splenectomy.

Interfering factors
● Failure to fill the collection tube completely, to use the appropriate anticoagulant, to adequately mix the sample and the anticoagulant, or to send the sample to the laboratory immediately
● Antimalarials, furazolidone (in infants), nitrofurantoin, phenacetin, procarbazine, sulfonamides (possible false-positive)
● Recent blood transfusion

IRON AND TOTAL IRONBINDING CAPACITY

Iron is essential to the formation and function of hemoglobin, as well as many other heme and nonheme compounds. After iron is absorbed by the intestine, it's distributed to various body compartments for synthesis, storage, and transport. Serum iron concentration is normally highest in the morning and declines progressively during the day; thus, the sample should be drawn in the morning.

An iron assay is used to measure the amount of iron bound to transferrin in blood plasma. Total iron-binding capacity (TIBC) measures the amount of iron that would appear in plasma if all the transferrin were saturated with iron.

Serum iron and TIBC are of greater diagnostic usefulness when performed with the serum ferritin assay, but together these tests may not accurately reflect the state of other iron compartments, such as myoglobin iron and the labile iron pool. Bone marrow or liver biopsy, and iron absorption or excretion studies may yield more information.

Purpose
● To estimate total iron storage
● To aid diagnosis of hemochromatosis
● To help distinguish iron deficiency anemia from anemia of chronic disease (For information on another test used to differentiate anemias, see *Siderocyte stain*.)
● To help evaluate nutritional status

Patient preparation
● Explain to the patient that this test evaluates the body's capacity to store iron.
● Tell him that a blood sample will be taken. Explain who will perform the venipuncture and when.
● Reassure him that drawing a blood sample will take less than 3 minutes.
● Explain that he may feel slight discomfort from the tourniquet pressure and the needle puncture.
● Review the patient's drug history for medications that may interfere with test results; withhold chloramphenicol, corticotropin, iron supplements, and

SIDEROCYTE STAIN

Siderocytes are red blood cells (RBCs) containing particles of non-hemoglobin iron known as siderocytic granules. In newborn infants, siderocytic granules are normally present in normoblasts and reticulocytes during hemoglobin synthesis. However, the spleen removes most of these granules from normal RBCs, and they disappear rapidly with age.

In adults, an elevated siderocyte level usually indicates abnormal erythropoiesis, which may occur in congenital spherocytic anemia, chronic hemolytic anemias (such as the thalassemias), pernicious anemia, hemochromatosis, toxicities (such as lead poisoning), infection, or severe burns. Elevated levels may also follow splenectomy because the spleen normally removes siderocytic granules.

Performing the test

The siderocyte stain test measures the number of circulating siderocytes. Venous blood is drawn into a 7-ml *lavender-top* tube or, for infants and children, collected in a Microtainer or a pipette and smeared directly on a 3″ × 1″ glass slide. When the blood smear is stained, siderocytic granules appear as purple-blue specks clustered around the periphery of mature erythrocytes. Cells containing these granules are counted as a percentage of total RBCs. The results aid differential diagnosis of the anemias and hemochromatosis and help detect toxicities.

Interpreting results

Normally, newborn infants have a slightly elevated siderocyte level that reaches the normal adult value of 0.5% of total RBCs in 7 to 10 days. In patients with pernicious anemia, the siderocyte level is 8% to 14%; in chronic hemolytic anemia, 20% to 100%; in lead poisoning, 10% to 30%; and in hemochromatosis, 3% to 7%. A high siderocyte level calls for additional testing (including bone marrow examination) to determine the cause of abnormal erythropoiesis.

---

oral contraceptives. If such medications must be continued, note this on the laboratory slip.
• Inform the patient that food or fluids need not be restricted before the test.

Procedure and posttest care

• Perform a venipuncture, collecting the sample in a 7-ml *red-top* tube.
• If a hematoma develops at the venipuncture site, apply warm soaks.
• Resume administration of medications withheld before the test.

Precautions

• Handle the sample gently to prevent hemolysis; send it to the laboratory immediately.

Reference values

Normal serum iron and TIBC values are as follows:
• *serum iron*
– Males: 50 to 150 µg/dl
– Females: 35 to 145 µg/dl
• *TIBC*
– Males and females: 250 to 400 µg/dl
• *saturation*
– Males and females: 14% to 50%

Abnormal findings

In iron deficiency, serum iron levels decrease and TIBC increases, decreasing saturation. In cases of chronic inflammation (such as in rheumatoid arthritis), serum iron may be low in the presence of adequate body stores, but TIBC may remain unchanged or may decrease to preserve normal saturation. Iron overload may not alter serum levels until relatively late but, in general, serum iron increases and TIBC remains the same, which increases the saturation.

Interfering factors

• Hemolysis due to rough handling of the sample or failure to send the sample to the laboratory immediately
• Chloramphenicol and oral contraceptives (possible false-positive)
• Corticotropin (possible false-negative)
• Iron supplements (possible false-positive serum iron values but false-negative TIBC)

FERRITIN

Ferritin, a major iron-storage protein, normally appears in small quantities in serum. In healthy adults, serum ferritin levels are directly related to the amount of available iron stored in the body and can be measured accurately by radioimmunoassay.

Purpose

• To screen for iron deficiency and iron overload
• To measure iron storage
• To distinguish between iron deficiency (a condition of low iron storage)

and chronic inflammation (a condition of normal storage)

Patient preparation

• Explain to the patient that this test is used to assess the available iron stored in the body.
• Tell him that a blood sample will be taken. Explain who will perform the venipuncture and when.
• Reassure him that drawing a blood sample will take less than 3 minutes.
• Explain that he may feel slight discomfort from the tourniquet pressure and the needle puncture.
• Review the patient's history for transfusion within the past 4 months.
• Inform the patient that food or fluids need not be restricted before the test.

Procedure and posttest care

• Perform a venipuncture, collecting the sample in a 10-ml *red-top* tube.
• If a hematoma develops at the venipuncture site, apply warm soaks.

Reference values

Normal serum ferritin values vary with age, as follows:
• neonates: 25 to 200 μg/ml
• infants up to age 1 month: 200 to 600 μg/ml
• infants ages 2 to 5 months: 50 to 200 μg/ml
• children ages 6 months to 15 years: 7 to 142 μg/ml
• adult males: 20 to 300 μg/ml
• adult females: 20 to 120 μg/ml.

Abnormal findings

High serum ferritin levels may indicate acute or chronic hepatic disease, iron overload, leukemia, acute or chronic infection or inflammation, Hodgkin's disease, or chronic hemolytic anemias. In these disorders, iron stores in the bone marrow may be normal or significantly increased. Serum ferritin levels are characteristically normal or slightly elevated in patients with chronic renal disease.

Low serum ferritin levels indicate chronic iron deficiency.

Interfering factor
• Recent blood transfusion (possible false-high)

METHEMOGLOBIN

Methemoglobin (MetHb, Hb M) is a structural hemoglobin (Hb) variant, which is formed when the heme portion of deoxygenated Hb is oxidized to a ferric state. When this occurs, the heme is incapable of combining with oxygen and transporting it to the tissues, and the patient becomes cyanotic.

Purpose
• To detect acquired methemoglobinemia, which is caused by excessive radiation or the toxic effects of chemicals or drugs
• To detect congenital methemoglobinemia

Patient preparation
• Obtain a history of the patient's hematologic status and hemoglobin disorder, conditions that produce nitrite, plus exposure to sources of nitrites in drugs.
• Explain to the patient that this test is used to detect abnormal Hb in the blood.
• Tell him that a blood sample will be taken. Explain who will perform the venipuncture and when.
• Reassure him that drawing a blood sample will take less than 3 minutes.

• Explain that he may feel slight discomfort from the tourniquet pressure and the needle puncture.
• Tell the patient to avoid medications that can interfere with test results.

Procedure and posttest care
• Perform a venipuncture, and collect sample in a 7-ml *green-top* tube.
• If a hematoma develops at the venipuncture site, apply warm soaks.

Precautions
• Completely fill the collection tube, and invert it gently several times.
• To avoid hemolysis, do not shake the tube vigorously.
• Place the collection tube on ice and send it to the laboratory immediately.

Reference values
Normal Met Hb levels are 0% to 1.5% of total Hb.

Abnormal findings
Increased MetHb levels may indicate acquired or hereditary methemoglobinemia, or carbon monoxide poisoning. These levels can also be caused by use of certain drugs or exposure to certain substances.

Decreased MetHb levels may occur in pancreatitis.

Interfering factors
• Acetanilid, aniline dyes, nitroglycerin, benzocaine, chlorates, lidocaine, nitrates, nitrites, phenacetin, sulfonamides, radiation, primaquine, and resorcinol (possible increase)
• Nitrite toxicity in breast-feeding infants as (increase due to conversion of inorganic nitrate to nitrite ion)

WHITE BLOOD CELLS

WHITE BLOOD CELL COUNT

A white blood cell (WBC) count, also called a leukocyte count, is part of a complete blood count. It indicates the number of white cells in a microliter (μl, or cubic millimeter) of whole blood.

WBC counts may vary by as much as 2,000 on any given day, due to strenuous exercise, stress, or digestion. The WBC count may increase or decrease significantly in certain diseases, but is diagnostically useful only when the patient's white cell differential and clinical status are considered.

Purpose
- To determine infection or inflammation
- To determine the need for further tests, such as the WBC differential or bone marrow biopsy
- To monitor response to chemotherapy or radiation therapy

Patient preparation
- Explain to the patient that the test is used to detect an infection or inflammation.
- Tell him that a blood sample will be taken. Explain who will perform the venipuncture and when.
- Reassure him that drawing a blood sample will take less than 3 minutes.
- Explain that he may feel slight discomfort from the tourniquet pressure and the needle puncture.

- Inform the patient that he should avoid strenuous exercise for 24 hours before the test. Also tell him that he should avoid ingesting a heavy meal before the test.
- If the patient is being treated for an infection, advise him that this test will be repeated to monitor his progress.
- Review the patient's medication history for drugs that may affect test results, including antineoplastics, anti-infectives, anticonvulsants, thyroid hormone antagonists, and nonsteroidal anti-inflammatory drugs (NSAIDs). Note the use of such medications on the laboratory slip.

Procedure and posttest care
- Perform a venipuncture, and collect the sample in a 7-ml *lavender-top* tube.
- If a hematoma develops at the venipuncture site, apply warm soaks.
- Tell the patient that he may resume normal activity that was discontinued before the test.
- A patient with severe leukopenia may have little or no resistance to infection and requires protective isolation.

Precautions
- Completely fill the sample collection tube, and invert it gently several times to mix the sample and the anticoagulant.

Reference values
The WBC count ranges from 4,000 to 10,000/μl.

Abnormal findings
An elevated WBC count (leukocytosis) often signals infection, such as an abscess, meningitis, appendicitis, or tonsillitis. A high count may also result from leukemia and tissue necrosis due to burns, myocardial infarction, or gangrene.

A low WBC count (leukopenia) indicates bone marrow depression that may result from viral infections or from toxic reactions, such as those following treatment with antineoplastics, ingestion of mercury or other heavy metals, or exposure to benzene or arsenicals. Leukopenia characteristically accompanies influenza, typhoid fever, measles, infectious hepatitis, mononucleosis, and rubella.

Interfering factors
- Hemolysis due to rough handling of the sample
- Exercise, stress, or digestion
- Most antineoplastics; anti-infectives, such as metronidazole and flucytosine; anticonvulsants, such as phenytoin derivatives; thyroid hormone antagonists; and NSAIDs such as indomethacin (decrease)

White blood cell differential

The white blood cell (WBC) differential is used to evaluate the distribution and morphology of WBCs, providing more specific information about a patient's immune system than the WBC count alone.

WBCs are classified as one of five major types of leukocytes — neutrophils, eosinophils, basophils, lymphocytes, and monocytes — and the percentage of each type is determined. The differential count is the percentage of each type of WBC in the blood. The total number of each type of WBC is obtained by multiplying the percentage of each type by the total WBC count.

High levels of these leukocytes are associated with various allergic diseases and reactions to parasites. An eosinophil count is sometimes ordered as a follow-up test when an elevated or depressed eosinophil level is reported. (See *Interpreting WBC differential values,* page 104, and *Influence of disease on blood cell count,* pages 105 and 106.)

Purpose
- To evaluate the body's capacity to resist and overcome infection
- To detect and identify various types of leukemia
- To determine the stage and severity of an infection
- To detect allergic reactions
- To assess the severity of allergic reactions (eosinophil count)
- To detect parasitic infections

Patient preparation
- Explain to the patient that this test is used to evaluate the immune system.
- Review the patient's history for use of medications that may interfere with test results, including methysergide, desipramine, indomethacin, procainamide, anticonvulsants, capreomycin, cephalosporins, D-penicillamine, gold compounds, isoniazid, nalidixic acid, novobiocin, para-aminosalicylic acid, paromomycin, penicillins, phenothiazines, rifampin, streptomycin, sulfonamides, and tetracyclines. If these medications must be continued, note this on the laboratory slip.
- Tell the patient that a blood sample will be taken. Explain who will perform the venipuncture and when.
- Inform the patient that he needn't restrict food or fluids but should refrain from strenuous exercise for 24 hours before the test.

(Text continues on page 106.)

INTERPRETING WBC DIFFERENTIAL VALUES

The differential count measures the types of white blood cells (WBCs) as a percentage of the total WBC count (the relative value). The absolute value is obtained by multiplying the relative value of each cell type by the total WBC count. Both the relative and absolute values must be considered to obtain an accurate diagnosis.

For example, consider a patient whose WBC count is 6,000/µl and whose differential shows 30% neutrophils and 70% lymphocytes. His relative lymphocyte count seems to be quite high (lymphocytosis), but when this figure is multiplied by his WBC count (6,000 x 70% = 4,200 lymphocytes/µl), it's well within the normal range.

However, this patient's neutrophil count (30%) is low; when this figure is multiplied by the WBC count (6,000 x 30% = 1,800 neutrophils/µl), the result is a low absolute number, which may mean depressed bone marrow.

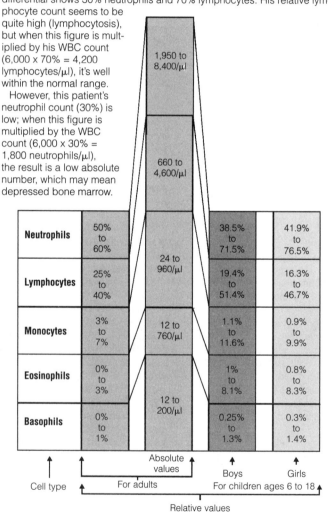

Cell type	For adults	Absolute values	For children ages 6 to 18 Boys	For children ages 6 to 18 Girls
Neutrophils	50% to 60%	1,950 to 8,400/µl	38.5% to 71.5%	41.9% to 76.5%
Lymphocytes	25% to 40%	660 to 4,600/µl	19.4% to 51.4%	16.3% to 46.7%
Monocytes	3% to 7%	24 to 960/µl	1.1% to 11.6%	0.9% to 9.9%
Eosinophils	0% to 3%	12 to 760/µl	1% to 8.1%	0.8% to 8.3%
Basophils	0% to 1%	12 to 200/µl	0.25% to 1.3%	0.3% to 1.4%

Relative values

INFLUENCE OF DISEASE ON BLOOD CELL COUNT

CELL TYPE	HOW AFFECTED

Neutrophils

Increased by:
- infections: osteomyelitis, otitis media, salpingitis, septicemia, gonorrhea, endocarditis, smallpox, chickenpox, herpes, Rocky Mountain spotted fever
- ischemic necrosis due to myocardial infarction, burns, carcinoma
- metabolic disorders: diabetic acidosis, eclampsia, uremia, thyrotoxicosis
- stress response due to acute hemorrhage, surgery, excessive exercise, emotional distress, third trimester of pregnancy, childbirth
- inflammatory disease: rheumatic fever, rheumatoid arthritis, acute gout, vasculitis and myositis.

Decreased by:
- bone marrow depression due to radiation or cytotoxic drugs
- infections: typhoid, tularemia, brucellosis, hepatitis, influenza, measles, mumps, rubella, infectious mononucleosis
- hypersplenism: hepatic disease and storage diseases
- collagen vascular disease, such as systemic lupus erythematosus
- deficiency of folic acid or vitamin B_{12}.

Eosinophils

Increased by:
- allergic disorders: asthma, hay fever, food or drug sensitivity, serum sickness, angioneurotic edema
- parasitic infections: trichinosis, hookworm, roundworm, amebiasis
- skin diseases: eczema, pemphigus, psoriasis, dermatitis, herpes
- neoplastic diseases: chronic myelocytic leukemia, Hodgkin's disease, metastases and necrosis of solid tumors
- miscellaneous: collagen vascular disease, adrenocortical hypofunction, ulcerative colitis, polyarteritis nodosa, post-splenectomy, pernicious anemia, scarlet fever, excessive exercise, sickle cell disease.

Decreased by:
- stress response due to trauma, shock, burns, surgery, mental distress
- Cushing's syndrome, infectious mononucleosis.

Basophils

Increased by:
- chronic myelocytic leukemia, polycythemia vera, some chronic hemolytic anemias, Hodgkin's disease, systemic mastocytosis, myxedema, ulcerative colitis, chronic hypersensitivity states, nephrosis.

Decreased by:
- hyperthyroidism
- ovulation, pregnancy
- stress.

(continued)

Iɴꜰʟᴜᴇɴᴄᴇ ᴏꜰ ᴅɪsᴇᴀsᴇ ᴏɴ ʙʟᴏᴏᴅ ᴄᴇʟʟ ᴄᴏᴜɴᴛ *(continued)*

CELL TYPE	HOW AFFECTED
Lymphocytes	*Increased by:* • infections: pertussis, brucellosis, syphilis, tuberculosis, hepatitis, infectious mononucleosis, mumps, rubella, cytomegalovirus • thyrotoxicosis, hypoadrenalism, ulcerative colitis, immune diseases, lymphocytic leukemia, Addison's disease. *Decreased by:* • severe debilitating illness, such as heart failure, renal failure, and advanced tuberculosis • defective lymphatic circulation, high levels of adrenal corticosteroids, immunodeficiency due to immunosuppressives.
Monocytes	*Increased by:* • infections: subacute bacterial endocarditis, tuberculosis, hepatitis, malaria, Rocky Mountain spotted fever • collagen vascular disease: systemic lupus erythematosus, rheumatoid arthritis, polyarteritis nodosa • carcinomas • monocytic leukemia • lymphomas. *Decreased by:* • hairy cell leukemia • HIV infection • rheumatoid arthritis • prednisone therapy.

• Reassure the patient that drawing a blood sample will take less than 3 minutes.

• Explain that he may feel slight discomfort from the tourniquet pressure and the needle puncture.

Procedure and posttest care
• Perform a venipuncture, collecting the sample in a 7-ml *lavender-top* tube.
• If a hematoma develops at the venipuncture site, apply warm soaks.

Precautions
• Completely fill the collection tube; invert it gently several times to thoroughly mix the sample and the anticoagulant; to prevent hemolysis, do not shake the tube.

Reference values
For normal values for the five types of WBCs classified in the differential for adults and children, see the chart on page 104. For an accurate diagnosis, differential test results must always be interpreted in relation to the total WBC count.

Abnormal findings
Abnormal differential patterns provide evidence for a wide range of disease states and other conditions.

Interfering factors
• Failure to completely fill the collection tube, to use the proper anticoagulant, or to adequately mix the sample and the anticoagulant

- Hemolysis due to rough handling of the sample
- Methysergide, desipramine, indomethacin, procainamide, anticonvulsants, capreomycin, cephalosporins, D-penicillamine, gold compounds, isoniazid, nalidixic acid, novobiocin, para-aminosalicylic acid, paromomycin, penicillins, phenothiazines, rifampin, streptomycin, sulfonamides, and tetracyclines

PLATELET ACTIVITY

BLEEDING TIME

Bleeding time is used to measure the duration of bleeding after a measured skin incision. Bleeding time may be measured by one of three methods: template, Ivy, or Duke. The template method is the most commonly used and the most accurate because the incision size is standardized. Bleeding time depends on the elasticity of the blood vessel wall and on the number and functional capacity of platelets.

Although this test is usually performed on patients with a personal or family history of bleeding disorders, it's also useful — along with a platelet count — for preoperative screening. The test is usually not recommended for patients with a platelet count of less than 75,000/µl.

Purpose
- To assess overall hemostatic function (platelet response to injury and functional capacity of vasoconstriction)
- To detect congenital and acquired platelet function disorders

Patient preparation
- Explain to the patient this test is used to measure the time required to form a clot and stop bleeding.
- Tell him who will perform the test and when it will take place.
- Inform him that he need not restrict food or fluids before the test.
- Reassure the patient that, although he may feel some discomfort from the incisions, the antiseptic, and the tightness of the blood pressure cuff, the test takes only 10 to 20 minutes to perform. Advise the patient that the incisions will leave two small, hairline scars that should be barely visible when healed.
- Check the patient's history for recent use of drugs that prolong bleeding time, including sulfonamides, thiazide diuretics, antineoplastics, anticoagulants, nonsteroidal anti-inflammatory drugs, aspirin and aspirin compounds, and some nonnarcotic analgesics. If the patient has taken such drugs, check with the laboratory for special instructions. If the test is being used to identify a suspected bleeding disorder, it should be postponed and the drugs discontinued. If the test is being used preoperatively to assess hemostatic function, it should proceed as scheduled.

Equipment
Blood pressure cuff, disposable lancet, template with 9-mm slits (template method), 70% alcohol or povidone-iodine solution, filter paper, small pressure bandage, stopwatch

Procedure and posttest care
- Template method: Wrap the pressure cuff around the upper arm and inflate the cuff to 40 mm Hg. Select an area on the forearm with no superficial veins, and clean it with antiseptic. Allow the skin to dry completely before making the incision. Apply the appropriate template lengthwise to the fore-

arm. Use the lancet to make two incisions, 1 mm deep and 9 mm long. Start the stopwatch. Without touching the cuts, gently blot the drops of blood with filter paper every 30 seconds, until the bleeding stops in both cuts. Average the time of the two cuts, and record the result.

• Ivy method: After applying the pressure cuff and preparing the test site, make three small punctures with a disposable lancet. Start the stopwatch immediately. Taking care not to touch the punctures, blot each site with filter paper every 30 seconds, until the bleeding stops. Average the bleeding time of the three punctures, and record the result.

• Duke method: Drape the patient's shoulder with a towel. Clean the earlobe, and let the skin air-dry. Then make a puncture wound 2 to 4 mm deep on the earlobe with a disposable lancet. Start the stopwatch. Being careful not to touch the ear, blot the site with filter paper every 30 seconds, until bleeding stops. Record bleeding time.

• In a patient with a bleeding tendency (hemophilia, for example), maintain a pressure bandage over the incision for 24 to 48 hours to prevent further bleeding; check the test area frequently; keep the edges of the cuts aligned to minimize scarring.

• In other patients, a piece of gauze held in place by an adhesive bandage is sufficient.

• Resume administration of medications discontinued before the test.

Precautions
• Be sure to maintain a cuff pressure of 40 mm Hg throughout the test.
• If the bleeding does not diminish after 15 minutes, discontinue the test.

Reference values
The normal range of bleeding time is from 3 to 6 minutes in the template method; from 3 to 6 minutes in the Ivy method; and from 1 to 3 minutes in the Duke method.

Abnormal findings
Prolonged bleeding time may indicate the presence of disorders associated with thrombocytopenia, such as Hodgkin's disease, acute leukemia, disseminated intravascular coagulation, hemolytic disease of the newborn, Schönlein-Henoch purpura, severe hepatic disease (cirrhosis, for example), or severe deficiency of factors I, II, V, VII, VIII, IX, and XI. Prolonged bleeding time in a person with a normal platelet count suggests a platelet function disorder (thrombasthenia, thrombocytopathia) and requires further investigation with clot retraction, prothrombin consumption, and platelet aggregation tests.

Interfering factors
• Sulfonamides, thiazide diuretics, antineoplastics, anticoagulants, nonsteroidal anti-inflammatory drugs, aspirin and aspirin compounds, and some nonnarcotic analgesics (prolonged bleeding time)

PLATELET COUNT

Platelets, or thrombocytes, are the smallest formed elements in blood. They promote coagulation and the formation of a hemostatic plug in vascular injury.

Platelet count is one of the most important screening tests of platelet function. Accurate counts are vital.

Purpose
- To evaluate platelet production
- To assess effects of chemotherapy or radiation therapy on platelet production
- To diagnose and monitor severe thrombocytosis or thrombocytopenia
- To confirm a visual estimate of platelet number and morphology from a stained blood film

Patient preparation
- Explain to the patient that this test is used to determine if the patient's blood clots normally.
- Tell him that a blood sample will be taken. Explain who will perform the venipuncture and when.
- Inform the patient that food or fluids need not be restricted before the test.
- Reassure the patient that drawing a blood sample will take less than 3 minutes.
- Explain that he may feel slight discomfort from the tourniquet pressure and the needle puncture.
- Check the patient's history for use of medications that may affect test results, including acetazolamide, acetohexamide, antineoplastics, brompheniramine maleate, carbamazepine, chloramphenicol, ethacrynic acid, furosemide, gold salts, hydroxychloroquine, indomethacin, isoniazid, mephenytoin, mefenamic acid, methazolamide, methimazole, methyldopa, oral diazoxide, oxyphenbutazone, penicillamine, penicillin, phenylbutazone, phenytoin, pyrimethamine, quinidine sulfate, quinine, salicylates, streptomycin, sulfonamides, thiazide and thiazide-like diuretics, and tricyclic antidepressants. Check also for heparin, which causes transient, reversible thrombocytopenia. Notify the laboratory if such drugs have been used.

Procedure and posttest care
- Perform a venipuncture and collect the sample in a 7-ml *lavender-top* tube.
- If a hematoma develops at the venipuncture site, apply warm soaks.

Precautions
- To prevent hemolysis, avoid excessive probing at the venipuncture site and handle the sample gently.
- Completely fill the collection tube, and invert it gently several times to mix the sample and the anticoagulant thoroughly.

Reference values
Normal platelet counts range from 140,000 to 400,000/μl.

Abnormal findings
A decreased platelet count (thrombocytopenia) can result from aplastic or hypoplastic bone marrow; infiltrative bone marrow disease, such as carcinoma, leukemia, or disseminated infection; megakaryocytic hypoplasia; ineffective thrombopoiesis due to folic acid or vitamin B_{12} deficiency; pooling of platelets in an enlarged spleen; increased platelet destruction due to drugs or immune disorders; disseminated intravascular coagulation; Bernard-Soulier syndrome; or mechanical injury to platelets.

A platelet count that falls below 50,000/μl can cause spontaneous bleeding. When it drops below 5,000, fatal central nervous system bleeding or massive GI hemorrhage is possible.

An increased platelet count (thrombocytosis) can result from hemorrhage, infectious disorders, malignant disease, iron deficiency anemia, recent surgery, pregnancy, splenectomy, or inflammatory disorders such as collagen vascular disease. In such cases, the platelet count returns to normal after the patient recovers from the primary disorder. However, the count remains elevated in primary thrombocythemia, myelofibrosis with myeloid metaplasia, polycythemia vera, and chronic myelogenous leukemia.

When the platelet count is abnormal, diagnosis usually requires further studies, such as complete blood count, bone marrow biopsy, direct antiglobulin test (direct Coombs' test), and serum protein electrophoresis.

Interfering factors
• Failure to use the proper anticoagulant, or to mix the sample and anticoagulant promptly and adequately
• Hemolysis due to rough handling of the sample or excessive probing at the venipuncture site
• Heparin (decrease)
• Acetazolamide, acetohexamide, antineoplastics, brompheniramine maleate, carbamazepine, chloramphenicol, ethacrynic acid, furosemide, gold salts, hydroxychloroquine, indomethacin, isoniazid, mephenytoin, mefenamic acid, methazolamide, methimazole, methyldopa, oral diazoxide, oxyphenbutazone, penicillamine, penicillin, phenylbutazone, phenytoin, pyrimethamine, quinidine sulfate, quinine, salicylates, streptomycin, sulfonamides, thiazide and thiazide-like diuretics, and tricyclic antidepressants (possible decrease)
• High altitudes, persistent cold temperatures, strenuous exercise, or excitement (increase)
• Menstruation (possible decrease just before onset)
• Testing delayed more than 3 hours after sample collection
• White blood cell count > 100,000/μl

CAPILLARY FRAGILITY

Also called the tourniquet test, the capillary fragility test is a nonspecific method for evaluating bleeding tendencies. A positive-pressure test, used to measure the capillaries' ability to remain intact under increased intracapillary pressure, is controlled by a blood pressure cuff around the patient's upper arm.

Purpose
• To assess the fragility of capillary walls
• To identify a platelet deficiency (thrombocytopenia)

Patient preparation
• Explain to the patient that this test is used to identify abnormal bleeding tendencies.
• Tell him who will perform the procedure and when.
• Inform him that food or fluids need not be restricted.
• Explain that he may feel discomfort from the pressure of the blood pressure cuff.

Procedure and posttest care
• The patient's skin temperature and the room temperature should be normal to ensure accurate results.
• Select and mark a 2″ (5-cm) space on the patient's forearm. Ideally, the site should be free of petechiae; otherwise, record the number of petechiae present on the site before starting the test.
• Fasten the cuff around the arm, and raise the pressure to a point midway between the systolic and diastolic blood pressures (approximately 100 mm Hg). Maintain this pressure for 5 minutes; then release the cuff.

- Count the number of petechiae that appear in the 2″ space.
- Record test results.
- Encourage the patient to open and close his hand a few times to hasten return of blood to the forearm.

Precautions
- Do not repeat this test on the same arm within 1 week.
- This test is contraindicated in patients with disseminated intravascular coagulation (DIC) or other bleeding disorders, and in those with significant petechiae already present.

Reference values
A few petechiae may normally be present before the test. Less than 10 petechiae on the forearm 5 minutes after the test is considered normal, or negative; more than 10 petechiae is considered a positive result. The following scale may also be used to report test results.

NUMBER OF PETECHIAE/5 CM	SCORE
A few on anterior forearm	1+
Many on anterior forearm	2+
Many on whole arm and top of hand	3+
Confluent petechiae on all areas of arm and top of hand	4+

Abnormal findings
A positive finding (more than 10 petechiae, or a score of 2+ to 4+) indicates weakness of the capillary walls (vascular purpura) or a platelet defect. It may occur in such conditions as thrombocytopenia, thrombasthenia, purpura senilis, scurvy, DIC, von

Willebrand's disease, vitamin K deficiency, dysproteinemia, and polycythemia vera and in severe deficiencies of factor VII, fibrinogen, or prothrombin. Conditions unrelated to bleeding defects, such as scarlet fever, measles, influenza, chronic renal disease, hypertension, and diabetes with coexistent vascular disease, may also increase capillary fragility. An abnormal number of petechiae sometimes appear before menstruation and at other times in some healthy persons, especially in women over age 40.

Interfering factors
- Decreasing estrogen levels in postmenopausal women (possible increase)
- Glucocorticoids (possible decrease)
- Repeating the test on the same arm within 1 week, causing errors in counting the number of petechiae
- Overinflation or underinflation of the cuff

PLATELET AGGREGATION

After vascular injury, platelets gather at the injury site and clump together to form an aggregate or plug that helps maintain hemostasis and promotes healing. The platelet aggregation test, an in vitro procedure, is used to measure the rate at which the platelets in a plasma sample form a clump after the addition of an aggregating reagent.

Purpose
- To assess platelet aggregation
- To detect congenital and acquired platelet bleeding disorders

Patient preparation
• Explain to the patient that this test is used to determine if blood clots properly.
• Tell him that the test requires a blood sample. Explain who will perform the venipuncture and when.
• Reassure him that drawing a blood sample will take less than 3 minutes.
• Explain that he may feel slight discomfort from the tourniquet pressure and the needle puncture.
• Instruct the patient to fast or to maintain a nonfat diet for 8 hours before the test, because lipemia can affect the test results.
• Withhold aspirin and aspirin compounds for 14 days, and phenylbutazone, sulfinpyrazone, phenothiazines, antihistamines, tricyclic antidepressants, and anti-inflammatory drugs for 48 hours. If these medications must be continued, note this on the laboratory slip.

Procedure and posttest care
• Perform a venipuncture, and collect the sample in a 7-ml *blue-top* siliconized tube.
• Completely fill the collection tube, and invert it gently several times to mix the sample and the anticoagulant thoroughly.
• Maintain the sample at 71.6° F (22° C) to 98.6° F (37°C) to prevent aggregation.
• Apply pressure to the venipuncture site for 5 minutes, or until bleeding stops.
• Resume diet and administration of medications withheld before the test.
• If a hematoma develops at the venipuncture site, apply warm soaks.

Precautions
• Because the list of medications known to alter the results of this test is long and continually growing, the patient should be as free of drugs as possible before the test.
• If the patient has taken aspirin within the past 14 days and the test cannot be postponed, ask the laboratory to verify the presence of aspirin in the plasma. If test results are abnormal for such a sample, the use of aspirin must be discontinued and the test repeated in 2 weeks.
• Avoid excessive probing at the venipuncture site.
• Remove the tourniquet promptly to avoid bruising.
• Handle the sample gently to prevent hemolysis.

Reference values
Normal aggregation occurs in 3 to 5 minutes, but findings are temperature-dependent and vary with the laboratory. Aggregation curves obtained by using different reagents help to distinguish various qualitative platelet defects.

Abnormal findings
Abnormal findings may indicate von Willebrand's disease, Bernard-Soulier syndrome, storage pool disease, Glanzmann's thrombasthenia, or polycythemia vera.

Interfering factors
• Failure to observe pretest restrictions
• Failure to use the proper anticoagulant or to adequately mix the sample and the anticoagulant
• Hemolysis due to rough handling of the sample or to excessive probing at the venipuncture site
• Aspirin and aspirin compounds, phenylbutazone, sulfinpyrazone, phenothiazines, anti-inflammatory drugs, antihistamines, and tricyclic antidepressants (decrease)

COAGULATION

ACTIVATED PARTIAL THROMBOPLASTIN TIME

The activated partial thromboplastin time (APTT) is used to evaluate all the clotting factors of the intrinsic pathway — except platelets — by measuring the time required for formation of a fibrin clot after the addition of calcium and phospholipid emulsion to a plasma sample. An activator, such as kaolin, is used to shorten clotting time.

Purpose
● To aid preoperative screening for bleeding tendencies
● To screen for congenital coagulation deficiencies of the clotting factors
● To monitor heparin therapy

Patient preparation
● Explain to the patient that this test is used to determine if blood clots normally.
● Tell him that a blood sample will be taken. Explain who will perform the venipuncture and when.
● Reassure him that drawing a blood sample will take less than 3 minutes.
● Explain that he may feel slight discomfort from the tourniquet pressure and the needle puncture.
● When appropriate, tell the patient receiving heparin therapy that this test may be repeated at regular intervals to assess the response to treatment.
● Inform the patient that food or fluids need not be restricted before the test.

Procedure and posttest care
● Perform a venipuncture, and collect the sample in a 7-ml *blue-top* tube.
● If a hematoma develops at the venipuncture site, apply warm soaks.

Precautions
● Completely fill the collection tube, invert it gently several times, and send it to the laboratory on ice.
● To prevent hemolysis, avoid excessive probing at the venipuncture site and handle the sample gently.
● For a patient on anticoagulant therapy, additional pressure may be needed at the venipuncture site to control bleeding.

Reference values
Normally, a fibrin clot forms 21 to 35 seconds after addition of reagents. For a patient on anticoagulant therapy, ask the attending doctor to specify the reference values for the therapy being delivered.

Abnormal findings
Prolonged APTT may indicate a deficiency of certain plasma clotting factors, the presence of heparin, or the presence of fibrin split products, fibrinolysins, or circulating anticoagulants that are antibodies to specific clotting factors.

Interfering factors
● Failure to fill the collection tube completely, to use the proper anticoagulant, or to adequately mix the sample and the anticoagulant
● Hemolysis due to rough handling of the sample or to excessive probing at the venipuncture site

• Failure to send the sample to the laboratory immediately or to place it on ice

PROTHROMBIN TIME

Prothrombin time (PT) measures the time required for a fibrin clot to form in a citrated plasma sample after addition of calcium ions and tissue thromboplastin (factor III).

Purpose
• To provide an overall evaluation of extrinsic coagulation factors V, VII, and X and of prothrombin and fibrinogen
• To monitor response to oral anticoagulant therapy

Patient preparation
• Explain to the patient that this test is used to determine if the blood clots normally.
• Check the patient's history for use of medications that may affect test results, including antihistamines, chloral hydrate, corticosteroids, digitalis glycosides, diuretics, glutethimide, griseofulvin, progestin-estrogen combinations, pyrazinamide, vitamin K, and xanthines. Notify the laboratory if such drugs have been used.
• Tell the patient that a blood sample will be taken. Explain who will perform the venipuncture and when.
• Reassure him that drawing a blood sample will take less than 3 minutes.
• Explain that he may feel slight discomfort from the tourniquet pressure and the needle puncture.
• When appropriate, explain that this test is used to monitor the effects of oral anticoagulants; the test will be performed daily when therapy begins

and will be repeated at longer intervals when medication levels stabilize.
• Inform the patient that food or fluids need not be restricted before the test.

Procedure and posttest care
• Perform a venipuncture, and collect the sample in a 7-ml *blue-top* tube.
• If a hematoma develops at the venipuncture site, apply warm soaks.

Precautions
• Completely fill the collection tube, and invert it gently several times to mix the sample and the anticoagulant thoroughly. If the tube is not filled to the correct volume, an excess of citrate appears in the sample.
• To prevent hemolysis, avoid excessive probing during venipuncture and handle the sample gently.
• Promptly send the sample on ice to the laboratory.

Reference values
Normally, PT values range from 11 to 13 seconds. Values vary, however, depending on the source of tissue thromboplastin and the type of sensing devices used to measure clot formation. In a patient receiving oral anticoagulants, PT is usually maintained between 2 and 2.5 times the normal control value.

Abnormal findings
Prolonged PT may indicate deficiencies in fibrinogen; prothrombin; factors V, VII, or X (specific assays can pinpoint such deficiencies); or vitamin K as well as hepatic disease. It may also result from ongoing oral anticoagulant therapy. Prolonged PT that exceeds two and one-half times the control value is commonly associated with abnormal bleeding.

Interfering factors

- Failure to fill the collection tube completely (possible false-high)
- Failure to adequately mix the sample and the anticoagulant, or to send the sample to the laboratory promptly
- Hemolysis due to rough handling of the sample
- Salicylates, more than 1 g/day (increase)
- Fibrin or fibrin split products in the sample or plasma fibrinogen levels < 100 mg/dl (possible prolonged PT)
- Antihistamines, chloral hydrate, corticosteroids, digitalis glycosides, diuretics, glutethimide, griseofulvin, progestin-estrogen combinations, pyrazinamide, vitamin K, and xanthines, such as caffeine and theophylline (possible decrease)
- Corticotropin, anabolic steroids, cholestyramine resin, heparin I.V. (within 5 hours of sample collection), indomethacin, mefenamic acid, para-aminosalicylic acid, methimazole, oxyphenbutazone, phenylbutazone, phenytoin, propylthiouracil, quinidine, quinine, thyroid hormones, vitamin A, or alcohol in excess (possible increase)
- Antibiotics, barbiturates, hydroxyzine, sulfonamides, mineral oil, or clofibrate (possible increase or decrease)

ACTIVATED CLOTTING TIME

Activated clotting time, or automated coagulation time (ACT), measures whole blood clotting time. This test is commonly performed during procedures that require extracorporeal circulation, such as cardiopulmonary bypass, ultrafiltration, hemodialysis, and extracorporeal membrane oxygenation (ECMO).

Purpose

- To monitor the effect of heparin
- To monitor the effect of protamine sulfate in heparin neutralization
- To detect severe deficiencies in clotting factors (except factor VII)

Patient preparation

- Explain to the patient that this test is used to monitor the effect of heparin on the blood's ability to coagulate.
- Tell him that the test requires a blood sample, which is usually drawn from an existing vascular access site; therefore, no venipuncture will be needed.
- Explain who will perform the test and that the test is usually done at the bedside.
- Explain that two blood samples will be drawn. The first one will be discarded so that any heparin in the tubing doesn't interfere with the results.
- If the sample is drawn from a line with a continuous infusion, stop the infusion before drawing the sample.

Procedure and posttest care

- Withdraw 5 to 10 ml of blood from the line and discard it.
- Withdraw a clean sample of blood into the special tube containing celite provided with the activated clotting time unit.
- Activate the activated clotting time unit and wait for the signal to insert the tube.
- Flush the vascular access site according to your facility's protocol.

Precautions

- Guard against contamination with heparin if drawn from an access site containing heparin.

Reference values

In a non-anticoagulated patient, normal activated clotting time is 107 seconds plus or minus 13 seconds. During cardiopulmonary bypass, heparin is titrated to maintain an activated clotting time between 400 and 600 seconds. During ECMO, heparin is titrated to maintain the activated clotting time between 220 and 260 seconds.

Interfering factors

• Failure to fill the collection tube completely, to use the proper anticoagulant, to adequately mix the sample and the anticoagulant, or to send the sample to the laboratory immediately or place it on ice

• Hemolysis due to rough handling of the sample or to excessive probing at the venipuncture site

• Failure to draw at least 5 ml waste to avoid sample contamination when drawing sample from a venous access device that's used for heparin infusion

ONE-STAGE FACTOR ASSAY: EXTRINSIC COAGULATION SYSTEM

When prothrombin time (PT) and activated partial thromboplastin time (APTT) are prolonged, a one-stage assay is used to detect a deficiency of factor II, factor V, or factor X. If PT is abnormal but APTT is normal, factor VII may be deficient.

Purpose

• To identify a specific factor deficiency in persons with prolonged PT or APTT

• To study patients with congenital or acquired coagulation defects

• To monitor the effects of blood component therapy in factor-deficient patients

Patient preparation

• Explain to the patient that this test is used to assess the function of the blood coagulation mechanism.

• Tell him that a blood sample will be taken. Explain who will perform the venipuncture and when.

• Reassure him that drawing a blood sample will take less than 3 minutes.

• Explain that he may feel slight discomfort from the tourniquet pressure and the needle puncture.

• When the patient is factor deficient and receiving blood component therapy, tell him that he may need a series of tests.

• Withhold oral anticoagulants before the test. If they must be continued, note this on the laboratory slip.

• Inform the patient that food or fluids need not be restricted before the test.

Procedure and posttest care

• Perform a venipuncture, and collect the sample in a 7-ml *blue-top* tube.

• If a hematoma develops at the venipuncture site, apply warm soaks.

• A patient with a bleeding disorder may require a pressure bandage to stop bleeding at the venipuncture site.

Precautions

• If the patient has a suspected coagulation defect, avoid excessive probing during venipuncture; don't leave the tourniquet on too long (it will cause bruising); and apply pressure to the puncture site for 5 minutes or until the bleeding stops.

• Completely fill the collection tube, and invert it gently several times to mix the sample and the anticoagulant.

• Handle the sample gently to prevent hemolysis, and send it to the laboratory immediately, or place it on ice.

Reference values
Diluted samples of the patient's plasma are added to a substrate plasma deficient in a single factor. The activity of this mixture is compared with normal activity. The reference ranges for the factors are as follows:
• factor II: 80% to 120% of normal
• factor V: 50% to 150% of normal
• factor VII: 65% to 140% of normal
• factor X: 45% to 155% of normal.

Abnormal findings
If the clotting time for the substrate mixture is prolonged compared to normal, the patient may be deficient in the factor being tested. Deficiency of factor II, factor VII, or factor X may indicate hepatic disease or vitamin K deficiency. Deficiency of factor X may also indicate disseminated intravascular coagulation (DIC). Factor V deficiency suggests severe hepatic disease, DIC, or fibrinogenolysis. Deficiencies of all four factors may be congenital; absence of factor II is lethal.

Interfering factors
• Failure to mix the sample and the anticoagulant adequately, or to send the sample to the laboratory immediately or place it on ice
• Hemolysis due to rough handling of the sample
• Oral anticoagulants (possible increase due to inhibition of vitamin K-dependent synthesis and activation of clotting factors II, VII, and X, which form in the liver)

ONE-STAGE FACTOR ASSAY: INTRINSIC COAGULATION SYSTEM

When prothrombin time (PT) is normal but activated partial thromboplastin time (APTT) is abnormal, a one-stage assay is used to identify a deficiency in the intrinsic coagulation system: factor VIII, factor IX, factor XI, or factor XII.

Purpose
• To identify a specific factor deficiency
• To study patients with congenital or acquired coagulation defects
• To monitor the effects of blood component therapy in factor-deficient patients

Patient preparation
• Explain to the patient that this test is used to assess the function of the blood coagulation mechanism.
• Tell him that a blood sample will be taken. Explain who will perform the venipuncture and when.
• Reassure him that drawing a blood sample will take less than 3 minutes.
• Explain that he may feel slight discomfort from the tourniquet pressure and the needle puncture.
• Withhold oral anticoagulants before the test. If such medications must be continued, note this on the laboratory slip.
• When the patient is factor deficient and receiving blood component therapy, tell him that a series of tests may be needed to monitor therapeutic progress.
• Inform the patient that food or fluids need not be restricted before the test.

Procedure and posttest care
• Perform a venipuncture, and collect the sample in a 7-ml *blue-top* tube.

• If a hematoma develops at the venipuncture site, apply warm soaks.
• A patient with a bleeding disorder may require a pressure bandage to stop bleeding at the venipuncture site.
• Resume administration of medications discontinued before the test.

Precautions
• If a coagulation defect is suspected, avoid excessive probing during venipuncture, don't leave the tourniquet on too long (it will cause bruising), and apply pressure to the puncture site for 5 minutes, or until the bleeding stops.
• Completely fill the collection tube, and invert it gently several times to mix the sample and the anticoagulant thoroughly.
• Handle the sample gently to prevent hemolysis, and send it to the laboratory immediately or place it on ice.

Reference values
Diluted samples of the patient's plasma are added to a substrate plasma deficient in a single factor. The activity of this mixture is compared with normal activity. Reference ranges for the factors are as follows:
• factor VIII: 45% to 185% of normal
• factor IX: 60% to 140% of normal
• factor XI: 65% to 135% of normal
• factor XII: 50% to 150% of normal.

Abnormal findings
If the clotting time for the substrate mixture is prolonged compared to normal, the patient may be deficient in the factor being tested. Factor VIII deficiency may indicate hemophilia A, von Willebrand's disease, or a factor VIII inhibitor. An acquired deficiency of factor VIII may result from disseminated intravascular coagulation or fibrinolysis. Factor VIII antigen and ristocetin cofactor tests distinguish between hemophilia A (and its carrier state) and von Willebrand's disease.

Factor IX deficiency may suggest hemophilia B, or it may be acquired as a result of hepatic disease, a factor IX inhibitor, vitamin K deficiency, or coumarin therapy. Factor VIII and IX inhibitors occur after blood transfusions in patients deficient in either factor and are antibodies specific to each factor.

Factor XI deficiency may appear after the stress of trauma or surgery, or transiently in neonates. Factor XII deficiency may be inherited or acquired (as in nephrosis) and may also appear transiently in neonates.

Interfering factors
• Failure to adequately mix the sample and the anticoagulant or to send the sample to the laboratory immediately
• Hemolysis due to rough handling of the sample
• Oral anticoagulants (decrease in factor IX)
• Pregnancy (increase in factor VIII)

PLASMA THROMBIN TIME

Plasma thrombin time, or thrombin clotting time, measures how quickly a clot forms when a standard amount of bovine thrombin is added to a platelet-poor plasma sample from the patient and to a normal plasma control sample. After thrombin is added, the clotting time for each sample is compared and recorded. This test allows a quick but imprecise estimation of plasma fibrinogen levels.

Purpose
• To detect fibrinogen deficiency or defect
• To aid diagnosis of disseminated intravascular coagulation (DIC) and hepatic disease
• To monitor the effectiveness of treatment with heparin or thrombolytic agents

Patient preparation
• Explain to the patient that this test is used to determine if blood clots normally.
• If possible, withhold heparin therapy before the test. If heparin must be continued, note this on the laboratory slip.
• Tell the patient that a blood sample will be taken. Explain who will perform the venipuncture and when.
• Reassure him that drawing a blood sample will take less than 3 minutes.
• Explain that he may feel slight discomfort from the tourniquet pressure and the needle puncture.
• Inform the patient that food or fluids need not be restricted before the test.

Procedure and posttest care
• Perform a venipuncture, and collect the sample in a 7-ml *blue-top* tube.
• If a hematoma develops at the venipuncture site, apply warm soaks.

Precautions
• If the tube isn't filled to the correct volume, an excess of citrate appears in the sample. Completely fill the collection tube, and invert it gently several times to mix the sample and the anticoagulant thoroughly.
• To prevent hemolysis, avoid excessive probing during venipuncture and rough handling of the sample.
• Immediately send the sample on ice to the laboratory.

Reference values
Normal thrombin times range from 7 to 12 seconds. Test results are usually reported with a normal control value.

Abnormal findings
A prolonged thrombin time may indicate heparin therapy, hepatic disease, DIC, hypofibrinogenemia, or dysfibrinogenemia. Patients with prolonged thrombin times may require measurement of fibrinogen levels; in suspected DIC, the test for fibrin split products is also necessary.

Interfering factors
• Failure to use the proper anticoagulant, to adequately mix the sample and the anticoagulant, or to send the sample to the laboratory immediately
• Hemolysis due to rough handling of the sample or to excessive probing at the venipuncture site
• Fibrinogen level < 100 mg/dl (prolonged thrombin time)
• Fibrinogen inhibitors, such as streptokinase, urokinase, and tissue plasminogen activators (increase)
• Heparin (possible increase)

PLASMA FIBRINOGEN

Fibrinogen (factor I) originates in the liver and is converted to fibrin during clotting. Because fibrin is necessary for clot formation, fibrinogen deficiency can produce mild-to-severe bleeding disorders.

This test is used to determine the amount of fibrinogen present in a blood sample. Note that fibrinogen deficiency may also be indicated by prolonged activated partial thromboplastin time, prothrombin time, and thrombin time.

Purpose
● To aid the diagnosis of suspected clotting or bleeding disorders caused by fibrinogen abnormalities

Patient preparation
● Explain to the patient that this test is used to determine if blood clots normally.
● Tell him that a blood sample will be taken. Explain who will perform the venipuncture and when.
● Reassure him that drawing a blood sample will take less than 3 minutes.
● Explain that he may feel slight discomfort from the tourniquet pressure and the needle puncture.
● Check patient history for use of heparin or oral contraceptives and notify the laboratory if these drugs are in use.
● Inform the patient that food or fluids need not be restricted before the test.

Procedure and posttest care
● Perform a venipuncture, and collect the sample in a 7-ml *blue-top* tube.
● Completely fill the collection tube, invert it gently several times, and send it to the laboratory immediately, or place it on ice.
● Avoid excessive probing during venipuncture, and handle the sample gently.
● If a hematoma develops at the venipuncture site, apply warm soaks.

Precautions
● This test is contraindicated in patients with active bleeding and acute infection or illness, and in those who have received blood transfusions within 4 weeks.

Reference values
Fibrinogen levels normally range from 175 to 350 mg/dl.

Abnormal findings
Depressed fibrinogen levels may indicate congenital afibrinogenemia; hypofibrinogenemia or dysfibrinogenemia; disseminated intravascular coagulation; fibrinolysis; severe hepatic disease; cancer of the prostate, pancreas, or lung; or bone marrow lesions. Obstetric complications or trauma may cause low levels.

Markedly decreased fibrinogen levels impede the accurate interpretation of coagulation tests that have a fibrin clot as an end point.

Elevated levels may indicate cancer of the stomach, breast, or kidney, or inflammatory disorders, such as pneumonia or membranoproliferative glomerulonephritis.

Interfering factors
● Failure to fill the collection tube completely, to adequately mix the sample and anticoagulant, or to send the sample to the laboratory promptly
● Hemolysis due to excessive probing at the venipuncture site or to rough handling of the sample
● Third trimester of pregnancy and postoperative status (possible increase)
● Fibrinogen inhibitors, such as streptokinase
● Acute infection
● Transfusion of whole blood, plasma, or fractions within 4 weeks before the test

FIBRIN SPLIT PRODUCTS

After a fibrin clot forms in response to vascular injury, the clot is eventually degraded by plasmin, a fibrin-dissolving enzyme. The resulting fragments are known as fibrin split products (FSP), or fibrinogen degradation products. In this test, FSP are detected in the diluted serum that is left in a blood sample after clotting.

Purpose
• To detect FSP in the circulation
• To help determine the presence and the approximate severity of a hyperfibrinolytic state (such as disseminated intravascular coagulation [DIC]) that may result in primary fibrinogenolysis or hypercoagulability

Patient preparation
• Explain to the patient that this test is used to determine if blood clots normally.
• Tell him that a blood sample will be taken. Explain who will perform the venipuncture and when.
• Reassure him that drawing a blood sample will take less than 3 minutes.
• Explain that he may feel slight discomfort from the tourniquet pressure and the needle puncture.
• Check patient history for use of any medications (especially heparin) that may interfere with accurate determination of test results.
• Inform the patient that food or fluids need not be restricted before the test.

Procedure and posttest care
• Perform a venipuncture, and then draw 2 ml of blood into a plastic syringe.
• Transfer the sample to the tube provided by the laboratory, which contains a soybean trypsin inhibitor and bovine thrombin.
• If a hematoma develops at the venipuncture site, apply warm soaks.

Precautions
• Draw the sample before administering heparin to avoid false-positive test results.
• Gently invert the collection tube several times to mix the contents thoroughly.
• The blood clots within 2 seconds and then must be sent immediately to the laboratory, to be incubated at 98.6° F (37° C) for 30 minutes before testing proceeds.

Reference values
Serum contains less than 10 μg/ml of FSP. A quantitative assay shows levels of less than 3 μg/ml.

Abnormal findings
FSP levels increase in primary fibrinolytic states, due to increased levels of circulating profibrinolysin; in secondary states, due to DIC and subsequent fibrinolysis; and in alcoholic cirrhosis, preeclampsia, abruptio placentae, congenital heart disease, sunstroke, burns, intrauterine death, pulmonary embolus, deep-vein thrombosis (transient increase), and myocardial infarction (after 1 or 2 days). FSP levels usually exceed 100 μg/ml in active renal disease or renal transplant rejection.

Interfering factors
• Pretest administration of heparin (false-high)
• Failure to fill the collection tube completely, to adequately mix the sample and additive, or to send the sample to the laboratory immediately
• Hemolysis due to rough handling of the sample
• Fibrinolytic drugs, such as urokinase and streptokinase, and large doses of barbiturates (increase)

Plasma Plasminogen

Plasma plasminogen testing is used to assess plasminogen levels in a plasma sample. During fibrinolysis, plasmin dissolves fibrin clots to prevent excessive coagulation and impaired blood flow. Plasmin doesn't circulate in active form, however, so it can't be directly measured. Its circulating precursor, plasminogen, can be measured and used to evaluate the fibrinolytic system.

Purpose
- To assess fibrinolysis
- To detect congenital and acquired fibrinolytic disorders

Patient preparation
- Explain to the patient that this test is used to evaluate blood clotting.
- Tell him that a blood sample will be taken. Explain who will perform the venipuncture and when.
- Reassure him that drawing a blood sample will take less than 3 minutes.
- Explain that he may feel slight discomfort from the tourniquet pressure and the needle puncture.
- Check patient history for use of thrombolytic drugs, such as streptokinase or urokinase, and oral contraceptives, which may cause inaccurate test results. If these drugs must be continued, note this on the laboratory slip.
- Inform the patient that food or fluids need not be restricted before the test.

Procedure and posttest care
- Perform a venipuncture and collect the sample in a 7-ml *blue-top* tube.
- If a hematoma develops at the venipuncture site, apply warm soaks.

- Resume medications withheld before the test.

Precautions
- Collect the sample as quickly as possible to prevent stasis, which can slow blood flow, causing coagulation and plasminogen activation.
- To prevent hemolysis, avoid excessive probing during venipuncture and rough handling of the sample.
- Immediately after collection, invert the tube gently several times and send the sample to the laboratory. If testing must be delayed, plasma must be separated and frozen at $-94°$ F ($-70°$ C).

Reference values
Normal plasminogen activity is 80% to 123 mg/dl. Plasminogen activity: 80% to 123%.

Abnormal findings
Diminished plasminogen levels can result from disseminated intravascular coagulation, tumors, preeclampsia, and eclampsia, which accelerate plasminogen conversion to plasmin and increase fibrinolysis. Some liver diseases prevent formation of sufficient plasminogen, decreasing fibrinolysis.

Interfering factors
- Failure to use the proper collection tube, to adequately mix the sample and the citrate, to send the sample to the laboratory immediately, or to have the sample separated and frozen
- Hemolysis due to excessive probing during venipuncture or to rough handling of the sample
- Hemoconcentration due to prolonged tourniquet use before venipuncture (possible false-low)
- Oral contraceptives (possible slight increase)
- Thrombolytic drugs, such as streptokinase and urokinase (possible decrease)

• Transfusion of whole blood, plasma, or fractions within 4 weeks of the test

PROTEIN C

Vitamin K-dependent, protein C is produced in the liver and circulates in the plasma. It acts as a potent anticoagulant by suppressing activated factors V and VIII. Deficiencies of protein C may be acquired or congenital.

If a deficiency of protein C is identified, further immunologic tests may be needed to determine the type of deficiency. Identifying the role of protein C deficiency in idiopathic venous thrombosis may help prevent thromboembolism.

Purpose
• To investigate the cause of otherwise unexplained thrombosis and to establish inheritance patterns

Patient preparation
• Explain to the patient that this test evaluates blood clotting.
• Tell him that a blood sample will be taken. Explain who will perform the venipuncture and when.
• Reassure him that drawing a blood sample will take less than 3 minutes.
• Explain that he may feel slight discomfort from the tourniquet pressure and the needle puncture.
• Inform the patient that food or fluids need not be restricted before the test.
• If the patient is receiving anticoagulant therapy, note this on the laboratory slip.

Procedure and posttest care
• Perform a venipuncture. Collect a 3-ml sample in a *blue-top* vacuum specimen tube or in a special syringe with anticoagulant provided by the laboratory.
• If a hematoma develops at the venipuncture site, apply warm soaks.

Precautions
• Avoid excessive probing during venipuncture.
• Completely fill the collection tube, and invert it several times to mix the sample and anticoagulant thoroughly; handle the sample gently.
• Send the sample to the laboratory immediately.

Reference values
The normal range is 70% to 130%.

Abnormal findings
Rare, homozygous protein C deficiency is characterized by rapidly fatal thrombosis in the perinatal period, a condition known as purpura fulminans.

The more common heterozygous deficiency is associated with genetic susceptibility to venous thromboembolism before age 30 and continuing throughout life. The patient may require long-term treatment with warfarin therapy or protein C supplements from plasma fractions.

Interfering factors
• Hemolysis due to excessive probing at the venipuncture site or to rough handling of the sample
• Anticoagulant therapy

EUGLOBULIN LYSIS TIME

Euglobulin lysis time measures the interval between clot formation and clot dissolution in plasma. A precipitated plasma extract is clotted with thrombin, and the time required for the clot to lyse is measured.

Purpose
- To assess the fibrinolytic system
- To help detect abnormal fibrinolytic states

Patient preparation
- Explain to the patient that this test is used to evaluate the blood clotting mechanism.
- Tell him that a blood sample will be taken. Explain who will perform the venipuncture and when.
- Reassure him that drawing a blood sample will take less than 3 minutes.
- Explain that he may feel slight discomfort from the tourniquet pressure and the needle puncture.
- Inform the patient that food or fluids need not be restricted before the test.

Procedure and posttest care
- Perform a venipuncture. Collect a 4.5-ml sample in a *blue-top* tube or in a chilled tube with 0.5-ml sodium oxalate.
- If a hematoma develops at the venipuncture site, apply warm soaks.

Precautions
- When drawing the sample, be careful not to rub the area over the vein too vigorously, pump the fist excessively, or leave the tourniquet in place too long.
- Avoid excessive probing during venipuncture, and handle the sample gently.
- If a *blue-top* tube is used, mix the sample and anticoagulant thoroughly. If a chilled tube containing 0.5 ml sodium oxalate is used, mix the sample and preservative thoroughly, pack the sample in ice, and send it to the laboratory immediately.

Reference values
Normal lysis of the plasma clot at 98.6° F (37° C) is 120 minutes.

Abnormal findings
Clot lysis within 1 hour indicates increased plasminogen activator activity. In pathologic fibrinolysis, lysis time may be as brief as 5 to 10 minutes.

Interfering factors
- Prolonged tourniquet constriction, vigorous vein preparation, or excessive pumping of the fist (decrease)
- Hemolysis due to excessive probing at the venipuncture site or to rough handling of the sample
- Failure to place the collection tube and sample on ice
- Fibrinogen level < 100 mg/dl (possible decrease)

D-DIMER

A D-dimer is an asymmetrical carbon compound fragment formed after thrombin converts fibrinogen to fibrin, factor XIIIa stabilizes it into a clot, and plasma acts on the cross-linked, or clotted, fibrin. The test is specific for fibrinolysis because it confirms the presence of fibrin split products.

Purpose
- To diagnose disseminated intravascular coagulation (DIC)
- To differentiate subarachnoid hemorrhage from a traumatic lumbar puncture in spinal fluid analysis

Patient preparation
- Obtain the patient's history of hematologic diseases, recent surgery, and the results of other tests performed.

- Explain to the patient that the test is used to determine if the blood is clotting normally.
- Tell him that the test requires a blood sample. Explain who will perform the venipuncture and when.
- Reassure him that drawing a blood sample will take less than 3 minutes.
- Explain that he may feel slight discomfort from the tourniquet pressure and the needle puncture.

Procedure and posttest care
- Perform a venipuncture and collect the sample in a 5-ml *blue-top* tube.
- For a spinal fluid analysis, the sample is collected during a lumbar puncture and placed in a plastic vial. See "CSF analysis" in chapter 7 for details of the procedure.
- Apply pressure to the venipuncture site for 5 minutes or until bleeding stops.
- If a hematoma develops at the venipuncture site, apply warm soaks.

Precautions
- Completely fill the collection tube, invert it gently several times, and send it to the laboratory immediately.
- For a patient with coagulation problems, you may need to apply additional pressure at the venipuncture site to control bleeding.

Reference values
Normal D-dimer test results are negative or < 250 μg/ml).

Abnormal findings
Increased D-dimer values may indicate DIC, pulmonary embolism, arterial or venous thrombosis, neoplastic disease, pregnancy (late and postpartum), surgery occurring up to 2 days before testing, subarachnoid hemorrhage (spinal fluid only), or secondary fibrinolysis.

Interfering factors
- Failure to fill the collection tube completely or to send the sample to laboratory immediately
- Hemolysis due to rough handling of the sample
- High rheumatoid factor titers or increased CA-125 levels (possible false-positive)
- Spinal fluid analysis in infants under age 6 months (possible false-negative)

INTERNATIONAL NORMALIZED RATIO

The international normalized ratio (INR) system is viewed as the best means of standardizing measurement of prothrombin time to monitor oral anticoagulant therapy. It isn't used as a screening test for coagulopathies.

Purpose
- To evaluate effectiveness of oral anticoagulant therapy

Patient preparation
- Explain to the patient that this test is used to determine the effectiveness of his oral anticoagulant therapy.
- Tell the patient that a blood sample will be taken. Explain who will perform the venipuncture and when.
- Reassure him that drawing a blood sample will take less than 3 minutes.
- Explain that he may feel slight discomfort from the tourniquet pressure and the needle puncture.

Procedure and posttest care
- Perform a venipuncture, and collect the sample in a 7-ml *blue-top* tube.
- If a hematoma develops at the venipuncture site, apply warm soaks.

Precautions
• Completely fill the collection tube; otherwise, an excess of citrate appears in the sample.
• Gently invert the tube several times to thoroughly mix the sample and the anticoagulant.
• To prevent hemolysis, avoid excessive probing during venipuncture and handle the sample gently.
• Put the sample on ice, and send it to the laboratory promptly.

Reference values
Normal INR for those receiving warfarin therapy is 2.0 to 3.0. For those with mechanical prosthetic heart valves, an INR of 2.5 to 3.5 is suggested.

Abnormal findings
Increased INR values may indicate disseminated intravascular coagulation, cirrhosis, hepatitis, vitamin K deficiency, salicylate intoxication, uncontrolled oral anticoagulation, or massive blood transfusion.

Interfering factors
• Failure to fill the collection tube completely, to adequately mix the sample and the anticoagulant, or to send the sample to the laboratory immediately
• Hemolysis due to excessive probing at the venipuncture site or to rough handling of the sample

CHAPTER 2

Blood Chemistry Tests

ARTERIAL BLOOD GASES			129
129	Arterial blood gas analysis	131	Total carbon dioxide content

ELECTROLYTES			132
132	Calcium	137	Potassium
133	Chloride	138	Sodium
134	Magnesium	139	Anion gap
135	Phosphates		

CARDIAC ENZYMES AND PROTEINS			141
141	Creatine kinase	145	Myoglobins
143	Lactate dehydrogenase		

HEPATIC ENZYMES AND PROTEINS			145
145	Alpha$_1$-antitrypsin	150	Leucine aminopeptidase
146	Aspartate aminotransferase	151	Gamma glutamyl transferase
148	Alanine aminotransferase	152	5′-Nucleotidase
149	Alkaline phosphatase		

PANCREATIC ENZYMES			153
153	Amylase	154	Lipase

SPECIAL ENZYMES			155
155	Acid phosphatase	161	Pyruvate kinase
156	Prostate-specific antigen	162	Hexosaminidase A and B
157	Plasma renin activity	163	Uroporphyrinogen I synthase
159	Cholinesterase	164	Galactose-1-phosphate uridyl
160	Glucose-6-phosphate		transferase
	dehydrogenase	165	Angiotensin-converting enzyme

LIPIDS AND LIPOPROTEINS			166
166	Triglycerides	169	Lipoprotein-cholesterol fraction-
167	Total cholesterol		ation
168	Phospholipids	170	Lipoprotein phenotyping

PROTEINS AND PROTEIN METABOLITES · 173

173 Protein electrophoresis
175 Ceruloplasmin
175 Haptoglobin
176 Transferrin
177 Plasma amino acid screening
178 Phenylalanine screening
179 Plasma ammonia
180 Blood urea nitrogen
181 Creatinine
181 Uric acid

PIGMENTS · 182

182 Bilirubin
183 Fractionated erythrocyte porphyrins

CARBOHYDRATES · 184

184 Fasting plasma glucose
186 Two-hour postprandial plasma glucose
188 Oral glucose tolerance test
190 β-Hydroxybutyrate
191 Glycosylated hemoglobin
191 Oral lactose tolerance test
193 Lactic acid and pyruvic acid

ARTERIAL BLOOD GASES

ARTERIAL BLOOD GAS ANALYSIS

Arterial blood gas (ABG) analysis is used to measure the partial pressures of oxygen (Pao_2) and carbon dioxide ($Paco_2$), and the pH of an arterial sample. Oxygen content (O_2CT), oxygen saturation (Sao_2), and bicarbonate (HCO_3^-) values are also measured. A blood sample for ABG analysis may be drawn by percutaneous arterial puncture or from an arterial line.

Purpose
• To evaluate gas exchange in the lungs
• To assess integrity of the ventilatory control system
• To determine the acid-base level of the blood
• To monitor respiratory therapy

Patient preparation
• Explain to the patient that this test is used to evaluate how well the lungs are delivering oxygen to blood and eliminating carbon dioxide.
• Tell him that the test requires a blood sample. Explain who will perform the arterial puncture and when and which site — radial, brachial, or femoral artery — has been selected for the puncture.
• Inform him that he needn't restrict food or fluids.
• Instruct the patient to breathe normally during the test, and warn him that he may experience a brief cramping or throbbing pain at the puncture site.

Procedure and posttest care
• Perform an arterial puncture.
• After applying pressure to the puncture site for 3 to 5 minutes, tape a gauze pad firmly over it. (If the puncture site is on the arm, don't tape the entire circumference; this may restrict circulation.)
• If the patient is receiving anticoagulants or has a coagulopathy, hold the puncture site longer than 5 minutes if necessary.
• Monitor vital signs, and observe for signs of circulatory impairment, such as swelling, discoloration, pain, numbness, and tingling in the bandaged arm or leg.
• Watch for bleeding from the puncture site.

Precautions
• Wait at least 15 minutes before drawing arterial blood when starting, changing, or discontinuing oxygen therapy.
• Before sending the sample to the laboratory, note on the laboratory slip whether the patient was breathing room air or receiving oxygen therapy when the sample was collected.
• If the patient was receiving oxygen therapy, note the flow rate. If he is on a ventilator, note the fraction of inspired oxygen and tidal volume.
• Note the patient's rectal temperature and respiratory rate.

Reference values
Normal ABG values fall within the following ranges:
• Pao_2: 75 to 100 mm Hg
• $Paco_2$: 35 to 45 mm Hg
• pH: 7.35 to 7.45
• O_2CT: 15% to 22%
• Sao_2: 95% to 100%
• HCO_3^-: 24 to 28 mEq/L.

Acid-Base Disorders

DISORDERS AND A.B.G. FINDINGS	POSSIBLE CAUSES	SIGNS AND SYMPTOMS
Respiratory acidosis (excess CO_2 retention) pH < 7.35 HCO_3^- > 28 mEq/L (if compensating) $Paco_2$ > 45 mm Hg	• CNS depression from drugs, injury, or disease • Asphyxia • Hypoventilation due to pulmonary, cardiac, musculoskeletal, or neuromuscular disease	• Diaphoresis, headache, tachycardia, confusion, restlessness, apprehension
Respiratory alkalosis (excess CO_2 excretion) pH > 7.45 HCO_3^- < 24 mEq/L (if compensating) $Paco_2$ < 35 mm Hg	• Hyperventilation due to anxiety, pain, or improper ventilator settings • Respiratory stimulation caused by drugs, disease, hypoxia, fever, or high room temperature • Gram-negative bacteremia	• Rapid, deep breathing; paresthesia; light-headedness; twitching; anxiety; fear
Metabolic acidosis (HCO_3^- loss, acid retention) pH < 7.35 HCO_3^- < 24 mEq/ $Paco_2$ > 35 mm Hg (if compensating)	• HCO_3^- depletion due to renal disease, diarrhea, or small-bowel fistulas • Excessive production of organic acids due to hepatic disease; endocrine disorders, including diabetes mellitus, hypoxia, shock, and drug intoxication	• Rapid, deep breathing; fruity breath; fatigue; headache; lethargy; drowsiness; nausea; vomiting; coma (if severe)
Metabolic alkalosis (HCO_3^- retention, acid loss) pH > 7.45 HCO_3^- > 28 mEq/L $Paco_2$ > 45 mm Hg	• Inadequate excretion of acids due to renal disease • Loss of hydrochloric acid from prolonged vomiting or gastric suctioning • Loss of potassium due to increased renal excretion (as in diuretic therapy) or steroid overdose • Excessive alkali ingestion	• Slow, shallow breathing; hypertonic muscles; restlessness; twitching; confusion; irritability; apathy; tetany; seizures; coma (if severe)

Abnormal findings

Low Pao_2, O_2CT, and Sao_2 levels and a high $Paco_2$ may result from conditions that impair respiratory function, such as respiratory muscle weakness or paralysis, respiratory center inhibition (from head injury, brain tumor, or drug abuse, for example), and airway obstruction (possibly from mucus plugs or a tumor). Similarly, low readings may result from bronchiole obstruction caused by asthma or emphysema, from an abnormal ventilation-perfusion ratio due to partially blocked alveoli or pulmonary capillaries, or from alveoli that are damaged or filled with fluid because of disease, hemorrhage, or near-drowning.

When inspired air contains insufficient oxygen, PaO_2, O_2CT, and SaO_2 decrease, but $PaCO_2$ may be normal. Such findings are common in pneumothorax, impaired diffusion between alveoli and blood (due to interstitial fibrosis, for example), or an arteriovenous shunt that permits blood to bypass the lungs.

Low O_2CT — with normal PaO_2, SaO_2 and, possibly, $PaCO_2$ values — may result from severe anemia, decreased blood volume, and reduced hemoglobin oxygen-carrying capacity.

In addition to clarifying blood oxygen disorders, ABG values can give considerable information about acid-base disorders. (See *Acid-base disorders*.)

Interfering factors

● Failure to heparinize syringe, place sample in an iced bag, or send the sample to the laboratory immediately (possible altered PaO_2 and $PaCO_2$ because metabolic processes continue after sample is drawn)
● Exposing the sample to air (increase or decrease in PaO_2 and $PaCO_2$)
● Venous blood in the sample (possible decrease in PaO_2 and increase in $PaCO_2$)
● Bicarbonate, ethacrynic acid, hydrocortisone, metolazone, prednisone, and thiazides (possible increase in $PaCO_2$)
● Acetazolamide, methicillin, nitrofurantoin, and tetracycline (possible decrease in $PaCO_2$)
● Fever (possible false-high PaO_2 and $PaCO_2$)

● Hypothermia (possible false-low PaO_2 and $PaCO_2$)

TOTAL CARBON DIOXIDE CONTENT

When carbon dioxide (CO_2) pressure in red blood cells exceeds 40 mm Hg, CO_2 spills out of the cells and dissolves in plasma. There it may combine with water to form carbonic acid, which in turn may dissociate into hydrogen and bicarbonate ions.

This test is used to measure the total concentration of all forms of CO_2 in serum, plasma, or whole blood samples. It's commonly ordered for patients with respiratory insufficiency and is usually included in an assessment of electrolyte balance. Test results are most significant when considered with pH and arterial blood gas values.

Purpose
● To help evaluate acid-base balance

Patient preparation
● Explain to the patient that this test is performed to measure the amount of CO_2 in the blood.
● Tell him that the test requires a blood sample. Explain who will perform the venipuncture and when.
● Explain that he may experience discomfort from the needle puncture and the tourniquet but that collecting the sample usually takes less than 3 minutes.
● Inform the patient that he needn't restrict food or fluids before the test.
● Check the patient's history for use of medications that may affect test results, including corticotropin, cortisone, thiazide diuretics, salicylates, paraldehyde, methicillin, dimercaprol, ammo-

nium chloride, and acetazolamide.
Also note excessive ingestion of alkalis
or licorice or accidental ingestion of
ethylene glycol or methyl alcohol.

Procedure and posttest care
• Perform a venipuncture.
• When CO_2 content is measured
along with electrolytes, a 7-ml *red-marble-top* tube may be used.
• When this test is performed alone, a
green-top (heparinized) tube is appropriate.
• If a hematoma develops at the
venipuncture site, apply warm soaks.

Precautions
• Fill the tube completely to prevent
diffusion of CO_2 into the vacuum.

Reference values
Normally, total CO_2 levels range from
23 to 30 mEq/L. Levels may vary, depending on sex and age.

Abnormal findings
High CO_2 levels may occur in metabolic alkalosis, respiratory acidosis, primary aldosteronism, and Cushing's
syndrome. CO_2 levels may also increase after excessive loss of acids, as
in severe vomiting and continuous gastric drainage.

Decreased CO_2 levels are common
in metabolic acidosis. Decreased total
CO_2 levels in metabolic acidosis also
result from loss of bicarbonate. Levels
may decrease in respiratory alkalosis.

Interfering factors
• Excessive use of corticotropin, cortisone, or thiazide diuretics; excessive
ingestion of alkalis or licorice (increase)
• Salicylates, paraldehyde, methicillin,
dimercaprol, ammonium chloride, and
acetazolamide; ingestion of ethylene
glycol or methyl alcohol (decrease)

ELECTROLYTES

CALCIUM

This test is used to measure serum levels of calcium, the most abundant mineral in the body. More than 98% of the
body's calcium is found in bones and
teeth, but relative concentrations in
those structures may vary as the body
maintains calcium balance. For example, when calcium concentrations in
the blood fall below normal, calcium
ions move out of the bones and teeth to
restore the blood's calcium level. Because the body excretes calcium daily,
regular ingestion of calcium in food (at
least 1 g/day) is necessary for normal
calcium balance.

Purpose
• To aid diagnosis of neuromuscular,
skeletal, and endocrine disorders; arrhythmias; blood-clotting deficiencies;
and acid-base imbalance

Patient preparation
• Explain to the patient that this test is
used to determine blood calcium levels.
• Tell him that the test requires a blood
sample. Explain who will perform the
venipuncture and when.
• Explain that he may experience
slight discomfort from the needle
puncture and the tourniquet but that
collecting the sample usually takes less
than 3 minutes.
• Inform him that he needn't restrict
food or fluids before the test.

Procedure and posttest care
• Perform a venipuncture (without a
tourniquet if possible), and collect the

sample in a 7-ml *red-top* or *red-marble-top* tube.
- If a hematoma develops at the venipuncture site, apply warm soaks.

Reference values

Normally, serum calcium levels range from 8.9 to 10.1 mg/dl in adults age 19 and older. Serum calcium levels are higher in children and can rise during phases of rapid bone growth.

Abnormal findings

Abnormally high serum calcium levels (hypercalcemia) may occur in hyperparathyroidism and parathyroid tumors, Paget's disease of the bone, multiple myeloma, metastatic carcinoma, multiple fractures, and prolonged immobilization. Elevated levels may also result from inadequate excretion of calcium, as in adrenal insufficiency and renal disease; from excessive calcium ingestion; and from overuse of antacids such as calcium carbonate.

CLINICAL ALERT Observe the patient with hypercalcemia for deep bone pain, flank pain due to renal calculi, and muscle hypotonicity. Hypercalcemic crisis begins with nausea, vomiting, and dehydration, leading to stupor and coma, and can end in cardiac arrest.

Low calcium levels (hypocalcemia) may result from hypoparathyroidism, total parathyroidectomy, and malabsorption. Decreased serum calcium levels may also occur with Cushing's syndrome, renal failure, acute pancreatitis, and peritonitis.

In a patient with hypocalcemia, be alert for circumoral and peripheral numbness and tingling, muscle twitching, Chvostek's sign (facial muscle spasm), tetany, muscle cramping, Trousseau's sign (carpopedal spasm), seizures, and arrhythmias.

Interfering factors

- Venous stasis due to prolonged tourniquet application (possible false-high)
- Excessive ingestion of vitamin D or its derivatives (dihydrotachysterol, calcitriol); use of androgens, calciferol-activated calcium salts, progestins-estrogens, and thiazide diuretics (possible increase)
- Acetazolamide, corticosteroids, mithramycin, chronic laxative use, excessive transfusions of citrated blood (possible increase or decrease)
- Increased or decreased serum protein levels
- Active bone growth and formation in childhood (increase)

CHLORIDE

This test is used to measure serum levels of chloride, the major extracellular fluid anion. Chloride helps maintain osmotic pressure of blood and, therefore, helps regulate blood volume and arterial pressure. Chloride levels also affect acid-base balance. This mineral is absorbed from the intestines and excreted primarily by the kidneys.

Purpose

- To detect acid-base imbalance (acidosis or alkalosis) and to aid evaluation of fluid status and extracellular cation-anion balance

Patient preparation

- Explain to the patient that the test is used to evaluate the chloride content of blood.
- Tell him that the test requires a blood sample. Explain who will perform the venipuncture and when.

• Explain that he may experience slight discomfort from the needle puncture and the tourniquet but that collecting the sample usually takes less than 3 minutes.
• Inform him that he needn't restrict food or fluids before the test.
• Check the patient's history for use of drugs that may increase chloride levels, such as ammonium chloride, cholestyramine, boric acid, oxyphenbutazone, phenylbutazone, and excessive I.V. infusion of sodium chloride. Serum chloride levels are decreased by thiazides, furosemide, ethacrynic acid, bicarbonates, and prolonged I.V. infusion of dextrose 5% in water.

Procedure and posttest care
• Perform a venipuncture, and collect the sample in a 7-ml *red-top* or *red-marble-top* tube.
• If a hematoma develops at the venipuncture site, apply warm soaks.

Precautions
• Handle the sample gently to prevent hemolysis.

Reference values
Normally, serum chloride levels range from 98 to 106 mEq/L in adults.

Abnormal findings
Chloride levels are inversely related to bicarbonate levels, reflecting acid-base balance. Excessive loss of gastric juices or other secretions containing chloride may cause hypochloremic metabolic alkalosis; excessive chloride retention or ingestion may lead to hyperchloremic metabolic acidosis.

Elevated serum chloride levels (hyperchloremia) may result from severe dehydration, complete renal shutdown, head injury (producing neurogenic hyperventilation), and primary aldosteronism.

Low chloride levels (hypochloremia) are usually associated with low sodium and potassium levels. Possible underlying causes include prolonged vomiting, gastric suctioning, intestinal fistula, chronic renal failure, and Addison's disease. Heart failure or edema resulting in excess extracellular fluid can cause dilutional hypochloremia.

▶ **CLINICAL ALERT** Observe a patient with hypochloremia for hypertonicity of muscles, tetany, and depressed respirations. In a patient with hyperchloremia, be alert for signs of developing stupor, rapid deep breathing, and weakness that may lead to coma.

Interfering factors
• Hemolysis due to rough handling of the sample
• Use of ammonium chloride, cholestyramine, boric acid, oxyphenbutazone, or phenylbutazone and excessive I.V. infusion of sodium chloride (possible increase)
• Use of thiazide diuretics, ethacrynic acid, furosemide, or bicarbonates and prolonged I.V. infusion of dextrose 5% in water (decrease)

MAGNESIUM

This test is used to measure serum levels of magnesium, an electrolyte that is vital to neuromuscular function. Most magnesium is found in bone and intracellular fluid; a small amount is found in extracellular fluid. Magnesium is absorbed by the small intestine and excreted in the urine and stool.

Purpose
• To evaluate electrolyte status
• To assess neuromuscular and renal function

Patient preparation

- Explain to the patient that this test is used to determine the magnesium content of the blood.
- Instruct him not to use magnesium salts (such as milk of magnesia or Epsom salt) for at least 3 days before the test, but tell him that he needn't restrict food or fluids.
- Tell the patient that the test requires a blood sample. Explain who will perform the venipuncture and when.
- Explain that he may experience transient discomfort from the needle puncture, but reassure him that collecting the sample takes only a few minutes.

Procedure and posttest care

- Perform a venipuncture, without a tourniquet if possible, and collect the sample in a 7-ml *red-top* or *red-marble-top* tube.
- If a hematoma develops at the venipuncture site, apply warm soaks.

Precautions

- Handle the sample gently to prevent hemolysis.

Reference values

Serum magnesium levels range from 1.7 to 2.1 mEq/L.

Abnormal findings

Elevated serum magnesium levels (hypermagnesemia) most commonly occur in renal failure, when the kidneys excrete inadequate amounts of magnesium. Adrenal insufficiency (Addison's disease) can also increase serum magnesium levels.

In suspected or confirmed hypermagnesemia, observe the patient for lethargy; flushing; diaphoresis; decreased blood pressure; slow, weak pulse; muscle weakness; diminished deep tendon reflexes; and slow, shallow respirations.

Decreased serum magnesium levels (hypomagnesemia) most commonly result from chronic alcoholism. Other causes include malabsorption syndrome, diarrhea, faulty absorption after bowel resection, prolonged bowel or gastric aspiration, acute pancreatitis, primary aldosteronism, severe burns, hypercalcemic conditions (including hyperparathyroidism), and certain diuretic therapy.

In hypomagnesemia, watch for leg and foot cramps, hyperactive deep tendon reflexes, arrhythmias, muscle weakness, seizures, twitching, tetany, and tremors.

Interfering factors

- Venous stasis due to tourniquet use
- Obtaining a sample above an I.V. site that's receiving a solution containing magnesium
- Excessive use of antacids or cathartics or excessive infusion of magnesium sulfate (increase)
- Prolonged I.V. infusions without magnesium; excessive use of diuretics (decrease)
- I.V. administration of calcium gluconate (possible false-low if measured using the Titan yellow method)
- Hemolysis (false-high)

PHOSPHATES

This test is used to measure serum levels of phosphates, the primary anion in intracellular fluid. About 85% of the body's phosphates are found in bone. The intestines absorb most phosphates from dietary sources; the kidneys excrete phosphates and serve as a regulatory mechanism. Abnormal concentrations of serum phosphates usually result from improper excretion rather than faulty ingestion or absorption from dietary sources.

Normally, calcium and phosphates have an inverse relationship; if one is increased, the other is decreased.

Purpose
• To aid diagnosis of renal disorders and acid-base imbalance
• To detect endocrine, skeletal, and calcium disorders

Patient preparation
• Explain to the patient that this test is used to measure phosphate levels in the blood.
• Tell him that the test requires a blood sample. Explain who will perform the venipuncture and when.
• Explain that he may experience slight discomfort from the needle puncture and the tourniquet but that collecting the sample usually takes less than 3 minutes.
• Inform him that he needn't restrict food or fluids before the test.
• Check the patient's medication history for drugs that alter phosphate levels, such as vitamin D, anabolic steroids, androgens, phosphate-binding antacids, acetazolamide, insulin, and epinephrine.

Procedure and posttest care
• Perform a venipuncture, without using a tourniquet if possible, and collect the sample in a 7-ml *red-top* or *red-marble-top* tube.
• If a hematoma develops at the venipuncture site, apply warm soaks.

Precautions
• Handle the sample gently to prevent hemolysis.

Reference values
Normally, serum phosphate levels in adults range from 2.5 to 4.5 mg/dl. Children have higher serum phosphate levels than adults. Phosphate levels rise during periods of increased bone growth.

Abnormal findings
Because serum phosphate values alone are of limited diagnostic use (only a few rare conditions directly affect phosphate metabolism), they should be interpreted in light of serum calcium results.

Decreased phosphate levels (hypophosphatemia) may result from malnutrition, malabsorption syndromes, hyperparathyroidism, renal tubular acidosis, and treatment of diabetic ketoacidosis. In children, hypophosphatemia can suppress normal growth.

Increased levels (hyperphosphatemia) may result from skeletal disease, healing fractures, hypoparathyroidism, acromegaly, diabetic ketoacidosis, high intestinal obstruction, and renal failure. Hyperphosphatemia is seldom clinically significant, but it can alter bone metabolism in prolonged cases.

Interfering factors
• Venous stasis due to tourniquet use
• Sample obtained above an I.V. site that's receiving a solution containing phosphate
• Excessive vitamin D intake or therapy with anabolic steroids or androgens (possible increase)
• Use of acetazolamide, insulin, epinephrine, or phosphate-binding antacids; excessive excretion due to prolonged vomiting or diarrhea; vitamin D deficiency; extended I.V. infusion of dextrose 5% in water (possible decrease)
• Hemolysis of the sample (false-high)

POTASSIUM

This test is used to measure serum levels of potassium, the major intracellular cation. Potassium helps to maintain cellular osmotic equilibrium and to regulate muscle activity, enzyme activity, and acid-base balance. It also influences renal function.

The body has no efficient method for conserving potassium; the kidneys excrete nearly all ingested potassium, even when the body's supply is depleted. Potassium deficiency can develop rapidly and is quite common. Dietary intake of at least 40 mEq/day is essential.

Purpose
● To evaluate clinical signs of potassium excess (hyperkalemia) or potassium depletion (hypokalemia)
● To monitor renal function, acid-base balance, and glucose metabolism
● To evaluate neuromuscular and endocrine disorders
● To detect the origin of arrhythmias

Patient preparation
● Explain to the patient that this test is used to determine the potassium content of blood.
● Tell him that the test requires a blood sample. Explain who will perform the venipuncture and when.
● Explain that he may experience slight discomfort from the needle puncture and the tourniquet but that collecting the sample usually takes less than 3 minutes.
● Inform him that he needn't restrict food or fluids before the test.
● Check the patient's history for use of drugs that may influence test results. They include diuretics, penicillin G potassium, amphotericin B, methi-

cillin, tetracycline, insulin, and glucose. If these medications must be continued, note this on the laboratory slip.

Procedure and posttest care
● Perform a venipuncture, and collect the sample in a 7-ml *red-top* or *red-marble-top* tube.
● If a hematoma develops at the venipuncture site, apply warm soaks.

Precautions
● Draw the sample immediately after applying the tourniquet because a delay may increase the potassium level by allowing intracellular potassium to leak into the serum.
● Handle the sample gently to avoid hemolysis.

Reference values
Normally, serum potassium levels range from 3.8 to 5.5 mEq/L.

Abnormal findings
Abnormally high serum potassium levels are common in conditions in which excess cellular potassium enters the blood, such as burn injuries, crush injuries, diabetic ketoacidosis, and myocardial infarction. Hyperkalemia may also indicate reduced sodium excretion, possibly due to renal failure (preventing normal exchange of sodium and potassium) or Addison's disease (due to potassium buildup and sodium depletion).

CLINICAL ALERT Observe a patient with hyperkalemia for weakness, malaise, nausea, diarrhea, colicky pain, muscle irritability progressing to flaccid paralysis, oliguria, and bradycardia. The electrocardiogram (ECG) reveals a prolonged PR interval; wide QRS complex; tall, tented T wave; and ST-segment depression. Cardiac arrest may occur without warning.

Below-normal potassium values often result from aldosteronism or Cushing's syndrome, loss of body fluids (as in long-term diuretic therapy), and excessive licorice ingestion. Although serum values and clinical symptoms can indicate a potassium imbalance, an ECG allows a definitive diagnosis.

▶ **CLINICAL ALERT** Observe a patient with hypokalemia for decreased reflexes; a rapid, weak, irregular pulse; mental confusion; hypotension; anorexia; muscle weakness; and paresthesia. ECG shows a flattened T wave, ST-segment depression, and U wave elevation. In severe cases, ventricular fibrillation, respiratory paralysis, and cardiac arrest can develop.

Interfering factors
● Repeated clenching of the fist before venipuncture (possible increase)
● Delay in drawing blood after applying a tourniquet or excessive hemolysis of the sample (increase)
● Excessive or rapid potassium infusion, spironolactone or penicillin G potassium therapy, and renal toxicity from administration of amphotericin B, methicillin, or tetracycline (increase)
● Insulin and glucose administration; diuretic therapy (especially with thiazides but not with triamterene, amiloride, or spironolactone); I.V. infusions without potassium (decrease)

SODIUM

This test is used to measure serum levels of sodium in relation to the amount of water in the body. Sodium, the major extracellular cation, affects body water distribution, maintains osmotic pressure of extracellular fluid, and helps promote neuromuscular function. It also helps maintain acid-base balance and influences chloride and potassium levels.

Purpose
● To evaluate fluid-electrolyte and acid-base balance and related neuromuscular, renal, and adrenal functions

Patient preparation
● Explain to the patient that this test is used to determine the sodium content of blood.
● Tell him that the test requires a blood sample. Explain who will perform the venipuncture and when.
● Explain that he may experience slight discomfort from the needle puncture and the tourniquet but that collecting the sample usually takes less than 3 minutes.
● Inform him that he needn't restrict food or fluids before the test.
● Check the patient's medication history for use of drugs that influence sodium levels, including most diuretics, lithium, chlorpropamide, vasopressin, corticosteroids, and antihypertensives (such as methyldopa, hydralazine, and reserpine). If these medications must be continued, note this on the laboratory slip.

Procedure and posttest care
● Perform a venipuncture, and collect the sample in a 7-ml *red-top* or *red-marble-top* tube.
● If a hematoma develops at the venipuncture site, apply warm soaks.

Precautions
● Handle the sample gently to prevent hemolysis.

Reference values
Normally, serum sodium levels range from 135 to 145 mEq/L.

Abnormal findings

Sodium imbalance can result from a loss or gain of sodium or from a change in the patient's state of hydration. Increased serum sodium levels (hypernatremia) may be due to inadequate water intake, water loss in excess of sodium (as in diabetes insipidus, impaired renal function, prolonged hyperventilation and, occasionally, severe vomiting or diarrhea), and sodium retention (as in aldosteronism). Hypernatremia can also result from excessive sodium intake.

CLINICAL ALERT In a patient with hypernatremia and associated loss of water, observe for signs of thirst, restlessness, dry and sticky mucous membranes, flushed skin, oliguria, and diminished reflexes. If increased total body sodium causes water retention, observe for hypertension, dyspnea, edema, and heart failure.

Abnormally low serum sodium levels (hyponatremia) may result from inadequate sodium intake or excessive sodium loss due to profuse sweating, GI suctioning, diuretic therapy, diarrhea, vomiting, adrenal insufficiency, burns, and chronic renal insufficiency with acidosis. Urine sodium determinations are usually more sensitive to early changes in sodium balance and should be evaluated simultaneously with serum sodium findings.

CLINICAL ALERT In a patient with hyponatremia, watch for apprehension, lassitude, headache, decreased skin turgor, abdominal cramps, and tremors that may progress to seizures.

Interfering factors

- Hemolysis due to rough handling of the sample
- Most diuretics (decrease by promoting sodium excretion)
- Lithium, chlorpropamide, and vasopressin (decrease by inhibiting water excretion)
- Corticosteroids (increase by promoting sodium retention)
- Antihypertensives, such as methyldopa, hydralazine, and reserpine (possible increase due to sodium and water retention)
- Continuous infusion of normal saline solution (increase)
- Infusion of dextrose 5% in water (decrease)
- High triglyceride or low protein levels (false-low)

ANION GAP

Total concentrations of cations and anions are normally equal, making serum electrically neutral. Measuring the gap between measured cation and anion levels provides information about the level of anions (including sulfate, phosphate, organic acids such as ketone bodies and lactic acid, and proteins) that are not routinely measured in laboratory tests. In metabolic acidosis, measuring the anion gap helps to identify the type of acidosis and possible causes. Further tests are usually needed to determine the specific cause of metabolic acidosis.

Purpose

- To distinguish types of metabolic acidosis
- To monitor renal function and total parenteral nutrition

Patient preparation

- Explain to the patient that this test is used to determine the cause of acidosis.

- Tell him that the test requires a blood sample. Explain who will perform the venipuncture and when.
- Explain that he may experience slight discomfort from the needle puncture and the tourniquet but that collecting the sample usually takes less than 3 minutes.
- Inform him that he needn't restrict food or fluids before the test.
- Check the patient's history for use of medications that may influence sodium, chloride, and bicarbonate blood levels (such as diuretics, corticosteroids, and antihypertensives). If these medications must be continued, note this on the laboratory slip.

Procedure and posttest care
- Perform a venipuncture, and collect the sample in a 7-ml *red-top* or *red-marble-top* tube.
- If a hematoma develops at the venipuncture site, apply warm soaks.
- Instruct the patient to resume use of medications discontinued before the test.

Precautions
- Handle the sample gently to prevent hemolysis.

Reference values
Normally, the anion gap is at least 12 mEq/L.

Abnormal findings
A normal anion gap does not rule out metabolic acidosis. It may occur in hyperchloremic acidoses, renal tubular acidosis, and severe bicarbonate-wasting conditions, such as biliary or pancreatic fistulas and poorly functioning ileal loops.

When acidosis results from loss of bicarbonate in the urine or other body fluids, the anion gap remains unchanged. This is known as *normal anion gap acidosis.*

An increased anion gap indicates an increase in one or more of the unmeasured anions (sulfate, phosphates, organic acids such as ketone bodies and lactic acid, and proteins). This may occur with acidoses that are characterized by excessive organic or inorganic acids, such as lactic acidosis or ketoacidosis.

When acidosis results from an accumulation of metabolic acids — as occurs in lactic acidosis, for example — the anion gap increases (above 12 mEq/L) with the increase in unmeasured anions. Metabolic acidosis caused by such an accumulation is known as *high anion gap acidosis.*

A decreased anion gap is rare but may occur with hypermagnesemia and paraproteinemic states, such as multiple myeloma and Waldenström's macroglobulinemia.

Interfering factors
- Hemolysis due to rough handling of the sample
- Diuretics, lithium, chlorpropamide, and vasopressin (possible decrease due to decreased serum sodium levels)
- Corticosteroids and antihypertensives (possible increase due to increased serum sodium levels)
- Salicylates, paraldehyde, methicillin, dimercaprol, ammonium chloride, acetazolamide, ethylene glycol, and methyl alcohol (possible increase due to decreased serum bicarbonate levels)
- Corticotropin, cortisone, mercurial or chlorthiazide diuretics, and excessive ingestion of alkalis or licorice (possible decrease due to increased serum bicarbonate levels)
- Ammonium chloride, cholestyramine, boric acid, oxyphenbutazone, phenylbutazone, and excessive I.V. infusion of sodium chloride (possible decrease due to increased serum chloride levels)

• Thiazide diuretics, ethacrynic acid, furosemide, bicarbonates, and prolonged I.V. infusion of dextrose 5% in water (possible increase due to decreased serum chloride levels)
• Iodine absorption from wounds packed with povidone-iodine or excessive use of magnesium-containing antacids, especially by patients with renal failure (possible false-low)

CARDIAC ENZYMES AND PROTEINS

CREATINE KINASE

Creatine kinase (CK) is an enzyme that catalyzes the creatine-creatinine metabolic pathway in muscle cells and brain tissue. Because of its intimate role in energy production, CK reflects normal tissue catabolism; increased serum levels indicate trauma to cells.

Fractionation and measurement of three distinct CK isoenzymes — CK-BB (CK_1), CK-MB (CK_2), and CK-MM (CK_3) — have replaced the use of total CK levels to accurately localize the site of increased tissue destruction. CK-BB is most often found in brain tissue. CK-MM and CK-MB are found primarily in skeletal and heart muscle. In addition, subunits of CK-MB and CK-MM, called isoforms or isoenzymes, can be assayed to increase the test's sensitivity.

Purpose

• To detect and diagnose acute myocardial infarction (MI) and reinfarction (CK-MB primarily used)
• To evaluate possible causes of chest pain and to monitor the severity of

myocardial ischemia after cardiac surgery, cardiac catheterization, and cardioversion (CK-MB primarily used)
• To detect musculoskeletal disorders that are not neurogenic in origin, such as Duchenne muscular dystrophy (total CK primarily used), rhabdomyolysis, and early dermatomyositis

Patient preparation

• Explain to the patient that this test is used to assess myocardial and musculoskeletal function and that multiple blood samples are required to detect fluctuations in serum levels.
• Tell him who will perform the venipunctures and when.
• Explain that he may experience some discomfort from the needle or tourniquet but that collecting each sample usually takes less than 3 minutes.
• Inform him that he needn't restrict food or most fluids before the test.
• If the patient is being evaluated for musculoskeletal disorders, advise him to avoid exercising for 24 hours before the test.
• Before the test, withhold alcohol, aminocaproic acid, and lithium. If these substances must be continued, note this on the laboratory slip.

Procedure and posttest care

• Perform a venipuncture, and collect the sample in a 7-ml *red-top* tube.
• If a hematoma develops at the venipuncture site, apply warm soaks.
• Instruct the patient that he can resume exercising and the use of substances discontinued before the test.

Precautions

• Draw the sample before giving or 1 hour after giving I.M. injections because muscle trauma increases total CK level.
• Obtain the sample on schedule. Note on the laboratory slip the time the sam-

SERUM ENZYME AND ISOENZYME LEVELS AFTER MI

Because they're released by damaged tissue, serum enzymes and isoenzymes (catalytic proteins that vary in concentration in specific organs) can help identify the compromised organ and assess the extent of damage. The serum enzyme and isoenzyme determinations listed below are most significant in myocardial infarction (MI).

Isoenzymes
• Creatine kinase-MB (CK-MB): in the heart muscle and a small amount in skeletal muscle
• Lactate dehydrogenase 1 and 2 (LD_1, LD_2): in the heart, brain, kidneys, liver, skeletal muscles, and red blood cells (RBCs)

Enzymes
• Hydroxybutyric dehydrogenase (HBD): an indirect measurement of LD_1, LD_2
• Aspartate aminotransferase (AST): heart muscle and liver and less extensively in skeletal muscle, kidneys, pancreas, and RBCs

ple was drawn and the hours elapsed since onset of chest pain.
• Handle the sample gently to prevent hemolysis.
• Send the sample to the laboratory immediately because CK activity diminishes significantly after 2 hours at room temperature.

Reference values
Total CK values determined by ultraviolet or kinetic measurement range from 40 to 175 U/L for men and from 25 to 140 U/L for women. CK levels may be significantly higher in muscular people. Infants up to age 1 have levels two to four times higher than adult levels, possibly reflecting birth trauma and striated muscle develop-

ment. Normal ranges for isoenzyme levels are as follows: CK-BB, undetectable; CK-MB, undetectable to 7 U/L; CK-MM, 5 to 7 U/L.

Abnormal findings

CK-MM makes up 99% of total CK normally present in serum. Detectable CK-BB isoenzyme may indicate but does not confirm a diagnosis of brain tissue injury, widespread malignant tumors, severe shock, or renal failure.

CK-MB levels greater than 5% of total CK (or more than 10 U/L) indicate MI, especially if the lactate dehydrogenase isoenzyme ratio (LD_1/LD_2) is greater than 1 (flipped LD). In acute MI and after cardiac surgery, CK-MB begins to increase within 2 to 4 hours, peaks within 12 to 24 hours, and usually returns to normal within 24 to 48 hours; persistent elevations and increasing levels indicate ongoing myocardial damage. Total CK follows roughly the same pattern but increases slightly later. CK-MB levels may not increase in heart failure or during angina pectoris not accompanied by myocardial cell necrosis. Serious skeletal muscle injury that occurs in certain muscular dystrophies, polymyositis, and severe myoglobinuria may produce a mild CK-MB increase because a small amount of this isoenzyme is present in some skeletal muscles.

Increasing CK-MM values follow skeletal muscle damage from trauma, such as surgery and I.M. injections, and from diseases, such as dermatomyositis and muscular dystrophy (values may be 50 to 100 times normal). A moderate increase in CK-MM levels develops in patients with hypothyroidism; sharp increases occur with muscle activity caused by agitation, such as during an acute psychotic episode.

Total CK levels may be increased in patients with severe hypokalemia, carbon monoxide poisoning, malignant hyperthermia, and alcoholic cardiomyopathy. They may also be increased after seizures and, occasionally, in patients who have suffered pulmonary or cerebral infarctions. (See *Serum enzyme and isoenzyme levels after MI.*)

Interfering factors

● Hemolysis due to rough handling of the sample

● Failure to send the sample to the laboratory immediately or to refrigerate the serum if testing will be delayed more than 2 hours (possible decrease in concentration)

● Failure to draw the samples at the scheduled time (may miss peak levels)

● Halothane and succinylcholine, alcohol, lithium, large doses of aminocaproic acid, I.M. injections, cardioversion, invasive diagnostic procedures, recent vigorous exercise or muscle massage, severe coughing, and trauma (increase in total CK)

● Surgery through skeletal muscle (increase in total CK)

LACTATE DEHYDROGENASE

Lactate dehydrogenase (LD) catalyzes the reversible conversion of muscle lactic acid into pyruvic acid, an essential step in the metabolic processes that ultimately produce cellular energy. Because LD is present in almost all body tissues, cellular damage increases total serum LD, limiting the diagnostic usefulness of LD.

Five tissue-specific isoenzymes can be identified and measured: LD_1 and LD_2 appear primarily in the heart, red blood cells (RBCs), and kidneys; LD_3 is primarily in the lungs; and LD_4 and

LD_5 are in the liver, skin, and the skeletal muscles.

Purpose
● To aid differential diagnosis of myocardial infarction (MI), pulmonary infarction, anemias, and hepatic disease
● To support creatine kinase (CK) isoenzyme test results in diagnosing MI, or to provide diagnosis when CK-MB samples are drawn too late to display increase
● To monitor patient response to some forms of chemotherapy

Patient preparation
● Explain to the patient that this test is used primarily to detect tissue alterations.
● Tell him that the test requires a blood sample. Explain who will perform the venipuncture and when.
● Explain that he may experience slight discomfort from the needle puncture and the tourniquet but that collecting the sample usually takes less than 3 minutes.
● Inform him that he needn't restrict food or fluids before the test.
● If MI is suspected, tell him that the test will be repeated on the next two mornings to monitor progressive changes.

Procedure and posttest care
● Perform a venipuncture, and collect the sample in a 7-ml *red-top* tube.
● If a hematoma develops at the venipuncture site, apply warm soaks.

Precautions
● Draw the samples on schedule to avoid missing peak levels, and mark the collection time on the laboratory slip.
● Handle the sample gently to prevent artifact blood sample hemolysis because RBCs contain LD_1.

● Send the sample to the laboratory immediately or, if transport is delayed, keep the sample at room temperature. Changes in temperature reportedly inactivate LD_5, thus altering isoenzyme patterns.

Reference values
Total LD levels normally range from 94 to 257 U/L in adults and from 108 to 540 U/L in children. Normal distribution is as follows:
● LD_1: 17.5% to 28.3% of total
● LD_2: 30.4% to 36.4% of total
● LD_3: 19.2% to 24.8% of total
● LD_4: 9.6% to 15.6% of total
● LD_5: 5.5% to 12.7% of total.

Abnormal findings
Because many common diseases increase total LD levels, isoenzyme electrophoresis is usually necessary for diagnosis. In some disorders, total LD may be within normal limits, but abnormal proportions of each enzyme indicate specific organ tissue damage. For instance, in acute MI, the LD_1/LD_2 isoenzyme ratio is typically greater than 1 within 12 to 48 hours after onset of symptoms (known as flipped LD).

Midzone fractions (LD_2, LD_3, LD_4) can be increased in granulocytic leukemia, lymphomas, and platelet disorders.

Interfering factors
● Hemolysis due to rough handling of the sample
● For diagnosis of acute MI, failure to draw the sample on schedule
● Failure to send the sample to the laboratory immediately (may obscure LD isoenzyme patterns)
● Failure to centrifuge the sample and separate the cells from the serum
● Recent surgery or pregnancy (possible increase)
● Prosthetic heart valve (possible increase due to chronic hemolysis)

• Anabolic steroids, anesthetics, alcohol, narcotics, and procainamide (increase)

MYOGLOBINS

Myoglobin, which is normally found in skeletal and cardiac muscle, functions as an oxygen-binding muscle protein. It's released into the bloodstream in ischemia, trauma, and inflammation of the muscle.

Purpose
• As a nonspecific test, to estimate damage to skeletal or cardiac muscle tissue
• To predict flareups of polymyositis
• Specifically, to determine if myocardial infarction (MI) has occurred

Patient preparation
• Explain the purpose of the test to the patient.
• Obtain a patient history, including disorders that may be associated with increased myoglobin levels.
• Tell the patient who will perform the venipuncture and when. Explain that he may experience slight discomfort from the needle puncture and the tourniquet but that collecting the sample usually takes less than 3 minutes.
• Inform the patient that the results need to be correlated with other tests for a definitive diagnosis.

Procedure and posttest care
• Perform a venipuncture, and collect the sample in a 5-ml *red-top* tube.
• If a hematoma develops at the venipuncture site, apply warm soaks.

Precautions
• Expect to collect blood samples 4 to 8 hours after the onset of an acute MI.

• Handle the sample gently to avoid hemolysis.
• Send the sample to the laboratory immediately.

Reference values
Normal myoglobin values are 0 to 0.09 µg/ml.

Abnormal findings
Besides MI, increased myoglobin levels may occur in acute alcohol intoxication, dermatomyositis, hypothermia (with prolonged shivering), muscular dystrophy, polymyositis, severe burn injuries, trauma, severe renal failure, and systemic lupus erythematosus.

Interfering factors
• Hemolysis or radioactive scans performed within 1 week of the test
• Recent angina, cardioversion, or improper timing of the test (possible increase)
• I.M. injection (possible false-positive)

HEPATIC ENZYMES AND PROTEINS

ALPHA$_1$-ANTITRYPSIN

A protein produced by the liver, alpha$_1$-antitrypsin (also known as AAT or α_1-AT) is believed to inhibit the release of protease into body fluids by dying cells and is a major component of alpha$_1$-globulin. AAT is measured using radioimmunoassay or isoelectric focusing. Congenital absence or deficiency of AAT has been linked to high susceptibility to emphysema.

Purpose

● To screen for high-risk emphysema patients

● As a nonspecific method of detecting inflammation, severe infection, and necrosis

● To test for congenital AAT deficiency

Patient preparation

● Explain to the patient that this test is used to diagnose respiratory or liver disease as well as inflammation, infection, or necrosis.

● Tell the patient to avoid smoking because irritants in tobacco stimulate leukocytes in the lungs to release protease.

● Tell the patient to avoid oral contraceptives and steroids for 24 hours before the test.

● Tell the patient to fast for at least 8 hours before the test.

● Tell the patient who will perform the venipuncture and when.

● Explain that he may experience slight discomfort from the needle puncture and the tourniquet but that collecting the sample usually takes less than 3 minutes.

Procedure and posttest care

● Perform a venipuncture, and collect the sample in a 7-ml *red-top* tube.

Precautions

● Handle the sample gently to avoid hemolysis.

● Send the sample to the laboratory promptly.

● If clinically indicated, patients with AAT levels lower than 125 mg/dl should be phenotyped to confirm homozygous and heterozygous deficiencies. (Heterozygous patients don't seem to be at increased risk for early emphysema.)

Reference values

AAT levels vary by age, but the normal range is 110 to 200 mg/dl.

Abnormal findings

Decreased AAT levels may occur in early-onset emphysema and cirrhosis, nephrotic syndrome, malnutrition, congenital alpha$_1$-globulin deficiency and, transiently, in the neonate.

Increased AAT levels can occur in chronic inflammatory disorders, necrosis, pregnancy, acute pulmonary infections, hyaline membrane disease in infants, hepatitis, systemic lupus erythematosus, and rheumatoid arthritis.

Interfering factors

● Oral contraceptives and steroids (possible false-high)

● Failure to fast for 8 hours before the test (possible false-high)

● Smoking

ASPARTATE AMINOTRANSFERASE

Aspartate aminotransferase (AST) is one of two enzymes that catalyze the conversion of the nitrogenous portion of an amino acid to an amino acid residue. It is essential to energy production in the Krebs cycle. AST is found in the cytoplasm and mitochondria of many cells, primarily in the liver, heart, skeletal muscles, kidneys, pancreas, and red blood cells. It's released into serum in proportion to cellular damage. The change in AST values over time is a reliable monitoring mechanism.

Purpose

● To aid detection and differential diagnosis of acute hepatic disease

• To monitor patient progress and prognosis in cardiac and hepatic diseases

• To aid diagnosis of myocardial infarction in correlation with creatine kinase and lactate dehydrogenase levels

Patient preparation

• Explain to the patient that this test is used to assess heart and liver function.

• Inform him that the test usually requires three venipunctures on 3 consecutive days.

• Tell the patient that he needn't restrict food or fluids.

• Reassure him that discomfort from the needle puncture and the tourniquet is transient and that collecting each sample takes less than 3 minutes.

• Withhold morphine, codeine, meperidine, chlorpropamide, methyldopa, and antitubercular drugs (isoniazid, para-aminosalicylates, and pyrazinamide). If these medications must be continued, note this on the laboratory slip.

Procedure and posttest care

• Perform a venipuncture, and collect the sample in a 7-ml *red-top* tube.

• If a hematoma develops, apply warm soaks.

• Instruct the patient to resume medications discontinued before the test.

Precautions

• To avoid missing peak AST levels, draw serum samples at the same time each day.

• Handle the sample gently to prevent hemolysis, and send it to the laboratory immediately.

Reference values

AST levels range from 5 to 40 U/L. Normal values for infants are as high as four times those of adults.

Abnormal findings

AST levels fluctuate in response to the extent of cellular necrosis, being transiently and minimally increased early in the disease process and extremely increased during the most acute phase. Depending on when the initial sample is drawn, AST levels may increase, indicating increasing disease severity and tissue damage, or decrease, indicating disease resolution and tissue repair.

Maximum elevations (more than 20 times normal) may indicate acute viral hepatitis, severe skeletal muscle trauma, extensive surgery, drug-induced hepatic injury, or severe passive liver congestion.

High levels (10 to 20 times normal) may indicate severe myocardial infarction, severe infectious mononucleosis, or alcoholic cirrhosis. High levels also occur during the prodromal or resolving stages of conditions that cause maximum elevations.

Moderate to high levels (5 to 10 times normal) may indicate dermatomyositis, Duchenne's muscular dystrophy, or chronic hepatitis. Moderate to high levels also occur during prodromal and resolving stages of diseases that cause high elevations.

Low to moderate levels (2 to 5 times normal) occur at some time during the preceding conditions or diseases or may indicate hemolytic anemia, metastatic hepatic tumors, acute pancreatitis, pulmonary emboli, delirium tremens, or fatty liver. AST levels rise slightly after the first few days of biliary duct obstruction.

Interfering factors

• Hemolysis due to rough handling of the sample

• Failure to draw the sample as scheduled (may miss peak)

• Chlorpropamide, opioids, methyldopa, erythromycin, sulfonamides, pyridoxine, dicumarol, and antitubercular agents; large doses of acetaminophen, salicylates, or vitamin A; and many other drugs known to affect the liver (increase)

● Strenuous exercise and muscle trauma due to I.M. injections (increase)

ALANINE AMINOTRANSFERASE

This test is used to measure serum levels of alanine aminotransferase (ALT), one of two enzymes that catalyze a reversible amino group transfer reaction in the Krebs cycle. ALT is necessary for tissue energy production. ALT is found primarily in the liver, with lesser amounts in the kidneys, heart, and skeletal muscles, and is a sensitive indicator of acute hepatocellular disease.

Purpose
● To detect and evaluate treatment of acute hepatic disease, especially hepatitis and cirrhosis without jaundice
● To distinguish between myocardial and hepatic tissue damage (used with aspartate aminotransferase)
● To assess hepatotoxicity of some drugs

Patient preparation
● Explain to the patient that this test is used to assess liver function.
● Tell him that the test requires a blood sample. Explain who will perform the venipuncture and when.
● Explain that he may experience slight discomfort from the needle puncture and the tourniquet but that collecting the sample usually takes less than 3 minutes.

● Inform him that he needn't restrict food or fluids before the test.
● Withhold hepatotoxic and cholestatic drugs, such as methotrexate, chlorpromazine, salicylates, and narcotic analgesics. If these medications must be continued, note this on the laboratory slip.

Procedure and posttest care
● Perform a venipuncture, and collect the sample in a 7-ml *red-top* tube.
● If a hematoma develops at the venipuncture site, apply warm soaks.
● Resume administration of medications that were withheld before the test.

Precautions
● Handle the sample gently to prevent hemolysis.
● ALT activity is stable in serum for up to 3 days at room temperature.

Reference values
Serum ALT levels range from 7 to 56 U/L.

Abnormal findings
Very high ALT levels (up to 50 times normal) suggest viral or severe drug-induced hepatitis or other hepatic disease with extensive necrosis. Moderate to high levels may indicate infectious mononucleosis, chronic hepatitis, intrahepatic cholestasis or cholecystitis, early or improving acute viral hepatitis, or severe hepatic congestion due to heart failure.

Slight to moderate elevations of ALT may appear in any condition that produces acute hepatocellular injury, such as active cirrhosis and drug-induced or alcoholic hepatitis. Marginal elevations occasionally occur in acute myocardial infarction, reflecting secondary hepatic congestion or the release of small amounts of ALT from myocardial tissue.

Interfering factors

• Hemolysis due to rough handling of the sample

• Barbiturates, griseofulvin, isoniazid, nitrofurantoin, methyldopa, phenothiazines, phenytoin, salicylates, methotrexate, tetracycline, chlorpromazine, para-aminosalicylic acid, and other drugs that cause hepatic injury by competitively interfering with cellular metabolism (false-high)

• Narcotic analgesics, such as morphine, codeine, and meperidine (possible false-high due to increased intrabiliary pressure)

• Ingestion of lead or exposure to carbon tetrachloride (sharp increase due to direct injury to hepatic cells)

ALKALINE PHOSPHATASE

This test is used to measure serum levels of alkaline phosphatase (ALP), an enzyme that influences bone calcification as well as lipid and metabolite transport. ALP measurements reflect the combined activity of several ALP isoenzymes found in the liver, bones, kidneys, intestinal lining, and placenta. Bone and liver ALP are always present in adult serum, with liver ALP most prominent except during the third trimester of pregnancy (when the placenta originates about half of all ALP). The intestinal variant of ALP can be a normal component (in less than 10% of normal patterns; almost exclusively in the sera of blood groups B and O), or it can be an abnormal finding associated with hepatic disease.

Purpose

• To detect and identify skeletal diseases primarily characterized by marked osteoblastic activity

• To detect focal hepatic lesions causing biliary obstruction, such as tumor or abscess

• To assess response to vitamin D in the treatment of rickets

• To supplement information from other liver function studies and GI enzyme tests; additional liver function studies are usually required to identify hepatobiliary disorders

Patient preparation

• Explain to the patient that this test is used to assess liver and bone function.

• Instruct him to fast for at least 8 hours before the test because fat intake stimulates intestinal ALP secretion.

• Tell him that this test requires a blood sample. Explain who will perform the venipuncture and when.

• Inform the patient that he may experience slight discomfort from the needle puncture and the tourniquet but that collecting the sample usually takes less than 3 minutes.

Procedure and posttest care

• Perform a venipuncture, and collect the sample in a 7-ml *red-top* tube.

• If a hematoma develops at the venipuncture site, apply warm soaks.

• Tell the patient that he may resume his usual diet.

Precautions

• Handle the sample gently to prevent hemolysis.

• Send the sample to the laboratory immediately; ALP activity increases at room temperature because of a rise in pH.

Reference values

Total ALP levels, when measured by chemical inhibition, range from 98 to

251 U/L for men ages 19 and older. For women ages 24 to 45, total ALP levels range from 81 to 213 U/L; for women over age 45, the range widens to 84 to 309 U/L.

Abnormal findings

Although significant ALP elevations are possible with diseases that affect many organs, they usually indicate skeletal disease or extrahepatic or intrahepatic biliary obstruction causing cholestasis. Many acute hepatic diseases cause ALP elevations before they affect serum bilirubin levels.

Moderate increases in ALP levels may reflect acute biliary obstruction from hepatocellular inflammation in active cirrhosis, mononucleosis, and viral hepatitis. Moderate increases are also seen in osteomalacia and deficiency-induced rickets.

CLINICAL ALERT Sharp elevations of ALP levels may indicate complete biliary obstruction by malignant or infectious infiltrations or fibrosis, most common in Paget's disease and, occasionally, in biliary obstruction, extensive bone metastasis, and hyperparathyroidism. Metastatic bone tumors resulting from pancreatic cancer raise ALP levels without a concomitant rise in serum alanine aminotransferase levels.

Isoenzyme fractionation and additional enzyme tests (gamma glutamyl transferase, lactate dehydrogenase, 5'-nucleotidase, and leucine aminopeptidase) are sometimes performed when the cause of ALP elevations is in doubt. Rarely, low levels of serum ALP are associated with hypophosphatasia and protein or magnesium deficiency.

Interfering factors

• Hemolysis due to rough handling of the sample
• Failure to analyze the sample within 4 hours

• Recent ingestion of vitamin D (possible increase due to effect on osteoblastic activity)
• Recent infusion of albumin prepared from placental venous blood (marked increase)
• Drugs that influence liver function or cause cholestasis, such as barbiturates, chlorpropamide, oral contraceptives, isoniazid, methyldopa, phenothiazines, phenytoin, and rifampin (possible mild increase)
• Halothane sensitivity (possible drastic increase)
• Clofibrate (decrease)
• Healing long-bone fractures and third trimester of pregnancy (possible increase)
• Age and sex (increase in infants, children, adolescents, and women over age 45)

LEUCINE AMINOPEPTIDASE

This test is used to measure serum levels of leucine aminopeptidase (LAP), an isoenzyme of alkaline phosphatase (ALP) that is widely distributed in body tissues. The greatest concentrations appear in the hepatobiliary tissues, pancreas, and small intestine. Serum levels of LAP parallel serum ALP levels in hepatic disease.

Purpose

• To provide information about suspected liver, pancreatic, and biliary diseases
• To differentiate skeletal disease from hepatobiliary or pancreatic disease
• To evaluate neonatal jaundice

Patient preparation

- Explain to the patient that this test is used to evaluate liver and pancreatic function.
- Tell him to fast for at least 8 hours before the test.
- Instruct the patient to stop taking drugs containing estrogen and progesterone.
- Tell the patient that this test requires a blood sample. Explain who will perform the venipuncture and when.
- Explain that he may experience slight discomfort from the needle puncture and the tourniquet but that collecting the sample usually takes less than 3 minutes.

Procedure and posttest care

- Perform a venipuncture, and collect the sample in a 7-ml *red-top* tube.
- Tell the patient that he may resume his usual diet and medications.

Precautions

- Handle the sample gently to avoid hemolysis.
- Transport the sample to the laboratory immediately.

Reference values

Normal values are 80 to 200 U/ml in men and 75 to 185 U/ml in women.

Abnormal findings

Elevated levels can occur in biliary obstruction, tumors, strictures, and atresia; advanced pregnancy; and therapy with drugs containing estrogen or progesterone.

Interfering factors

- Advanced pregnancy (false-high)
- Estrogen or progesterone (false-high)

GAMMA GLUTAMYL TRANSFERASE

Also called gamma glutamyl transpeptidase, gamma glutamyl transferase (GGT) participates in the transfer of amino acids across cellular membranes and, possibly, in glutathione metabolism. The highest concentrations of GGT exist in the renal tubules, but the enzyme also appears in the liver, biliary tract epithelium, pancreas, lymphocytes, brain, and testes. This test is used to measure serum GGT levels.

Purpose

- To provide information about hepatobiliary diseases, to assess liver function, and to detect alcohol ingestion
- To distinguish between skeletal disease and hepatic disease when serum alkaline phosphatase level is elevated (a normal GGT level suggests that such elevation stems from skeletal disease)

Patient preparation

- Explain to the patient that this test is used to evaluate liver function.
- Tell him that the test requires a blood sample. Explain who will perform the venipuncture and when.
- Explain that he may experience slight discomfort from the needle puncture and the tourniquet but that collecting the sample usually takes less than 3 minutes.
- Inform him that he needn't restrict food or fluids before the test.

Procedure and posttest care

- Perform a venipuncture, and collect the sample in a 7-ml *red-top* tube.
- If a hematoma develops, apply warm soaks.

Precautions
- Handle the sample gently to prevent hemolysis.
- GGT activity is stable in serum at room temperature for 2 days.

Reference values
Serum GGT values vary with the assay method used (kinetic or end-point method). Normal levels range from 7 to 48 U/L in males and from 6 to 29 U/L in females.

Abnormal findings
Serum GGT levels rise in any acute hepatic disease because enzyme production increases in response to hepatocellular injury. Moderate increases occur in acute pancreatitis, renal disease, and prostatic metastases; postoperatively; and in some patients with epilepsy or brain tumors. Levels also increase after alcohol ingestion because of enzyme induction. The sharpest elevations occur in patients with obstructive jaundice and hepatic metastatic infiltrations.

GGT levels may also increase 5 to 10 days after acute myocardial infarction, either as a result of tissue granulation and healing or as an indication of the effects of cardiac insufficiency on the liver.

Interfering factors
- Hemolysis due to rough handling of the sample
- Clofibrate, oral contraceptives, and late pregnancy (decrease)
- Aminoglycosides, barbiturates, and phenytoin (increase)
- Moderate intake of alcohol (increase for at least 60 hours)

5'-NUCLEOTIDASE

The enzyme 5'-nucleotidase (5'NT) is a phosphatase formed almost entirely in the hepatobiliary tract. Unlike alkaline phosphatase (ALP), it hydrolyzes nucleoside 5'-phosphate groups only. Measurement of serum 5'NT levels helps to determine whether ALP elevation is due to skeletal or hepatic disease. Because 5'NT remains normal in skeletal disease and pregnancy, it's more specific for assessing hepatic dysfunction than ALP or leucine aminopeptidase.

Purpose
- To distinguish between hepatobiliary and skeletal disease when the source of increased ALP levels is uncertain
- To help differentiate biliary obstruction from acute hepatocellular damage
- To detect hepatic metastasis in the absence of jaundice

Patient preparation
- Explain to the patient that this test is used to evaluate liver function.
- Tell him that the test requires a blood sample. Explain who will perform the venipuncture and when.
- Explain that he may experience slight discomfort from the needle puncture and the tourniquet but that collecting the sample usually takes less than 3 minutes.
- Tell him that he needn't restrict food or fluids before the test.

Procedure and posttest care
- Perform a venipuncture, and collect the sample in a 7-ml *red-top* tube.
- If a hematoma develops at the venipuncture site, apply warm soaks.

Precautions
● Handle the sample gently to prevent hemolysis.

Reference values
Serum 5'NT values for adults range from 4 to 11.5 U/L; values for children may be lower.

Abnormal findings
Extremely high levels of 5'NT occur in common bile duct obstruction by calculi or tumors in diseases that cause severe intrahepatic cholestasis, such as neoplastic infiltrations of the liver. Slight to moderate increases may reflect acute hepatocellular damage or active cirrhosis.

Interfering factors
● Hemolysis due to rough handling of the sample
● Cholestatic drugs, such as phenothiazines, morphine, meperidine, and codeine (increase)

PANCREATIC ENZYMES

AMYLASE

An enzyme that is synthesized primarily in the pancreas and salivary glands, amylase (alpha-amylase or AML) helps to digest starch and glycogen in the mouth, stomach, and intestine. In cases of suspected acute pancreatic disease, measurement of serum or urine AML is the most important laboratory test.

Purpose
● To diagnose acute pancreatitis

● To distinguish between acute pancreatitis and other causes of abdominal pain that require immediate surgery
● To evaluate possible pancreatic injury caused by abdominal trauma or surgery

Patient preparation
● Explain to the patient that this test is used to assess pancreatic function.
● Inform him that he needn't fast before the test but must abstain from alcohol.
● Tell him that this test requires a blood sample. Explain who will perform the venipuncture and when.
● Inform the patient that he may experience transient discomfort from the needle puncture and the tourniquet but that collecting the sample takes less than 3 minutes.
● Withhold drugs that may elevate AML levels. They include aspirin, asparaginase, azathioprine, corticosteroids, cyproheptadine, narcotic analgesics, oral contraceptives, rifampin, sulfasalazine, and thiazide or loop diuretics. If these drugs must be continued, note this on the laboratory slip.

Procedure and posttest care
● Perform a venipuncture, and collect the sample in a 7-ml *red-top* tube.
● If a hematoma develops at the venipuncture site, apply warm soaks.
● Resume administration of drugs discontinued before the test.

Precautions
● If the patient has severe abdominal pain, draw the sample before diagnostic or therapeutic intervention. For accurate results, it's important to obtain an early sample.
● Handle the sample gently to prevent hemolysis.

Reference values
Normal serum amylase levels range from 25 to 160 U/L. (More than 20 methods of measuring serum AML exist, with different ranges of normal values. Test values cannot always be converted to a standard measurement.)

Abnormal findings
After the onset of acute pancreatitis, AML levels begin to rise within 2 hours, peak within 12 to 48 hours, and return to normal within 3 to 4 days. Determination of urine levels should follow normal serum AML results to rule out pancreatitis. Moderate serum elevations may accompany obstruction of the common bile duct, pancreatic duct, or ampulla of Vater; pancreatic injury from a perforated peptic ulcer; pancreatic cancer; and acute salivary gland disease. Impaired kidney function may increase serum levels.

Levels may be slightly elevated in a patient who is asymptomatic or responding unusually to therapy. An AML fractionation test is used to determine the source of the AML and the need for additional tests.

Decreased levels can occur in chronic pancreatitis, pancreatic cancer, cirrhosis, hepatitis, and eclampsia.

Interfering factors
• Hemolysis due to rough handling of the sample
• Ingestion of ethyl alcohol (possible false-high)
• Aminosalicylic acid, asparaginase, azathioprine, corticosteroids, cyproheptadine, narcotic analgesics, oral contraceptives, pentazocine, rifampin, secretin, sulfasalazine, and thiazide or loop diuretics (possible false-high)
• Recent peripancreatic surgery, perforated ulcer or intestine, abscess, spasm of the sphincter of Oddi or, rarely, macroamylasemia (possible false-high)

• High blood glucose levels associated with diabetes or administration of I.V. glucose solutions (possible decrease)

LIPASE

Lipase is produced in the pancreas and secreted into the duodenum, where it converts triglycerides and other fats into fatty acids and glycerol. The destruction of pancreatic cells, which occurs in acute pancreatitis, causes large amounts of lipase to be released into the blood. This test is used to measure serum lipase levels; it's most useful when performed with a serum or urine amylase test.

Purpose
• To aid diagnosis of acute pancreatitis

Patient preparation
• Explain to the patient that this test is used to evaluate pancreatic function.
• Instruct him to fast overnight before the test.
• Tell him that the test requires a blood sample. Explain who will perform the venipuncture and when. Inform him that he may experience transient discomfort but that collecting the sample takes less than 3 minutes.
• Withhold cholinergics, codeine, meperidine, and morphine. If these drugs must be continued, note this on the laboratory slip.

Procedure and posttest care
• Perform a venipuncture, and collect the sample in a 7-ml *red-top* tube.
• If a hematoma develops at the venipuncture site, apply warm soaks.
• Resume administration of drugs discontinued before the test.

Precautions
● Handle the sample gently to prevent hemolysis.

Reference values
Serum levels are method-dependent and range from 56 to 239 U/L.

Abnormal findings
High lipase levels suggest acute pancreatitis or pancreatic duct obstruction. After an acute attack, levels remain elevated for up to 14 days. Lipase levels may also increase in other pancreatic injuries, such as perforated peptic ulcer with chemical pancreatitis due to gastric juices, and in patients with high intestinal obstruction, pancreatic cancer, or renal disease with impaired excretion.

Interfering factors
● Hemolysis due to rough handling of the sample
● Cholinergics, codeine, meperidine, and morphine (false-high due to spasm of the sphincter of Oddi)
● Heparin (possible increase)
● Protamine and I.V. infusions of saline solutions (possible decrease)

SPECIAL ENZYMES

ACID PHOSPHATASE

Acid phosphatase (ACP) — a group of phosphatase enzymes most active at a pH of about 5.0 — is found primarily in the prostate gland and semen and, to a lesser extent, in the liver, spleen, red blood cells, bone marrow, and platelets. This test is used to measure total ACP and the prostatic fraction in serum.

Purpose
● To detect prostate cancer
● To monitor response to therapy for prostate cancer; successful treatment decreases ACP levels

Patient preparation
● Explain to the patient that this test is used to evaluate prostate function.
● Tell him that the test requires a blood sample. Explain who will perform the venipuncture and when.
● Explain that he may experience slight discomfort from the needle puncture and the tourniquet but that collecting the sample usually takes less than 3 minutes.
● Inform him that he needn't restrict food or fluids before the test.
● Withhold fluorides, phosphates, and clofibrate. If they must be continued, note this on the laboratory slip.

Procedure and posttest care
● Perform a venipuncture, and collect the sample in a 7-ml *red-top* tube.
● If a hematoma develops at the venipuncture site, apply warm soaks.
● Resume administration of medications discontinued before the test.

Precautions
● Don't draw the sample within 48 hours of prostate manipulation (rectal examination).
● Handle the sample gently to prevent hemolysis.
● Send the sample to the laboratory immediately. ACP levels decrease by 50% within 1 hour if the sample remains at room temperature without a preservative or is not packed in ice.

Reference values
Serum values for total ACP depend on the assay method and range from 0 to 3.7 ng/ml.

Abnormal findings

High prostatic ACP levels generally indicate the presence of a tumor that has spread beyond the prostatic capsule. If the tumor has metastasized to bone, high ACP levels are accompanied by high alkaline phosphatase (ALP) levels, reflecting increased osteoblastic activity.

ACP levels rise moderately in prostatic infarction, Paget's disease (some patients), Gaucher's disease and, occasionally, other conditions, such as multiple myeloma. False results may occur if ALP levels are high because ACP and ALP are similar, differing mainly in their optimum pH ranges.

Interfering factors

- Hemolysis due to rough handling of the sample or improper sample storage
- Delayed delivery of the sample to the laboratory (possible false-low or false-normal)
- Fluorides, phosphates, and oxalates (possible false-low)
- Clofibrate (possible false-high)
- Androgens in females (increase)
- Prostate massage, catheterization, or rectal examination within 48 hours of the test

PROSTATE-SPECIFIC ANTIGEN

Prostate-specific antigen (PSA) appears in normal, benign hyperplastic, and malignant prostatic tissue as well as in metastatic prostatic carcinoma. Serum PSA levels are used to monitor the spread of recurrence of prostate cancer and to evaluate the patient's response to treatment. This test is not a suitable screening procedure for prostate cancer.

Purpose

- To monitor the course of prostate cancer and aid evaluation of treatment

Patient preparation

- Explain to the patient that this test is used to monitor prostate cancer and the patient's response to treatment.
- Tell him that the test requires a blood sample. Explain who will perform the venipuncture and when.
- Explain that he may experience slight discomfort from the needle puncture and the tourniquet but that collecting the sample usually takes less than 3 minutes.
- Inform him that he needn't restrict food or fluids before the test.

Procedure and posttest care

- Perform a venipuncture, and collect the sample in a 7-ml *red-top* tube.
- Place the sample on ice, and send it to the laboratory immediately.
- If a hematoma develops at the venipuncture site, apply warm soaks.

Precautions

- Collect the sample either before digital prostate examination or at least 48 hours after examination to avoid falsely elevated PSA levels.
- Handle the sample gently to prevent hemolysis.

Reference values

Normal serum values for PSA should not exceed 2 ng/ml in males age 40 and younger and 4 ng/ml in men ages 41 to 61. In men over age 61, values should not exceed 7 ng/ml.

Abnormal findings

About 80% of patients with prostate cancer have pretreatment PSA values greater than 4 ng/ml. However, PSA results alone don't confirm a diagnosis of prostate cancer. About 20% of patients with benign prostatic hyperplasia also have levels greater than 4 ng/ml. Further assessment and testing, including tissue biopsy, are needed to confirm cancer.

Interfering factors

- Hemolysis due to rough handling of the sample
- Excessive doses of chemotherapeutic drugs, such as cyclophosphamide, diethylstilbestrol, and methotrexate (possible increase or decrease)
- Digital prostate examination (false-high)

PLASMA RENIN ACTIVITY

Renin secretion from the kidneys is the first stage of the renin-angiotensin-aldosterone cycle, which controls the body's sodium-potassium balance, fluid volume, and blood pressure. Renin is released into the renal veins in response to sodium depletion and blood loss. This test is a screening procedure for renovascular hypertension but does not unequivocally confirm it.

Purpose

- To screen for renal origin of hypertension
- To help plan treatment of essential hypertension, a genetic disease often aggravated by excess sodium intake
- To help identify hypertension linked to unilateral (sometimes bilateral) renovascular disease by renal vein catheterization
- To help identify primary aldosteronism (Conn's syndrome) resulting from aldosterone-secreting adrenal adenoma
- To confirm primary aldosteronism (sodium-depleted plasma renin test)

Patient preparation

- Explain to the patient that this test is used to determine the cause of hypertension.
- Tell the patient to discontinue or hold the use of diuretics, antihypertensives, vasodilators, oral contraceptives, and licorice as ordered by the doctor and to maintain a normal sodium diet (3 g/day) during this period.
- For the sodium-depleted plasma renin test, tell the patient that he'll receive furosemide (or, if he has angina or cerebrovascular insufficiency, chlorthiazide) and will follow a specific low-sodium diet for 3 days.
- The patient should not receive radioactive treatments for several days before the test.
- Tell him that the test requires a blood sample. Explain who will perform the venipuncture and when.
- Explain that he may experience slight discomfort from the needle puncture and the tourniquet but that collecting the sample usually takes less than 3 minutes. Collect a morning sample, if possible.
- If a recumbent sample is ordered, instruct the patient to remain in bed at least 2 hours before the sample is obtained. (Posture influences renin secretion.) If an upright sample is ordered, instruct him to stand or sit upright for 2 hours before the test is performed.
- If renal vein catheterization is ordered, make sure the patient has signed an informed consent form. Tell him that the procedure will be done in the X-ray department and that he'll receive a local anesthetic.

Procedure and posttest care

Peripheral vein sample

- Perform a venipuncture, and collect the sample in a 7-ml *lavender-top* tube.
- Note on the laboratory slip if the patient was fasting and whether he was

upright or supine during sample collection.
- If a hematoma develops at the peripheral venipuncture site, apply warm soaks.

Renal vein catheterization
- A catheter is advanced to the kidneys through the femoral vein under fluoroscopic control, and samples are obtained from both renal veins and the vena cava.
- After renal vein catheterization, apply pressure to the catheterization site for 10 to 20 minutes to prevent extravasation.
- Monitor vital signs, and check the catheterization site every 30 minutes for 2 hours and then every hour for 4 hours to ensure that the bleeding has stopped. Check distal pulse for signs of thrombus formation and arterial occlusion (cyanosis, loss of pulse, coolness of skin).

Both methods
- Tell the patient he may resume his usual diet.
- Resume administration of medications that were discontinued before the test.

Precautions
- Because renin is unstable, the sample must be drawn into a chilled syringe and collection tube, placed on ice, and sent to the laboratory immediately.
- Completely fill the collection tube, and invert it gently several times to mix the sample and the anticoagulant.

Reference values
Levels of plasma renin activity and aldosterone decrease with advancing age, as follows:
- *Sodium-depleted, upright, peripheral vein:* For ages 18 to 39, the range is from 2.9 to 24 ng/ml/hour; mean, 10.8 ng/ml/hour. For age 40 and over, range is from 2.9 to 10.8 ng/ml/hour; mean, 5.9 ng/ml/hour.

- *Sodium-replete, upright, peripheral vein:* For ages 18 to 39, range is from 0.6 to 4.3 ng/ml/hour; mean, 1.9 ng/ml/hour. For age 40 and over, the range is from 0.6 to 3 ng/ml/hour; the mean is 1 ng/ml/hour.

Abnormal findings
Elevated renin levels may occur in essential hypertension (uncommon), malignant and renovascular hypertension, cirrhosis, hypokalemia, hypovolemia due to hemorrhage, renin-producing renal tumors (Bartter's syndrome), and adrenal hypofunction (Addison's disease). High renin levels may also be found in chronic renal failure with parenchymal disease, end-stage renal disease, and transplant rejection.

Decreased renin levels may indicate hypervolemia due to a high-sodium diet, salt-retaining steroids, primary aldosteronism, Cushing's syndrome, licorice ingestion syndrome, or essential hypertension with low renin levels.

High serum and urine aldosterone levels with low plasma renin activity help identify primary aldosteronism. In the sodium-depleted renin test, low plasma renin confirms this and differentiates it from secondary aldosteronism (characterized by increased renin).

Interfering factors
- Failure to observe pretest restrictions
- Improper patient positioning during test
- Failure to use the proper anticoagulant in the collection tube, to completely fill it, or to adequately mix the sample and the anticoagulant (EDTA helps preserve angiotensin I; heparin does not)
- Failure to chill the collection tube, syringe, and sample or to send the sample to the laboratory immediately
- Salt intake, severe blood loss, ingestion of licorice, oral contraceptives, pregnancy, and therapy with diuretics,

antihypertensives, or vasodilators (increase)

• Salt-retaining steroid therapy and antidiuretic therapy (decrease)

• Radioisotope use within several days before the test

CHOLINESTERASE

The cholinesterase test is used to measure the amounts of two similar enzymes that hydrolyze acetylcholine: acetylcholinesterase and pseudocholinesterase. Acetylcholinesterase is present in nerve tissue, red cells of the spleen, and the gray matter of the brain. Pseudocholinesterase is produced primarily in the liver and appears in small amounts in the pancreas, intestines, heart, and white matter of the brain.

When poisoning by an organophosphate (used by the military in nerve gases and common in many insecticides) is suspected, either cholinesterase may be measured. For technical reasons, pseudocholinesterase is generally tested, although this analysis is less sensitive than the one for acetylcholinesterase.

In suspected poisoning by muscle relaxant, the patient lacks adequate pseudocholinesterase, which normally inactivates the muscle relaxant. In this case, measurement of pseudocholinesterase is required.

Purpose

• To evaluate before surgery or electroconvulsive therapy the patient's potential response to succinylcholine, which is hydrolyzed by cholinesterase

• To detect patients who may have adverse reactions to muscle relaxants

• To assess overexposure to insecticides containing organophosphate compounds

• To assess liver function and aid diagnosis of hepatic disease (a rare purpose)

Patient preparation

• Explain to the patient that this test is used to assess muscle function or the extent of poisoning.

• Tell him that the test requires a blood sample. Explain who will perform the venipuncture and when.

• Explain that he may experience slight discomfort from the needle puncture and the tourniquet but that collecting the sample usually takes less than 3 minutes.

• Inform him that he needn't restrict food or fluids before the test.

• Withhold drugs and other substances that affect serum cholinesterase levels, such as cyclophosphamide, echothiophate iodide, monoamine oxidase (MAO) inhibitors, succinylcholine, neostigmine, quinine, quinidine, chloroquine, caffeine, theophylline, epinephrine, ether, barbiturates, atropine, morphine, codeine, phenothiazines, vitamin K, and folic acid. If such substances must be continued, note this on the laboratory slip.

Procedure and posttest care

• Perform a venipuncture, and collect the sample in a 7-ml *red-top* tube.

• If a hematoma develops at the venipuncture site, apply warm soaks.

• Resume administration of medications that were discontinued before the test.

Precautions

• Handle the sample gently to prevent hemolysis.

• If the sample can't be sent to the laboratory within 6 hours after being drawn, refrigerate it.

Reference values

Pseudocholinesterase levels vary, based on age, but range from 8 to 25 U/ml (when determined by kinetic colorimetric technique).

Abnormal findings

Severely decreased pseudocholinesterase levels suggest a congenital deficiency or organophosphate insecticide poisoning; levels near zero necessitate emergency treatment.

Pseudocholinesterase levels are usually normal in early extrahepatic obstruction and variably decreased in hepatocellular diseases, such as hepatitis and cirrhosis (especially cirrhosis with ascites and jaundice). Levels also drop in acute infections, chronic malnutrition, anemia, myocardial infarction, obstructive jaundice, and metastasis.

Interfering factors

• Hemolysis due to rough handling of the sample
• Pregnancy or recent surgery
• Cyclophosphamide, echothiophate iodide, MAO inhibitors, succinylcholine, neostigmine, quinine, quinidine, chloroquine, caffeine, theophylline, epinephrine, ether, barbiturates, atropine, morphine, codeine, phenothiazines, vitamin K, and folic acid (possible false-low)

GLUCOSE-6-PHOSPHATE DEHYDROGENASE

An enzyme found in most body cells, glucose-6-phosphate dehydrogenase (G6PD) is involved in metabolizing glucose. This test is used to detect G6PD deficiency, a hereditary, sex-linked condition that impairs stability of the red cell membrane and allows red cells to be destroyed by strong oxidizing agents.

About 10% of black males in the United States inherit a mild G6PD deficiency; some people of Mediterranean origin inherit a severe deficiency. In some whites, fava beans may produce hemolytic episodes. Although a deficiency of G6PD provides partial immunity to falciparum malaria, it precipitates an adverse reaction to antimalarials.

Purpose

• To detect hemolytic anemia caused by G6PD deficiency
• To aid differential diagnosis of hemolytic anemia

Patient preparation

• Explain to the patient that this test is used to detect an inherited enzyme deficiency that may affect red blood cells.
• Tell him that the test requires a blood sample. Explain who will perform the venipuncture and when.
• Explain that he may experience slight discomfort from the needle puncture and the tourniquet but that collecting the sample usually takes less than 3 minutes.
• Inform him that he needn't restrict food or fluids before the test.
• Check patient history, and report recent blood transfusion or ingestion of aspirin, sulfonamides, nitrofurantoin, vitamin K derivatives, antimalarials, or fava beans, which cause hemolysis in people who are G6PD-deficient.

Procedure and posttest care

• Perform a venipuncture, and collect the sample in a 7-ml *lavender-top* tube.
• If a hematoma develops at the venipuncture site, apply warm soaks.

Precautions

• Completely fill the collection tube, and invert it gently several times to mix the sample and the anticoagulant.

• Handle the sample gently to prevent hemolysis.

• Refrigerate the sample if you can't send it to the laboratory immediately.

Reference values

Serum values of G6PD vary with the measurement method used and may be reported as normal or abnormal.

Abnormal findings

Fluorescent spot testing or staining for Heinz bodies or erythrocytes can test for G6PD deficiency. If results are positive, the kinetic quantitative assay for G6PD may be performed. Electrophoretic techniques assess genetic variants of deficiencies (which may cause lifelong, mild, or asymptomatic anemia). Some variants are symptomatic only when the patient experiences stress or illness or has been exposed to drugs or agents that elicit hemolytic episodes.

Interfering factors

• Performing the test after a hemolytic episode or a blood transfusion (possible false-negative)

• Failure to use the proper anticoagulant or to adequately mix the sample and the anticoagulant

• Hemolysis due to rough handling of the sample

• Aspirin, sulfonamides, nitrofurantoin, vitamin K derivatives, primaquine, and fava beans (decrease G6PD enzyme activity and precipitate hemolytic episode)

PYRUVATE KINASE

An erythrocyte enzyme, pyruvate kinase (PK) takes part in the anaerobic metabolism of glucose. An abnormally low PK level is an inherited autosomal recessive trait that may cause a red cell membrane defect associated with congenital hemolytic anemia. PK assay confirms PK deficiency when red cell enzyme deficiency is the suspected cause of anemia.

Purpose

• To differentiate PK-deficient hemolytic anemia from other congenital hemolytic anemias or from acquired hemolytic anemia

• To detect PK deficiency in asymptomatic, heterozygous inheritance

Patient preparation

• Explain to the patient that this test is used to detect inherited enzyme deficiencies.

• Tell him that the test requires a blood sample. Explain who will perform the venipuncture and when.

• Explain that he may experience slight discomfort from the needle puncture and the tourniquet but that collecting the sample usually takes less than 3 minutes.

• Inform him that he needn't restrict food or fluids before the test, but should avoid fava beans.

• Check the patient's history for recent blood transfusion, and note it on the laboratory slip.

• Tell him to avoid aspirin, sulfonamides, nitrofurantoin, vitamin K derivatives, and antimalarials as ordered by the doctor.

Procedure and posttest care

• Perform a venipuncture, and collect the sample in a 7-ml *lavender-top* tube.

• If a hematoma develops at the venipuncture site, apply warm soaks.

Precautions

• Completely fill the collection tube, and invert it *gently* several times to mix the sample and the anticoagulant without causing hemolysis.

● Refrigerate the sample if you can't send it to the laboratory immediately.

Reference values
Serum PK levels range from 9 to 22 U/g of hemoglobin.

Abnormal findings
Low serum PK levels confirm a diagnosis of PK deficiency and allow differentiation between PK-deficient hemolytic anemia and other inherited disorders.

Interfering factors
● Failure to use the proper anticoagulant or to adequately mix the sample and the anticoagulant
● Hemolysis due to rough handling of the sample
● Failure to remove white cells from sample (possible false results)
● Recent blood transfusion or recent hemolytic event
● Aspirin, sulfonamides, nitrofurantoin, vitamin K derivatives, antimalarials, fava beans (possible hemolysis)

HEXOSAMINIDASE A AND B

Hexosaminidase is a group of enzymes that are necessary for metabolism of gangliosides, water-soluble glycolipids found primarily in brain tissue. This test is used to measure the hexosaminidase A and B content of serum and amniotic fluid.

Deficiency of hexosaminidase A indicates Tay-Sachs disease, which affects people of eastern European Jewish ancestry about 100 times more often than the general population. Both parents must carry the defective gene to transmit Tay-Sachs disease to their children. Sandhoff's disease, which results from deficiency of both hexosaminidase A and B, is uncommon and not prevalent in any ethnic group.

Purpose
● To confirm or rule out Tay-Sachs disease in neonates
● To screen for Tay-Sachs carriers
● To establish prenatal diagnosis of hexosaminidase A deficiency

Patient preparation
● Explain to the patient that this test is used to identify carriers of Tay-Sachs disease.
● Tell him that the test requires a blood sample. Explain who will perform the venipuncture and when.
● Explain that he may experience slight discomfort from the needle puncture and the tourniquet but that collecting the sample usually takes less than 3 minutes.
● Inform the patient that he needn't restrict food or fluids before the test.
● When testing a neonate, explain to the parents that this test is used to detect Tay-Sachs disease. Tell them that blood will be drawn from the baby's arm, neck, or umbilical cord; that the procedure is safe and quickly performed; and that the infant will have a small bandage on the venipuncture site. Inform them that no pretest restrictions of food or fluid are needed .
● If the test is being performed prenatally, advise the patient of preparations for amniocentesis.

Procedure and posttest care
● Perform a venipuncture, collect cord blood, or assist with amniocentesis, as appropriate. Collect the sample in a 7-ml *red-top* tube.
● If a hematoma develops at the venipuncture site, apply warm soaks.

• If both partners are carriers of Tay-Sachs disease, refer them for genetic counseling.

• When testing a neonate, follow laboratory procedure for collecting serum samples.

Precautions

• Handle the sample gently to prevent hemolysis.

• This test can't be done on a pregnant woman's serum (but her leukocytes or amniotic fluid may be tested, if necessary); if the father's blood test result is negative, Tay-Sachs disease won't be transmitted to the child.

Reference values

Total serum levels of hexosaminidase range from 10.4 to 23.8 U/L; hexosaminidase A accounts for 56% to 80% of the total.

Abnormal findings

Absence of hexosaminidase A indicates Tay-Sachs disease (total hexosaminidase levels can be normal). Absence of both hexosaminidase A and B indicates Sandhoff's disease, an uncommon, virulent variant of Tay-Sachs disease in which deterioration occurs more rapidly.

Interfering factors

• Hemolysis due to rough handling of the sample

• Oral contraceptives (false-high)

• Pregnancy

UROPORPHYRINOGEN I SYNTHASE

This test is used to measure blood levels of uroporphyrinogen I synthase, an enzyme involved in heme biosynthesis.

This enzyme is normally present in erythrocytes, fibroblasts, lymphocytes, hepatic cells, and amniotic fluid cells. A hereditary deficiency that can reduce uroporphyrinogen I synthase levels by 50% or more results in acute intermittent porphyria (AIP). This disorder can be latent indefinitely until certain factors (some sex hormones and drugs, a low-carbohydrate diet, or an infection) precipitate active disease.

Purpose

• To aid diagnosis of latent or active AIP

• To differentiate AIP from other types of porphyria

Patient preparation

• Explain to the patient that this test is used to detect a red blood cell disorder.

• Inform him that he'll need to fast for 12 to 14 hours before the test and to abstain from alcohol for 24 hours but that he may drink water.

• Tell him that the test requires a blood sample. Explain who will perform the venipuncture and when.

• Explain that he may experience slight discomfort from the needle puncture and the tourniquet but that collecting the sample usually takes less than 3 minutes.

• If the patient's hematocrit is available, record this on the laboratory slip.

• Check the patient's medication history. Withhold drugs that may decrease uroporphyrinogen I synthase levels, such as steroid hormones, estrogens, barbiturates, sulfonamides, phenytoin, griseofulvin, chlordiazepoxide, meprobamate, glutethimide, and ergot alkaloids. If they must be continued, note this on the laboratory slip.

Procedure and posttest care

• Perform a venipuncture, and collect the sample in a 10-ml *green-top* tube.

• If a hematoma develops at the venipuncture site, apply warm soaks.
• Instruct the patient to resume usual diet and medications.
• If AIP is present, refer the patient for nutrition and genetic counseling. Advise him to avoid low-carbohydrate diets, alcohol, and drugs that may trigger an acute episode and to seek care promptly for all infections.

Precautions
• Handle the sample gently to prevent hemolysis.
• Place the sample on ice, and send it to the laboratory immediately.

Reference values
Normal values for uroporphyrinogen I synthase are greater than or equal to 7 nmol/sec/L.

Abnormal findings
Decreased uroporphyrinogen I synthase levels generally indicate latent or active AIP; symptoms differentiate these phases. Levels that are below 6 nmol/sec/L confirm AIP. Levels between 6 and 6.9 nmol/sec/L are indeterminate, in which case urine and stool tests for the porphyrin precursors aminolevulinic acid and porphobilinogen may be ordered to support the diagnosis.

Interfering factors
• Failure to observe pretest restrictions (false-positive)
• Hemolysis due to rough handling of the sample
• Hemolytic and hepatic diseases (possible increase)
• Alcohol and use of drugs such as steroid hormones, estrogens, barbiturates, sulfonamides, phenytoin, griseofulvin, chlordiazepoxide, meprobamate, glutethimide, and ergot alkaloids (possible decrease)

GALACTOSE-1-PHOSPHATE URIDYL TRANSFERASE

This enzyme is involved in the conversion of galactose to glucose during lactose metabolism. Deficiency may lead to galactosemia, a hereditary disorder marked by elevated serum galactose levels and decreased serum glucose levels. Unless detected and treated soon after birth, galactosemia can impair eye, brain, and liver development, causing irreversible cataracts, mental retardation, and cirrhosis.

The qualitative test, a simple screening test for deficiency of galactose-1-phosphate uridyl transferase, is required in some facilities for all neonates. Prenatal testing of amniotic fluid can also detect transferase deficiency but is seldom performed.

Purpose
• To screen infants for galactosemia
• To detect heterozygous carriers of galactosemia

Patient preparation
• When testing a neonate, explain to the parents that the test screens for galactosemia, a potentially dangerous enzyme deficiency.
• If a blood sample was not taken from the umbilical cord at birth, tell the parents that a small amount of blood will be drawn from their infant's heel. Explain that the procedure is safe and quickly performed.
• When testing an adult, explain that this test is used to identify carriers of galactosemia, a genetic disorder that may be transmitted to offspring.

• Tell him that the test requires a blood sample. Explain who will perform the venipuncture and when.
• Explain that he may experience slight discomfort from the needle puncture and the tourniquet but that collecting the sample usually takes less than 3 minutes.
• Inform him that he needn't restrict food or fluids before the test.

Procedure and posttest care
• For a qualitative (screening) test, collect cord blood or blood from a heel-stick on special filter paper, saturating all three circles.
• For a quantitative test, perform a venipuncture, and collect a 4-ml sample in a *green-top* or *lavender-top* tube, depending on the laboratory method used.
• Indicate the patient's age on the laboratory slip.
• Check his history for a recent exchange transfusion. Note this on the laboratory slip or postpone the test.
• If a hematoma develops at the venipuncture site, apply warm soaks.
• If test results indicate galactosemia, refer the parents for nutrition counseling, and provide a galactose- and lactose-free diet for their infant. A soybean- or meat-based formula may be substituted for formulas based on cow's milk.

Precautions
• Handle the sample gently to prevent hemolysis.
• Send the sample to the laboratory on wet ice.

Reference values
Normally, the qualitative test is negative. The normal range for the quantitative test is 18.5 to 28.5 U/g of hemoglobin; confirm the normal range with the laboratory in case a different method is used.

Abnormal findings
A positive qualitative test may indicate a transferase deficiency. A follow-up quantitative test should be performed as soon as possible. Quantitative test results showing less than 5 U/g of hemoglobin indicate galactosemia. Levels between 5 and 18.5 U/g of hemoglobin may indicate a carrier state.

Interfering factors
• Hemolysis due to rough handling of the sample
• Failure to use the proper collection tube or to send the sample to the laboratory on wet ice (possible false-positive because heat inactivates transferase)
• Total exchange transfusion (transient false-negative because normal blood contains enzyme)

ANGIOTENSIN-CONVERTING ENZYME

This test is used to measure serum levels of angiotensin-converting enzyme (ACE), which is found in lung capillaries and, in lesser concentrations, blood vessels and kidney tissue. Its primary function is to help regulate arterial pressure by converting angiotensin I to angiotensin II. Measurement of ACE is of little use in diagnosing hypertension.

Purpose
• To aid diagnosis of sarcoidosis, especially pulmonary sarcoidosis
• To monitor response to therapy in sarcoidosis
• To help confirm Gaucher's disease and leprosy

Patient preparation

- Explain to the patient that this test is used to diagnose sarcoidosis, Gaucher's disease, and leprosy and to check response to treatment for sarcoidosis.
- Tell him that the test requires a blood sample. Explain who will perform the venipuncture and when.
- Explain that he may experience slight discomfort from the needle puncture and the tourniquet but that collecting the sample usually takes less than 3 minutes.
- Inform the patient that he must fast for 12 hours before the test.
- Note the patient's age on the laboratory slip. If the patient is under age 20, the test may have to be postponed because patients under age 20 have variable ACE levels.

Procedure and posttest care

- Perform a venipuncture, and collect the sample in a 7-ml *red-top* tube.
- If a hematoma develops at the venipuncture site, apply warm soaks.

Precautions

- Avoid using a *lavender-top* tube or contaminating the sample with EDTA because this can decrease ACE levels, thereby altering test results.
- Handle the sample gently to prevent hemolysis.
- Send the sample to the laboratory immediately, or freeze it and place it on dry ice until the test can be performed.

Reference values

In the colorimetric assay, normal values for serum ACE in patients age 20 and older range from 6.1 to 21.1 U/L.

Abnormal findings

Elevated serum ACE levels may indicate sarcoidosis, Gaucher's disease, or leprosy, but results must be correlated with the patient's clinical condition. In some patients, elevated ACE levels may result from hyperthyroidism, diabetic retinopathy, or hepatic disease.

Serum ACE levels decline as the patient responds to steroid or prednisone therapy for sarcoidosis.

Interfering factors

- Failure to fast before the test (may cause significant lipemia of the sample)
- Use of a lavender-top collection tube or other EDTA contamination (possible decrease)
- Hemolysis due to excessive agitation of the sample
- Failure to send the sample to the laboratory at once or to freeze it and place it on dry ice (possible false-low due to ACE degradation)

LIPIDS AND LIPOPROTEINS

TRIGLYCERIDES

Serum triglyceride analysis provides quantitative analysis of triglycerides — the main storage form of lipids — which constitute about 95% of fatty tissue. Although not in itself diagnostic, this test permits early identification of hyperlipidemia and the risk of coronary artery disease (CAD).

Purpose

- To screen for hyperlipidemia
- To help identify nephrotic syndrome
- To determine the risk of CAD

Patient preparation

- Explain to the patient that this test is used to detect disorders of fat metabolism.

• Tell him that the test requires a blood sample. Explain who will perform the venipuncture and when.

• Explain that he may experience slight discomfort from the needle puncture and the tourniquet but that collecting the sample usually takes less than 3 minutes.

• Instruct him to fast for at least 12 hours before the test and to abstain from alcohol for 24 hours. Tell him that he can drink water.

• Withhold medications that may interfere with the accuracy of test results, including antilipemics, corticosteroids, estrogen, and some diuretics. If these medications can't be discontinued, note them on the laboratory slip.

Procedure and posttest care

• Perform a venipuncture, and collect a sample in a 7-ml *lavender-top* tube.

• If a hematoma develops at the venipuncture site, apply warm soaks.

• Tell the patient that he may resume his usual diet.

• Resume the administration of medications discontinued before the test.

Precautions

• Send the sample to the laboratory immediately.

• Some redistribution may occur among lipids.

Reference values

Triglyceride values vary with age and sex. There is some controversy about the most appropriate normal ranges, but values of 40 to 160 mg/dl for men and 35 to 135 mg/dl for women over age 20 are widely accepted.

Abnormal findings

Increased or decreased serum triglyceride levels suggest a clinical abnormality; additional tests are required for a definitive diagnosis.

A mild to moderate increase in serum triglyceride levels indicates biliary obstruction, diabetes mellitus, nephrotic syndrome, endocrinopathies, or overconsumption of alcohol. Markedly increased levels without an identifiable cause reflect congenital hyperlipoproteinemia and necessitate lipoprotein phenotyping to confirm the diagnosis.

Decreased serum triglyceride levels are rare and occur mainly in malnutrition and abetalipoproteinemia.

Interfering factors

• Failure to observe pretest restrictions

• Use of glycol-lubricated collection tube

• Failure to send the sample to the laboratory immediately

• Antilipemics (decrease serum lipid levels)

• Cholestyramine and colestipol (decrease cholesterol levels but increase or have no effect on triglyceride levels)

• Corticosteroids (long-term use), oral contraceptives, estrogen, ethyl alcohol, furosemide, and miconazole (increase)

• Clofibrate, dextrothyroxine, gemfibrozil, and niacin (decrease cholesterol and triglyceride levels)

• Probucol (decreases cholesterol levels but has variable effect on triglyceride levels)

TOTAL CHOLESTEROL

This test, the quantitative analysis of serum cholesterol, is used to measure the circulating levels of free cholesterol and cholesterol esters; it reflects the level of the two forms in which this biochemical compound appears in the body. High serum cholesterol levels may be associated with an increased risk of coronary artery disease (CAD).

Purpose
- To assess the risk of CAD
- To evaluate fat metabolism
- To aid diagnosis of nephrotic syndrome, pancreatitis, hepatic disease, hypothyroidism, and hyperthyroidism

Patient preparation
- Explain to the patient that this test is used to assess the body's fat metabolism.
- Tell him that the test requires a blood sample. Explain who will perform the venipuncture and when.
- Explain that he may experience slight discomfort from the needle puncture and the tourniquet but that collecting the sample usually takes less than 3 minutes.
- Instruct the patient not to eat or drink for 12 hours before the test.
- Withhold drugs that influence cholesterol levels. They may include cholestyramine, clofibrate, colestipol, dextrothyroxine, haloperidol, neomycin, niacin, chlortetracycline, epinephrine, chlorpromazine, trifluoperazine, oral contraceptives, trimethadione, and androgens.

Procedure and posttest care
- Perform a venipuncture, and collect the sample in a 7-ml *lavender-top* tube.
- If a hematoma develops at the venipuncture site, apply warm soaks.
- Tell the patient that he may resume his usual diet.
- Resume administration of medications discontinued before the test.

Precautions
- Send the sample to the laboratory immediately.

Reference values
Total cholesterol concentrations vary with age and sex. The desirable range is 140 to 199 mg/dl. Levels exceeding 240 mg/dl are considered elevated.

Abnormal findings
Elevated serum cholesterol levels (hypercholesterolemia) may indicate a risk of CAD as well as incipient hepatitis, lipid disorders, bile duct blockage, nephrotic syndrome, obstructive jaundice, pancreatitis, and hypothyroidism.

Low serum cholesterol levels (hypocholesterolemia) are commonly associated with malnutrition, cellular necrosis of the liver, and hyperthyroidism. Abnormal cholesterol levels frequently necessitate further testing to pinpoint the cause.

Interfering factors
- Failure to observe pretest restrictions
- Failure to send the sample to the laboratory immediately
- Cholestyramine, clofibrate, colestipol, dextrothyroxine, haloperidol, neomycin, niacin, and chlortetracycline (decrease)
- Epinephrine, chlorpromazine, trifluoperazine, oral contraceptives, and trimethadione (increase)
- Androgens (possible variable effect)

PHOSPHOLIPIDS

This test is a quantitative analysis of phospholipids, the major form of lipids in cell membranes. Phospholipids are involved in cellular membrane composition and permeability and help control enzyme activity within the membrane. They aid transport of fatty acids and lipids across the intestinal barrier and from the liver and other fat depots to other body tissues. Phospholipids are essential for pulmonary gas exchange.

Purpose
- To aid in the evaluation of fat metabolism
- To aid diagnosis of hypothyroidism, diabetes mellitus, nephrotic syndrome,

chronic pancreatitis, obstructive jaundice, and hypolipoproteinemia

Patient preparation
• Explain to the patient that this test is used to determine how the body metabolizes fats.
• Tell him that the test requires a blood sample. Explain who will perform the venipuncture and when.
• Explain that he may experience slight discomfort from the needle puncture and the tourniquet but that collecting the sample usually takes less than 3 minutes.
• Instruct him to abstain from drinking alcohol for 24 hours before the test and not to eat or drink anything after midnight before the test.
• Tell the patient to withhold or discontinue medications that may alter test results, such as antilipemics, estrogens, epinephrine, and phenothiazines, as ordered.

Procedure and posttest care
• Perform a venipuncture, and collect the sample in a 10- to 15-ml *red-top* tube.
• If a hematoma develops at the venipuncture site, apply warm soaks.
• Tell the patient that he may resume his usual diet.
• Resume administration of medications discontinued before the test.

Precautions
• Send the sample to the laboratory immediately because spontaneous redistribution may occur among plasma lipids.

Reference values
Normal phospholipid levels range from 180 to 320 mg/dl. Although men usually have higher levels than women, values in pregnant women exceed those of men.

Abnormal findings
Elevated phospholipid levels may indicate hypothyroidism, diabetes mellitus, nephrotic syndrome, chronic pancreatitis, or obstructive jaundice. Decreased levels may indicate primary hypolipoproteinemia.

Lack of phospholipids in premature infants leads to neonatal respiratory distress syndrome.

Interfering factors
• Failure to observe pretest restrictions
• Failure to send the sample to the laboratory immediately
• Clofibrate and other antilipemics (possible decrease)
• Estrogens, epinephrine, and some phenothiazines (increase)

LIPOPROTEIN-CHOLESTEROL FRACTIONATION

Cholesterol fractionation tests are used to isolate and measure the types of cholesterol in serum, low-density lipoproteins (LDLs) and high-density lipoproteins (HDLs). The HDL level is inversely related to the risk of coronary artery disease (CAD); the higher the HDL level, the lower the incidence of CAD. Conversely, the higher the LDL level, the higher the incidence of CAD.

Purpose
• To assess the risk of CAD

Patient preparation
• Tell the patient that this test is used to determine the risk of CAD.
• Tell him that the test requires a blood sample. Explain who will perform the venipuncture and when.

• Explain that he may experience slight discomfort from the needle puncture and the tourniquet but that collecting the sample usually takes less than 3 minutes.

• Instruct him to maintain his normal diet for 2 weeks before the test, to abstain from alcohol for 24 hours before the test, and to fast and avoid exercise for 12 to 14 hours before the test.

• Withhold thyroid hormones, oral contraceptives, and antilipemics.

Procedure and posttest care

• Perform a venipuncture, and collect the sample in a 7-ml *red-top* or *red-marble-top* tube.

• If a hematoma develops at the venipuncture site, apply warm soaks.

• Tell the patient that he may resume his usual diet.

• Resume administration of medications discontinued before the test.

Precautions

• Send the sample to the laboratory immediately to avoid spontaneous redistribution among the lipoproteins.

• If the sample can't be transported immediately, refrigerate it but don't freeze it.

Reference values

Normal lipoprotein values vary by age, sex, geographic area, and ethnic group; check the laboratory for reference values. Normal HDL levels range from 37 to 70 mg/dl for males and from 40 to 85 mg/dl for females; normal LDL levels are less than 130 mg/dl.

Abnormal findings

High LDL levels increase the risk of CAD. Elevated HDL levels generally reflect a healthy state but can also indicate chronic hepatitis, early-stage primary biliary cirrhosis, and alcohol consumption. Rarely, a sharp rise (to as high as 100 mg/dl) in a second type of HDL (alpha$_2$-HDL) may signal CAD.

Interfering factors

• Failure to observe pretest restrictions

• Concurrent illness, especially if accompanied by fever, recent surgery, or myocardial infarction

• Collecting the sample in a heparinized tube (possible false-high due to activation of the enzyme lipase, which causes release of fatty acids from triglycerides)

• Failure to send the sample to the laboratory immediately

• Antilipemic medications, such as clofibrate, cholestyramine, colestipol, dextrothyroxine, niacin, probucol, and gemfibrozil (decrease)

• Oral contraceptives, disulfiram, alcohol, miconazole, and high doses of phenothiazines (possible increase)

• Estrogens (possible increase or decrease)

LIPOPROTEIN PHENOTYPING

Lipoprotein phenotyping is used to determine levels of the four major lipoproteins: chylomicrons, very low-density (prebeta) lipoproteins (VLDLs), low-density (beta) lipoproteins (LDLs), and high-density (alpha) lipoproteins (HDLs). (See *Familial hyperlipoproteinemias.*) Detecting altered lipoprotein patterns is essential in identifying hyperlipoproteinemia and hypolipoproteinemia.

Purpose

• To determine classification of hyperlipoproteinemia and hypolipoproteinemia

FAMILIAL HYPERLIPOPROTEINEMIAS

TYPE	CAUSES AND INCIDENCE	CLINICAL SIGNS	LABORATORY FINDINGS
I	• Deficient lipoprotein lipase, resulting in increased chylomicrons • May be induced by alcoholism • Incidence: rare	• Eruptive xanthomas • Lipemia retinalis • Abdominal pain	• Increased chylomicron, total cholesterol, and triglyceride levels • Normal or slightly increased very low-density lipoproteins (VLDLs) • Normal or decreased low-density lipoproteins (LDLs) and high-density lipoproteins (HDLs) • Cholesterol-triglyceride ratio under 0.2
IIa	• Deficient cell receptor, resulting in increased LDL and excessive cholesterol synthesis • May be induced by hypothyroidism • Incidence: common	• Premature coronary artery disease (CAD) • Arcus cornea • Xanthelasma • Tendinous and tuberous xanthomas	• Increased LDL • Normal VLDL • Cholesterol-triglyceride ratio over 2.0
IIb	• Deficient cell receptor, resulting in increased LDL and excessive cholesterol synthesis • May be induced by dysgammaglobulinemia, hypothyroidism, uncontrolled diabetes mellitus, and nephrotic syndrome • Incidence: common	• Premature CAD • Obesity • Possible xanthelasmas	• Increased LDL, VLDL, total cholesterol, and triglycerides
III	• Unknown cause, resulting in deficient VLDL-to-LDL conversion • May be induced by hypothyroidism, uncontrolled diabetes mellitus, and paraproteinemia • Incidence: rare	• Premature CAD • Arcus cornea • Eruptive tuberous xanthomas	• Increased total cholesterol, VLDL, and triglycerides • Normal or decreased LDL • Cholesterol-triglyceride ratio of VLDL over 0.4 • Broad beta band observed on electrophoresis

(continued)

FAMILIAL HYPERLIPOPROTEINEMIAS *(continued)*

TYPE	CAUSES AND INCIDENCE	CLINICAL SIGNS	LABORATORY FINDINGS
IV	• Unknown cause, resulting in decreased levels of lipoprotein lipase • May be induced by uncontrolled diabetes mellitus, alcoholism, pregnancy, steroid or estrogen therapy, dysgammaglobulinemia, and hyperthyroidism • Incidence: common	• Possible premature CAD • Obesity • Hypertension • Peripheral neuropathy	• Increased VLDL and triglycerides • Normal LDL • Cholesterol-triglyceride ratio of VLDL under 0.25
V	• Unknown cause, resulting in defective triglyceride clearance • May be induced by alcoholism, dysgammaglobulinemia, uncontrolled diabetes mellitus, nephrotic syndrome, pancreatitis, and steroid therapy • Incidence: rare	• Premature CAD • Abdominal pain • Lipemia retinalis • Eruptive xanthomas • Hepatosplenomegaly	• Increased VLDL, total cholesterol, and triglyceride levels • Chylomicrons present • Cholesterol-triglyceride ratio under 0.6

Patient preparation

• Explain to the patient that this test is used to determine how the body metabolizes fats.

• Tell him that the test requires a blood sample. Explain who will perform the venipuncture and when.

• Explain that he may experience slight discomfort from the needle puncture and the tourniquet but that collecting the sample usually takes less than 3 minutes.

• Instruct him to abstain from alcohol for 24 hours before the test and to fast after midnight before the test. Provide a low-fat meal the night before the test.

• Check the patient's drug history for use of heparin. Withhold antilipemics, such as cholestyramine, about 2 weeks before the test.

• Notify the laboratory if the patient is receiving treatment for any other condition that might significantly alter lipo-protein metabolism, such as diabetes mellitus, nephrosis, or hypothyroidism.

Procedure and posttest care

• Perform a venipuncture, and collect the sample in a 7-ml *lavender-top* tube.

• If a hematoma develops at the venipuncture site, apply warm soaks.

• Instruct the patient to resume his normal diet.

• Resume administration of medications withheld before the test.

Precautions

• When drawing multiple samples, collect the sample for lipoprotein phenotyping first because venous obstruction for 2 minutes can affect test results.

• Fill the collection tube completely, and invert it gently several times to mix the sample and anticoagulant thoroughly.

• Handle the sample gently to prevent hemolysis.

Findings
The types of hyperlipoproteinemias and hypolipoproteinemias are identified by characteristic electrophoretic patterns.

Familial lipoprotein disorders are classified as either hyperlipoproteinemias or hypolipoproteinemias. There are six types of hyperlipoproteinemias: I, IIa, IIb, III, IV, and V. Types IIa, IIb, and IV are relatively common. All hypolipoproteinemias are rare, including hypobetalipoproteinemia, abetalipoproteinemia, and alpha-lipoprotein deficiency.

Interfering factors
• Recent use of antilipemics
• Failure to observe pretest restrictions
• Hemolysis due to rough handling of the sample
• Administration of heparin (which activates the enzyme lipase, producing fatty acids from triglycerides) or collection of the sample in a heparinized tube (possible false-high)

PROTEINS AND PROTEIN METABOLITES

PROTEIN ELECTROPHORESIS

This test is used to measure serum albumin and globulins, the major blood proteins, by separating the proteins into five distinct fractions: albumin and alpha$_1$, alpha$_2$, beta, and gamma proteins.

Purpose
• To aid diagnosis of hepatic disease, protein deficiency, renal disorders, and GI and neoplastic diseases

Patient preparation
• Explain to the patient that this test is used to determine the protein content of blood.
• Tell him that the test requires a blood sample. Explain who will perform the venipuncture and when.
• Explain that he may experience slight discomfort from the needle puncture and the tourniquet but that collecting the sample usually takes less than 3 minutes.
• Inform him that he needn't restrict food or fluids before the test.
• Check the patient's medication history for drugs that may influence serum protein levels, such as alkylating agents, antimetabolites, antibiotic antineoplastic agents, and antineoplastics that alter hormone balance. If they must be continued, note this on the laboratory slip.

Procedure and posttest care
• Perform a venipuncture, and collect the sample in a 7-ml *red-top* or *red-marble-top* tube.
• If a hematoma develops at the venipuncture site, apply warm soaks.

Precautions
• This test must be performed on a serum sample to avoid measuring the fibrinogen fraction.

Reference values
Normally, total serum protein levels range from 6.3 to 7.9 g/dl, and the albumin fraction ranges from 3.4 to 4.8 g/dl. The alpha$_1$-globulin fraction ranges from 0.1 to 0.4 g/dl; alpha$_2$globulin

CLINICAL IMPLICATIONS OF ABNORMAL PROTEIN LEVELS

	Total proteins	Albumin	Globulins
INCREASED LEVELS	• Chronic inflammatory disease (such as rheumatoid arthritis or early-stage Laënnec's cirrhosis) • Dehydration • Diabetic ketoacidosis • Fulminating and chronic infections • Multiple myeloma • Monocytic leukemia • Vomiting, diarrhea	• Multiple myeloma	• Chronic syphilis • Collagen diseases • Diabetes mellitus • Hodgkin's disease • Levels variable in neoplastic and renal diseases, hepatic dysfunction, and blood dyscrasias • Multiple myeloma • Rheumatoid arthritis • Subacute bacterial endocarditis • Systemic lupus erythematosus • Tuberculosis
DECREASED LEVELS	• Benzene and carbon tetrachloride poisoning • Blood dyscrasias • Essential hypertension • GI disease • Heart failure • Hepatic dysfunction • Hemorrhage • Hodgkin's disease • Hyperthyroidism • Malabsorption • Malnutrition • Nephrosis • Severe burns • Surgical and traumatic shock • Toxemia of pregnancy • Uncontrolled diabetes mellitus	• Acute cholecystitis • Collagen diseases • Diarrhea • Essential hypertension • Hepatic disease • Hyperthyroidism • Hypogammaglobulinemia • Malnutrition • Metastatic carcinoma • Nephritis, nephrosis • Peptic ulcer • Plasma loss from burns • Rheumatoid arthritis • Sarcoidosis • Systemic lupus erythematosus	• Levels variable in neoplastic and renal diseases, hepatic dysfunction, and blood dyscrasias

ranges from 0.5 to 1.1 g/dl. Beta globulin ranges from 0.6 to 1.2 g/dl; gamma globulin ranges from 0.7 to 1.7 g/dl.

Abnormal findings

For common findings, see *Clinical implications of abnormal protein levels.*

Interfering factors

• Pretest administration of a contrast agent, such as sulfobromophthalein (false-high total protein)
• Pregnancy or cytotoxic drugs (possible decrease in serum albumin)
• Use of plasma instead of serum
• High serum lipid levels

CERULOPLASMIN

This test is used to measure serum levels of ceruloplasmin, an alpha$_2$-globulin that binds about 95% of serum copper, usually in the liver. Ceruloplasmin is thought to regulate iron uptake by transferrin, making iron available to reticulocytes for heme synthesis.

Purpose

• To aid diagnosis of Wilson's disease, Menkes' syndrome, and copper deficiency from total parenteral nutrition (TPN)

Patient preparation

• Explain to the patient that this test is used to determine the copper content of blood.
• Tell him that the test requires a blood sample. Explain who will perform the venipuncture and when.
• Explain that he may experience slight discomfort from the needle puncture and the tourniquet but that collecting the sample usually takes less than 3 minutes.

• Check the patient's history for drugs that may influence ceruloplasmin levels, such as estrogen, methadone, and phenytoin.

Procedure and posttest care

• Perform a venipuncture, and collect the sample in a 7-ml *red-top* or *red-marble-top* tube.
• If a hematoma develops at the venipuncture site, apply warm soaks.

Precautions

• Send the sample to the laboratory immediately.

Reference values

Serum ceruloplasmin levels normally range from 22.9 to 43.1 mg/dl in adults.

Abnormal findings

Low ceruloplasmin levels usually indicate Wilson's disease. Low levels may also occur in Menkes' syndrome, nephrotic syndrome, and copper deficiency caused by TPN. Elevated levels may indicate certain hepatic diseases and infections.

Interfering factors

• Estrogen, methadone, phenytoin, and pregnancy (possible increase)
• Failure to send the sample to the laboratory immediately

HAPTOGLOBIN

This test is used to measure serum levels of haptoglobin, a glycoprotein produced in the liver. In acute intravascular hemolysis, haptoglobin concentration decreases rapidly and may remain low for 5 to 7 days, until the liver synthesizes more glycoprotein.

Purpose

● To serve as an index of hemolysis
● To distinguish between hemoglobin and myoglobin in plasma; haptoglobin binds with free hemoglobin but doesn't bind with myoglobin
● To investigate hemolytic transfusion reactions
● To establish proof of paternity, using genetic (phenotypic) variations in haptoglobin structure

Patient preparation

● Explain to the patient that this test is used to determine the condition of red blood cells.
● Tell him that the test requires a blood sample. Explain who will perform the venipuncture and when.
● Explain that he may experience slight discomfort from the needle puncture and the tourniquet but that collecting the sample usually takes less than 3 minutes.
● Inform him that he needn't restrict food or fluids before the test.
● Check the patient's history for drugs that may influence haptoglobin levels, such as steroids and androgens.

Procedure and posttest care

● Perform a venipuncture, and collect the sample in a 7-ml *red-top* or *red-marble-top* tube.
● If a hematoma develops at the venipuncture site, apply warm soaks.

Precautions

● Handle the sample gently to prevent hemolysis.

Reference values

Normally, serum haptoglobin concentrations, measured in terms of the protein's hemoglobin-binding capacity, range from 25 to 200 mg/dl. Nephelometric procedures yield lower results.

Haptoglobin is absent in 90% of neonates, but in most cases, levels gradually increase to normal by age 4 months.

Abnormal findings

Markedly decreased serum haptoglobin levels are characteristic in acute and chronic hemolysis, severe hepatocellular disease, infectious mononucleosis, and transfusion reactions. Hepatocellular disease inhibits the synthesis of haptoglobin. In hemolytic transfusion reactions, haptoglobin levels begin decreasing after 6 to 8 hours and drop to 40% of pretransfusion levels after 24 hours.

If serum haptoglobin values are very low, watch for symptoms of hemolysis: chills, fever, back pain, flushing, distended neck veins, tachycardia, tachypnea, and hypotension.

In about 1% of the population, including 4% of African-Americans, haptoglobin is permanently absent; this disorder is known as congenital ahaptoglobinemia.

Strikingly elevated serum haptoglobin levels occur in diseases marked by chronic inflammatory reactions or tissue destruction, such as rheumatoid arthritis and malignant neoplasms.

Interfering factors

● Hemolysis due to rough handling of the sample
● Steroids and androgens (possible increase; may mask hemolysis)

TRANSFERRIN

A quantitative analysis of serum transferrin (siderophilin) levels is used to evaluate iron metabolism. Transferrin is a glycoprotein that is formed in the liver. It transports circulating iron obtained from dietary sources or the breakdown of red blood cells by reticuloendothelial cells to bone marrow for use in hemoglobin synthesis or to the liver, spleen, and bone marrow for storage. A serum iron level is usually obtained simultaneously.

Purpose
- To determine the iron-transporting capacity of the blood
- To evaluate iron metabolism in iron deficiency anemia

Patient preparation
- Explain to the patient that this test is used to determine the cause of anemia.
- Tell him that the test requires a blood sample. Explain who will perform the venipuncture and when.
- Explain that he may experience slight discomfort from the needle puncture and the tourniquet but that collecting the sample usually takes less than 3 minutes.
- Inform him that he needn't restrict food or fluids before the test.
- Check the patient's history for drugs that may influence transferrin levels, such as oral contraceptives.

Procedure and posttest care
- Perform a venipuncture, and collect the sample in a 7-ml *red-top* or *red-marble-top* tube.
- If a hematoma develops at the venipuncture site, apply warm soaks.

Precautions
- Handle the sample gently to prevent hemolysis, and send it to the laboratory immediately.

Reference values
Normal serum transferrin values range from 200 to 400 µg/dl.

Abnormal findings
Inadequate transferrin levels may lead to impaired hemoglobin synthesis and, possibly, anemia. Low serum levels may indicate inadequate production of transferrin due to hepatic damage or excessive protein loss from renal disease. Decreased transferrin levels may also result from acute or chronic infection and cancer.

Increased serum transferrin levels may indicate severe iron deficiency.

Interfering factors
- Hemolysis due to rough handling of the sample
- Blood transfusions within 4 weeks of testing
- Oral contraceptives and late pregnancy (possible increase)
- Failure to send the sample to the laboratory immediately

PLASMA AMINO ACID SCREENING

Plasma and amino acid screening is a qualitative screen for inborn errors of amino acid metabolism. Amino acids are the chief component of all proteins and polypeptides. The body contains at least 20 amino acids; 10 of these aren't formed in the body and must be acquired by diet. Certain congenital enzyme deficiencies interfere with normal metabolism of these amino acids, resulting in amino acid accumulation or deficiency.

Purpose
- To screen for inborn errors of amino acid metabolism

Patient preparation
- Explain to the parents that this test is used to determine how well their infant metabolizes amino acids.

• The infant must fast for 4 hours before the test.
• Tell the parents that a small amount of blood will be drawn from the infant's heel but that collecting the sample only takes a few minutes.

Procedure and posttest care
• Perform a heelstick, and collect 0.1 ml of blood in a heparinized capillary tube.
• If a hematoma develops at the heelstick site, apply warm soaks.
• Tell the parents to resume their infant's usual diet.

Precautions
• Handle the sample gently to prevent hemolysis.

Normal findings
Chromatography shows a normal plasma amino acid pattern.

Abnormal findings
Excessive accumulation of amino acids typically produces overflow aminoacidurias. Congenital abnormalities of the amino acid transport system in the kidneys produce a second group of disorders called renal aminoacidurias. Comparisons of blood and urine chromatography can help distinguish between the two types of aminoacidurias. The plasma amino acid pattern is normal in renal aminoacidurias and abnormal in overflow aminoacidurias.

Interfering factors
• Failure to observe pretest restrictions
• Hemolysis due to rough handling of the sample

PHENYLALANINE SCREENING

Also called the Guthrie screening test, this test is used to screen infants for elevated serum phenylalanine levels, a possible indication of phenylketonuria (PKU). Phenylalanine is a naturally occurring amino acid essential to growth and nitrogen balance; an accumulation of this amino acid may indicate a serious enzyme deficiency. This test detects abnormal phenylalanine levels through the growth rate of *Bacillus subtilis*, an organism that needs phenylalanine to thrive. To ensure accurate results, the test must be performed after 3 full days (preferably 4 days) of milk or formula feeding.

Purpose
• To screen infants for possible PKU

Patient preparation
• Explain to the parents that the test is a routine screening measure for possible PKU and is required in many states.
• Tell them that a small amount of blood will be drawn from the infant's heel but that collecting the sample only takes a few minutes.

Procedure and posttest care
• Perform a heelstick, and collect three drops of blood — one in each circle — on the filter paper.
• Reassure the parents of a child who may have PKU that although this disease is a common cause of congenital mental deficiency, early detection and continuous treatment with a low-phenylalanine diet can prevent permanent mental retardation.

Precautions

• Note the infant's name and birth date and the date of the first milk or formula feeding on the laboratory slip, and send the sample to the laboratory immediately.

Reference values

A negative test result indicates normal phenylalanine levels (< 2 mg/dl) and no appreciable danger of PKU.

Abnormal findings

At birth, an infant with PKU usually has normal phenylalanine levels, but after milk or formula feeding begins, levels gradually increase because of a deficiency of the liver enzyme that converts phenylalanine to tyrosine. A positive test result suggests the *possibility* of PKU. A definitive diagnosis requires exact serum phenylalanine measurement and urine testing. A positive test result may also indicate hepatic disease, galactosemia, or delayed development of certain enzyme systems. (See *Confirming PKU.*)

Interfering factors

• Performing the test before the infant has received at least 3 full days of milk or formula feeding (false-negative)

PLASMA AMMONIA

This test measures plasma levels of ammonia, a nonprotein nitrogen compound that helps maintain acid-base balance. In diseases such as cirrhosis of the liver, ammonia can bypass the liver and accumulate in the blood. Plasma ammonia levels may help indicate the severity of hepatocellular damage.

CONFIRMING PKU

If phenylalanine screening detects the possible presence of phenylketonuria (PKU), serum phenylalanine and tyrosine levels are measured to confirm the diagnosis. Phenylalanine hydroxylase is the enzyme that converts phenylalanine to tyrosine. If this enzyme is absent, increasing phenylalanine levels and falling tyrosine levels indicate PKU.

Samples are obtained by venipuncture (femoral or external jugular) and measured by fluorometry. Elevated serum phenylalanine levels (> 15 mg/dl) and decreased tyrosine levels (< 5 mg/dl) — with urinary excretion of phenylpyruvic acid — confirm the diagnosis of PKU.

Purpose

• To help monitor the progression of severe hepatic disease and the effectiveness of therapy
• To recognize impending or established hepatic coma

Patient preparation

• Explain to the patient (or to a family member if the patient is comatose) that this test is used to evaluate liver function.
• Tell him that the test requires a blood sample. Explain who will perform the venipuncture and when.
• Inform him that he may experience transient discomfort from the needle puncture and the tourniquet, but reassure him that collecting the sample takes only a few minutes.
• Check the patient's history for drugs that influence plasma ammonia levels. They include acetazolamide, thiazides, ammonium salts, furosemide, lactulose, neomycin, and kanamycin.

Procedure and posttest care
● Perform a venipuncture, and collect the sample in a 10-ml *green-marble-top* (heparinized) tube.
● Make sure bleeding has stopped before removing pressure from the venipuncture site.
● If a hematoma develops at the puncture site, apply warm soaks.
● Watch for signs of impending or established hepatic coma if plasma ammonia levels are high.

Precautions
● Notify the laboratory before performing the venipuncture so that preliminary preparations can begin.
● Handle the sample gently to prevent hemolysis, pack it in ice, and send it to the laboratory immediately.
● *Do not* use a chilled container.

Reference values
Normally, plasma ammonia levels in adults range from 9 to 33 µmol/L.

Abnormal findings
Elevated plasma ammonia levels are common in severe hepatic disease, such as cirrhosis and acute hepatic necrosis, and can lead to hepatic coma. Elevated levels may also occur in Reye's syndrome, severe heart failure, GI hemorrhage, and erythroblastosis fetalis.

Interfering factors
● Hemolysis due to rough handling of the sample
● Delay in testing
● Acetazolamide, thiazides, ammonium salts, and furosemide (increase)
● Parenteral nutrition or a portacaval shunt (possible increase)
● Lactulose, neomycin, and kanamycin (decrease)
● Smoking, poor venipuncture technique, and exposure to ammonia cleaners in the laboratory (possible increase)

BLOOD UREA NITROGEN

This test is used to measure the nitrogen fraction of urea, the chief end product of protein metabolism. Formed in the liver from ammonia and excreted by the kidneys, urea constitutes 40% to 50% of the blood's nonprotein nitrogen. The blood urea nitrogen (BUN) level reflects protein intake and renal excretory capacity but is a less reliable indicator of uremia than the serum creatinine level.

Purpose
● To evaluate kidney function and aid diagnosis of renal disease
● To aid assessment of hydration

Patient preparation
● Tell the patient that this test is used to evaluate kidney function.
● Inform him that he needn't restrict food or fluids but should avoid a diet high in meat.
● Tell him that the test requires a blood sample. Explain who will perform the venipuncture and when.
● Explain that he may experience slight discomfort from the needle puncture and the tourniquet.
● Reassure him that collecting the sample takes only a few minutes and that test results should be available the next day.
● Check the patient's history for drugs that influence BUN levels, such as chloramphenicol.

Procedure and posttest care
● Perform a venipuncture, and collect the sample in a 7-ml *red-top* or *red-marble-top* tube.
● If a hematoma develops at the venipuncture site, apply warm soaks.

Precautions
• Handle the sample gently to prevent hemolysis.

Reference values
BUN values normally range from 8 to 20 mg/dl, with slightly higher values in elderly patients.

Abnormal findings
Elevated BUN levels occur in renal disease, reduced renal blood flow (due to dehydration, for example), urinary tract obstruction, and increased protein catabolism (as in burn injuries).

Low BUN levels occur in severe hepatic damage, malnutrition, and overhydration.

Interfering factors
• Hemolysis due to rough handling of the sample
• Chloramphenicol (possible decrease)

CREATININE

Analysis of serum creatinine levels provides a more sensitive measure of renal damage than blood urea nitrogen levels. Creatinine is a nonprotein end product of creatine metabolism that appears in serum in amounts proportional to the body's muscle mass.

Purpose
• To assess glomerular filtration
• To screen for renal damage

Patient preparation
• Explain to the patient that this test is used to evaluate kidney function.
• Tell him that the test requires a blood sample. Explain who will perform the venipuncture and when.
• Explain that he may experience slight discomfort from the needle puncture and the tourniquet but that collecting the sample usually takes less than 3 minutes.
• Instruct him not to eat or drink for about 8 hours before the test.
• Check whether he has received ascorbic acid, barbiturates, or diuretics within the past 24 hours.

Procedure and posttest care
• Perform a venipuncture, and collect the sample in a 7-ml *red-top* or *red-marble-top* tube.
• If a hematoma develops at the venipuncture site, apply warm soaks.

Precautions
• Handle the sample gently, and send it to the laboratory immediately.

Reference values
Creatinine concentrations normally range from 0.6 to 1.3 mg/dl.

Abnormal findings
Elevated serum creatinine levels generally indicate renal disease that has seriously damaged 50% or more of the nephrons. Elevated levels may also be associated with gigantism and acromegaly.

Interfering factors
• Ascorbic acid, barbiturates, and diuretics (possible increase)
• Exceptionally large muscle mass, as in athletes (possible increase despite normal renal function)
• Hemolysis due to rough handling of the sample

URIC ACID

This test is used to measure serum levels of uric acid, the major end metabolite of purine. Disorders of purine metabolism, rapid destruction of nucleic acids, and conditions marked by impaired renal excretion characteristically raise serum uric acid levels.

Purpose
- To confirm diagnosis of gout
- To help detect renal dysfunction

Patient preparation
- Explain to the patient that this test is used to detect gout and kidney dysfunction.
- Tell him that the test requires a blood sample. Explain who will perform the venipuncture and when.
- Explain that he may experience slight discomfort from the needle puncture and the tourniquet. Reassure him that collecting the sample takes only a few minutes.
- Instruct him to fast for 8 hours before the test.
- Check his medication history for the use of loop diuretics, ethambutol, vincristine, pyrazinamide, thiazides, aspirin, acetaminophen, ascorbic acid, and levodopa.

Procedure and posttest care
- Perform a venipuncture, and collect the sample in a 7-ml *red-top* or *red-marble-top* tube.
- If a hematoma develops at the venipuncture site, apply warm soaks.

Precautions
- Handle the sample gently to prevent hemolysis.

Reference values
Uric acid concentrations in men normally range from 3.5 to 7.2 mg/dl; in women, normal levels range from 2.6 to 6 mg/dl.

Abnormal findings
Increased uric acid levels may indicate gout or impaired kidney function. Lev-

els may also rise in heart failure, glycogen storage disease, infections, hemolytic and sickle cell anemia, polycythemia, neoplasms, and psoriasis.

Low uric acid levels may indicate defective tubular absorption (as in Fanconi's syndrome) or acute hepatic atrophy.

Interfering factors
- Failure to observe pretest restrictions
- Loop diuretics, ethambutol, vincristine, pyrazinamide, thiazides, and low doses of aspirin (possible increase)
- Acetaminophen, ascorbic acid, and levodopa (possible false-high if using colorimetric method)
- Aspirin in high doses (possible decrease)
- Starvation, high-purine diet, stress, and alcohol abuse (possible increase)

PIGMENTS

BILIRUBIN

This test is used to measure serum levels of bilirubin, the predominant pigment in bile. Bilirubin is the major product of hemoglobin catabolism. Serum bilirubin measurements are especially significant in neonates because elevated unconjugated bilirubin can accumulate in the brain, causing irreparable damage.

Purpose
- To evaluate hepatobiliary and erythropoietic functions
- To aid differential diagnosis of jaundice and monitor its progress
- To aid diagnosis of biliary obstruction and hemolytic anemia

• To determine whether a neonate requires an exchange transfusion or phototherapy because of dangerously high unconjugated bilirubin levels

Patient preparation
• Explain to the patient that this test is used to evaluate liver function and the condition of red blood cells.
• Tell him that the test requires a blood sample. Explain who will perform the venipuncture and when.
• Explain that he may experience slight discomfort from the needle puncture and the tourniquet but that collecting the sample usually takes less than 3 minutes.
• Inform the adult patient that he needn't restrict fluids but should fast for at least 4 hours before the test. (Fasting isn't necessary for neonates.)
• If the patient is an infant, tell the parents that a small amount of blood will be drawn from his heel.
• Tell them who will perform the heelstick and when.

Procedure and posttest care
• If the patient is an adult, perform a venipuncture, and collect the sample in a 7-ml *red-top* or *red-marble-top* tube.
• If the patient is an infant, perform a heelstick, and fill the microcapillary tube to the designated level with blood.
• If a hematoma develops at the venipuncture or heelstick site, apply warm soaks.

Precautions
• Protect the sample from strong sunlight and ultraviolet light.
• Handle the sample gently, and send it to the laboratory immediately.

Reference values
In adults, normal indirect serum bilirubin levels are 1 mg/dl or less, and direct serum bilirubin levels are less than 0.2 mg/dl. In neonates, total serum bilirubin levels are 1 to 10 mg/dl.

Abnormal findings
Elevated indirect serum bilirubin levels usually indicate hepatic damage. High levels of indirect bilirubin are also likely in severe hemolytic anemia. If hemolysis continues, both direct and indirect bilirubin levels may rise. Other causes of elevated indirect bilirubin levels include congenital enzyme deficiencies, such as Gilbert's disease.

Elevated direct serum bilirubin levels usually indicate biliary obstruction. If obstruction continues, both direct and indirect bilirubin levels may rise. In severe chronic hepatic damage, direct bilirubin concentrations may return to normal or near-normal levels, but indirect bilirubin levels remain elevated.

In neonates, total bilirubin levels of 18 mg/dl or more indicate the need for an exchange transfusion.

Interfering factors
• Failure to observe pretest restrictions
• Exposure of the sample to direct sunlight or ultraviolet light (possible decrease)
• Hemolysis due to rough handling of the sample
• Failure to send sample to laboratory immediately

FRACTIONATED ERYTHROCYTE PORPHYRINS

This test is used to measure erythrocyte porphyrins (also called erythropoietic porphyrins): protoporphyrin, coproporphyrin, and uroporphyrin. Porphyrins are present in all protoplasm and are significant in energy storage and use. They are produced during heme biosynthesis and normally appear in small amounts in blood, urine, and stool. The production and excretion of porphyrins or their precursors increase in porphyria.

Purpose
• To aid diagnosis of congenital and acquired erythropoietic porphyrias
• To help confirm diagnosis of disorders affecting red blood cell activity

Patient preparation
• Explain to the patient that this test is used to detect red blood cell disorders.
• Tell him that the test requires a blood sample. Explain who will perform the venipuncture and when.
• Explain that he may experience slight discomfort from the needle puncture and the tourniquet but that collecting the sample usually takes less than 3 minutes.

Procedure and posttest care
• Perform a venipuncture, collect the sample in a 5-ml or larger *green-top* tube, and send it to the laboratory immediately.
• Protect the sample from light and place it on ice.
• If a hematoma develops at the venipuncture site, apply warm soaks.

Precautions
• Handle the sample gently to prevent hemolysis.
• Send the sample to the laboratory promptly.

Reference values
Total porphyrin levels range from 16 to 60 µg/dl of packed red blood cells. Protoporphyrin levels range from 16 to 60 µg/dl. Coproporphyrin and uroporphyrin levels are normally less than 2 µg/dl.

Abnormal findings
Elevated total porphyrin levels suggest the need for further enzyme testing to identify the specific porphyria. Elevated protoporphyrin levels may indicate erythropoietic protoporphyria, infection, increased erythropoiesis, thalassemia, sideroblastic anemia, iron deficiency anemia, or lead poisoning.

Increased coproporphyrin levels may indicate congenital erythropoietic porphyria, erythropoietic protoporphyria or coproporphyria, or sideroblastic anemia.

Elevated uroporphyrin levels may indicate congenital erythropoietic porphyria or erythropoietic protoporphyria.

Interfering factors
• Hemolysis due to rough handling of the sample
• Exposure of the sample to direct sunlight or ultraviolet light

CARBOHYDRATES

FASTING PLASMA GLUCOSE

The fasting plasma glucose (or fasting blood sugar) test is used to measure plasma glucose levels after a 12- to 14-hour fast. This test is commonly used to screen for diabetes mellitus, in which absence or deficiency of insulin allows persistently high glucose levels.

Purpose
• To screen for diabetes mellitus
• To monitor drug or diet therapy in patients with diabetes mellitus

Patient preparation

- Explain to the patient that this test is used to detect disorders of glucose metabolism and aids diagnosis of diabetes.
- Tell him that the test requires a blood sample. Explain who will perform the venipuncture and when.
- Explain that he may experience slight discomfort from the needle puncture and the tourniquet but that collecting the sample usually takes less than 3 minutes.
- Instruct him to fast for 12 to 14 hours before the test.
- Withhold drugs that may affect test results, such as acetaminophen, chlorthalidone, thiazide diuretics, furosemide, triamterene, oral contraceptives, benzodiazepines, phenytoin, phenothiazines, lithium, epinephrine, arginine, phenolphthalein, dextrothyroxine, diazoxide, nicotinic acid (large doses), corticosteroids, I.V. glucose (note recent infusions), beta-adrenergic blockers, ethanol, clofibrate, insulin, oral antidiabetic agents, monoamine oxidase (MAO) inhibitors, and ethacrynic acid. If these medications must be continued, note this on the laboratory slip. Tell the patient with diabetes that he'll receive his medication after the test.
- Alert the patient to the symptoms of hypoglycemia (weakness, restlessness, nervousness, hunger, and sweating), and tell him to report such symptoms immediately.

Procedure and posttest care

- Perform a venipuncture, and collect the sample in a 5-ml *gray-top* tube.
- If a hematoma develops at the venipuncture site, apply warm soaks.
- Provide a balanced meal or a snack.
- Resume administration of medications withheld before the test.

Precautions

- Send the sample to the laboratory immediately. If transport is delayed, refrigerate the sample.
- Note on the laboratory slip when the patient last ate, the sample collection time, and when the last pretest dose of insulin or oral antidiabetic drug (if applicable) was given.

Reference values

The normal range for fasting plasma glucose varies according to the laboratory procedure. However, the American Diabetes Association's guidelines, revised in 1998, call for normal blood glucose levels of less than 126 mg/dl.

Abnormal findings

Confirmation of diabetes mellitus requires fasting plasma glucose levels of 126 mg/dl or more obtained on two or more occasions. In patients with borderline or transient elevated levels, a 2-hour postprandial plasma glucose test or oral glucose tolerance test may be performed to confirm diagnosis.

Increased fasting plasma glucose levels can also result from pancreatitis, recent acute illness (such as myocardial infarction), Cushing's syndrome, acromegaly, and pheochromocytoma. Hyperglycemia may also stem from hyperlipoproteinemia (especially type III, IV, or V), chronic hepatic disease, nephrotic syndrome, brain tumor, sepsis, or gastrectomy with dumping syndrome and is typical in eclampsia, anoxia, and seizure disorder.

Low plasma glucose levels can result from hyperinsulinism, insulinoma, von Gierke's disease, functional and reactive hypoglycemia, myxedema, adrenal insufficiency, congenital adrenal hyperplasia, hypopituitarism, malabsorption syndrome, and some cases of hepatic insufficiency.

Interfering factors

- Failure to observe pretest restrictions (possible increase)
- Recent illness, infection, or pregnancy (possible increase)
- Glycolysis due to failure to refrigerate the sample or to send it to the laboratory immediately (possible false-negative)
- Acetaminophen, if using the glucose oxidase or hexokinase method (possible false-positive)
- Chlorthalidone, thiazide diuretics, furosemide, triamterene, oral contraceptives, benzodiazepines, phenytoin, phenothiazines, lithium, epinephrine, arginine, phenolphthalein, dextrothyroxine, diazoxide, large doses of nicotinic acid, corticosteroids, and recent I.V. glucose infusions (increase)
- Ethacrynic acid (may cause hyperglycemia); large doses in patients with uremia (can cause hypoglycemia)
- Beta-adrenergic blockers, ethanol, clofibrate, insulin, oral antidiabetic agents, and MAO inhibitors (possible decrease)
- Strenuous exercise (decrease)
- Elevated urea levels (possible false-high)

Two-hour Postprandial Plasma Glucose

Also called the 2-hour postprandial blood sugar test, this procedure is a valuable screening tool for detecting diabetes mellitus. It's performed when the patient demonstrates symptoms of diabetes (polydipsia and polyuria) or when results of the fasting plasma glucose test suggest diabetes.

Purpose

- To aid diagnosis of diabetes mellitus
- To monitor drug or diet therapy in patients with diabetes mellitus

Patient preparation

- Explain to the patient that this test is used to evaluate glucose metabolism and to detect diabetes.
- Tell him that the test requires a blood sample. Explain who will perform the venipuncture and when.
- Explain that he may experience slight discomfort from the needle puncture and the tourniquet but that collecting the sample usually takes less than 3 minutes.
- Tell him to eat a balanced meal or one containing 100 g of carbohydrates before the test and then to fast for 2 hours. Instruct him to avoid smoking and strenuous exercise after the meal.
- Withhold any medications that may alter glucose levels, such as acetaminophen, chlorthalidone, thiazide diuretics, triamterene, oral contraceptives, benzodiazepines, and lithium.

Procedure and posttest care

- Perform a venipuncture, and collect the sample in a 5-ml *gray-top* tube.
- If a hematoma develops at the venipuncture site, apply warm soaks.
- Tell the patient to resume his usual diet and normal activity.
- Resume administration of medications discontinued before the test.

Precautions

- Send the sample to the laboratory immediately or refrigerate it.
- Specify on the laboratory slip when the patient last ate, the sample collection time, and when the last pretest dose of insulin or oral antidiabetic drug was given.
- If the sample is to be drawn by a technician, tell him the exact time the venipuncture must be performed.

Two-hour Postprandial Plasma Glucose Levels by Age

The greatest difference in normal and diabetic insulin responses, and thus in plasma glucose concentration, occurs about 2 hours after a glucose challenge. Values of this test can fluctuate according to the patient's age. After age 50, for example, normal levels rise markedly and steadily, sometimes reaching 160 mg/dl or higher. In younger patients, glucose concentration over 145 mg/dl suggests incipient diabetes and requires further evaluation.

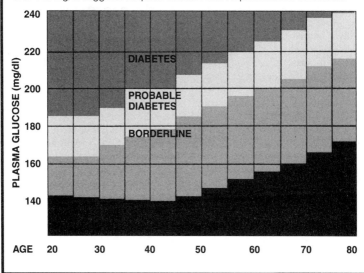

Reference values

In a person who doesn't have diabetes, postprandial glucose values are 65 to 139 mg/dl by the glucose oxidase or hexokinase method; levels are slightly elevated in people over age 87. (See *Two-hour postprandial plasma glucose levels by age.*)

Abnormal findings

Two 2-hour postprandial blood glucose values of 200 mg/dl or above indicate diabetes mellitus. High levels may also occur with pancreatitis, Cushing's syndrome, acromegaly, and pheochromocytoma. Hyperglycemia may also be caused by hyperlipoproteinemia (especially type III, IV, or V), chronic hepatic disease, nephrotic syndrome, brain tumor, sepsis, gastrectomy with dumping syndrome, eclampsia, anoxia, and seizure disorders.

Low glucose levels occur in hyperinsulinism, insulinoma, von Gierke's disease, functional and reactive hypoglycemia, myxedema, adrenal insufficiency, congenital adrenal hyperplasia, hypopituitarism, malabsorption syndrome, and some cases of hepatic insufficiency.

Interfering factors

● Recent illness, infection, or pregnancy (possible increase)

- Acetaminophen, if using the glucose oxidase or hexokinase method (possible false-positive)
- Chlorthalidone, thiazide diuretics, furosemide, triamterene, oral contraceptives, benzodiazepines, phenytoin, phenothiazines, lithium, epinephrine, arginine, phenolphthalein, dextrothyroxine, diazoxide, large doses of nicotinic acid, corticosteroids, and recent I.V. glucose infusions (increase)
- Ethacrynic acid (possible increase); large doses in patients with uremia (possible decrease)
- Beta-adrenergic blockers, amphetamines, ethanol, clofibrate, insulin, oral antidiabetic drugs, and monoamine oxidase inhibitors (possible decrease)
- Strenuous exercise or stress (possible decrease)
- Glycolysis caused by failure to refrigerate the sample or to send it to the laboratory immediately (possible decrease)

ORAL GLUCOSE TOLERANCE TEST

The oral glucose tolerance test is the most sensitive method of evaluating borderline cases of diabetes mellitus. Plasma and urine glucose levels are monitored for 3 hours after ingestion of a challenge dose of glucose to assess insulin secretion and the body's ability to metabolize glucose.

The oral glucose tolerance test is not generally used in patients with fasting plasma glucose values greater than 140 mg/dl or postprandial plasma glucose values greater than 200 mg/dl.

Purpose
- To confirm diabetes mellitus in selected patients

- To aid diagnosis of hypoglycemia and malabsorption syndrome (requires monitoring for an additional 2 to 3 hours to aid diagnosis, which is contraindicated when insulinoma is strongly suspected because prolonged fasting may lead to fainting and coma)

Patient preparation
- Explain to the patient that this test is used to evaluate glucose metabolism.
- Instruct him to maintain a high-carbohydrate diet for 3 days and then to fast for 12 to 16 hours, as instructed by the doctor, before the test.
- Tell him not to smoke, drink coffee or alcohol, or exercise strenuously for 8 hours before or during the test.
- Tell him that this test requires five blood samples and usually five urine samples. Explain who will perform the venipunctures and when and that he may experience transient discomfort from the needle punctures and the tourniquet.
- Suggest that he bring a book or other quiet diversions with him to the test because the procedure usually takes 3 hours but can last as long as 6 hours.
- Withhold drugs that may affect test results. They may include chlorthalidone, thiazide diuretics, furosemide, triamterene, oral contraceptives, benzodiazepines, phenytoin, phenothiazines, lithium, epinephrine, phenolphthalein, caffeine, arginine, dextrothyroxine, diazoxide, nicotinic acid (large doses), corticosteroids, I.V. glucose (note recent infusions), beta-adrenergic blockers, amphetamines, ethanol, clofibrate, insulin, oral antidiabetic drugs, and monoamine oxidase (MAO) inhibitors. If these drugs must be continued, note this on the laboratory slip.
- Alert the patient to the symptoms of hypoglycemia (weakness, restlessness, nervousness, hunger, and sweating), and tell him to report such symptoms immediately.

Procedure and posttest care

• Between 7 a.m. and 9 a.m., perform a venipuncture to obtain a fasting blood sample. Draw this sample into a 7-ml *gray-top* tube.

• Collect a urine sample at the same time, if your facility includes this as part of the test.

• After collecting these samples, administer the test load of oral glucose, and record the time of ingestion. Encourage the patient to drink the entire glucose solution within 5 minutes.

• Draw blood samples 30 minutes, 1 hour, 2 hours, and 3 hours after giving the loading dose, using 7-ml *gray-top* tubes.

• Collect urine samples at the same intervals.

• Tell the patient to lie down if he feels faint from the numerous venipunctures.

• Encourage him to drink water throughout the test to promote adequate urine excretion.

• If a hematoma develops at the venipuncture site, apply warm soaks.

• Provide a balanced meal or a snack, but observe for a hypoglycemic reaction.

• Resume administration of medications withheld before the test.

Precautions

• Send blood and urine samples to the laboratory immediately or refrigerate them.

• Specify when the patient last ate and the blood and urine sample collection times.

• As appropriate, record the time the patient received his last pretest dose of insulin or oral antidiabetic drug.

• If the patient develops severe hypoglycemia, notify the doctor. Draw a blood sample, record the time on the laboratory slip, and discontinue the test. Have the patient drink a glass of orange juice with sugar added, or administer glucose I.V. to reverse the reaction.

Reference values

Normal plasma glucose levels peak at 110 to 170 mg/dl within 30 minutes to 1 hour after administration of an oral glucose test dose and return to fasting levels or lower within 2 to 3 hours. Urine glucose tests remain negative throughout.

Abnormal findings

Decreased glucose tolerance, in which levels peak sharply before falling slowly to fasting levels, may confirm diabetes mellitus or may result from Cushing's disease, hemochromatosis, pheochromocytoma, or central nervous system lesions.

Increased glucose tolerance, in which levels may peak at less than normal, may indicate insulinoma, malabsorption syndrome, adrenocortical insufficiency (Addison's disease), hypothyroidism, or hypopituitarism.

Interfering factors

• Recent infection, fever, pregnancy, or acute illness, such as myocardial infarction (possible increase)

• Failure to observe pretest restrictions

• Carbohydrate deprivation before the test (may cause a diabetic response [abnormal increase with a delayed decrease] because the pancreas is unaccustomed to responding to high-carbohydrate load)

• Failure to consume the entire test load of oral glucose

• Chlorthalidone, thiazide diuretics, furosemide, triamterene, oral contraceptives, benzodiazepines, phenytoin, phenothiazines, lithium, epinephrine, phenolphthalein, caffeine, arginine, dextrothyroxine, diazoxide, corticosteroids, large doses of nicotinic acid, and recent I.V. glucose infusions (possible increase)

• Beta-adrenergic blockers, amphetamines, ethanol, clofibrate, insulin, oral antidiabetic drugs, and MAO inhibitors (possible decrease)
• Age 50 or older (decreasing carbohydrate tolerance, which causes increasing glucose tolerance to upper limits of about 1 mg/dl for every year over age 50)

β-HYDROXYBUTYRATE

This test is used to measure serum levels of ß-hydroxybutyric acid (ß-hydroxybutyrate), one of three ketone bodies. The other two ketone bodies are acetoacetate and acetone. An accumulation of all three ketone bodies is referred to as *ketosis*; excessive formation of ketone bodies in the blood is called *ketonemia*.

Purpose
• To diagnose carbohydrate deprivation, which may result from starvation, digestive disturbances, dietary imbalances, or frequent vomiting
• To aid diagnosis of diabetes mellitus resulting from decreased utilization of carbohydrates
• To aid diagnosis of glycogen storage diseases, specifically von Gierke's disease
• To monitor the effect of insulin therapy during treatment of diabetic ketoacidosis
• To monitor patient status during emergency management of hypoglycemia, acidosis, excessive alcohol ingestion, or an unexplained increase in the anion gap

Patient preparation
• Explain to the patient that this test is used to evaluate ketones in the blood.

• Tell him that the test requires a blood sample. Explain who will perform the venipuncture and when.
• Explain that he may experience slight discomfort from the needle puncture and the tourniquet but that collecting the sample usually takes less than 3 minutes.
• Inform him that he needn't restrict food or fluids before the test.

Procedure and posttest care
• Perform a venipuncture, and collect the sample in a 5-ml *red-top* tube.
• Allow the sample to clot.
• Centrifuge and remove the serum.
• If an acetone level is requested, have this analysis performed first.
• Serum ß-hydroxybutyrate remains stable for at least 1 week at 35.6° to 46.4° F (2° to 8° C). Plasma is also an acceptable sample for analysis of ß-hydroxybutyrate.
• If a hematoma develops at the venipuncture site, apply warm soaks.

Precautions
• Send the sample to the laboratory immediately.

Reference values
The normal value for serum or plasma ß-hydroxybutyrate levels is less than 0.4 mmol/L.

Abnormal findings
Elevated ß-hydroxybutyrate levels may suggest worsening of ketosis. Reference values greater than 2 mmol/L should be reported to the patient's doctor immediately.

Interfering factors
• Presence of both lactate dehydrogenase at high concentrations and lactic acid at concentrations greater than 10 mmol/L (possible increase)

- Sodium fluoride at concentrations greater than 2.5 nmol/L (possible decrease)
- Fasting (increase with extended fasting time)

GLYCOSYLATED HEMOGLOBIN

Also called total fasting hemoglobin, the glycosylated hemoglobin test is a tool for monitoring diabetes therapy. Measurement of glycosylated hemoglobin levels provides information about the average blood glucose level during the preceding 2 to 3 months. This test requires only one venipuncture every 6 to 8 weeks and can, therefore, be used for evaluating long-term effectiveness of diabetes therapy.

Purpose
- To assess control of diabetes mellitus

Patient preparation
- Explain to the patient that this test is used to evaluate diabetes therapy.
- Tell him that the test requires a blood sample. Explain who will perform the venipuncture and when.
- Explain that he may experience slight discomfort from the needle puncture and the tourniquet but that collecting the sample usually takes less than 3 minutes.
- Inform him that he needn't restrict food or fluids, and instruct him to maintain his prescribed medication and diet regimens.

Procedure and posttest care
- Perform a venipuncture, and collect the sample in a 5-ml *lavender-top* tube.
- If a hematoma develops at the venipuncture site, apply warm soaks.

- Schedule the patient for an appointment in 6 to 8 weeks for appropriate follow-up testing.

Precautions
- Completely fill the collection tube, and invert it gently several times to mix the sample and anticoagulant adequately.

Reference values
Glycosylated hemoglobin values are reported as a percentage of the total hemoglobin within an erythrocyte. Glycosylated hemoglobin accounts for 4% to 7%.

Abnormal findings
In diabetes, the patient has good control of blood glucose concentrations when the glycosylated hemoglobin value is less than 8%. A glycosylated hemoglobin value greater than 10% indicates poor control.

Interfering factors
- Failure to adequately mix the sample and the anticoagulant
- Hemolytic anemia

ORAL LACTOSE TOLERANCE TEST

The oral lactose tolerance test is used to measure plasma glucose levels after ingestion of a challenge dose of lactose. It's used to screen for lactose intolerance due to lactase deficiency.

Absence or deficiency of lactase causes undigested lactose to remain in the intestinal lumen, producing such symptoms as abdominal cramps and watery diarrhea. True congenital lactase deficiency is rare. Usually, lactose intolerance is acquired because lactase levels generally decrease with age.

Purpose
• To detect lactose intolerance

Patient preparation
• Explain to the patient that this test is used to determine if his symptoms are due to an inability to digest lactose.
• Instruct him to fast and to avoid strenuous activity for 8 hours before the test.
• Inform him that this test requires four blood samples. Tell him who will perform the venipunctures and when.
• Explain that he may experience transient discomfort from the needle punctures and the tourniquet but that collecting each blood sample takes less than 3 minutes. Tell him that the entire procedure may take up to 2 hours.
• Tell him that this test may also require a stool sample.
• Withhold drugs that may affect plasma glucose levels, including thiazide diuretics, oral contraceptives, benzodiazepines, propranolol, and insulin. If these drugs must be continued, note this on the laboratory slip.

Procedure and posttest care
• After the patient has fasted for 8 hours, perform a venipuncture and collect a blood sample in a 7-ml *gray-top* tube.
• Administer the test load of lactose: for an adult, 50 g of lactose dissolved in 400 ml of water; for a child, 50 g/m^2 of body surface area. Record the time of ingestion.
• Draw a blood sample 30, 60, and 120 minutes after giving the loading dose, using 7-ml *gray-top* tubes.
• If ordered, collect a stool sample 5 hours after giving the loading dose.
• If a hematoma develops at the venipuncture site, apply warm soaks.

• Instruct the patient to resume his usual diet and activity.
• Resume administration of medications withheld before the test.

Precautions
• Send blood and stool samples to the laboratory immediately, or refrigerate them if transport is delayed.
• Specify the collection time on the laboratory slips.
• Watch for symptoms of lactose intolerance — abdominal cramps, nausea, bloating, flatulence, and watery diarrhea — caused by the loading dose.

Reference values
Normally, plasma glucose levels rise more than 30 mg/dl over fasting levels within 15 to 60 minutes after ingestion of the lactose loading dose. Stool sample analysis shows normal pH (7.0 to 8.0) and low glucose content (< 1+ on a glucose-indicating dipstick).

Abnormal findings
A rise in plasma glucose of less than 20 mg/dl indicates lactose intolerance, as does stool acidity (pH of 5.5 or less) and high glucose content (> 1+ on the dipstick). Accompanying signs and symptoms provoked by the test also suggest but do not confirm the diagnosis because such symptoms may appear in patients with normal lactase activity after a loading dose of lactose. Small-bowel biopsy with lactase assay may be performed to confirm the diagnosis.

Interfering factors
• Failure to observe pretest restrictions
• Failure to ingest the complete test load of lactose
• Thiazide diuretics, oral contraceptives, benzodiazepines, propranolol, and insulin (possible false-low)
• Delayed emptying of stomach contents (possible decrease)
• Glycolysis (possible false-negative)

LACTIC ACID AND PYRUVIC ACID

Lactic acid, present in blood as lactate ion, is derived primarily from muscle cells and erythrocytes. It's an intermediate product of carbohydrate metabolism and is normally metabolized by the liver. Blood lactate concentration depends on the rates of production and metabolism; levels may increase significantly during exercise.

Lactate and pyruvate together form a reversible reaction that's regulated by oxygen supply. When oxygen levels are deficient, pyruvate converts to lactate; when they're adequate, lactate converts to pyruvate. When the hepatic system fails to metabolize lactose sufficiently or when excess pyruvate converts to lactate, lactic acidosis may result. Measurement of blood lactate levels is recommended for all patients with symptoms of lactic acidosis, such as Kussmaul's respiration.

Comparison of pyruvate and lactate levels provides reliable information about tissue oxidation, but measurement of pyruvate is technically difficult and infrequently performed.

Purpose
- To assess tissue oxidation
- To help determine the cause of lactic acidosis

Patient preparation
- Explain to the patient that this blood test is used to evaluate the oxygen level in tissues.
- Tell him that the test requires a blood sample. Explain who will perform the venipuncture and when.
- Explain that he may experience slight discomfort from the needle

puncture and the tourniquet but that collecting the sample usually takes less than 3 minutes.
- Withhold food overnight, and make sure the patient rests for at least 1 hour before the test.

Procedure and posttest care
- Perform a venipuncture, and collect the sample in a 5-ml *gray-top* tube.
- If a hematoma develops at the venipuncture site, apply warm soaks.
- Tell the patient that he may resume his normal diet.

Precautions
- Because venostasis may raise blood lactate levels, tell the patient that he must not clench his fist during the venipuncture.
- Because lactate and pyruvate are extremely unstable, place the sample container in an ice-filled cup, and send it to the laboratory immediately.

Reference values
Blood lactate values normally range from 0.5 to 1.6 mEq/L; pyruvate levels, from 0.08 to 0.16 mEq/L. The lactate-pyruvate ratio is normally less than 10:1.

Abnormal findings
Elevated blood lactate levels associated with hypoxia may result from strenuous muscle exercise, shock, hemorrhage, septicemia, myocardial infarction, pulmonary embolism, and cardiac arrest. When no reason for diminished tissue perfusion is apparent, increased lactate levels may result from systemic disorders, such as diabetes mellitus, leukemias and lymphomas, hepatic disease, and renal failure, or from enzymatic defects, such as von Gierke's disease (glycogen storage disease) and fructose 1,6-diphosphatase deficiency.

Lactic acidosis can follow ingestion of large doses of acetaminophen and

ethanol as well as I.V. infusion of epinephrine, glucagon, fructose, or sor-
bitol.

Interfering factors
● Failure to observe pretest restrictions
● Failure to pack the sample in ice and
to transport it to the laboratory immediately (possible increase)

CHAPTER 3

Hormone Tests

PITUITARY HORMONES		196

196	Corticotropin	205	Plasma luteinizing hormone
197	Rapid corticotropin test	207	Prolactin
199	Growth hormone	209	Thyroid-stimulating hormone
200	Growth hormone suppression test	210	Neonatal thyroid-stimulating hormone
201	Insulin tolerance test	212	Antidiuretic hormone
202	Arginine test	213	Alpha-subunit of pituitary glycoprotein hormones
204	Follicle-stimulating hormone		

THYROID AND PARATHYROID HORMONES		214

214	Thyroxine	219	Screening test for congenital hypothyroidism
215	Triiodothyronine	221	Plasma calcitonin
216	Thyroxine-binding globulin	222	Parathyroid hormone
217	T_3 uptake		
218	Free thyroxine and free triiodothyronine		

ADRENAL AND RENAL HORMONES		224

224	Aldosterone	229	Androstenedione
225	Plasma cortisol	230	Erythropoietin
227	Plasma catecholamines	231	Plasma atrial natriuretic factor

PANCREATIC AND GASTRIC HORMONES		232

232	Insulin	235	Plasma glucagon
233	Gastrin		

GONADAL HORMONES		235

235	Estrogens	238	Testosterone
237	Plasma progesterone		

PLACENTAL HORMONES		240

240	Human chorionic gonadotropin	241	Human placental lactogen

PITUITARY HORMONES

CORTICOTROPIN

This test measures the plasma levels of corticotropin (also known as adreno-corticotropic hormone or ACTH) by radioimmunoassay. Corticotropin stimulates the adrenal cortex to secrete cortisol and, to a lesser degree, androgens and aldosterone. It also has some melanocyte-stimulating activity, increases the uptake of amino acids by muscle cells, promotes lipolysis by fat cells, stimulates pancreatic beta cells to secrete insulin, and may contribute to the release of growth hormone. Corticotropin levels vary diurnally, peaking between 6 a.m. and 8 a.m. and ebbing between 6 p.m. and 11 p.m.

The corticotropin test may be ordered for patients with signs of adrenal hypofunction (insufficiency) or hyperfunction (Cushing's syndrome). Corticotropin suppression or stimulation testing is usually necessary to confirm diagnosis. The instability and unavailability of corticotropin greatly limit this test's diagnostic significance and reliability.

Purpose

• To facilitate differential diagnosis of primary and secondary adrenal hypofunction
• To aid differential diagnosis of Cushing's syndrome

Patient preparation

• Explain to the patient that this test helps determine if his hormonal secretion is normal.

• Advise him that he must fast and limit his physical activity for 10 to 12 hours before the test.
• Tell him that the test requires a blood sample, and explain who will perform the venipuncture and when.
• Inform him that he may experience some transient discomfort from the needle puncture and the tourniquet but that collecting the sample takes only a few minutes.
• Check the patient's drug history for the use of medications that may affect the accuracy of test results, such as corticosteroids, and medications that affect cortisol levels, such as estrogens, amphetamines, spironolactone, lithium carbonate, calcium gluconate, and alcohol (ethanol). Withhold these medications for 48 hours or longer before the test. If they must be continued, note this on the laboratory slip.
• Arrange with the dietary department to provide a low-carbohydrate diet for 2 days before the test. This requirement may vary, depending on the laboratory.

Procedure and posttest care

• For a patient with suspected adrenal hypofunction, perform the venipuncture for a baseline level between 6 a.m. and 8 a.m. (peak secretion).
• For a patient with suspected Cushing's syndrome, perform the venipuncture between 6 p.m. and 11 p.m. (low secretion).
• Collect the sample in a plastic tube (corticotropin may adhere to glass) or in a *lavender-top* tube. The tube must be full because excess anticoagulant will affect results.
• Pack the sample in ice, and send it to the laboratory immediately, where plasma must be rapidly separated from blood cells at 39.2° F (4° C). The collection technique may vary, depending on the laboratory.

• If a hematoma develops at the venipuncture site, apply warm soaks.

• Resume diet and administration of medications that were discontinued before the test.

Precautions

• Because proteolytic enzymes in plasma degrade corticotropin, a temperature of 39.2° F (4° C) is necessary to retard enzyme activity. Immediate transfer of the sample, packed in ice, to the laboratory is essential for reliable test results.

Reference values

Mayo Medical Laboratories sets baseline values at less than 60 pg/ml, but these values may vary, depending on the laboratory.

Abnormal findings

A higher-than-normal corticotropin level may indicate primary adrenal hypofunction (Addison's disease), in which the pituitary gland attempts to compensate for the unresponsiveness of the target organ by releasing excessive corticotropin. The underlying cause of adrenocortical hypofunction may be idiopathic atrophy of the adrenal cortex or partial destruction of the gland by granuloma, neoplasm, amyloidosis, or inflammatory necrosis.

A low-normal corticotropin level suggests secondary adrenal hypofunction resulting from pituitary or hypothalamic dysfunction. The primary determinant may be panhypopituitarism, absence of corticotropin-releasing hormone in the hypothalamus, or chronic blunting of corticotropin levels by long-term corticosteroid therapy.

In suspected Cushing's syndrome, an elevated corticotropin level suggests Cushing's disease, in which pituitary dysfunction (due to adenoma) causes continuous hypersecretion of corticotropin and, consequently, continuously elevated cortisol levels without diurnal variations. Moderately elevated corticotropin levels suggest pituitary-dependent adrenal hyperplasia and nonadrenal tumors, such as oat cell carcinoma of the lungs.

A low-normal corticotropin level implies adrenal hyperfunction due to adrenocortical tumor or hyperplasia.

Interfering factors

• Failure to observe pretest restrictions

• Corticosteroids, including cortisone and its analogues (decrease)

• Drugs that increase endogenous cortisol secretion, such as estrogens, calcium gluconate, amphetamines, spironolactone, and ethanol (decrease)

• Lithium carbonate (decreases cortisol levels and may interfere with corticotropin secretion)

• Menstrual cycle and pregnancy

• Radioactive scan performed within 1 week before the test

• Acute stress (including hospitalization and surgery) and depression (increase)

RAPID CORTICOTROPIN TEST

The rapid corticotropin test (also known as the rapid ACTH test or cosyntropin test) is gradually replacing the 8-hour corticotropin stimulation test as the most effective diagnostic tool for evaluating adrenal hypofunction. Using cosyntropin, the rapid corticotropin test provides faster results and causes fewer allergic reactions than the 8-hour test, which uses natural corticotropin from animal sources.

This test requires prior determination of baseline cortisol levels to evaluate the effect of cosyntropin administration on cortisol secretion. An unequivocally high morning cortisol level rules out adrenal hypofunction and makes further testing unnecessary.

Purpose
• To aid in identification of primary and secondary adrenal hypofunction

Patient preparation
• Explain to the patient that this test helps determine if his condition is due to a hormonal deficiency.
• Inform him that he may be required to fast for 10 to 12 hours before the test and must be relaxed and resting quietly for 30 minutes before the test.
• Tell him that the test takes at least 1 hour to perform.
• If the patient is in a facility, withhold corticotropin and all steroid medications before the test as ordered. If he is an outpatient, tell him to refrain from taking these drugs, if instructed by his doctor. If the drugs must be continued, note this on the laboratory slip.
• Inform the patient that he may experience transient discomfort from the needle puncture and the tourniquet.

Procedure and posttest care
• Draw 5 ml of blood for a baseline value. Collect the sample in a 5-ml *green-top* (heparinized) tube. Label this sample "preinjection," and send it to the laboratory.
• Inject 250 µg (0.25 mg) of cosyntropin I.V. or I.M. (I.V. administration provides more accurate results because ineffective absorption after I.M. administration may cause wide variations in response.) Direct I.V. injection should take about 2 minutes.

• Draw another 5 ml of blood at 30 and 60 minutes after the cosyntropin injection. Collect the samples in 5-ml *green-top* (heparinized) tubes. Label the samples "30 minutes postinjection" and "60 minutes postinjection," and send them to the laboratory. Include the actual collection times on the laboratory slip.
• If a hematoma develops at the venipuncture sites, apply warm soaks.
• Observe the patient for signs of a rare allergic reaction to cosyntropin, such as hives, itching, and tachycardia.
• Instruct the patient to resume his normal diet.
• Resume administration of medications discontinued before the test.

Precautions
• Handle the samples gently to prevent hemolysis. They require no special precautions other than avoiding stasis.

Reference values
Normally, cortisol levels rise 7 µg/dl or more above the baseline value to a peak of 18 µg/dl or more 60 minutes after the cosyntropin injection. Generally, a doubling of the baseline value indicates a normal response.

Abnormal findings
A normal result excludes adrenal hypofunction (insufficiency). In patients with primary adrenal hypofunction (Addison's disease), cortisol levels remain low. Thus, the rapid corticotropin test provides an effective method of screening for adrenal hypofunction. If test results show subnormal increases in cortisol levels, prolonged stimulation of the adrenal cortex may be required to differentiate between primary and secondary adrenal hypofunction.

Interfering factors
- Failure to observe pretest restrictions
- Hemolysis due to rough handling of the sample
- Estrogens and amphetamines (increase in plasma cortisol)
- Smoking and obesity (possible increase in plasma cortisol)
- Lithium carbonate (decrease in plasma cortisol)
- Radioactive scan performed within 1 week before the test

GROWTH HORMONE

Human growth hormone (hGH), also called somatotropin, is a protein secreted by acidophils of the anterior pituitary gland. It's the primary regulator of human growth. Unlike other pituitary hormones, hGH has no easily defined feedback mechanism or single target gland — it affects many body tissues. Like insulin, hGH promotes protein synthesis and stimulates amino acid uptake by cells. Hyposecretion or hypersecretion of this hormone may induce pathologic states (such as dwarfism and gigantism, respectively). Altered hGH levels are common in patients with pituitary dysfunction.

This test, a quantitative analysis of plasma hGH levels, is usually performed as part of an anterior pituitary stimulation or suppression test. Such testing is crucial because clinical manifestations of an hGH deficiency can seldom be reversed by therapy.

Purpose
- To aid differential diagnosis of dwarfism because growth retardation can result from pituitary or thyroid hypofunction
- To confirm diagnosis of acromegaly and gigantism
- To aid diagnosis of pituitary and hypothalamic tumors
- To help evaluate hGH therapy

Patient preparation
- Explain to the patient, or to his parents if the patient is a child, that this test measures hormone levels and helps determine the cause of abnormal growth.
- Instruct him to fast and limit physical activity for 10 to 12 hours before the test.
- Tell him that the test requires a blood sample, and explain who will perform the venipuncture and when.
- Reassure him that although he may experience some discomfort from the needle puncture and tourniquet, collecting the sample takes less than 3 minutes.
- Inform him that another sample may have to be drawn the next day for comparison.
- Withhold all medications that affect hGH levels, such as pituitary-based steroids. If they must be continued, note this on the laboratory slip.
- Make sure the patient is relaxed and recumbent for 30 minutes before the test because stress and physical activity elevate hGH levels.

Procedure and posttest care
- Between 6 a.m. and 8 a.m. on 2 consecutive days, or as ordered, perform a venipuncture and collect at least 7 ml of blood in a 10-ml *red-top* tube.
- If a hematoma develops at the venipuncture site, apply warm soaks.
- Instruct the patient to resume his normal diet and medications that were discontinued before the test.

Precautions
• Handle the sample gently to prevent hemolysis.
• Send it to the laboratory immediately because hGH has a half-life of only 20 to 25 minutes.

Reference values
Normal hGH levels for males range from undetectable to 5 ng/ml; for females, from undetectable to 10 ng/ml.

Abnormal findings
Increased hGH levels may indicate a pituitary or hypothalamic tumor, frequently an adenoma, which causes gigantism in children and acromegaly in adults and adolescents. Some patients with diabetes mellitus have elevated hGH levels without acromegaly. Suppression testing is necessary to confirm diagnosis.

Pituitary infarction, metastatic disease, and tumors may decrease hGH levels. Dwarfism may be due to low hGH levels, although only 15% of all cases of growth failure relate to endocrine dysfunction. Confirmation of diagnosis requires stimulation testing with arginine or insulin.

Interfering factors
• Failure to observe pretest restrictions
• Hemolysis due to rough handling of the sample
• Arginine, beta blockers such as propranolol, and estrogens (increase)
• Amphetamines, bromocriptine, levodopa, dopamine, pituitary-based steroids, methyldopa, and histamine (increase)
• Insulin (induced hypoglycemia), glucagon, and nicotinic acid (increase)
• Phenothiazines (such as chlorpromazine) and corticosteroids (decrease)
• Radioactive scan performed within 1 week before the test

GROWTH HORMONE SUPPRESSION TEST

Also called glucose loading, this test evaluates excessive baseline levels of human growth hormone (hGH) from the anterior pituitary. Normally, a glucose load should suppress hGH secretion. In a patient with excessive hGH levels, failure of suppression indicates anterior pituitary dysfunction and confirms diagnosis of acromegaly and gigantism.

Purpose
• To assess elevated baseline levels of hGH
• To confirm diagnosis of gigantism in children and acromegaly in adults and adolescents

Patient preparation
• Explain to the patient, or to his parents if the patient is a child, that this test helps determine the cause of his abnormal growth.
• Instruct him to fast and limit physical activity for 10 to 12 hours before the test.
• Tell him that two blood samples will be drawn. Warn him that he may experience nausea after drinking the glucose solution and some discomfort from the needle punctures and tourniquet.
• Withhold all steroids and other pituitary-based hormones. If they or other medications must be continued, note this on the laboratory slip.
• Tell the patient to lie down and relax for 30 minutes before the test.

Procedure and posttest care
• Perform a venipuncture and collect 6 ml of blood (basal sample) in a 10- to 15-ml *red-top* tube.

- Administer 100 g of glucose solution by mouth. To prevent nausea, advise the patient to drink the glucose slowly.
- After 30 minutes and again after 2 hours, collect another 6 ml of blood in a second 10- to 15-ml *red-top* tube. Label the tubes appropriately, and send them to the laboratory.
- If a hematoma develops at the venipuncture sites, apply warm soaks.
- Instruct the patient to resume his normal diet and medications discontinued before the test.

Precautions
- Handle the samples gently to prevent hemolysis.
- Send each sample to the laboratory immediately because hGH has a half-life of only 20 to 25 minutes.

Reference values
Normally, glucose suppresses hGH to levels ranging from undetectable to 3 ng/ml in 30 minutes to 2 hours. In children, rebound stimulation may occur after 2 to 5 hours.

Abnormal findings
In a patient with active acromegaly, elevated baseline hGH levels (75 ng/ml) are not suppressed to less than 5 ng/ml during the test. Unchanged or rising hGH levels in response to glucose loading indicate hGH hypersecretion and may confirm suspected acromegaly and gigantism. This response may be verified by repeating the test after a 1-day rest.

Interfering factors
- Failure to observe pretest restrictions
- Hemolysis due to rough handling of the sample
- Corticosteroids and phenothiazines such as chlorpromazine (possible decrease in hGH secretion)

- Arginine, levodopa, amphetamines, glucagon, niacin, and estrogens (possible increase in hGH secretion)
- Radioactive scan performed within 1 week before the test
- Exercise and excitement (false-high)
- Failure to consume entire volume of glucose for test

INSULIN TOLERANCE TEST

This test measures serum levels of human growth hormone (hGH) and corticotropin after administration of a loading dose of insulin and is more reliable than direct measurement of hGH and corticotropin. Insulin-induced hypoglycemia stimulates hGH and corticotropin secretion. Failure of stimulation indicates anterior pituitary or adrenal hypofunction and helps confirm an hGH or a corticotropin insufficiency.

Purpose
- To aid diagnosis of hGH and corticotropin deficiency
- To identify pituitary dysfunction
- To aid differential diagnosis of primary and secondary adrenal hypofunction

Patient preparation
- Explain to the patient, or to his parents if the patient is a child, that this test evaluates hormonal secretion.
- Instruct him to fast and restrict physical activity for 10 to 12 hours before the test.
- Explain that the test involves I.V. infusion of insulin and the collection of multiple blood samples.
- Warn him that he may experience an increased heart rate, diaphoresis,

hunger, and anxiety after administration of insulin. Reassure him that these symptoms are transient, and that if they become severe, the test will be discontinued.

• Tell him to lie down and relax for 90 minutes before the test.

Procedure and posttest care

• Between 6 a.m. and 8 a.m., perform a venipuncture and collect three 5-ml samples of blood for basal levels: one in a *gray-top* tube (for blood glucose) and two in *green-top* tubes (for hGH and corticotropin).

• Administer an I.V. bolus of U-100 regular insulin (0.15 U/kg, or as ordered) over 1 to 2 minutes.

• Use an indwelling venous catheter to avoid repeated venipunctures. Collect additional blood samples 15, 30, 45, 60, 90, and 120 minutes after administration of insulin. At each interval, collect three samples: one in a *gray-top* tube and two in *green-top* tubes. Label the tubes appropriately, and send them to the laboratory immediately.

• If a hematoma develops at the I.V. or venipuncture site, apply warm soaks.

• Instruct the patient to resume his normal diet and activity and medications discontinued before the test.

Precautions

• This test is not recommended for patients with cardiovascular or cerebrovascular disorders, epilepsy, or low basal cortisol levels.

• Be sure to have concentrated glucose solution readily available in the event that the patient has a severe hypoglycemic reaction to insulin.

• Label the tubes appropriately, including the collection times on the laboratory slip, and send all samples to the laboratory immediately.

• Handle the samples gently to prevent hemolysis.

Reference values

Normally, blood glucose falls to 50% of the fasting level 20 to 30 minutes after insulin administration. This stimulates a 10- to 20-ng/dl increase in baseline values for both hGH and corticotropin, with peak levels occurring 60 to 90 minutes after insulin administration.

Abnormal findings

Failure of stimulation or a blunted response suggests dysfunction of the hypothalamic-pituitary-adrenal axis. An hGH increase of less than 10 ng/dl above baseline suggests hGH deficiency. A definitive diagnosis of hGH deficiency requires a supplementary stimulation test, such as the arginine test. Additional testing is necessary to determine the site of the abnormality.

An increase in corticotropin levels of less than 10 ng/dl above baseline suggests adrenal insufficiency. The metyrapone or corticotropin stimulation test then confirms the diagnosis and determines whether the insufficiency is primary or secondary.

Interfering factors

• Failure to observe pretest restrictions

• Hemolysis due to rough handling of the sample

• Steroids and pituitary-based drugs (increase in hGH)

• Glucocorticoids and beta blockers (decrease in hGH)

• Glucocorticoids, estrogens, calcium gluconate, amphetamines, methamphetamines, spironolactone, and ethanol (decrease in corticotropin)

ARGININE TEST

This test, also known as the human growth hormone (hGH) stimulation test and the GH stimulation with arginine test, measures hGH levels after I.V. administration of arginine, an amino acid that normally stimulates hGH secretion. It's commonly used to identify pituitary dysfunction in infants and children with growth retardation and to confirm hGH deficiency. This test may be performed concomitantly with an insulin tolerance test or after administration of other hGH stimulants, such as glucagon, vasopressin, and levodopa.

Purpose
• To aid diagnosis of pituitary tumors
• To confirm hGH deficiency in infants and children with low baseline levels

Patient preparation
• Explain to the patient, or to his parents if the patient is a child, that this test identifies hGH deficiency.
• Instruct him to fast and limit physical activity for 10 to 12 hours before the test.
• Explain that this test requires I.V. infusion of a drug and collection of several blood samples. Tell him that the test takes at least 2 hours to perform and that results are available in 2 days.
• Withhold all steroid medications, including pituitary-based hormones. If they must be continued, record this on the laboratory slip.
• Tell the patient to lie down and relax for at least 90 minutes before the test.

Procedure and posttest care
• Between 6 a.m. and 8 a.m., perform a venipuncture and collect 6 ml of blood (basal sample) in a *red-top* tube.
• Use of an indwelling venous catheter avoids repeated venipunctures and minimizes stress and anxiety. Start I.V. infusion of arginine (0.5 g/kg of body weight) in normal saline solution, and continue for 30 minutes.

• Discontinue the I.V. infusion, and then draw a total of three 6-ml samples at 30-minute intervals. Collect each sample in a *red-top* tube, and label it appropriately.
• If a hematoma develops at the I.V. or venipuncture site, apply warm soaks.
• Instruct the patient to resume his normal diet, activities, and medications discontinued before the test.

Precautions
• Collect each sample at the scheduled time, and specify the collection time on the laboratory slip.
• Send each sample to the laboratory immediately because hGH has a half-life of only 20 to 25 minutes.
• Handle the samples gently to prevent hemolysis.

Reference values
Arginine should raise hGH levels to more than 10 ng/ml in men, more than 15 ng/ml in women, and more than 48 ng/ml in children. Such an increase may appear in the first sample collected 30 minutes after arginine infusion is discontinued or in the samples collected 60 and 90 minutes afterward.

Abnormal findings
Levels that are elevated during fasting or that rise during sleep help to rule out hGH deficiency. Failure of hGH levels to rise after arginine infusion indicates decreased anterior pituitary hGH reserve. In children, this deficiency causes dwarfism; in adults, it can indicate panhypopituitarism. When hGH levels fail to reach 10 ng/ml, retesting is required at the same time of day as the original test.

Interfering factors
• Failure to observe pretest restrictions
• Hemolysis due to rough handling of the sample

- Radioactive scan performed within 1 week before the test
- Steroid medications

FOLLICLE-STIMULATING HORMONE

This test of gonadal function, performed more often on women than on men, measures follicle-stimulating hormone (FSH) levels and is vital in infertility studies. Plasma levels fluctuate widely in females; to obtain a true baseline level, daily testing may be necessary for 3 to 5 days.

Purpose
- To aid in the diagnosis and treatment of infertility and disorders of menstruation, such as amenorrhea
- To aid in the diagnosis of precocious puberty in girls (before age 9) and in boys (before age 10)
- To aid in the differential diagnosis of hypogonadism

Patient preparation
- Explain to the patient, or to her parents if she's a minor, that this test helps determine if her hormonal secretion is normal.
- Tell her that a blood sample will be collected and that she may experience some discomfort from the needle puncture and tourniquet.
- Withhold medications, such as steroids, before obtaining baseline levels. If they must be continued (for example, for infertility treatment), note this on the laboratory slip.
- Make sure the patient is relaxed and recumbent for 30 minutes before the test.

Procedure and posttest care
- Perform a venipuncture, preferably between 6 a.m. and 8 a.m., and collect the sample in a 7-ml *red-top* tube. Send the sample to the laboratory immediately.
- If a hematoma develops at the venipuncture site, apply warm soaks.
- Resume administration of medications discontinued before the test.

Precautions
- Handle the sample gently to prevent hemolysis.
- If the patient is female, indicate the phase of her menstrual cycle on the laboratory slip. If she is menopausal, note this on the laboratory slip.

Reference values
Reference values vary greatly, depending on the patient's age, stage of sexual development, and — for a female — phase of her menstrual cycle. For menstruating females, approximate FSH values are as follows:
- Prepuberty: < 2 IU/L
- Follicular phase: 1 to 10 IU/L
- Midcycle peak: 6 to 30 IU/L
- Luteal phase: 1 to 8 IU/L.

Approximate FSH values for men range from 1 to 10 IU/L; for prepubertal males, less than 2 IU/L; and for menopausal women, 30 to 100 IU/L.

Abnormal findings
Decreased FSH levels may cause male or female infertility: aspermatogenesis in men and anovulation in women. Low FSH levels may indicate secondary hypogonadotropic states, which can result from anorexia nervosa, panhypopituitarism, or hypothalamic lesions.

High FSH levels in women may indicate ovarian failure associated with Turner's syndrome (primary hypogonadism) or Stein-Leventhal syndrome (polycystic ovary syndrome). Elevated levels may occur in patients with precocious puberty (idiopathic or with central nervous system lesions) and in postmenopausal women. In men, abnormally high FSH levels may indicate destruction of the testes (from mumps orchitis or X-ray exposure), testicular failure, seminoma, or male climacteric. Congenital absence of the gonads and early-stage acromegaly may cause FSH levels to rise in both sexes.

Interfering factors
- Failure to observe pretest restrictions
- Hemolysis due to rough handling of the sample
- Ovarian steroid hormones, such as estrogen and progesterone, related compounds, and phenothiazines, such as chlorpromazine (possible decrease through negative feedback by inhibiting FSH flow from hypothalamus and pituitary)
- Radioactive scan performed within 1 week before the test
- Failure to send the sample to the laboratory immediately

PLASMA LUTEINIZING HORMONE

This test, usually ordered for anovulation and infertility studies on women, is a quantitative analysis of plasma luteinizing hormone (LH) or interstitial cell-stimulating hormone levels. In women, cyclic LH secretion (with folicle-stimulating hormone [FSH]) causes ovulation and transforms the ovarian follicle into the corpus luteum, which in turn secretes progesterone. (See *LH secretion peaks at ovulation,* page 206.) In males, continuous LH

secretion stimulates the interstitial (Leydig) cells of the testes to release testosterone, which stimulates and maintains spermatogenesis (with FSH).

Purpose
- To detect ovulation
- To assess male or female infertility
- To evaluate amenorrhea
- To monitor therapy designed to induce ovulation

Patient preparation
- Explain to the patient that this test helps determine if her secretion of female hormones is normal.
- Because there is no evidence that LH levels are affected by fasting, eating, or exercise, such pretest restrictions may be unnecessary.
- Tell the patient that this test requires a blood sample. Explain who will perform the venipuncture and when.
- Inform the patient that she may experience some discomfort from the needle puncture and the tourniquet but that collecting the sample takes only a few minutes.
- Withhold drugs that may interfere with plasma LH levels, such as steroids (including estrogens and progesterone), for 48 hours before the test. If they must be continued, note this on the laboratory slip.

Procedure and posttest care
- Perform a venipuncture, and collect the sample in a 7-ml *red-top* tube.
- If a hematoma develops at the venipuncture site, apply warm soaks.
- Resume administration of medications discontinued before the test.

Precautions
- Handle the sample gently to prevent hemolysis.
- If the patient is a female, indicate the phase of her menstrual cycle on the

LH SECRETION PEAKS AT OVULATION

The menstrual cycle is divided into three distinct phases: the menstrual phase (days 1 to 5); the proliferative, or follicular, phase (days 6 to 13); and, after ovulation on day 14, the secretory, or luteal, phase (days 15 to 28).

The menstrual phase
This phase of the normal cycle is characterized by endometrial sloughing, corpus luteum degenera-

tion, and new follicle growth. During this stage, the concentration of both estrogen and progesterone is low, triggering increased follicle-stimulating hormone (FSH) and luteinizing hormone (LH) secretion.

The follicular phase
During the follicular phase, the follicle stimulated by FSH reaches full size and increases its secretion of estrogen. Simultaneously with in-

(continued)

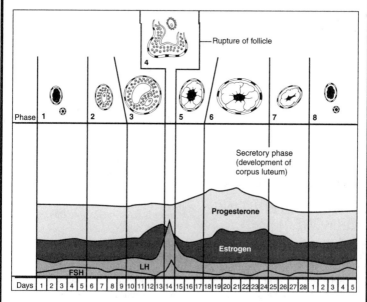

1. Menstrual phase (degeneration of corpus luteum)
2. Early follicular phase (development of follicle)
3. Late follicular phase (development of follicle)
4. Ovulation at midcycle (rupture of follicle)

5. Early luteal phase (development of corpus luteum)
6. Midluteal phase (development of corpus luteum)
7. Late luteal phase (development of corpus luteum)
8. Menstrual phase (degeneration of corpus luteum)

LH SECRETION PEAKS AT OVULATION *(continued)*

================

creased estrogen, FSH decreases while LH increases slowly but steadily. During the late follicular phase, LH rises sharply and FSH rises slightly. At about the 14th day, within hours of this abrupt surge in LH, estrogen levels in the plasma drop and ovulation occurs. After ovulation, the concentration of both LH and FSH falls rapidly.

The secretory phase
During the final, or luteal, phase, the follicle reorganizes as the corpus luteum secretes progesterone and estrogen. Within 7 or 8 days after ovulation, if fertilization has not occurred, the corpus luteum regresses and progesterone and estrogen levels decrease. The endometrium sloughs, and the menstrual cycle begins again.

---

laboratory slip. Make a note if the patient is menopausal.

Reference values
Normal values may have a wide range, as follows:
• Postmenopausal females: 12 to 55 IU/L
• Premenopausal females: Reference values vary, depending on the phase of the patient's menstrual cycle. During the follicular phase, values are 1 to 18 IU/L; during midcycle (ovulation), 20 to 80 IU/L; during the luteal phase, 0.5 to 18 IU/L.
• Prepubertal females: < 1 IU/L
• Males: 1 to 9 IU/L
• Prepubertal males: < 1 IU/L.

Abnormal findings
In women, absence of a midcycle peak in LH secretion may indicate anovulation. Decreased or low-normal LH levels may indicate hypogonadism; these findings are commonly associated with amenorrhea. High LH levels may indicate congenital absence of ovaries or ovarian failure associated with Stein-Leventhal syndrome (polycystic ovary syndrome), Turner's syndrome (ovarian dysgenesis), menopause, or early-stage acromegaly. Infertility can result from

primary or secondary gonadal dysfunction.

In men, low LH values may indicate secondary gonadal dysfunction (of hypothalamic or pituitary origin); high values may indicate testicular failure (primary hypogonadism) or destruction or congenital absence of testes.

Interfering factors
• Failure to observe pretest restrictions
• Hemolysis due to rough handling of the sample
• Steroids, including estrogens, progesterone, and testosterone (possible decrease)
• Radioactive scan performed within 1 week before the test

PROLACTIN

Prolactin is essential for the development of the mammary glands for lactation during pregnancy and for stimulating and maintaining lactation postpartum. Like human growth hormone, prolactin acts directly on tissues, and its levels rise in response to sleep and physical or emotional stress.

This radioimmunoassay is a quantitative analysis of serum prolactin levels, which normally rise 10- to 20-fold during pregnancy, corresponding to concomitant elevations in human placental lactogen levels. After delivery, prolactin secretion falls to basal levels in mothers who don't breast-feed. However, prolactin secretion increases during breast-feeding, apparently as a result of a stimulus triggered by suckling that curtails the release of prolactin-inhibiting factor by the hypothalamus. This in turn allows transient elevations of prolactin secretion by the pituitary.

This test is considered useful in patients suspected of having pituitary tumors, which are known to secrete prolactin in excessive amounts.

Purpose
• To facilitate diagnosis of pituitary dysfunction, possibly due to pituitary adenoma
• To aid in the diagnosis of hypothalamic dysfunction regardless of cause
• To evaluate secondary amenorrhea and galactorrhea

Patient preparation
• Tell the patient that this test helps evaluate hormonal secretion.
• Advise her that she needn't restrict food or fluids or limit physical activity, but encourage her to relax for about 30 minutes before the test.
• Tell the patient that this test requires a blood sample. Inform her who will perform the venipuncture and when.
• Explain that she may experience some discomfort from the needle puncture and tourniquet but that collecting the sample takes just a few minutes.
• Withhold drugs that may interfere with test results, such as ethanol, morphine, methyldopa, estrogens, apomorphine, ergot alkaloids, and levodopa. If

they must be continued, note this on the laboratory slip.

Procedure and posttest care
• Perform a venipuncture at least 2 hours after the patient wakes; samples collected earlier are likely to show sleep-induced peak levels. Collect the sample in a 7-ml *red-top* tube.
• If a hematoma develops at the venipuncture site, apply warm soaks.
• Resume administration of medications discontinued before the test.

Precautions
• Handle the sample gently to prevent hemolysis.

Reference values
Normal values may have a wide range, as follows:
Males
• 0 to 1 month: 0 to 90 ng/ml
• 1 to 12 months: 0 to 30 ng/ml
• 1 to 18 years: 1 to 15 ng/ml
• > 18 years: 4 to 23 ng/ml
Females
• 0 to 1 month: 0 to 90 ng/ml
• 1 to 12 months: 0 to 30 ng/ml
• 1 to 18 years: 1 to 15 ng/ml
• > 18 years: 4 to 30 ng/ml

Abnormal findings
Abnormally high prolactin levels (100 to 300 ng/ml) suggest autonomous prolactin production by a pituitary adenoma, especially when amenorrhea or galactorrhea is present (Forbes-Albright syndrome). Rarely, hyperprolactinemia may also result from severe endocrine disorders, such as hypothyroidism. Idiopathic hyperprolactinemia may be associated with anovulatory infertility. Confirm slight elevations with repeat measurements on two other occasions.

Decreased prolactin levels in a lactating mother cause failure of lactation and may be associated with postpartum pituitary infarction (Sheehan's syndrome). Abnormally low prolactin levels have also been found in some patients with empty-sella syndrome. In these patients, a flattened pituitary gland makes the pituitary fossa look empty.

Interfering factors

• Failure to take into account physiologic variations related to sleep or stress

• Ethanol, morphine, methyldopa, and estrogens (increase)

• Apomorphine, ergot alkaloids, and levodopa (decrease)

• Radioactive scan performed within 1 week before the test or recent surgery

• Breast stimulation

• Hemolysis due to rough handling of the sample

THYROID-STIMULATING HORMONE

Thyroid-stimulating hormone (TSH), or thyrotropin, promotes increases in the size, number, and activity of thyroid cells and stimulates the release of triiodothyronine and thyroxine. These hormones affect total body metabolism and are essential for normal growth and development.

This test measures serum TSH levels by radioimmunoassay. It can detect primary hypothyroidism and determine whether the hypothyroidism results from thyroid gland failure or from pituitary or hypothalamic dysfunction. Normal serum TSH levels rule out primary hypothyroid-ism. This test may not distinguish between low-normal and subnormal levels, especially in secondary hypothyroidism.

Purpose

• To confirm or rule out primary hypothyroidism and distinguish it from secondary hypothyroidism

• To monitor drug therapy in patients with primary hypothyroidism

Patient preparation

• Explain to the patient that this test helps assess thyroid gland function.

• Tell him that the test requires a blood sample, and inform him who will perform the venipuncture and when.

• Explain that he may experience discomfort from the needle puncture and tourniquet but that collecting the sample takes only a few minutes.

• Withhold steroids, thyroid hormones, aspirin, and other medications that may influence test results. If they must be continued, note this on the laboratory slip.

• Keep the patient relaxed and recumbent for 30 minutes before the test.

Procedure and posttest care

• Between 6 a.m. and 8 a.m., perform a venipuncture, and collect the sample in a 5-ml *red-top* tube.

• If a hematoma develops at the venipuncture site, apply warm soaks.

• Resume administration of medications discontinued before the test.

Precautions

• Handle the sample gently to prevent hemolysis.

Reference values

Normal TSH values range from 0.3 to 5 mIU/L.

Abnormal findings

TSH levels may be slightly elevated in euthyroid patients with thyroid cancer. Extremely high levels suggest primary hypothyroidism or, possibly, endemic goiter.

TRH STIMULATION TEST

This test evaluates hypothalamic dysfunction and pituitary tumors by stimulating the release of prolactin. The procedure is as follows: perform a venipuncture in the basal state to obtain a baseline prolactin level, and then place the patient in the supine position. Administer an I.V. bolus dose (500 µg) of synthetic thyrotropin-releasing hormone (TRH) over 15 to 30 seconds. Take blood samples at 15- and 30-minute intervals to measure prolactin.

A baseline prolactin reading greater than 200 ng/ml indicates a pituitary tumor, but levels between 30 and 200 ng/ml are also consistent with this condition. Normally, patients show at least a twofold increase in prolactin after injection with TRH. If the prolactin level fails to rise, hypothalamic dysfunction or adenoma of the pituitary gland is likely.

NEONATAL THYROID-STIMULATING HORMONE

This immunoassay confirms congenital hypothyroidism after an initial screening test detects low thyroxine (T_4) levels. Normally, thyroid-stimulating hormone (TSH) levels surge after birth, triggering a rise in thyroid hormone that's essential for neurologic development. In primary congenital hypothyroidism, the thyroid gland doesn't respond to TSH stimulation, resulting in diminished thyroid hormone levels and elevated TSH levels. Early detection and treatment of congenital hypothyroidism is critical to prevent mental retardation and cretinism.

Purpose
● To confirm diagnosis of congenital hypothyroidism

Patient preparation
● Explain to the infant's parents that this test helps confirm the diagnosis of congenital hypothyroidism. Emphasize the importance of detecting the disorder early so that prompt therapy can prevent irreversible brain damage.

Equipment
For a filter paper sample: alcohol or povidone-iodine swabs, sterile lancet, specially marked filter paper, 2″ × 2″ sterile gauze pads, adhesive bandage, labels, gloves

For a serum sample: venipuncture equipment

Procedure and posttest care
For a filter paper sample
● Assemble the necessary equipment, wash your hands thoroughly, and put on gloves.

Low or undetectable TSH levels may be normal but occasionally indicate secondary hypothyroidism (with inadequate secretion of TSH or thyrotropin-releasing hormone [TRH]). Low TSH levels may also result from hyperthyroidism (Graves' disease) and thyroiditis; both are marked by hypersecretion of thyroid hormones, which suppresses TSH release. Provocative testing with TRH is necessary to confirm the diagnosis. (See *TRH stimulation test* and *TRH challenge test*.)

Interfering factors
● Failure to observe pretest restrictions
● Hemolysis due to rough handling of the sample
● Steroids, thyroid hormones, and aspirin

- Wipe the infant's heel with an alcohol or povidone-iodine swab, and then dry it thoroughly with a gauze pad.
- Perform a heelstick.
- Squeezing the infant's heel gently, fill the circles on the filter paper with blood. Make sure the blood saturates the paper.
- Gently apply pressure with a gauze pad to ensure hemostasis at the puncture site.
- Allow the filter paper to dry, label it appropriately, and send it to the laboratory.

For a serum sample
- Perform a venipuncture, and collect the sample in a 5-ml *red-top* tube. Label the sample and send it to the laboratory immediately.
- If a hematoma develops at the venipuncture site, apply warm soaks. Heelsticks require no special care.

Precautions
- Handle the samples carefully to prevent hemolysis.

Reference values
Neonate TSH levels are normally 3 to 20 µU/ml by day 3 of life.

Abnormal findings
Neonatal TSH levels must be interpreted in light of T_4 concentrations. Elevated TSH levels accompanied by decreased T_4 levels indicates primary congenital hypothyroidism (thyroid gland dysfunction). Low TSH and T_4 levels may be present in secondary congenital hypothyroidism (pituitary or hypothalamic dysfunction). Normal TSH levels accompanied by low T_4 levels may indicate hypothyroidism due to a congenital defect in thyroxine-binding globulin or transient congenital hypothyroidism due to prematurity or prenatal hypoxia. A complete thy-

TRH CHALLENGE TEST

This test, which evaluates thyroid function and is the first direct test of pituitary reserve, is a reliable diagnostic tool in thyrotoxicosis (Graves' disease). The challenge test requires an injection of thyrotropin-releasing hormone (TRH).

One commonly accepted procedure is the following: After a venipuncture is performed to obtain a baseline thyroid-stimulating hormone (TSH) reading, synthetic TRH (protirelin) is administered by I.V. bolus in a dose of 200 to 500 µg. As many as five samples (5 ml each) are then drawn at 5, 10, 15, 20, and 60 minutes after the TRH injection to assess thyroid response. To facilitate blood collection, an indwelling catheter can be used to obtain the required samples.

A sudden spike above the baseline TSH reading indicates a normally functioning pituitary but suggests hypothalamic dysfunction. If the TSH level fails to rise or remains undetectable, pituitary failure is likely. In thyrotoxicosis and thyroiditis, TSH levels fail to rise when challenged by TRH.

roid workup must be done to confirm the cause of hypothyroidism before treatment can begin.

Interfering factors
- Failure to let a filter paper sample dry completely
- Hemolysis due to rough handling of the sample
- Corticosteroids, triiodothyronine, and T_4 (decrease)

• Lithium carbonate, potassium iodide, excessive topical resorcinol, and TSH injection (increase)

ANTIDIURETIC HORMONE

Antidiuretic hormone (ADH), also called vasopressin, promotes water reabsorption in response to increased osmolality (water deficiency with high concentration of sodium and other solutes). In response to decreased osmolality (water excess), reduced secretion of ADH allows increased excretion of water to maintain fluid balance. Along with aldosterone, ADH helps regulate sodium, potassium, and fluid balance. It also stimulates vascular smooth-muscle contraction, causing an increase in arterial blood pressure.

This relatively rare test, a quantitative analysis of serum ADH levels, may identify diabetes insipidus and other causes of severe homeostatic imbalance. It may be ordered as part of dehydration or hypertonic saline infusion testing, which determines the body's response to states of hyperosmolality.

Purpose
• To aid in the differential diagnosis of pituitary diabetes insipidus, nephrogenic diabetes insipidus (congenital or familial), and syndrome of inappropriate antidiuretic hormone (SIADH)

Patient preparation
• Explain to the patient that this test, used to measure hormonal secretion levels, may aid in identifying the cause of his symptoms.

• Instruct him to fast and limit physical activity for 10 to 12 hours before the test.
• Tell him that a blood sample will be collected. Inform him who will perform the venipuncture and when.
• Reassure him that although he may experience some discomfort from the needle puncture and tourniquet, collecting the sample takes only a few minutes.
• Make sure the patient is relaxed and recumbent for 30 minutes before the test.

Procedure and posttest care
• Perform a venipuncture, and collect the sample in a *red-top* plastic collection tube.
• Immediately send the sample to the laboratory, where serum must be separated from the clot within 10 minutes.
• Perform a serum osmolality test at the same time to facilitate interpretation of results.
• If a hematoma develops at the venipuncture site, apply warm soaks.
• Instruct the patient to resume his normal diet and medications discontinued before the test.

Precautions
• Make sure you use a syringe and collection tube made of plastic because the fragile ADH degrades on contact with glass.

Reference values
ADH values range from 1 to 4.7 pg/ml.

Abnormal findings
Absent or below-normal ADH levels indicate pituitary diabetes insipidus, resulting from a neurohypophyseal or hypothalamic tumor, viral infection, metastatic disease, sarcoidosis, tuberculosis, Hand-Schüller-Christian disease, syphilis, neurosurgical procedures, or head trauma.

Normal ADH levels in the presence of signs of diabetes insipidus (such as polydipsia, polyuria, and hypotonic urine) may indicate the nephrogenic form of the disease, marked by renal tubular resistance to ADH; however, levels may rise if the pituitary tries to compensate.

Elevated ADH levels may also indicate SIADH, possibly as a result of bronchogenic carcinoma, acute porphyria, hypothyroidism, Addison's disease, cirrhosis of the liver, infectious hepatitis, severe hemorrhage, or circulatory shock.

Interfering factors
- Failure to observe pretest restrictions
- Morphine, anesthetics, estrogen, oxytocin, chlorpropamide, vincristine, carbamazepine, cyclophosphamide, tranquilizers, hypnotics, lithium carbonate, and chlorothiazide (increase)
- Stress, pain, and positive-pressure ventilation (increase)
- Alcohol, beta-adrenergic agents, morphine antagonists, phenytoin, and negative-pressure ventilation (decrease)
- Radioactive scan performed within 1 week before the test

ALPHA-SUBUNIT OF PITUITARY GLYCOPROTEIN HORMONES

Using radioimmunoassay, this test measures the alpha-subunit of the pituitary glycoprotein hormones (alpha-PGH). These hormones — thyroid-stimulating hormone (TSH) and human chorionic gonadotropin — contain similar alpha-subunits but differ in their beta-subunits. Alpha-PGH

measurement assesses total pituitary production of these hormones.

Purpose
- To aid diagnosis of recurrent pituitary tumors in patients who have undergone resection

Patient preparation
- Explain to the patient that this test helps assess pituitary function.
- Inform him that he needn't fast.
- Tell him that this test requires a blood sample, and inform him who will perform the venipuncture and when.
- Explain that he may experience discomfort from the needle puncture and tourniquet but that the procedure takes only a few minutes.

Procedure and posttest care
- Perform a venipuncture, and collect the sample in a 5-ml *red-top* tube.
- Send the sample to the laboratory immediately.
- If a hematoma develops at the venipuncture site, apply warm soaks.

Precautions
- Handle the sample gently to prevent hemolysis.
- Indicate the patient's sex on the laboratory slip.

Reference values
Normal alpha-PGH values are up to 1.2 ng/ml.

Abnormal findings
Low levels of alpha-PGH appear in patients with inadequate pituitary hormone production. Hypopituitarism results in reduced follicle-stimulating hormone, luteinizing hormone, and TSH levels.

Elevated alpha-PGH levels indicate recurrent pituitary tumors or ineffective treatment.

Interfering factor
- Hemolysis due to rough handling of the sample

THYROID AND PARATHYROID HORMONES

THYROXINE

Thyroxine (T_4) is an amine secreted by the thyroid gland in response to thyroid-stimulating hormone (TSH) and, indirectly, thyrotropin-releasing hormone. The rate of secretion is normally regulated by a complex system of negative and positive feedback mechanisms.

Only a fraction of T_4 (about 0.05%) circulates freely in the blood; the rest binds strongly to plasma proteins, primarily thyroxine-binding globulin (TBG). This minute fraction is responsible for the clinical effects of thyroid hormone. TBG binds so tenaciously that T_4 survives in the plasma for a relatively long time, with a half-life of about 6 days. This immunoassay, one of the most common thyroid diagnostic tools, measures the total circulating T_4 level when TBG is normal. An alternative test is the Murphy-Pattee or $T_4(D)$, based on competitive protein binding.

Purpose
- To evaluate thyroid function
- To aid diagnosis of hyperthyroidism and hypothyroidism
- To monitor response to antithyroid medication in hyperthyroidism or to thyroid replacement therapy in hypothyroidism (TSH estimates are needed to confirm hypothyroidism)

Patient preparation
- Explain to the patient that this test helps evaluate thyroid gland function.
- Inform him that he needn't fast or restrict activity.
- Tell him that a blood sample is needed and that the procedure, which takes a few minutes, may cause some discomfort.
- Inform him who will perform the venipuncture and when.
- Withhold levothyroxine, methadone, heparin, iodides, liothyronine sodium, lithium, phenylbutazone, phenytoin, salicylates (high doses), propylthiouracil, steroids, sulfonamides, and sulfonylureas. If they must be continued, note this on the laboratory slip. If this test is being performed to monitor thyroid therapy, the patient should continue to receive daily thyroid supplements.

Procedure and posttest care
- Perform a venipuncture, and collect the sample in a 7-ml *red-top* tube.
- Send the sample to the laboratory immediately so that the serum can be separated.
- If a hematoma develops at the venipuncture site, apply warm soaks.
- Resume administration of medications discontinued before the test.

Precautions
- Handle the sample gently to prevent hemolysis.

Reference values
Normally, total T_4 levels range from 5 to 12.5 µg/dl.

Abnormal findings
Abnormally elevated T_4 levels are consistent with primary and secondary hyperthyroidism, including excessive T_4

(levothyroxine) replacement therapy (factitious or iatrogenic hyperthyroidism). Subnormal levels suggest primary or secondary hypothyroidism or may be due to T_4 suppression by normal, elevated, or replacement levels of triiodothyronine (T_3). In doubtful cases of hypothyroidism, TSH levels may be indicated.

Normal T_4 levels don't guarantee euthyroidism; for example, normal readings occur in T_3 toxicosis. Overt signs of hyperthyroidism require further testing.

Interfering factors

• Hemolysis due to rough handling of the sample
• Hereditary factors and hepatic disease (possible increase or decrease in TBG)
• Protein-wasting disease (such as nephrotic syndrome) and androgens (possible decrease in TBG)
• Estrogens, progestins, levothyroxine, and methadone (increase)
• Free fatty acids, heparin, iodides, liothyronine sodium, lithium, methylthiouracil, phenylbutazone, phenytoin, propylthiouracil, salicylates (high doses), steroids, sulfonamides, and sulfonylureas (decrease)
• Clofibrate (possible increase or decrease)

TRIIODOTHYRONINE

This highly specific radioimmunoassay measures total (bound and free) serum content of triiodothyronine (T_3) to investigate clinical indications of thyroid dysfunction. Like thyroxine (T_4) secretion, T_3 secretion occurs in response to thyroid-stimulating hormone (TSH) and, secondarily, thyrotropin-releasing hormone.

Although T_3 is present in the bloodstream in minute quantities and is metabolically active for only a short time, its impact on body metabolism dominates that of T_4. Another significant difference between the two major thyroid hormones is that T_3 binds less firmly to thyroxine-binding globulin. Consequently, T_3 persists in the bloodstream for a short time; half disappears in about 1 day, whereas half of T_4 disappears in 6 days.

Purpose

• To aid diagnosis of T_3 toxicosis
• To aid diagnosis of hypothyroidism and hyperthyroidism
• To monitor clinical response to thyroid replacement therapy in hypothyroidism

Patient preparation

• Explain to the patient that this test helps to evaluate thyroid gland function and determine the cause of his symptoms.
• Withhold medications, such as steroids, propranolol, and cholestyramine, that may influence thyroid function. If they must be continued, record this information on the laboratory slip.
• Tell him that a blood sample is needed and that the procedure, which takes a few minutes, may cause some discomfort.

Procedure and posttest care

• Perform a venipuncture, and collect the sample in a 7-ml *red-top* tube.
• Send the sample to the laboratory as soon as possible to avoid stasis and to allow early separation of serum from the clotted blood.
• If a hematoma develops at the venipuncture site, apply warm soaks.
• Resume administration of medications discontinued before the test.

Precautions
- Handle the sample gently to prevent hemolysis.
- If the patient must receive thyroid preparations such as T_3 (liothyronine), note the administration time on the laboratory slip. Otherwise, T_3 levels are not reliable.

Reference values
Serum T_3 levels vary by age:
- 1 to 14 years: 125 to 250 ng/dl
- 15 to 23 years: 100 to 220 ng/dl
- 24 years and older: 80 to 200 ng/dl.

Abnormal findings
Serum T_3 and serum T_4 levels usually rise and fall in tandem. However, in T_3 toxicosis, T_3 levels rise while total and free T_4 levels remain normal. T_3 toxicosis occurs in patients with Graves' disease, toxic adenoma, or toxic nodular goiter. T_3 levels also surpass T_4 levels in patients receiving thyroid replacement therapy containing more T_3 than T_4. In iodine-deficient areas, the thyroid may produce larger amounts of the more cellularly active T_3 than of T_4 in an effort to maintain the euthyroid state.

Generally, T_3 levels appear to be a more accurate diagnostic indicator of hyperthyroidism. Although both T_3 and T_4 levels are increased in about 90% of patients with hyperthyroidism, there's a disproportionate increase in T_3. In some patients with hypothyroidism, T_3 levels may fall within the normal range and not be diagnostically significant.

A rise in serum T_3 levels normally occurs during pregnancy. Low T_3 levels may appear in euthyroid patients with systemic illness (especially hepatic or renal disease), during severe acute illness, and after trauma or major surgery; in such patients, TSH levels are within normal limits. Low serum T_3 levels are found in some euthyroid patients with malnutrition.

Interfering factors
- Hemolysis due to rough handling of the sample
- Markedly increased or decreased TBG levels, regardless of cause
- Failure to take into account medications that affect T_3 levels, such as steroids, clofibrate, cholestyramine, and propranolol

THYROXINE-BINDING GLOBULIN

This test measures the serum level of thyroxine-binding globulin (TBG), the predominant protein carrier for circulating thyroxine (T_4).

Any condition that affects TBG levels and subsequent binding capacity also affects the amount of free T_4 (FT_4) in circulation. An underlying TBG abnormality renders tests for total triiodothyronine (T_3) and T_4 inaccurate but doesn't affect the accuracy of tests for free T_3 (FT_3) and FT_4.

Purpose
- To evaluate abnormal thyrometabolic states that don't correlate with thyroid hormone (T_3 or T_4) values; an example is a patient with overt signs of hypothyroidism and a low FT_4 level with a high total T_4 level due to a marked increase of TBG secondary to oral contraceptives
- To identify TBG abnormalities

Patient preparation
- Explain to the patient that this test helps evaluate thyroid function.

• Tell him that a blood sample is needed and that the procedure, which takes a few minutes, may cause some discomfort.

• Inform him who will perform the venipuncture and when.

• Withhold medications that may affect the accuracy of test results, such as estrogens, anabolic steroids, phenytoin, salicylates, or thyroid preparations. If they must be continued, note this on the laboratory slip. (They may be continued to determine if prescribed drugs are affecting TBG levels.)

Procedure and posttest care

• Perform a venipuncture, and collect the sample in a 10-ml *red-top* tube.

• If a hematoma develops at the venipuncture site, apply warm soaks.

• Resume administration of medications discontinued before the test.

Precautions

• Handle the sample gently to prevent hemolysis.

Reference values

Normal values vary by sex and age, as follows:

Males

• 1 to 6 years: 17 to 26 µg/ml
• 7 to 13 years: 15 to 24 µg/ml
• 14 to 18 years: 13 to 22 µg/ml
• 19 to 23 years: 11 to 20 µg/ml
• 24 years and older: 16 to 24 µg/ml

Females

• 1 to 6 years: 17 to 26 µg/ml
• 7 to 23 years: 15 to 26 µg/ml
• 24 years and older: 16 to 24 µg/ml

Abnormal findings

Elevated TBG levels may indicate hypothyroidism or congenital (genetic) excess, some forms of hepatic disease, or acute intermittent porphyria. TBG levels normally rise during pregnancy and are high in neonates. Suppressed levels may indicate hyperthyroidism or congenital deficiency and can occur in active acromegaly, nephrotic syndrome, and malnutrition associated with hypoproteinemia, acute illness, or surgical stress.

Patients with TBG abnormalities require additional testing, such as the serum FT_3 and serum T_4 tests, to evaluate thyroid function more precisely.

Interfering factors

• Hemolysis due to rough handling of the sample

• Estrogens, including oral contraceptives, and phenothiazines, such as perphenazine (increase)

• Androgens, prednisone, phenytoin, and high doses of salicylates (decrease)

T_3 UPTAKE

Also called triiodothyronine uptake, the T_3 uptake test indirectly measures free thyroxine (FT_4) levels by demonstrating the availability of serum protein-binding sites for T_4. The results of T_3 uptake are frequently combined with a T_4 radioimmunoassay or $T_4(D)$ (competitive protein-binding test) to determine the FT_4 index, a mathematical calculation that is thought to reflect FT_4 by correcting for thyroxine-binding globulin (TBG) abnormalities.

The T_3 uptake test has become less popular recently because rapid tests for T_3, T_4, and thyroid-stimulating hormone are readily available.

Purpose

• To aid diagnosis of hypothroidism and hyperthyroidism when TBG is normal

• To aid diagnosis of primary disorders of TBG levels

Patient preparation
• Explain to the patient that this test helps evaluate thyroid function.
• Tell him that a blood sample is needed and that the procedure, which takes a few minutes, may cause some discomfort.
• Inform him who will perform the venipuncture and when.
• Tell him the laboratory requires several days to complete the analysis.
• Withhold medications, such as estrogens, androgens, phenytoin, salicylates, and thyroid preparations, that may interfere with test results. If they must be continued, note this on the laboratory slip.

Procedure and posttest care
• Perform a venipuncture, and collect the sample in a 7-ml *red-top* tube.
• If a hematoma develops at the venipuncture site, apply warm soaks.
• Resume administration of medications discontinued before the test.

Precautions
• Handle the sample gently to prevent hemolysis.

Reference values
Normal T_3 uptake values are 25% to 35%.

Abnormal findings
A high T_3 uptake percentage in the presence of elevated T_4 levels indicates hyperthyroidism (implying few TBG free binding sites and high FT_4 levels). A low uptake percentage, together with low T_4 levels, indicates hypothyroidism (implying more TBG free binding sites and low FT_4 levels). Thus, in primary thyroid disease, T_4 and T_3 uptake vary in the same direction; availability of binding sites varies inversely.

Discordant variance in T_4 and T_3 uptake suggests abnormality of TBG. For example, a high T_3 uptake percentage and a low or normal FT_4 level suggest decreased TBG levels. Such decreased levels may result from protein loss (as in nephrotic syndrome), decreased production (due to androgen excess or genetic or idiopathic causes), or competition for T_4 binding sites by certain drugs (salicylates, phenylbutazone, and phenytoin). Conversely, a low T_3 uptake percentage and a high or normal FT_4 level suggest increased TBG levels. Such increased levels may be due to exogenous or endogenous estrogen (pregnancy) or result from idiopathic causes. Thus, in primary disorders of TBG levels, measured T_4 and free sites change in the same direction.

Interfering factors
• Radioisotope scans performed before sample collection
• Anabolic steroids, heparin, phenytoin, salicylates (high dose), thyroid preparations, and warfarin (possible increase in TBG and thyroxine-binding protein electrophoresis)
• Antithyroid agents, clofibrate, estrogen, oral contraceptives, and thiazide diuretics (decrease uptake)

FREE THYROXINE AND FREE TRIIODOTHYRONINE

These tests, often done simultaneously, measure serum levels of free thyroxine (FT_4) and free triiodothyronine (FT_3), the minute portions of T_4 and T_3 not bound to thyroxine-binding globulin (TBG) and other serum proteins. These unbound hormones are responsible for the thyroid's effects on cellular metabolism. Measurement of free hormone levels is the best indicator of thyroid function.

Because of disagreement as to whether FT_4 or FT_3 is the better indicator, laboratories commonly measure both. The disadvantages of these tests include a cumbersome and difficult laboratory method, inaccessibility, and cost. This test may be useful in the 5% of patients in whom the standard T_3 or T_4 tests fail to produce diagnostic results.

Purpose

• To measure the metabolically active form of the thyroid hormones
• To aid diagnosis of hyperthyroidism and hypothyroidism when TBG levels are abnormal

Patient preparation

• Explain to the patient that this special test helps evaluate thyroid function.
• Tell him that a blood sample is needed and that the procedure, which takes a few minutes, may cause some discomfort.
• Inform him who will perform the venipuncture and when.

Procedure and posttest care

• Perform a venipuncture, and collect the sample in a 7-ml *red-top* tube.
• If a hematoma develops at the venipuncture site, apply warm soaks.

Precautions

• Handle the sample gently to prevent hemolysis.

Reference values

Normal range for FT_4 is 0.7 to 2 ng/dl; for FT_3, 2.3 to 4.2 pmol/L. Values vary, depending on the laboratory.

Abnormal findings

Elevated FT_4 and FT_3 levels indicate hyperthyroidism, unless peripheral resistance to thyroid hormone is present. T_3 toxicosis, a distinct form of hyperthyroidism, yields high FT_3 levels with normal or low FT_4 values. Low FT_4 levels usually indicate hypothyroidism, except in patients receiving replacement therapy with T_3. Patients receiving thyroid therapy may have varying levels of FT_4 and FT_3, depending on the preparation used and the time of sample collection.

Interfering factors

• Hemolysis due to rough handling of the sample
• Thyroid therapy, depending on dosage (possible increase)

SCREENING TEST FOR CONGENITAL HYPOTHYROIDISM

This test measures serum thyroxine (T_4) levels in the neonate to detect congenital hypothyroidism. Characterized by low or absent levels of T_4, congenital hypothyroidism affects roughly 1 in 5,000 neonates, occurring in girls three times more often than in boys. This disorder can result from thyroid dysgenesis or hypoplasia, congenital goiter, or maternal use of thyroid inhibitors during pregnancy. If untreated, it can lead to irreversible brain damage by age 3 months.

Because clinical signs are few, in the past, most cases of congenital hypothyroidism went undetected until cretinism became apparent or death followed respiratory distress. Recently, radioimmunoassays for T_4 and thyroid-stimulating hormone (TSH) have been used effectively to screen neonates for congenital hypothyroidism. This test is now mandatory in some states.

Purpose
• To screen neonates for congenital hypothyroidism

Patient preparation
• Explain to the parents that although hypothyroidism is uncommon in infants, this screening test detects the disorder early enough to begin therapy before irreversible brain damage occurs.
• Tell the parents that the test will be performed before the infant is discharged from the facility and again 4 to 6 weeks later.
• Emphasize the importance of the screening and the need for following the test protocol.
• Because false-positive findings can result from variations in the test procedure or from a congenital thyroxine-binding globulin (TBG) defect, inform the parents that a second test may be done before the infant is discharged.

Equipment
Gloves, alcohol or povidone-iodine swabs, sterile lancet, specially marked filter paper, 2″ × 2″ sterile gauze pads, small adhesive bandage strip, labels for infant's and mother's names, doctor's name, room number, and date

Procedure and posttest care
• After assembling the necessary equipment and washing your hands, put on gloves.
• Wipe the infant's heel with an alcohol or a povidone-iodine swab, and then dry it thoroughly with a gauze pad.
• Perform a heelstick.

• Squeezing the heel gently, fill the circles on the filter paper with blood. Make sure the blood saturates the paper. Apply gentle pressure with a gauze pad to ensure hemostasis at the puncture site.
• When the filter paper is dry, label it appropriately and send it to the laboratory.
• Heelsticks heal readily and require no special care.
• If results of the screening test indicate congenital hypothyroidism, tell the parents that additional testing is necessary to determine the cause of the disorder.
• If diagnosis is confirmed, inform the parents that replacement therapy can restore normal thyroid gland function. Also tell them that such therapy is lifelong and that dosage will increase until the adult requirement is reached.
• If the sample isn't processed in the facility's laboratory, make sure the parents are notified when test results are available.

Reference values
Immediately after birth, neonatal T_4 levels are considerably higher than normal adult levels. By the end of the 1st week, T_4 values decrease markedly:
• 1 to 5 days: 4.9 µg/dl
• 6 to 8 days: 4 µg/dl
• 9 to 11 days: 3.5 µg/dl
• 12 to 120 days: 3 µg/dl.

Abnormal findings
Low serum T_4 levels in the neonate require TSH testing for clarification of the diagnosis. Decreased T_4 levels accompanied by elevated TSH readings (> 25 µU/ml) indicate primary congenital hypothyroidism (thyroid gland dysfunction). If T_4 and TSH levels are depressed, secondary congenital hypothyroidism (resulting from pituitary or

hypothalamic dysfunction) should be suspected.

If T_4 levels are subnormal in the presence of normal TSH readings, further testing is required. Serum TBG levels must be analyzed to identify infants with hypothyroidism resulting from congenital defects in TBG. This low T_4–normal TSH pattern also occurs in a transient form of congenital hypothyroidism, which may accompany prematurity, or prenatal hypoxia.

A complete thyroid workup, including serum T_3, TBG, and free T_4 levels, is necessary for unequivocal diagnosis of congenital hypothyroidism before treatment begins.

Interfering factor
• Failure to allow filter paper to dry completely

PLASMA CALCITONIN

This radioimmunoassay measures plasma levels of calcitonin (thyrocalcitonin). The exact role of calcitonin in normal human physiology hasn't been fully defined. However, calcitonin is known to act as an antagonist to parathyroid hormone and to lower serum calcium levels.

The usual clinical indication for this test is suspected medullary carcinoma of the thyroid, which causes hypersecretion of calcitonin (without associated hypocalcemia). Equivocal results require provocative testing with I.V. pentagastrin or calcium to rule out disease.

Purpose
• To aid diagnosis of thyroid medullary carcinoma and ectopic calcitonin-producing tumors (rare)

Patient preparation
• Explain to the patient that this test helps evaluate thyroid function.
• Instruct him to fast overnight because food may interfere with calcium homeostasis and, subsequently, calcitonin levels.
• Tell him that this test requires a blood sample. Inform him who will perform the venipuncture and when.
• Explain that he may experience transient discomfort from the needle puncture and tourniquet but that collecting the sample takes only a few minutes.
• Tell him that the laboratory requires several days to complete the analysis.

Procedure and posttest care
• Perform a venipuncture, and collect the sample in a 10-ml *green-top* (heparinized) tube.
• If a hematoma develops at the venipuncture site, apply warm soaks.
• Instruct the patient to resume his normal diet.

Precautions
• Handle the sample gently to prevent hemolysis, and send it to the laboratory immediately.

Reference values
Serum calcitonin levels (basal) normally are less than or equal to 19 pg/ml in men and less than or equal to 14 pg/ml in women.

Reference values after provocative testing with calcium infusion are as follows:
• Males: ≤ 190 pg/ml
• Females: ≤ 130 pg/ml.

Values after provocative testing with pentagastrin infusion are:
• Males: ≤ 110 pg/ml
• Females: ≤ 30 pg/ml.

Abnormal findings

Elevated serum calcitonin levels in the absence of hypocalcemia usually indicate medullary carcinoma of the thyroid. Transmitted as an autosomal dominant trait, thyroid medullary carcinoma may occur as part of multiple endocrine neoplasia. Occasionally, increased calcitonin levels may be due to ectopic calcitonin production by oat cell carcinoma of the lung or by breast carcinoma.

Interfering factors

• Failure to fast overnight before the test
• Hemolysis due to rough handling of the sample

PARATHYROID HORMONE

Parathyroid hormone (PTH) regulates plasma concentration of calcium and phosphorus. The overall effect of PTH is to raise plasma levels of calcium while lowering phosphorus levels.

Circulating PTH exists in three distinct molecular forms: the intact PTH molecule, which originates in the parathyroids, and two smaller circulating forms, N-terminal fragments and C-terminal fragments. Two radioimmunoassays are available to detect intact PTH and the N- and C-terminal fragments. Both tests can be used to confirm diagnosis of hyperparathyroidism and hypoparathyroidism.

Each test has other specific applications as well. The C-terminal PTH assay is more useful in diagnosing chronic disturbances in PTH metabolism, such as secondary and tertiary hyperparathyroidism; it also better differentiates ectopic from primary hyperparathyroidism. The assay for intact PTH and the N-terminal fragment (both forms are measured concomitantly) more accurately reflects acute changes in PTH metabolism and thus is useful in monitoring a patient's response to PTH therapy.

The clinical and diagnostic effects of PTH excess or deficiency are directly related to the effects of PTH on bone and the renal tubules and to its interaction with ionized calcium and biologically active vitamin D. Therefore, measuring serum calcium, phosphorus, and creatinine levels with serum PTH is helpful when trying to understand the causes and effects of pathologic parathyroid function. Suppression or stimulation tests may help confirm findings.

Purpose

• To aid the differential diagnosis of parathyroid disorders

Patient preparation

• Explain to the patient that this test helps evaluate parathyroid function.
• Instruct him to observe an overnight fast because food may affect PTH levels and interfere with the test results.
• Tell the patient that this test requires a blood sample. Inform him who will perform the venipuncture and when.
• Explain that although he may experience transient discomfort from the needle puncture and tourniquet, collecting the sample takes only a few minutes.

Procedure and posttest care

• Perform a venipuncture, and collect 3 ml of blood into two separate 7-ml *red-top* tubes.
• If a hematoma develops at the venipuncture site, apply warm soaks.
• Instruct the patient to resume his normal diet.

Clinical Implications of Abnormal Parathyroid Secretion

CONDITIONS	CAUSES	P.T.H. LEVELS	IONIZED CALCIUM LEVELS
Primary hyperparathyroidism	• Parathyroid adenoma or carcinoma	●	● *to* ○
Secondary hyperparathyroidism	• Chronic renal disease • Severe vitamin D deficiency • Calcium malabsorption • Pregnancy and lactation	●	○
Tertiary hyperparathyroidism	• Progressive secondary hyperparathyroidism leading to autonomous hyperparathyroidism	●	● *to* ○
Hypoparathyroidism	• Usually, accidental removal of the parathyroid glands during surgery • Occasionally, in association with autoimmune disease	○	○
Malignant tumors	• Squamous cell carcinoma of the lung • Renal, pancreatic, or ovarian carcinoma	● *to* ○	●

KEY:
High ●   Normal ○   Low ○

Precautions

• Handle the sample gently to prevent hemolysis. Send it to the laboratory immediately so the serum can be separated and frozen for assay.

Reference values

Normal serum PTH levels vary, depending on the laboratory, and must be interpreted in association with serum calcium levels. Typical values for intact PTH range from 10 to 65 pg/ml.

Abnormal findings

Measured concomitantly with serum calcium levels, abnormally elevated PTH values may indicate primary, sec-

ondary, or tertiary hyperparathyroidism. Abnormally low PTH levels may result from hypoparathyroidism and from certain malignant diseases. (See *Clinical implications of abnormal parathyroid secretion.*)

Interfering factors

• Failure to fast overnight before the test
• Hemolysis due to rough handling of the sample

ADRENAL AND RENAL HORMONES

ALDOSTERONE

This test measures serum aldosterone levels by quantitative analysis and radioimmunoassay. Aldosterone regulates ion transport across cell membranes to promote reabsorption of sodium and chloride in exchange for potassium and hydrogen ions. Consequently, it helps to maintain blood pressure and blood volume and to regulate fluid and electrolyte balance.

This test identifies aldosteronism and, when supported by plasma renin levels, distinguishes between the primary and secondary forms of this disorder.

Purpose
• To aid diagnosis of primary aldosteronism and potential causes of the disorder, including adrenal adenoma and adrenal hyperplasia
• To aid diagnosis of secondary hypoaldosteronism and commonly related conditions, such as salt-losing syndrome, potassium excess, heart failure with ascites, and other conditions that characteristically increase activity of the renin-angiotensin system

Patient preparation
• Explain to the patient that this test helps determine if symptoms are due to improper hormonal secretion.
• Tell him that the test requires a blood sample and that he may experience some discomfort from the needle puncture and tourniquet. Tell him who will perform the venipuncture and when.
• Instruct him to maintain a low-carbohydrate, normal-sodium diet (135 mEq or 3 g/day) for at least 2 weeks or, preferably, for 30 days before the test.
• Withhold all drugs that alter fluid, sodium, and potassium balance — especially diuretics, antihypertensives, steroids, oral contraceptives, and estrogens — for at least 2 weeks or, preferably, for 30 days before the test.
• Withhold all renin inhibitors (such as propranolol) for 1 week before the test. If they must be continued, note this on the laboratory slip.
• Tell the patient to avoid licorice for at least 2 weeks before the test because it produces an aldosterone-like effect.

Procedure and posttest care
• Perform a venipuncture while the patient is still supine after a night's rest.
• Collect the sample in a 7-ml *red-top* tube, and send it to the laboratory immediately.
• Draw another sample 4 hours later, while the patient is standing and after he has been up and about, to evaluate the effect of postural change.
• Collect the second sample in a 7-ml *red-top* tube, and send it to the laboratory immediately.
• If a hematoma develops at the venipuncture site, apply warm soaks.
• Instruct the patient to resume his normal diet and medications discontinued before the test.

Precautions
• Handle the sample gently to prevent hemolysis.
• Record on the laboratory slip whether the patient was supine or standing during the venipuncture.

- If the patient is a premenopausal female, specify the phase of her menstrual cycle because aldosterone levels may fluctuate during the menstrual cycle.
- Send the sample to the laboratory immediately.

Reference values
Laboratory values vary with the patient's age:
- 0 to 30 days: 16.5 to 154 ng/dl
- 1 to 11 months: 6.5 to 86 ng/dl
- 1 to 10 years: 3 to 39.5 ng/dl (supine), 3.5 to 124 ng/dl (upright)
- 11 years and older: 1 to 21 ng/dl

Abnormal findings
Excessive aldosterone secretion may indicate a primary or secondary disease. Primary aldosteronism (Conn's syndrome) may result from adrenocortical adenoma or carcinoma or from bilateral adrenal hyperplasia. Secondary aldosteronism can result from renovascular hypertension, heart failure, cirrhosis of the liver, nephrotic syndrome, idiopathic cyclic edema, and the third trimester of pregnancy.

Low serum aldosterone levels may indicate primary hypoaldosteronism, salt-losing syndrome, eclampsia, or Addison's disease.

Interfering factors
- Failure to observe pretest restrictions
- Hemolysis due to rough handling of the sample
- Some antihypertensives, such as methyldopa, that promote sodium and water retention (possible decrease)
- Diuretics (possible increase)
- Some corticosteroids, such as fludrocortisone, that mimic mineralocorticoid activity (possible decrease)
- Radioactive scan performed within 1 week before the test

PLASMA CORTISOL

Cortisol — the principal glucocorticoid secreted by the zona fasciculata of the adrenal cortex — helps metabolize nutrients, mediate physiologic stress, and regulate the immune system. Cortisol secretion normally follows a diurnal pattern: Levels rise during the early morning hours and peak around 8 a.m. and then decline to very low levels in the evening and during the early phase of sleep. Intense heat or cold, infection, trauma, exercise, obesity, and debilitating disease influence cortisol secretion.

This radioimmunoassay, a quantitative analysis of plasma cortisol levels, is usually ordered for patients with signs of adrenal dysfunction. Dynamic tests, suppression tests for hyperfunction, and stimulation tests for hypofunction are generally required for confirmation of diagnoses.

Purpose
- To aid in the diagnosis of Cushing's disease, Cushing's syndrome, Addison's disease, and secondary adrenal insufficiency

Patient preparation
- Explain to the patient that this test helps determine if his symptoms are due to improper hormonal secretion.
- Instruct him to maintain a normal salt diet (2 to 3 g/day) for 3 days before the test and to fast and limit physical activity for 10 to 12 hours before the test.
- Tell him that a blood sample is required. Inform him who will perform the venipuncture and when.
- Explain that he may feel some discomfort from the needle puncture and

tourniquet but that collecting the sample takes only a few minutes.

• Withhold all medications that may interfere with plasma cortisol levels, such as estrogens, androgens, and phenytoin, for 48 hours before the test. If the patient is receiving replacement therapy and is dependent on exogenous steroids for survival, note this on the laboratory slip as well as any other medications that must be continued.

• Make sure the patient is relaxed and recumbent for at least 30 minutes before the test.

Procedure and posttest care

• Perform a venipuncture between 6 a.m. and 8 a.m.

• Collect the sample in a *green-top* tube, label it appropriately, and send it to the laboratory immediately.

• For diurnal variation testing, draw another sample between 4 p.m. and 6 p.m.

• Collect the second sample in a *green-top* tube, label it appropriately, and send it to the laboratory immediately.

• If a hematoma develops at the venipuncture site, apply warm soaks.

• Instruct the patient to resume his normal diet and administration of medications discontinued before the test.

Precautions

• Handle the sample gently to prevent hemolysis.

• Record the collection time on the laboratory slip.

Reference values

Normally, plasma cortisol levels range from 7 to 25 µg/dl in the morning and from 2 to 14 µg/dl in the afternoon. The afternoon level is usually half the morning level.

Abnormal findings

Increased plasma cortisol levels may indicate adrenocortical hyperfunction in Cushing's disease (a rare disease due to basophilic adenoma of the pituitary gland) or Cushing's syndrome (glucocorticoid excess from any cause). In most patients with Cushing's syndrome, the adrenal cortex secretes independently of a natural rhythm. Thus, absence of diurnal variation in cortisol secretion is a significant finding in almost all patients with Cushing's syndrome; in these patients, little if any difference in values is found between morning samples and those taken in the afternoon. Diurnal variations may also be absent in otherwise healthy people who are under considerable emotional or physical stress.

Decreased cortisol levels may indicate primary adrenal hypofunction (Addison's disease), most often due to idiopathic glandular atrophy (a presumed autoimmune process). Tuberculosis, fungal invasion, and hemorrhage can cause adrenocortical destruction. Low cortisol levels resulting from secondary adrenal insufficiency may occur in conditions of impaired corticotropin secretion, such as hypophysectomy, postpartum pituitary necrosis, craniopharyngioma, and chromophobe adenoma.

Interfering factors

• Failure to observe pretest restrictions

• Hemolysis due to rough handling of the sample

• Pregnancy or use of oral contraceptives because of increase in cortisol-binding plasma proteins (false-high)

• Obesity, stress, and severe hepatic or renal disease (possible increase)

• Androgens and phenytoin due to decrease in cortisol-binding plasma proteins (possible decrease)

• Radioactive scan performed within 1 week before the test

PLASMA CATECHOLAMINES

This test, a quantitative (total or fractionated) analysis of plasma catecholamines, has clinical importance in patients with hypertension and signs of adrenal medullary tumor as well as in those with neural tumors that affect endocrine function. Elevated plasma catecholamine levels necessitate supportive confirmation by urinalysis.

Major catecholamines include the hormones epinephrine, norepinephrine, and dopamine. When secreted into the bloodstream, catecholamines produced in the adrenal medulla prepare the body for the fight-or-flight reaction. They increase heart rate and contractility, constrict blood vessels and redistribute circulating blood toward the skeletal and coronary muscles, mobilize carbohydrate and lipid reserves, and sharpen alertness. Excessive catecholamine secretion by tumors causes hypertension, weight loss, episodic sweating, headache, palpitations, and anxiety.

Plasma levels commonly fluctuate in response to temperature, stress, postural change, diet, smoking, anoxia, volume depletion, renal failure, obesity, and many drugs.

Purpose
• To rule out pheochromocytoma (adrenal medullary or extra-adrenal) in patients with hypertension

• To help identify neuroblastoma, ganglioneuroblastoma, and ganglioneuroma
• To distinguish between adrenal medullary tumors and other catecholamine-producing tumors through fractional analysis; urinalysis for catecholamine degradation products is recommended to support diagnosis
• To aid diagnosis of autonomic nervous system dysfunction, such as idiopathic orthostatic hypotension

Patient preparation
• Explain to the patient that this test helps determine if hypertension or other symptoms are related to improper hormonal secretion. Advise the patient to strictly follow pretest instructions for a reliable test result. Instruct him to refrain from using self-prescribed medications, especially cold and allergy remedies that may contain sympathomimetics, for 2 weeks before the test.
• Tell him to exclude amine-rich foods and beverages, such as bananas, avocados, cheese, coffee, tea, cocoa, beer, and Chianti, from his diet for 48 hours; to maintain vitamin C intake, which is necessary for formation of catecholamines; to abstain from smoking for 24 hours; and to fast for 10 to 12 hours before the test.
• Tell the patient that this test requires one or two blood samples, and inform him who will perform the venipunctures and when.
• Explain that he may experience some discomfort from the needle punctures and tourniquet but that collecting the samples takes less than 20 minutes.
• If the patient is in your facility, withhold medications that affect catecholamine levels, such as amphetamines, phenothiazines (chlorpromazine), sympathomimetics, and tricyclic antidepressants.

• Insert an indwelling venous catheter (heparin lock) 24 hours before the test because the stress of the venipuncture itself may significantly raise catecholamine levels.

• Make sure the patient is relaxed and recumbent for 45 to 60 minutes before the test.

• If necessary, provide blankets to keep him warm; low temperatures stimulate catecholamine secretion.

Procedure and posttest care

• Perform a venipuncture between 6 a.m. and 8 a.m.

• Collect the sample in a 10-ml chilled tube containing EDTA (sodium metabisulfite solution), which can be obtained from the laboratory on request.

• If a second sample is requested, have the patient stand for 10 minutes, and draw the sample into another tube exactly like the first.

• If a heparin lock is used, it may be necessary to discard the first 1 or 2 ml of blood. Check with the laboratory for the preferred procedure.

• If a hematoma develops at the venipuncture site, apply warm soaks.

• Instruct the patient to resume his normal diet and medications discontinued before the test.

Precautions

• After collecting each sample, roll the tube slowly between your palms to distribute the EDTA without agitating the blood.

• Pack the tube in crushed ice to minimize deactivation of catecholamines, and send it to the laboratory immediately.

• Indicate on the laboratory slip whether the patient was supine or standing during the venipuncture and the time the sample was drawn.

Reference values

In fractional analysis, catecholamine levels range as follows:

• Supine: epinephrine, undetectable to 110 pg/ml; norepinephrine, 70 to 750 pg/ml; dopamine, undetectable to 30 pg/ml

• Standing: epinephrine, undetectable to 140 pg/ml; norepinephrine, 200 to 1,700 pg/ml; dopamine, undetectable to 30 pg/ml (no postural change).

Abnormal findings

High catecholamine levels may indicate pheochromocytoma, neuroblastoma, ganglioneuroblastoma, or ganglioneuroma. Elevations are possible with but don't directly confirm thyroid disorders, hypoglycemia, and cardiac disease. Electroconvulsive therapy, shock resulting from hemorrhage, endotoxins, and anaphylaxis also raise catecholamine levels.

In the patient with normal or low baseline catecholamine levels, failure to show an increase in the sample taken after standing suggests autonomic nervous system dysfunction.

Fractional analysis helps identify the cause of elevated catecholamine levels. For example, adrenal medullary tumors secrete epinephrine, whereas ganglioneuromas, ganglioblastomas, and neuroblastomas secrete norepinephrine.

Interfering factors

• Failure to observe pretest restrictions

• Epinephrine, levodopa, amphetamines, phenothiazines, sympathomimetics, decongestants, and tricyclic antidepressants (increase)

• Reserpine (decrease)

• Radioactive scan performed within 1 week before the test

ANDROSTENEDIONE

The androstenedione test helps identify disorders related to altered hormone levels, such as female virilization syndromes and polycystic ovary (Stein-Leventhal) syndrome. Androstenedione is a precusrsor of cortisol, aldosterone, estrogen, and testosterone. Tumors of the ovaries or adrenal glands can secrete excessive amounts of androstenedione, which then converts to testosterone, resulting in virilizing symptoms, such as hirsutism and sterility.

Increased androstenedione production may induce premature sexual development in children. It may produce renewed ovarian stimulation, endometriosis, bleeding, and polycystic ovaries in postmenopausal women. In obese women, increased levels of estrogen can lead to menstrual irregularities. In men, overproduction of androstenedione may cause feminizing signs, such as gynecomastia.

Purpose
- To help determine the cause of gonadal dysfunction, menstrual or menopausal irregularities, virilizing symptoms, and premature sexual development

Patient preparation
- Explain to the patient that this test determines the cause of her symptoms.
- Tell her that the test requires a blood sample and who will perform the venipuncture and when.
- Explain that she may experience transient discomfort from the needle puncture and tourniquet.
- If appropriate, explain that the test should be done 1 week before or after her menstrual period and that it may be repeated.
- Withhold steroid and pituitary-based hormones. If they must be continued, note this on the laboratory slip.

Procedure and posttest care
- Perform a venipuncture, and collect a serum sample in a 10-ml *red-top* tube or collect a plasma sample in a *green-top* tube. (If a plasma sample is taken, refrigerate it or place it on ice.)
- Label the sample appropriately, and send it to the laboratory immediately.
- If a hematoma develops at the venipuncture site, apply warm soaks.
- Resume administration of medications discontinued before the test.

Precautions
- Handle the sample gently to prevent hemolysis.
- Refrigerate plasma samples or place them on ice.
- Record the patient's age, sex, and (if appropriate) phase of menstrual cycle on the laboratory slip.

Reference values
- Females age 18 and older: 0.2 to 3.1 ng/ml
- Males age 18 and older: 0.3 to 3.1 ng/ml

Abnormal findings
Elevated androstenedione levels are associated with polycystic ovary (Stein-Leventhal) syndrome; Cushing's syndrome; ovarian, testicular, and adrenocortical tumors; ectopic corticotropin-producing tumors; late-onset congenital adrenal hyperplasia; and ovarian stromal hyperplasia. Elevated levels result in increased estrone levels, causing premature sexual development in children; menstrual irregularities in premenopausal women; bleeding, endometriosis, and polycystic ovaries in

postmenopausal women; and feminizing signs, such as gynecomastia, in men. Decreased levels occur in hypogonadism.

Interfering factors
● Hemolysis due to rough handling of the sample
● Steroids and pituitary hormones (possible increase)

ERYTHROPOIETIN

This test of renal hormone production measures erythropoietin (EPO) by immunoassay. It's used to evaluate anemia, polycythemia, and kidney tumors. It's also used to evaluate abuse of commercially prepared EPO by athletes who believe that the drug enhances performance.

Purpose
● To aid diagnosis of anemia and polycythemia
● To aid diagnosis of kidney tumors
● To detect abuse of EPO by athletes

Patient preparation
● Explain to the patient that this test determines if hormonal secretion is causing changes in his red blood cells.
● Instruct him to fast for 8 to 10 hours before the test.
● Tell him that this test requires a blood sample, and inform him who will perform the venipuncture and when.
● Explain that although he may experience transient discomfort from the needle puncture and tourniquet, blood collection takes only a few minutes.
● Keep the patient relaxed and recumbent for 30 minutes before the test.

Procedure and posttest care
● Perform a venipuncture, and collect the sample in a 5-ml *red-top* tube.
● If requested, a hematocrit may be drawn at the same time by collecting an additional sample in a 2-ml *lavender-top* tube.
● If a hematoma develops at the venipuncture site, apply warm soaks.

Precautions
● Handle the sample gently to prevent hemolysis.

Reference values
The reference range for EPO is 4 to 24 mU/ml; in high altitudes, such as in Denver, the range is 4 to 48 mU/ml.

Abnormal findings
Low levels of EPO appear in anemic patients with inadequate or absent hormone production. Congenital absence of EPO can occur. Severe renal disease may decrease EPO production.

Elevated EPO levels occur in anemias as a compensatory mechanism in the reestablishment of homeostasis. Inappropriate elevations (when the hematocrit is normal to high) are seen in polycythemia and EPO-secreting tumors.

Some athletes use EPO to enhance performance. The increased red cell volume conveys additional oxygen-carrying capacity to the blood. Adverse reactions include clotting abnormalities, headache, seizures, hypertension, nausea, vomiting, diarrhea, and rash.

Interfering factors
● Failure to observe pretest restrictions
● Hemolysis due to rough handling of the sample
● Anabolic steroids and amphotericin B

PLASMA ATRIAL NATRIURETIC FACTOR

This radioimmunoassay measures the plasma level of atrial natriuretic factor (ANF), also known as atrionatriuretic peptides or atriopeptins. An extremely potent natriuretic agent and vasodilator, ANF rapidly produces diuresis and increases the glomerular filtration rate. ANF's role in regulating extracellular fluid volume, blood pressure, and sodium metabolism appears critical.

Patients with overt heart failure have highly elevated plasma levels of ANF. Patients with cardiovascular disease and elevated cardiac filling pressure but without heart failure also have markedly elevated ANF levels. ANF may provide a marker for early asymptomatic left ventricular dysfunction and increased cardiac volume.

Purpose
• To confirm heart failure
• To identify asymptomatic cardiac volume overload

Patient preparation
• As appropriate, explain the purpose of the test to the patient.
• Inform him that he must fast for 12 hours before the test.
• Tell him that this test requires a blood sample, and inform him who will perform the venipuncture and when.
• Reassure him that although he may experience transient discomfort from the needle puncture and tourniquet, collecting the sample takes less than 3 minutes.
• Explain that the test results will be available within 4 days.

• Check patient history for use of medications that can influence test results.
• Withhold beta blockers, calcium antagonists, diuretics, vasodilators, and digitalis glycosides for 24 hours before collection.

Procedure and posttest care
• Perform a venipuncture, and collect the sample in a prechilled potassium-EDTA tube.
• After chilled centrifugation, the EDTA plasma should be promptly frozen and sent to the laboratory.
• If a hematoma develops at the venipuncture site, apply warm soaks.
• Tell the patient that he may resume his normal diet and medications withheld before the test.

Precautions
• Handle the sample gently to prevent hemolysis.

Reference values
Normal ANF levels range from 20 to 77 pg/ml.

Abnormal findings
Markedly elevated levels of ANF occur in patients with frank heart failure and significantly elevated cardiac filling pressure.

Interfering factors
• Cardiovascular drugs, including beta blockers, calcium antagonists, diuretics, vasodilators, and digitalis glycosides
• Failure to observe pretest restrictions
• Failure to use proper procedure for obtaining, centrifuging, and freezing the sample

PANCREATIC AND GASTRIC HORMONES

INSULIN

This radioimmunoassay is a quantitative analysis of serum insulin levels. Insulin is usually measured concomitantly with glucose levels because glucose is the primary stimulus for insulin release.

Insulin regulates the metabolism and transport or mobilization of carbohydrates, amino acids, proteins, and lipids. Stimulated by increased plasma levels of glucose, insulin secretion reaches peak levels after meals, when metabolism and food storage are greatest.

Purpose
• To aid diagnosis of hyperinsulinemia as well as hypoglycemia resulting from tumor or hyperplasia of pancreatic islet cells, glucocorticoid deficiency, or severe hepatic disease
• To aid diagnosis of diabetes mellitus and insulin-resistant states

Patient preparation
• Explain to the patient that this test helps determine if the pancreas is functioning normally.
• Inform the patient that the test requires blood samples. Tell him who will perform the venipuncture and when.
• Instruct the patient to fast for 10 to 12 hours before the test.
• Explain that he may experience discomfort from the needle puncture and

tourniquet but that collecting the samples takes only a few minutes.
• Explain that questionable results may require a repeat test or a simultaneous glucose tolerance test, which requires that the patient drink a glucose solution.
• Withhold corticotropin, steroids (including oral contraceptives), thyroid supplements, epinephrine, and other medications that may interfere with test results. If they must be continued, note this on the laboratory slip.
• Make sure the patient is relaxed and recumbent for 30 minutes before the test.

Procedure and posttest care
• Perform a venipuncture, and collect one sample for insulin level in a 7-ml *lavender-top* tube.
• Collect a sample for glucose level in a *gray-top* tube, if requested.
• If a hematoma develops at the venipuncture site, apply warm soaks.
• Instruct the patient to resume his normal diet and medications discontinued before the test.

Precautions
• Pack the insulin sample in ice, and send it, along with the glucose sample, to the laboratory immediately.
• In the patient with an insulinoma, fasting for this test may precipitate dangerously severe hypoglycemia. Keep an ampule of dextrose 50% available to counteract possible hypoglycemia.
• Handle the samples gently to prevent hemolysis.

Reference values
Serum insulin levels normally are less than or equal to 20 µU/ml.

Abnormal findings
Insulin levels are interpreted in light of the prevailing glucose concentration. A

CONNECTING-PEPTIDE ASSAY

Connecting peptide (C-peptide) is a biologically inactive peptide chain formed during the proteolytic conversion of proinsulin to insulin in the pancreatic beta cells. It has no insulin effect either biologically or immunologically. This is important because circulating insulin is measured by immunologic assay. As insulin is released into the bloodstream, the C-peptide chain splits off from the hormone. Except in patients with islet cell tumors and, possibly, in obese patients, serum C-peptide levels generally parallel those of insulin. Normal values range between 170 and 900 pmol/L.

Purpose
A C-peptide assay may help to:
• determine the cause of hypoglycemia by distinguishing between endogenous hyperinsulinism or insulinoma (elevated C-peptide levels) and surreptitious insulin injection (decreased C-peptide levels)
• indirectly measure insulin secretion in the presence of circulating insulin antibodies, which interfere with insulin assays but not with C-peptide assays
• detect residual tissue (some C-peptide present) after total pancreatectomy for carcinoma
• indicate the remission phase (some C-peptide present) of diabetes mellitus
• determine beta cell function in patients with diabetes mellitus. Absence of C-peptide indicates no beta cell function; presence indicates residual beta cell function.

---

normal insulin level may be inappropriate for the glucose results. High insulin and low glucose levels after a significant fast suggest the presence of an insulinoma. Prolonged fasting or stimulation testing may be required to confirm the diagnosis. (See *Connecting-peptide assay.*) In insulin-resistant diabetes mellitus, insulin levels are elevated; in non-insulin-resistant diabetes, they're low.

Interfering factors
• Failure to observe pretest restrictions
• Patient's agitation and stress
• Hemolysis due to rough handling of the sample
• Failure to pack the insulin sample in ice and send it to the laboratory promptly
• Corticotropin, steroids (including oral contraceptives), thyroid hormones, and epinephrine (possible increase)
• Use of insulin by non-insulin-dependent patients (possible increase)
• High levels of insulin antibodies in patients with insulin-dependent diabetes mellitus

---

GASTRIN

Gastrin is a polypeptide hormone produced and stored primarily in the antrum of the stomach and to a lesser degree in the islets of Langerhans. Its main function is to facilitate digestion of food by triggering gastric acid secretion. It also stimulates the release of pancreatic enzymes and the gastric enzyme pepsin, increases gastric and intestinal motility, and stimulates bile flow from the liver. Abnormal secretion of gastrin can result from tumors (gastrinomas) and pathologic disorders that affect the stomach, pancreas and, less commonly, the esophagus and small bowel.

This radioimmunoassay, a quantitative analysis of gastrin levels, is especially useful in patients suspected of having gastrinomas (Zollinger-Ellison syndrome). In doubtful situations, provocative testing may be necessary.

Purpose
• To confirm a diagnosis of gastrinoma, the gastrin-secreting tumor in Zollinger-Ellison syndrome
• To aid differential diagnosis of gastric and duodenal ulcers and pernicious anemia (gastrin estimation has limited value in patients with duodenal ulcer)

Patient preparation
• Explain to the patient that this test helps determine the cause of GI symptoms.
• Instruct him to abstain from alcohol for at least 24 hours before the test and to fast and avoid caffeinated drinks for 12 hours before the test, although he may drink water.
• Tell him that the test requires a blood sample. Inform him who will perform the venipuncture and when.
• Reassure him that although he may experience transient discomfort from the needle puncture and tourniquet, collecting the sample takes only a few minutes.
• Withhold all drugs that may interfere with test results, especially insulin and anticholinergics, such as atropine and belladonna. If they must be continued, note this on the laboratory slip.
• Tell the patient to lie down and relax for at least 30 minutes before the test.

Procedure and posttest care
• Perform a venipuncture, and collect the sample in a 10- to 15-ml *red-top* tube.

• If a hematoma develops at the venipuncture site, apply warm soaks.
• Instruct the patient to resume his normal diet and medications discontinued before the test.

Precautions
• Handle the sample gently to avoid hemolysis.
• To prevent destruction of serum gastrin by proteolytic enzymes, immediately send the sample to the laboratory to have the serum separated and frozen.

Reference values
Normal serum gastrin levels are less than 200 pg/ml.

Abnormal findings
Strikingly high serum gastrin levels (> 1,000 pg/ml) confirm Zollinger-Ellison syndrome. (Levels as high as 450,000 pg/ml have been reported.)

Increased serum levels of gastrin may occur in a few patients with duodenal ulceration (< 1%) and in patients with achlorhydria (with or without pernicious anemia) or extensive stomach carcinoma (because of hyposecretion of gastric juices and hydrochloric acid).

Interfering factors
• Failure to observe pretest restrictions, including abstention from caffeine
• Hemolysis due to rough handling of the sample
• Amino acids (especially glycine), calcium carbonate, acetylcholine, calcium chloride, and ethanol (increase)
• Anticholinergics, such as atropine and belladonna, as well as hydrochloric acid and secretin, a strongly basic polypeptide (decrease)
• Insulin-induced hypoglycemia (increase)

PLASMA GLUCAGON

Glucagon, a polypeptide hormone, is secreted by alpha cells of the islets of Langerhans in the pancreas. It acts primarily on the liver to promote glucose production and control glucose. This test is a quantitative analysis of plasma glucagon by radioimmunoassay.

Purpose
• To aid diagnosis of glucagonoma and hypoglycemia due to chronic pancreatitis or idiopathic glucagon deficiency

Patient preparation
• Explain to the patient that this test helps to evaluate pancreatic function.
• Instruct the patient to fast for 10 to 12 hours before the test.
• Tell the patient that the test requires a blood sample. Inform him who will perform the venipuncture and when.
• Explain that he may experience transient discomfort from the needle puncture and tourniquet but that collecting the sample takes only a few minutes.
• Withhold insulin, catecholamines, and other drugs that could influence the test results, as ordered. If they must be continued, note this on the laboratory slip.
• Have the patient lie down and relax for 30 minutes before the test.

Procedure and posttest care
• Perform a venipuncture, and collect the sample in a chilled, 10-ml *lavender-top* tube.
• If a hematoma develops at the venipuncture site, apply warm soaks.
• Instruct the patient to resume his normal diet and medications withheld before the test.

Precautions
• Place the sample on ice, and send it to the laboratory immediately.
• Handle the sample gently to prevent hemolysis.

Reference values
Fasting glucagon levels are normally less than 60 pg/ml.

Abnormal findings
Elevated fasting glucagon levels (900 to 7,800 pg/ml) can occur in glucagonoma, diabetes mellitus, acute pancreatitis, and pheochromocytoma.

Abnormally low glucagon levels are associated with idiopathic glucagon deficiency and hypoglycemia due to chronic pancreatitis.

Interfering factors
• Failure to observe pretest restrictions
• Hemolysis due to rough handling of the sample
• Failure to pack the sample in ice and send it to the laboratory immediately
• Exercise, stress, prolonged fasting, insulin, or catecholamines (increase)
• Radioactive scans and tests performed within 48 hours of the test

GONADAL HORMONES

ESTROGENS

Estrogens (and progesterone) are secreted by the ovaries. They are responsible for the development of secondary female sexual characteristics and for normal menstruation. Levels are usual-

PREDICTING PREMATURE LABOR

A simple salivary test can now help determine whether a pregnant woman is at risk for premature labor, a complication that is detrimental to the health of the premature infant. The test, known as the SalEst test, measures salivary levels of estriol, an estrogen that increases 1,000-fold during pregnancy. For women determined to be at risk, the SalEst test is 98% accurate in ruling out premature labor and delivery.

The test is performed on women between weeks 22 and 36 of gestation, using their saliva and the SalEst test kit. Estriol has been found to increase 2 to 3 weeks before the spontaneous onset of labor and delivery. A positive test indicates that the patient is at risk for premature labor. With this knowledge and evaluation by a doctor, precautions can be instituted to decrease the risk of preterm labor and maintain fetal viability.

ly undetectable in children. These hormones are secreted by ovarian follicular cells during the first half of the menstrual cycle and by the corpus luteum during the luteal phase and during pregnancy. In menopause, estrogen secretion drops to a constant, low level.

This radioimmunoassay measures serum levels of estradiol, estrone, and estriol (the only estrogens that appear in serum in measurable amounts) and has diagnostic significance in evaluating female gonadal dysfunction. (See *Predicting premature labor.*) Tests of

hypothalamic-pituitary function may be required to confirm the diagnosis.

Purpose
- To determine sexual maturation and fertility
- To aid diagnosis of gonadal dysfunction, such as precocious or delayed puberty, menstrual disorders (especially amenorrhea), and infertility
- To determine fetal well-being
- To aid diagnosis of tumors known to secrete estrogen

Patient preparation
- Explain to the patient that this test helps determine if secretion of female hormones is normal and that the test may be repeated during the various phases of the menstrual cycle.
- Tell her that she needn't restrict food or fluids.
- Inform her that the test requires a blood sample, and tell her who will perform the venipuncture and when.
- Explain that she may experience transient discomfort from the needle puncture and tourniquet but that collecting the sample takes only a few minutes.
- Withhold all steroid and pituitary-based hormones. If they must be continued, note this on the laboratory slip.

Procedure and posttest care
Procedure and posttest care may vary slightly, depending on whether plasma or serum is being measured.
- Perform a venipuncture, and collect the sample in a 10-ml *red-top* tube.
- If the patient is premenopausal, indicate the phase of her menstrual cycle on the laboratory slip.
- If a hematoma develops at the venipuncture site, apply warm soaks.
- Resume administration of medications discontinued before the test.

Precautions
- Handle the sample gently to prevent hemolysis.
- Send the sample to the laboratory immediately.

Reference values
Normal serum estrogen levels for premenopausal women vary widely during the menstrual cycle, ranging from 30 to 400 pg/ml. The range for postmenopausal women is 0 to 30 pg/ml.

Serum estrogen levels in men range from 10 to 50 pg/ml. In children under age 6, the normal level of serum estrogen is less than 10 pg/ml.

Abnormal findings
Decreased estrogen levels may indicate primary hypogonadism, or ovarian failure, as in Turner's syndrome or ovarian agenesis; secondary hypogonadism, such as in hypopituitarism; or menopause.

Abnormally high estrogen levels may occur with estrogen-producing tumors, in precocious puberty, and in severe hepatic disease, such as cirrhosis, that prevents clearance of plasma estrogens. High levels may also result from congenital adrenal hyperplasia (increased conversion of androgens to estrogen).

Interfering factors
- Hemolysis due to rough handling of the sample
- Pregnancy and pretest use of estrogens, such as oral contraceptives (possible increase)
- Clomiphene, an estrogen antagonist (possible decrease)
- Steroids and pituitary-based hormones, such as dexamethasone

PLASMA PROGESTERONE

Progesterone, an ovarian steroid hormone secreted by the corpus luteum, causes thickening and secretory development of the endometrium in preparation for implantation of the fertilized ovum. Progesterone levels, therefore, peak during the midluteal phase of the menstrual cycle. If implantation does not occur, progesterone (and estrogen) levels drop sharply and menstruation begins about 2 days later.

During pregnancy, the placenta releases about 10 times the normal monthly amount of progesterone to maintain the pregnancy. Increased secretion begins toward the end of the first trimester and continues until delivery. Progesterone prevents abortion by decreasing uterine contractions. Along with estrogen, progesterone helps prepare the breasts for lactation.

This radioimmunoassay is a quantitative analysis of plasma progesterone levels and provides reliable information about corpus luteum function in fertility studies and placental function in pregnancy. Serial determinations are recommended. Although plasma levels provide accurate information, progesterone can also be monitored by measuring urine pregnanediol, a catabolite of progesterone.

Purpose
- To assess corpus luteum function as part of infertility studies
- To evaluate placental function during pregnancy
- To aid in confirming ovulation; test results support basal body temperature readings

Patient preparation

• Explain to the patient that this test helps determine if her female sex hormone secretion is normal.

• Inform her that she needn't restrict food or fluids.

• Tell her that the test requires a blood sample, and inform her who will perform the venipuncture and when.

• Reassure her that although she may experience transient discomfort from the needle puncture and tourniquet, collecting the sample takes only a few minutes.

• Inform her that the test may be repeated at specific times coinciding with phases of her menstrual cycle or with each prenatal visit.

• Check the patient's medication history to determine if she's taking any drugs that may interfere with test results, including progesterone and estrogen. Note your findings on the laboratory slip.

Procedure and posttest care

• Perform a venipuncture, and collect the sample in a 7-ml *green-top* (heparinized) tube.

• If a hematoma develops at the venipuncture site, apply warm soaks.

Precautions

• Handle the sample gently to prevent hemolysis.

• Completely fill the collection tube; then invert it gently at least 10 times to mix the sample and anticoagulant adequately.

• Indicate the date of the patient's last menstrual period and the phase of her cycle on the laboratory slip. If the patient is pregnant, also indicate the month of gestation.

• Send the sample to the laboratory immediately.

Reference values

During menstruation, normal progesterone values are as follows:

• Follicular phase: < 0.7 ng/ml
• Luteal phase: 2 to 20 ng/ml.

During pregnancy, normal progesterone values are as follows:

• First trimester: 9 to 47 ng/dl
• Second trimester: 16.8 to 146 ng/dl
• Third trimester: 55 to 255 ng/dl.

Abnormal findings

Elevated progesterone levels may indicate ovulation, luteinizing tumors, ovarian cysts that produce progesterone, or adrenocortical hyperplasias and tumors that produce progesterone along with other steroidal hormones.

Low progesterone levels are associated with amenorrhea due to several causes (such as panhypopituitarism and gonadal dysfunction), eclampsia, threatened abortion, and fetal death.

Interfering factors

• Hemolysis due to rough handling of the sample

• Progesterone or estrogen therapy

• Radioactive scans performed within 1 week of the test

TESTOSTERONE

The principal androgen secreted by the interstitial cells of the testes (Leydig cells), testosterone induces puberty in the male and maintains male secondary sex characteristics. Prepubertal levels of testosterone are low. Increased testosterone secretion during puberty stimulates growth of the seminiferous tubules and the production of sperm; it also contributes to the enlargement of external genitalia, accessory sex organs (such as prostate glands), and voluntary muscles and to the growth of facial, pubic, and axillary hair.

Testosterone production begins to increase at onset of puberty and continues to rise during adulthood. Production begins to taper off at about age 40 and eventually drops to about one-fifth the peak level by age 80. In women, the adrenal glands and ovaries secrete small amounts of testosterone.

This competitive protein-binding test measures plasma or serum testosterone levels. When combined with measurement of plasma gonadotropin levels (follicle-stimulating hormone and luteinizing hormone), it's a reliable aid in the evaluation of gonadal dysfunction in men and women.

Purpose

● To facilitate differential diagnosis of male sexual precocity in boys under age 10 (true precocious puberty must be distinguished from pseudoprecocious puberty)
● To aid differential diagnosis of hypogonadism; primary hypogonadism must be distinguished from secondary hypogonadism
● To evaluate male infertility or other sexual dysfunction
● To evaluate hirsutism and virilization in women

Patient preparation

● Explain to the patient that this test helps determine if male sex hormone secretion is adequate.
● Inform him that he needn't restrict food or fluids.
● Tell him that this test requires a blood sample, and inform him who will perform the venipuncture and when.
● Explain that he may experience some discomfort from the needle puncture and tourniquet but that collecting the sample takes only a few minutes.

Procedure and posttest care

● Perform a venipuncture, and collect the serum sample in a 7-ml *red-top* tube.
● If plasma is to be collected, use a *green-top* (heparinized) tube.
● Indicate the patient's age, sex, and history of hormone therapy on the laboratory slip.
● If a hematoma develops at the venipuncture site, apply warm soaks.

Precautions

● Handle the sample gently to prevent hemolysis, and send it to the laboratory promptly.
● The sample is stable and requires no refrigeration or preservative for up to 1 week. Frozen samples are stable for at least 6 months.

Reference values

Normal testosterone levels are as follows (laboratory values vary slightly):
● Males age 18 and older: 240 to 950 ng/dl
● Females age 18 and older: 20 to 80 ng/dl
● Prepubertal boys: < 200 ng/dl
● Prepubertal girls: < 75 ng/dl.

Abnormal findings

Elevated testosterone levels in prepubertal boys may indicate true sexual precocity due to excessive gonadotropin secretion or pseudoprecocious puberty due to male hormone production by a testicular tumor. They can also indicate congenital adrenal hyperplasia, which results in precocious puberty in boys (from ages 2 to 3), and pseudohermaphroditism and milder virilization in girls.

Increased testosterone levels can occur with a benign adrenal tumor or cancer, hyperthyroidism, and incipient puberty. In women with ovarian tumors or polycystic ovary syndrome, testosterone levels may rise, leading to hirsutism.

Low testosterone levels can indicate primary hypogonadism (as in Klinefelter's syndrome) or secondary hypogonadism (hypogonadotropic eunuchoidism) from hypothalamic-pituitary dysfunction. Low levels can also follow orchiectomy, testicular or prostate cancer, delayed male puberty, estrogen therapy, and cirrhosis.

Interfering factors
● Hemolysis due to rough handling of the sample
● Exogenous sources of estrogens and androgens, thyroid and growth hormones, and other pituitary-based hormones
● Estrogens (decrease free testosterone levels by increasing sex hormone-binding globulin, which binds testosterone)
● Androgens (possible increase)

PLACENTAL HORMONES

HUMAN CHORIONIC GONADOTROPIN

Human chorionic gonadotropin (hCG) is a glycoprotein hormone produced in the placenta. If conception occurs, a specific assay for hCG — commonly called the beta-subunit assay — may detect this hormone in the blood 9 days after ovulation. This interval coincides with the implantation of the fertilized ovum into the uterine wall. Although the precise function of hCG is still unclear, it appears that hCG, with progesterone, maintains the corpus luteum during early pregnancy.

Production of hCG increases steadily during the first trimester, peaking around the 10th week of gestation. Levels then fall to less than 10% of first-trimester peak levels during the remainder of the pregnancy. About 2 weeks after delivery, the hormone may no longer be detectable.

This serum immunoassay, a quantitative analysis of hCG beta-subunit level, is more sensitive (and costlier) than the routine pregnancy test using a urine sample.

Purpose
● To detect early pregnancy
● To determine adequacy of hormonal production in high-risk pregnancies (for example, habitual abortion)
● To aid diagnosis of trophoblastic tumors, such as hydatidiform moles and choriocarcinoma, and tumors that ectopically secrete hCG
● To monitor treatment for induction of ovulation and conception

Patient preparation
● Explain to the patient that this test determines if she's pregnant. If detection of pregnancy isn't the diagnostic objective, offer the appropriate explanation.
● Inform her that she needn't restrict food or fluids.
● Tell her that the test requires a blood sample, and inform her who will perform the venipuncture and when.
● Explain that she may experience transient discomfort from the needle puncture and tourniquet but that collecting the sample takes only a few minutes.

Procedure and posttest care
● Perform a venipuncture, and collect the sample in a 7-ml *red-top* tube.
● If a hematoma develops at the venipuncture site, apply warm soaks.

Precautions
● Handle the sample gently to prevent hemolysis, and send it to the laboratory immediately.

Reference values
Normally, hCG levels are less than 4 IU/L. During pregnancy, hCG levels vary widely, depending partly on the number of days after the last normal menstrual period.

Abnormal findings
Elevated hCG beta-subunit levels indicate pregnancy; significantly higher concentrations are present in a multiple pregnancy. Increased levels may also suggest hydatidiform mole, trophoblastic neoplasms of the placenta, and nontrophoblastic carcinomas that secrete hCG (including gastric, pancreatic, and ovarian adenocarcinomas). Low hCG beta-subunit levels can occur in ectopic pregnancy or pregnancy of less than 9 days. Beta-subunit levels cannot differentiate between pregnancy and tumor recurrence because they're high in both conditions.

Interfering factors
● Hemolysis due to rough handling of the sample
● Heparin anticoagulants and EDTA (decrease; ask laboratory whether test will be performed on plasma or serum)
● Injections of hCG, used in treating infertility and anovulation (possible false-positive, if drawn before 2 weeks)
● Failure to send the sample to the laboratory immediately

HUMAN PLACENTAL LACTOGEN

A polypeptide hormone, human placental lactogen (hPL) — also known as human chorionic somatomammotropin — displays lactogenic and somatotropic (growth hormone) properties in a pregnant female. In combination with prolactin, hPL prepares the breasts for lactation. It also indirectly provides energy for maternal metabolism and fetal nutrition. It facilitates protein synthesis and mobilization essential to fetal growth. Secretion is autonomous, beginning about the 5th week of gestation and declining rapidly after delivery. According to some evidence, this hormone may not be essential for a successful pregnancy.

This radioimmunoassay measures plasma hPL levels, which are roughly proportional to placental mass. Such assays may be required in high-risk pregnancies (patients with diabetes mellitus or hypertension) and suspected placental tissue dysfunction. Because values vary widely during the latter half of pregnancy, serial determinations over several days provide the most reliable test results.

Purpose
● To assess placental function and fetal well-being (combined with measurement of estriol levels)
● To aid diagnosis of hydatidiform moles and choriocarcinoma (human chorionic gonadotropin levels may be more useful in diagnosing these conditions)
● To aid diagnosis and monitor treatment of nontrophoblastic tumors that ectopically secrete hPL

Patient preparation

• Explain to the patient that this test helps assess placental function and fetal well-being. (If assessing fetal well-being isn't the diagnostic objective, offer an appropriate explanation.)
• Tell her that the test requires a blood sample, and inform her who will perform the venipuncture and when.
• Reassure her that although she may experience transient discomfort from the needle puncture and tourniquet, collecting the sample takes only a few minutes.
• Inform the pregnant patient that this test may be repeated during her pregnancy.

Procedure and posttest care

• Perform a venipuncture, and collect the sample in a 7-ml *red-top* tube.
• If a hematoma develops at the venipuncture site, apply warm soaks.

Precautions

• Handle the sample gently to prevent hemolysis, and send it to the laboratory without delay.

Reference values

For pregnant women, normal hPL levels slowly increase throughout pregnancy and reach 7 µg/ml at term. Testing for hPL usually begins after the 30th week of gestation, but a level of 1 µg/ml may be detected at 6 to 8 weeks.

Abnormal findings

For reliable interpretation, hPL levels must be correlated with gestational age; for example, after 30 weeks' gestation, levels below 4 µg/ml may indicate placental dysfunction. Low hPL concentrations are also characteristically associated with postmaturity syndrome, intrauterine growth retardation, preeclampsia, and eclampsia. Declining concentrations may help differentiate incomplete abortion from threatened abortion.

Be aware that low hPL concentrations don't confirm fetal distress. Conversely, concentrations over 4 µg/ml after 30 weeks' gestation don't guarantee fetal well-being because elevated levels have been reported after fetal death.

An hPL value above 6 µg/ml after 30 weeks' gestation may suggest an unusually large placenta, commonly occurring in patients with diabetes mellitus, multiple pregnancy, and Rh isoimmunization. The usefulness of this test in predicting fetal death in a patient with diabetes mellitus and in managing Rh isoimmunization during pregnancy is limited.

Below-normal concentrations of hPL may be associated with trophoblastic neoplastic disease, such as hydatidiform mole and choriocarcinoma. Abnormal concentrations of hPL have been found in the sera of patients with other neoplastic disorders, including bronchogenic carcinoma, hepatoma, lymphoma, and pheochromocytoma. In these patients, hPL levels are used as tumor markers for evaluating chemotherapy, monitoring tumor growth and recurrence, and detecting residual tissue after excision.

Interfering factor

• Hemolysis due to rough handling of the sample

CHAPTER 4

Vitamin and Trace Element Tests

VITAMINS — 244

244	Vitamin A and carotene	247	Vitamin C
245	Vitamin B_2	248	Vitamin D_3
246	Vitamin B_{12}	249	Folic acid

TRACE ELEMENTS — 250

250	Manganese	251	Zinc

VITAMINS

VITAMIN A AND CAROTENE

The vitamin A and carotene test measures serum levels of vitamin A (retinol) and its precursor, carotene. A fat-soluble vitamin normally supplied by diet, vitamin A is important for reproduction, vision (especially night vision), and epithelial tissue and bone growth. Vitamin A is found mostly in fruits, vegetables, eggs, poultry, meat, and fish. Carotene is present in leafy green vegetables and in yellow fruits and vegetables.

In this serum test, the color reactions produced by vitamin A and related compounds with various reagents provide both quantitative and qualitative information.

Purpose
• To investigate suspected vitamin A deficiency or toxicity
• To aid diagnosis of visual disturbances, especially night blindness and xerophthalmia
• To aid diagnosis of skin diseases, such as keratosis follicularis or ichthyosis
• To screen for malabsorption

Patient preparation
• Explain to the patient that this test measures the level of vitamin A in the blood.
• Instruct him to fast overnight, but that he needn't restrict water intake.

• Tell him that this test requires a blood sample. Explain who will perform the venipuncture and when.
• Reassure him that although he may feel some discomfort from the needle puncture and the pressure of the tourniquet, collecting the sample takes only a few minutes.

Procedure and posttest care
• Perform a venipuncture, and collect the sample in a 7-ml *red-top* or *royal-blue-top* tube.
• If a hematoma develops at the venipuncture site, apply warm soaks.
• Remove diet restrictions.

Precautions
• Protect the sample from light, because vitamin A characteristically absorbs light.
• Handle the sample gently, and send it to the laboratory immediately.

Reference values
Normal serum levels for carotene, the precursor to vitamin A, range from 48 to 200 µg/dl; for vitamin A (retinol), 360 to 1,200 µg/L.

Abnormal findings
Low serum levels of vitamin A (hypovitaminosis A) may indicate impaired fat absorption, as in celiac disease, infectious hepatitis, cystic fibrosis of the pancreas, or obstructive jaundice. Low levels are also associated with protein-calorie malnutrition (marasmic kwashiorkor). Similar decreases in vitamin A levels may also result from chronic nephritis.

Elevated vitamin A levels (hypervitaminosis A) usually indicate chronically excessive intake of vitamin A supplements or of foods high in vitamin A. Increased levels are also associated with hyperlipemia and hypercholesterolemia of uncontrolled diabetes mellitus.

Decreased serum carotene levels may indicate impaired fat absorption or, rarely, insufficient dietary intake of carotene. Carotene levels may also be suppressed during pregnancy. Elevated carotene levels indicate grossly excessive dietary intake.

Interfering factors
- Failure to observe pretest restrictions
- Hemolysis due to rough handling of the sample
- Mineral oil, neomycin, and cholestyramine (possible decrease)
- Glucocorticoids and oral contraceptives (possible increase)

VITAMIN B$_2$

The serum vitamin B$_2$ test evaluates serum levels of vitamin B$_2$ (riboflavin), a vitamin essential for growth and tissue function. The serum test is considered more reliable than the urine vitamin B$_2$ test, which can produce artificially high values in patients after surgery or prolonged fasting.

Purpose
- To detect vitamin B$_2$ deficiency

Patient preparation
- Explain to the patient that this test evaluates vitamin B$_2$ levels.
- Instruct him to maintain a normal diet before the test.
- Inform him that the test requires a blood sample. Tell him who will perform the venipuncture and when.

- Reassure him that although he may experience some discomfort from the needle puncture and the pressure of the tourniquet, collecting the sample takes only a few minutes.

Procedure and posttest care
- Perform a venipuncture, and collect the sample in a 7-ml *royal-blue-top* tube.
- If a hematoma develops at the venipuncture site, apply warm soaks.
- Inform the patient with vitamin B$_2$ deficiency that good dietary sources of vitamin B$_2$ are milk products, organ meats (liver and kidneys), fish, green leafy vegetables, and legumes.

Precautions
- Handle the sample gently to prevent hemolysis.
- Send the sample to the laboratory immediately.
- Don't refrigerate or freeze the sample.

Reference values
Normal test results are 3 to 15 µg/dl; 2 to 3 µg/dl is considered marginally low, and less than 2 µg/dl is considered significantly diminished.

Abnormal findings
Marginally low test results (< 3 µg/dl) indicate vitamin B$_2$ deficiency. Such deficiency can result from insufficient dietary intake of vitamin B$_2$, malabsorption syndrome, or conditions that increase metabolic demands such as stress.

Interfering factor
- Hemolysis due to rough handling of the sample

COBALT: CRITICAL TRACE ELEMENT

A trace element found mainly in the liver, cobalt is an essential component of vitamin B_{12} and therefore is a critical factor in hematopoiesis. A balanced diet supplies sufficient cobalt to maintain hematopoiesis, primarily through foods containing vitamin B_{12}.

However, excessive ingestion of cobalt may have toxic effects. Toxicity has occurred, for example, in individuals who consumed large quantities of beer containing cobalt as a stabilizer, resulting in heart failure from cardiomyopathy. Since quantitative analysis of cobalt alone is difficult because of the minute amount found in the body, cobalt is often measured by bioassay as part of vitamin B_{12}.

Normal cobalt reference values range from 0.007 to 6 µg/dl.

VITAMIN B_{12}

The vitamin B_{12} radioisotopic assay of competitive binding is a quantitative analysis of serum levels of vitamin B_{12} (also called cyanocobalamin, antipernicious anemia factor, or extrinsic factor). This test is usually performed concurrently with measurement of serum folic acid levels.

A water-soluble vitamin containing cobalt, vitamin B_{12} is essential to hematopoiesis, deoxyribonucleic acid synthesis and growth, myelin synthesis, and central nervous system (CNS) integrity. This vitamin is found almost exclusively in animal products, such as meat, shellfish, milk, and eggs. (See *Cobalt: Critical trace element.*)

Purpose
● To aid differential diagnosis of megaloblastic anemia, which may be due to a deficiency of vitamin B_{12} or folic acid
● To aid differential diagnosis of CNS disorders that are affecting peripheral and spinal myelinated nerves

Patient preparation
● Explain to the patient that this test determines the amount of vitamin B_{12} in the blood.
● Instruct the patient to observe an overnight fast before the test.
● Tell him that this test requires a blood sample. Explain who will perform the venipuncture and when.
● Reassure him that although he may feel some discomfort from the needle puncture and the pressure of the tourniquet, collecting the sample takes only a few minutes.

Procedure and posttest care
● Perform a venipuncture, and collect the sample in a 7-ml *royal-blue-top* tube.
● If a hematoma develops at the venipuncture site, apply warm soaks.
● Remove diet restrictions.

Precautions
● Handle the sample gently to prevent hemolysis, and send it to the laboratory immediately.

Reference values
Normally, serum vitamin B_{12} values range from 190 to 900 ng/L.

Abnormal findings

Decreased serum levels may indicate inadequate dietary intake, especially if the patient is a strict vegetarian. Low levels are also associated with malabsorption syndromes (such as celiac disease), isolated malabsorption of vitamin B_{12}, hypermetabolic states (such as hyperthyroidism), pregnancy, and CNS damage (posterolateral sclerosis or funicular degeneration, for example).

Elevated levels of serum vitamin B_{12} may result from excessive dietary intake; hepatic disease, such as cirrhosis or acute or chronic hepatitis; and myeloproliferative disorders such as myelocytic leukemia.

Interfering factors

- Failure to observe pretest restrictions
- Hemolysis due to rough handling of the sample
- Neomycin, metformin, anticonvulsants, and ethanol (possible decrease)
- Oral contraceptives (increase)

VITAMIN C

Vitamin C chemical assay measures plasma levels of vitamin C (ascorbic acid), a water-soluble vitamin required for collagen synthesis and cartilage and bone maintenance. Vitamin C also promotes iron absorption, influences folic acid metabolism, and may be necessary for withstanding the stresses of injury and infection.

This vitamin is present in generous amounts in citrus fruits, berries, tomatoes, raw cabbage, green peppers, and green leafy vegetables. Severe vitamin C deficiency, or scurvy, causes capillary fragility, joint abnormalities, and multiple systemic symptoms.

Purpose

- To aid diagnosis of scurvy, scurvy-like conditions, and metabolic disorders, such as malnutrition and malabsorption syndromes

Patient preparation

- Explain to the patient that this test detects the amount of vitamin C in the blood.
- Instruct him to observe an overnight fast before the test.
- Tell him that this test requires a blood sample. Explain who will perform the venipuncture and when.
- Reassure him that although he may feel some discomfort from the needle puncture and the pressure of the tourniquet, collecting the sample takes only a few minutes.

Procedure and posttest care

- Perform a venipuncture, and collect the sample in a 7-ml *green-top* (heparinized) tube.
- If a hematoma develops at the venipuncture site, apply warm soaks.
- Remove diet restrictions.

Precautions

- Avoid rough handling or excessive agitation of the sample to prevent hemolysis.
- Send the sample to the laboratory immediately.

Reference values

Normal plasma vitamin C levels range from 0.6 to 2 mg/dl.

Abnormal findings

Values less than 0.3 mg/dl indicate significant deficiency. Vitamin C levels diminish during pregnancy to a low point immediately postpartum. Depressed levels occur with infection, fever, and anemia. Severe deficiencies result in scurvy.

High plasma levels can indicate increased ingestion of vitamin C. Excess vitamin C is converted to oxalate, which is excreted in the urine. Excessive concentration of oxalate can produce urinary calculi.

Interfering factors
● Failure to observe pretest restrictions
● Hemolysis due to rough handling of the sample
● Failure to promptly send the sample to the laboratory
● Tetracycline (possible decrease in leukocyte absorbate and increase in urinary loss of vitamin C)

VITAMIN D$_3$

Vitamin D$_3$ (cholecalciferol), the major form of vitamin D, is endogenously produced in the skin by the sun's ultraviolet rays and occurs naturally in fish liver oils, egg yolks, liver, and butter.

This test, a competitive protein binding assay, determines serum levels of 25-hydroxycholecalciferol after chromatography has separated it from other vitamin D metabolites and contaminants. It's commonly combined with measurement of serum calcium and alkaline phosphatase levels.

Purpose
● To evaluate skeletal disease, such as rickets and osteomalacia
● To aid diagnosis of hypercalcemia
● To detect vitamin D toxicity
● To monitor therapy with vitamin D$_3$

Patient preparation
● Explain to the patient that this test measures vitamin D in the body.

● Tell the patient that he needn't restrict food or fluids.
● Inform him that the test requires a blood sample. Tell him who will perform the venipuncture and when.
● Reassure him that although he may feel discomfort from the needle and the tourniquet, collecting the sample takes less than 3 minutes.
● Check for drugs that alter test results (corticosteroids or anticonvulsants). If they must be continued, note this on the laboratory slip.

Procedure and posttest care
● Perform a venipuncture, and collect the sample in a 7-ml *royal-blue-top* tube.
● If a hematoma develops at the venipuncture site, apply warm soaks.

Precautions
● Handle the sample carefully to prevent hemolysis.

Reference values
In summer, the range for serum 25-hydroxycholecalciferol values is from 15 to 80 ng/ml; in winter, it's 14 to 42 ng/ml.

Abnormal findings
Low or undetectable levels may result from vitamin D deficiency, which can cause rickets or osteomalacia. Such deficiency may stem from poor diet, decreased exposure to the sun, or impaired absorption of vitamin D (secondary to hepatobiliary disease, pancreatitis, celiac disease, cystic fibrosis, or gastric or small-bowel resection). Low levels may also be related to various hepatic diseases that directly affect vitamin D metabolism.

Elevated levels (> 100 ng/ml) may indicate toxicity due to excessive self-medication or prolonged therapy.

Elevated levels associated with hypercalcemia may be due to hypersensitivity to vitamin D, as in sarcoidosis.

Interfering factors
• Hemolysis due to rough handling of the sample
• Anticonvulsants, isoniazid, mineral oil, corticosteroids, aluminum hydroxide, cholestyramine, and colestipol (possible decrease)

FOLIC ACID

The folic acid test is a quantitative analysis of serum levels of folic acid (also called pteroylglutamic acid, folacin, or folate) by radioisotopic assay of competitive binding. It's often performed concomitantly with measurement of serum vitamin B_{12} levels. Like vitamin B_{12}, folic acid is a water-soluble vitamin that influences hematopoiesis, deoxyribonucleic acid synthesis, and overall body growth.

Normally, diet supplies folic acid in liver, kidney, yeast, fruits, leafy vegetables, eggs, and milk. Inadequate dietary intake may cause a deficiency, especially during pregnancy. Because of folic acid's vital role in hematopoiesis, the usual indication for this test is a suspected hematologic abnormality.

Purpose
• To aid differential diagnosis of megaloblastic anemia, which may result from deficiency of folic acid or vitamin B_{12}
• To assess folate stores in pregnancy

Patient preparation
• Explain to the patient that this test determines the folic acid level in the blood.
• Instruct him to observe an overnight fast before the test.
• Tell him that the test requires a blood sample. Explain who will perform the venipuncture and when.
• Reassure him that although he may experience some discomfort from the needle puncture and the pressure of the tourniquet, collecting the sample takes only a few minutes.
• Check the patient's medication history for drugs that may affect test results, such as phenytoin or pyrimethamine.

Procedure and posttest care
• Perform a venipuncture, and collect the sample in a 7-ml *royal-blue-top* tube.
• If a hematoma develops at the venipuncture site, apply warm soaks.
• Remove diet restrictions.

Precautions
• Handle the sample gently to prevent hemolysis.
• Protect it from light.
• Send the sample to the laboratory immediately.

Reference values
Normally, serum folic acid values are greater than or equal to 3.5 µg/L.

Abnormal findings
Low serum levels may indicate hematologic abnormalities, such as anemia (especially megaloblastic anemia), leukopenia, and thrombocytopenia. The Schilling test is often performed to rule out vitamin B_{12} deficiency, which also causes megaloblastic anemia. Decreased folic acid levels can also result from hypermetabolic states (such as

hyperthyroidism), inadequate dietary intake, small-bowel malabsorption syndrome, chronic alcoholism, or pregnancy.

Serum levels greater than normal may indicate excessive dietary intake of folic acid or folic acid supplements. Even when taken in large doses, this vitamin is nontoxic.

Interfering factors
● Hemolysis due to rough handling of the sample
● Sample deterioration caused by exposure to light (possible decrease)
● Alcohol, phenytoin, pyrimethamine, anticonvulsants such as primidone, antineoplastics, antimalarials, and oral contraceptives (possible decrease)

TRACE ELEMENTS

MANGANESE

The manganese test, an analysis by atomic absorption spectroscopy, measures serum levels of manganese, a trace element. Although its function is only partially understood, manganese is known to activate several enzymes — including cholinesterase and arginase — that are essential to metabolism. Dietary sources of manganese include unrefined cereals, green leafy vegetables, and nuts.

Manganese toxicity may result from the inhalation of manganese dust or fumes — a hazard in the steel and dry-cell battery industries — or from ingestion of contaminated water.

Purpose
● To detect manganese toxicity

Patient preparation
● Explain to the patient that this test determines the level of manganese in the blood.
● Inform him that he needn't restrict food or fluids.
● Tell him that this test requires a blood sample. Explain who will perform the venipuncture and when.
● Reassure him that although he may feel some transient discomfort from the needle puncture and the pressure of the tourniquet, collecting the sample takes only a few minutes.
● Check patient history for use of medications that may influence serum manganese levels, such as estrogens and glucocorticoids.

Procedure and posttest care
● Perform a venipuncture, and collect the sample in a metal-free collection tube. Laboratories will supply a special kit for this test on request.
● If a hematoma develops at the venipuncture site, apply warm soaks.

Precautions
● Handle the sample gently to prevent hemolysis, and send it to the laboratory immediately.

Reference values
Normally, serum manganese values range from 0.4 to 0.85 ng/ml.

Abnormal findings
Significantly elevated serum levels indicate manganese toxicity, which requires prompt medical attention to prevent central nervous system deterioration. Depressed serum manganese levels may indicate deficient dietary

intake, although deficiency hasn't been linked to disease.

Interfering factors
- Failure to use metal-free collection tube
- Hemolysis due to rough handling of the sample
- High dietary intake of calcium and phosphorus (possible decrease due to interference with intestinal absorption of manganese)
- Estrogen (increase)
- Glucocorticoids (increase or decrease due to altered distribution of manganese in the body)

ZINC

The zinc test, an analysis by atomic absorption spectroscopy, measures serum levels of zinc. An important trace element, zinc is an integral component of more than 80 enzymes and proteins, and plays a critical role in enzyme catalytic reactions.

Zinc occurs naturally in water and in most foods; high concentrations are found in meat, seafood, dairy products, whole grains, nuts, and legumes. Zinc deficiency can seriously impair body metabolism, growth, and development.

Purpose
- To detect zinc deficiency or toxicity

Patient preparation
- Explain to the patient that this test determines the concentration of zinc in the blood.
- Inform him that he needn't restrict food or fluids.
- Tell him that the test requires a blood sample. Explain who will perform the venipuncture and when.

- Reassure him that although he may feel some discomfort from the needle and the pressure of the tourniquet, collecting the sample takes only a few minutes.

Procedure and posttest care
- Perform a venipuncture, and collect a 3-ml sample in a zinc-free collection tube.
- If a hematoma develops at the venipuncture site, apply warm soaks.

Precautions
- Handle the sample gently to prevent hemolysis, and send it to the laboratory immediately. Reliable analysis must begin before platelet disintegration can alter test results.

Reference values
Normally, plasma zinc values range from 0.66 to 1.10 µg/ml.

Abnormal findings
Decreased serum zinc levels may indicate an acquired deficiency (from insufficient dietary intake or due to an underlying disease) or a hereditary deficiency. Markedly depressed levels are common in leukemia and may be related to impaired zinc-dependent enzyme systems. Low serum zinc levels are commonly associated with alcoholic cirrhosis of the liver, myocardial infarction, ileitis, chronic renal failure, rheumatoid arthritis, and anemia (such as hemolytic or sickle cell anemia).

Elevated and potentially toxic serum zinc levels may result from accidental ingestion or industrial exposure.

Interfering factors
- Failure to use metal-free collection tube
- Hemolysis due to rough handling of the sample
- Delayed transport to laboratory

- Time of day and time of last meal (possible increase or decrease)
- Zinc-chelating agents, such as penicillinase, and corticosteroids (decrease)
- Estrogens, penicillamine, antineoplastics such as cisplatin, antimetabolites, and diuretics (possible decrease)

CHAPTER 5

Immunologic Tests

IMMUNOHEMATOLOGY · 255

255 ABO blood typing
256 Rh typing
257 Fetal-maternal erythrocyte
distribution
258 Crossmatching
260 Direct antiglobulin test
261 Antibody screening test
262 Leukoagglutinin test

GENERAL CELLULAR FUNCTION · 264

264 T- and B-lymphocyte assays
265 Lymphocyte transformation tests
267 Terminal deoxynucleotidyl
transferase test

GENERAL HUMORAL FUNCTION · 269

269 Quantitative immunoglobulins
G, A, and M
271 Immune complex assays
273 Raji cell assay
273 Complement assays
275 Radioallergosorbent test
275 Ham test
276 Human leukocyte antigen test

AUTOANTIBODIES · 277

277 Antinuclear antibodies
279 Extractable nuclear antigen
antibodies
280 Antimitochondrial antibodies
281 Anti-smooth-muscle antibodies
282 Antithyroid antibodies
282 Thyroid-stimulating
immunoglobulin
283 Cardiolipin antibodies
284 Rheumatoid factor
285 Cold agglutinins
286 Cryoglobulins
287 Acetylcholine receptor
antibodies
288 Anti-insulin antibodies
289 Anti-double-stranded DNA
antibodies

VIRUSES · 290

290 Rubella antibodies
291 Hepatitis B surface antigen
292 Heterophil antibody tests
294 Epstein-Barr virus antibodies
296 Respiratory syncytial virus
antibodies
297 Herpes simplex antibodies
298 Cytomegalovirus antibody
screen
299 Human immunodeficiency virus
antibodies
300 Parvovirus B-19 antibodies

BACTERIA AND FUNGI 301

301 Antistreptolysin-O test
302 Febrile agglutination tests
304 Fungal serology
306 *Candida* antibodies

307 Bacterial meningitis antigen
308 Lyme disease serology
309 *H. pylori* antibodies

MISCELLANEOUS TESTS 310

310 VDRL test
311 Fluorescent treponemal antibody absorption test
313 Carcinoembryonic antigen
314 Alpha-fetoprotein

315 TORCH test
316 Tuberculin skin tests

IMMUNO-HEMATOLOGY

ABO BLOOD TYPING

ABO blood typing classifies blood according to the presence of major antigens A and B on red cell surfaces and according to serum antibodies anti-A and anti-B. ABO blood typing using both forward and reverse methods is required before transfusion to prevent a lethal reaction.

In forward typing, the patient's red cells are mixed with anti-A serum, then with anti-B serum; the presence or absence of agglutination determines the blood group. In reverse typing, the results of the forward method are verified by mixing the patient's serum with known group A and group B cells. Blood group determination is confirmed when the results of forward and reverse typing match perfectly.

Purpose
● To establish blood group according to the ABO system
● To check compatibility of donor and recipient blood before transfusion

Patient preparation
● Tell the patient that this test determines his blood group.
● If he's scheduled for a transfusion, explain that once his blood group is known, it can be matched with the right donor blood.
● Inform him that he needn't fast before the test.

● Tell him that the test requires a blood sample and who will perform the venipuncture and when.
● Reassure him that although he may experience transient discomfort from the needle puncture and the tourniquet, collecting the sample takes only a few minutes.
● Check his history for recent administration of blood, dextran, or I.V. contrast media.

Procedure and posttest care
● Perform a venipuncture, and collect the sample in a 10-ml *lavender-top* or *red-top* tube.
● If a hematoma develops at the venipuncture site, apply warm soaks.

Precautions
● Before leaving the patient's bedside or dismissing the patient, label the sample with the patient's name, the hospital or blood bank number, the date, and the phlebotomist's initials.
● Handle the sample gently to prevent hemolysis, and send it to the laboratory immediately with a properly completed laboratory slip.
● The sample must be free from hemolysis due to traumatic phlebotomy.
● If you use a *red-top* tube for sample collection, the sample must be completely clotted before testing begins.
● Before the transfusion, compare current and past ABO typing and crossmatching to detect mistaken identification and prevent transfusion reaction.

Findings
In forward typing, if agglutination occurs when the patient's red cells are mixed with anti-A serum, the A antigen is present and the blood is typed A. If agglutination occurs when the patient's red cells are mixed with anti-B serum, the B antigen is present and the

blood is typed B. If agglutination occurs in both mixes, both A and B antigens are present and the blood is typed AB. If it doesn't occur in either mix, no antigens are present and the blood is typed O.

In reverse typing, if agglutination occurs when B cells are mixed with the patient's serum, anti-B is present and the blood is typed A. If agglutination occurs when A cells are mixed, anti-A is present and the blood is typed B. If agglutination occurs when both A and B cells are mixed, anti-A and anti-B are present and the blood is typed O. If agglutination doesn't occur when both A and B cells are mixed, neither anti-A nor anti-B is present and the blood is typed AB.

CLINICAL ALERT Donor blood may be transfused only when ABO compatibility has been confirmed with the recipient's blood. The transfusion of blood containing either A or B antigens to a recipient whose red cells lack these antigens can cause a potentially fatal reaction.

Interfering factors
• Recent administration of dextran or I.V. contrast media, causing cellular aggregation resembling antibody-mediated agglutination
• Hemolysis due to rough handling of the sample
• Blood transfusion or pregnancy in the past 3 months (possibility of lingering antibodies)

RH TYPING

The Rh system classifies blood by the presence or absence of antigen D, formerly known as Rh_o, on the surface of red blood cells (RBCs). In Rh typing, a patient's RBCs are mixed with serum containing anti-$Rh_o(D)$ antibodies and are observed for agglutination. If agglutination occurs, the $Rh_o(D)$ antigen is present and the patient's blood is typed Rh-positive; if agglutination doesn't occur, the antigen is absent and the patient's blood is typed Rh-negative.

Prospective blood donors are fully tested to exclude the D^u variant, a weak variant of the D antigen, before being classified as having Rh-negative blood. People who have this antigen are considered Rh-positive donors but are generally transfused as Rh-negative recipients.

Purpose
• To establish blood type according to the Rh system
• To help determine the compatibility of donor and recipient before transfusion
• To determine if the patient will require an Rh immune globulin (RhIG) injection

Patient preparation
• Explain to the patient that the test determines or verifies blood group to ensure safe transfusion.
• Inform him that he needn't fast before the test.
• Tell him that the test requires a blood sample and who will perform the venipuncture and when.
• Reassure him that although he may experience transient discomfort from the needle puncture and the tourniquet, collecting the sample takes only a few minutes.
• Check the patient's history for recent administration of dextran, I.V. contrast media, or drugs that may alter results.

Procedure and posttest care
● Perform a venipuncture, and collect the sample in a 10- to 15-ml *lavender-top* or *red-top* tube.
● If a hematoma develops at the venipuncture site, apply warm soaks.
● If necessary, give the pregnant patient a card identifying that she may need to receive RhIG.

Precautions
● Label the sample with the patient's name, the hospital or blood bank number, the date, and the phlebotomist's initials.
● Send it to the laboratory immediately with a properly completed laboratory slip.

Findings
Classified as Rh-positive or Rh-negative, donor blood may be transfused only if it's compatible with the recipient's blood.

If an Rh-negative woman delivers an Rh-positive baby or aborts a fetus whose Rh type is unknown, she should receive an RhIG injection within 72 hours to prevent hemolytic disease of the newborn in future births.

Interfering factors
● Recent administration of dextran or I.V. contrast media (cellular aggregation resembling antibody-mediated agglutination)
● Blood transfusion or pregnancy in the past 3 months (possibility of lingering antibodies)
● Methyldopa, cephalosporins, and levodopa (possible false-positive for the D^u antigen due to positive direct antiglobulin [Coombs'] test)
● Abnormal plasma and protein level or presence of a cold autoagglutinin (possible false-positive)

FETAL-MATERNAL ERYTHROCYTE DISTRIBUTION

Some transfer of red blood cells (RBCs) from the fetal to the maternal circulation occurs during most spontaneous or elective abortions and most normal deliveries. Usually, the amount of blood transferred is minimal and has no clinical significance. But transfer of significant amounts of blood from an Rh-positive fetus to an Rh-negative mother can result in maternal immunization to the D antigen and the development of anti-D antibodies in the maternal circulation.

During a subsequent pregnancy, the maternal immunization subjects an Rh-positive fetus to potentially fatal hemolysis and erythroblastosis. This test measures the number of fetal RBCs in the maternal circulation.

Purpose
● To detect and measure fetal-maternal blood transfer
● To determine the amount of Rh immune globulin (RhIG) needed to prevent maternal immunization to the D antigen

Patient preparation
● Explain to the patient that this test determines the amount of fetal blood transferred to the maternal circulation and helps determine the appropriate treatment, if necessary.
● Inform the patient that she needn't fast before the test.
● Tell her that the test requires a blood sample and who will perform the venipuncture and when.

• Reassure her that although she may experience transient discomfort from the needle and the tourniquet, collecting the sample takes only a few minutes.
• Check the patient's history for recent administration of dextran, I.V. contrast media, or drugs that may alter results.

Procedure and posttest care
• Perform a venipuncture, and collect the sample in a 10-ml *lavender-top* tube.
• If a hematoma develops at the venipuncture site, apply warm soaks.

Precautions
• Label the sample with the patient's name, the hospital or blood bank number, the date, and the phlebotomist's initials.
• Send the sample to the laboratory immediately with a properly completed laboratory slip.

Normal findings
Normal maternal whole blood contains no fetal RBCs.

Abnormal findings
An elevated fetal RBC volume in the maternal circulation necessitates administration of more than one dose of RhIG. The number of vials needed is determined by dividing the calculated fetomaternal hemorrhage by 30 (a single vial of RhIG provides protection against a 30-ml fetomaternal hemorrhage).

Administration of RhIG to an unsensitized Rh-negative mother as soon as possible (no later than 72 hours) after the birth of an Rh-positive infant or after a spontaneous or elective abortion prevents complications in subsequent pregnancies. Most clinicians are now administering RhIG prophylactically at 28 weeks' gestation to women who are Rh-negative but have no detectable Rh antibodies.

The following patients should be screened for Rh isoimmunization or irregular antibodies: all Rh-negative mothers during their first prenatal visit and at 28 weeks' gestation and all Rh-positive mothers with histories of transfusion, a jaundiced infant, stillbirth, cesarean delivery, or induced or spontaneous abortion.

Interfering factor
• Delay of testing for more than 72 hours after sample collection

CROSSMATCHING

Crossmatching (also known as compatibility testing) establishes compatibility or incompatibility of a donor's and a recipient's blood. It's the best antibody detection test available for avoiding lethal transfusion reactions. After the donor's and the recipient's ABO and Rh-factor type are determined, major crossmatching determines compatibility between the donor's red blood cells (RBCs) and the recipient's serum. Minor crossmatching determines compatibility between the donor's serum and the recipient's RBCs. Because the antibody-screening test is routinely performed on all blood donors, minor crossmatching is often omitted.

Because a complete crossmatch may take from 45 minutes to 2 hours, an incomplete (10-minute) crossmatch may be performed in an emergency, such as severe blood loss due to trauma. In an emergency, transfusion can begin with limited amounts of group O packed RBCs while crossmatching is completed. Incomplete typing and crossmatching increase the risk of complications.

After crossmatching, compatible units of blood are labeled and a compatibility record is completed.

⬛ **CLINICAL ALERT** The most carefully performed crossmatch may not detect all the possible sources of patient-donor incompatibility.

Purpose
• To serve as the final check for compatibility between a donor's and a recipient's blood

Patient preparation
• Explain to the patient that this test ensures that the blood he receives matches his own to prevent a transfusion reaction.
• Inform him that he needn't fast before the test.
• Tell him that the test requires a blood sample and who will perform the venipuncture and when.
• Reassure him that although he may experience transient discomfort from the needle puncture and the tourniquet, collecting the sample takes only a few minutes.
• Check the patient's history for recent administration of blood, dextran, or I.V. contrast media.

Procedure and posttest care
• Perform a venipuncture, and collect the sample in a 10-ml *red-top* tube. ABO typing, Rh typing, and crossmatching are all done together.
• If a hematoma develops at the venipuncture site, apply warm soaks.

Precautions
• Handle the sample gently to prevent hemolysis, which can mask hemolysis of the donor's RBCs.
• Label the sample with the patient's name, the hospital or blood bank number, the date, and the phlebotomist's initials.

• Indicate on the laboratory slip the amount and type of blood component needed.
• Send the sample to the laboratory immediately.
• If more than 72 hours have elapsed since an earlier transfusion, previously crossmatched donor blood must be recrossmatched with a new recipient serum sample to detect newly acquired incompatibilities before transfusion.
• If the patient is scheduled for surgery and has received blood during the past 3 months, his blood needs to be crossmatched again if his surgery is rescheduled to detect recently acquired incompatibilities.

Normal findings
Absence of agglutination indicates compatibility between the donor's and the recipient's blood, which means that the transfusion of donor blood can proceed. Note that this doesn't guarantee a safe transfusion.

Abnormal findings
A positive crossmatch indicates incompatibility between the donor's blood and the recipient's blood, which means that the donor's blood can't be transfused to the recipient. The sign of a positive crossmatch is agglutination, or clumping, when the donor's RBCs and the recipient's serum are correctly mixed and incubated. Agglutination indicates an undesirable antigen-antibody reaction. The donor's blood must be withheld and the crossmatch continued to determine the cause of the incompatibility and identify the antibody.

Interfering factors
• Recent administration of dextran or I.V. contrast media (causing cellular aggregation resembling antibody-mediated agglutination)

• Previous blood transfusion (possibility of new antibodies to donor blood)
• Hemolysis due to rough handling of the sample
• Delay of testing for more than 72 hours after sample collection

DIRECT ANTIGLOBULIN TEST

The direct antiglobulin test (or direct Coombs' test) detects immunoglobulins (antibodies) on the surface of red blood cells (RBCs). These immunoglobulins coat RBCs when they become sensitized to an antigen, such as the Rh factor.

In this test, antiglobulin (Coombs') serum added to saline-washed RBCs results in agglutination if immunoglobulins or complement is present. This test is "direct" because it requires only one step — the addition of Coombs' serum to washed cells.

Purpose
• To diagnose hemolytic disease of the newborn (HDN)
• To investigate hemolytic transfusion reactions
• To aid differential diagnosis of hemolytic anemias, which can result from an autoimmune reaction or drugs or be congenital

Patient preparation
• If the patient is a neonate, explain to the parents that this test helps diagnose HDN.
• If the patient is suspected of having hemolytic anemia, explain that the test determines whether the condition results from an abnormality in the body's

immune system, the use of certain drugs, or some unknown cause.
• Inform the adult patient that he need not fast before the test.
• Tell the patient (or a neonate's parents) that the test requires a blood sample and who will collect the blood or perform the venipuncture and when.
• Provide assurance that although the procedure may cause transient discomfort, collecting the sample takes only a few minutes.
• Withhold medications that may interfere with test results, including quinidine, methyldopa, cephalosporins, sulfonamides, chlorpromazine, diphenylhydantoin, ethosuximide, hydralazine, levodopa, mefenamic acid, melphalan, penicillin, procainamide, rifampin, streptomycin, tetracyclines, and isoniazid.

Procedure and posttest care
• For an adult, perform a venipuncture, and collect the sample in two 5-ml *lavender-top* tubes.
• For a neonate, draw 5 ml of cord blood into a *red-top* or *lavender-top* tube after the cord is clamped and cut.
• If a hematoma develops at the venipuncture site, apply warm soaks.
• Resume administration of medications withheld before the test.
• Tell the patient or the parents of the neonate with HDN that further tests will be necessary to monitor anemia.

Precautions
• Handle the sample gently to prevent hemolysis.
• Label the sample with the patient's full name, the hospital or blood bank number, the date, and the phlebotomist's initials.
• Send the sample to the laboratory immediately.

Normal findings

A negative test, in which neither antibodies nor complement appears on the RBCs, is normal.

Abnormal findings

A positive test on umbilical cord blood indicates that maternal antibodies have crossed the placenta and coated fetal RBCs, causing HDN. Transfusion of compatible blood lacking the antigens to these maternal antibodies may be necessary to prevent anemia.

In other patients, a positive test result may indicate hemolytic anemia and help differentiate between autoimmune and secondary hemolytic anemia, which can be drug-induced or associated with an underlying disease. A positive test can also indicate sepsis.

A weakly positive test may suggest a transfusion reaction in which the patient's antibodies react with transfused RBCs containing the corresponding antigen.

Interfering factors

● Hemolysis due to rough handling of the sample
● Quinidine, methyldopa, cephalosporins, sulfonamides, chlorpromazine, diphenylhydantoin, ethosuximide, hydralazine, levodopa, mefenamic acid, melphalan, penicillin, procainamide, rifampin, streptomycin, tetracyclines, and isoniazid (positive test results, possibly due to immune hemolysis)

ANTIBODY SCREENING TEST

Also called the indirect Coombs' test, the antibody screening test detects unexpected circulating antibodies in the patient's serum. After incubating the serum with group O red cells, which are unaffected by anti-A or anti-B antibodies, an antiglobulin (Coombs') serum is added. Agglutination occurs if the patient's serum contains an antibody to one or more antigens on the red cells.

The antibody screening test detects 95% to 99% of the circulating antibodies. After this screening procedure detects them, the antibody identification test can determine the specific identity of the antibodies present.

Purpose

● To detect unexpected circulating antibodies to red cell antigens in the recipient's or donor's serum before transfusion
● To determine the presence of anti-D antibody in maternal blood
● To evaluate the need for Rh immune globulin administration
● To aid diagnosis of acquired hemolytic anemia

Patient preparation

● Explain to the prospective blood recipient that the antibody screening test helps evaluate the possibility of a transfusion reaction.
● If the test is being performed because the patient is anemic, explain to him that it helps identify the specific type of anemia.
● Inform the patient that he needn't fast before the test.
● Tell him that the test requires a blood sample and who will perform the venipuncture and when.
● Reassure him that although he may experience discomfort from the needle puncture and the tourniquet, collecting the sample takes only a few minutes.
● Check the patient's history for recent administration of blood, dextran, or I.V. contrast media.

Procedure and posttest care
• Perform a venipuncture, and collect the sample in a 10-ml *red-top* or *lavender-top* tube. Some laboratories require 20 ml of clotted blood to perform this test.
• If a hematoma develops at the venipuncture site, apply warm soaks.

Precautions
• Handle the sample gently to prevent hemolysis.
• Label the sample with the patient's name, the hospital or blood bank number, the date, and the phlebotomist's initials. Be sure to include on the laboratory slip the patient's diagnosis and pregnancy status, any history of transfusions, and any current drug therapy.
• Send the sample to the laboratory immediately.

Normal findings
Normally, agglutination does not occur, indicating that the patient's serum contains no circulating antibodies other than anti-A or anti-B.

Abnormal findings
A positive result indicates the presence of unexpected circulating antibodies to red cell antigens. Such a reaction demonstrates donor and recipient incompatibility.

A positive result in a pregnant patient with Rh-negative blood may indicate the presence of antibodies to the Rh factor from an earlier transfusion with incompatible blood or from a previous pregnancy with an Rh-positive fetus.

A positive result indicates that the fetus may develop hemolytic disease of the newborn. As a result, repeated testing throughout the pregnancy is necessary to evaluate progressive development of circulating antibody levels.

Interfering factors
• Previous administration of dextran or I.V. contrast media (causing aggregation resembling agglutination)
• Hemolysis due to rough handling of the sample
• Blood transfusion or pregnancy within the past 3 months (possible presence of antibodies)

LEUKOAGGLUTININ TEST

This test detects leukoagglutinins — antibodies that react with white blood cells (WBCs) and may cause a transfusion reaction. These antibodies usually develop after exposure to foreign WBCs through transfusions, pregnancies, and allografts.

If a blood recipient has these antibodies, a febrile nonhemolytic reaction may occur 1 to 4 hours after the start of whole blood, red blood cell, platelet, or granulocyte transfusion. This nonhemolytic reaction (marked by fever and severe chills, sometimes with nausea, headache, and transient hypertension) must be distinguished from a true hemolytic reaction before further transfusion can proceed.

CLINICAL ALERT The presence of these antibodies in a recipient can cause immune-mediated platelet refractoriness, a condition characterized by failure of the platelet count to increase after platelet transfusion.

The technique used to detect leukoagglutinins is the microlymphocytotoxicity test. In this test, the recipient serum is tested against donor lymphocytes or against a panel of lymphocytes of known HLA phenotype. The antibodies in the recipient serum bind to the corresponding antigen present in the lymphocytes and cause cell membrane injury when the complement is added to the test system. Cell injury is detected by examining the lymphocytes under a microscope. If the lymphocytes don't absorb the added dye, the test is negative. If the lymphocytes show dye uptake, the test is positive.

Purpose
• To detect leukoagglutinins in blood recipients who develop transfusion reactions, thus differentiating between hemolytic and febrile nonhemolytic transfusion reactions
• To detect leukoagglutinins in blood donors after transfusion of donor blood causes a reaction

Patient preparation
• Explain to the patient that this test helps determine the cause of his transfusion reaction.
• Tell him that the test requires a blood sample and who will perform the venipuncture and when.
• Reassure him that although he may experience transient discomfort from the needle puncture and the tourniquet, collecting the sample takes only a few minutes.
• Check the patient's history for recent administration of blood, dextran, or I.V. contrast media.

Procedure and posttest care
• Perform a venipuncture, and collect a sample in a 10-ml *red-top* tube. The laboratory requires 3 to 4 ml of serum for testing.
• If a hematoma develops at the venipuncture site, apply warm soaks.
• If a transfusion recipient has a positive leukoagglutinin test, continued transfusions require premedication with acetaminophen 1 to 2 hours before the transfusion, specially prepared leukocyte-poor blood, or use of leukocyte removal blood filters to prevent further reactions.

Precautions
• Label the sample with the patient's name, the hospital or blood bank number, the date, and the phlebotomist's initials.
• Be sure to include on the laboratory slip the patient's suspected diagnosis and pregnancy status, any history of blood transfusions, and current drug therapy.
• Note that tests for these antibodies aren't useful in deciding which patients should receive leukocyte-poor blood components; the decision must be based on clinical experience.

Normal findings
Normally, test results are negative: Agglutination doesn't occur because the serum contains no antibodies.

Abnormal findings
A positive result in a transfusion recipient indicates the presence of leukoagglutinins in his blood, identifying his transfusion reaction as a febrile nonhemolytic reaction to these antibodies.

A positive result in a donor indicates the presence of leukoagglutinins in his blood, identifying the cause of a recipient's reaction as an acute, noncardiogenic pulmonary edema.

If a patient is determined to have antibodies or develops the immune-mediated destruction of transfused platelets, he may require special matched blood products for subsequent transfusions.

Interfering factor
• Previous administration of blood, dextran, or I.V. contrast media (causing aggregation resembling agglutination)

GENERAL CELLULAR FUNCTION

T- AND B-LYMPHOCYTE ASSAYS

Lymphocytes — key cells in the immune system — have the capacity to recognize antigens through special receptors found on their surfaces.

Cell separation is used to isolate lymphocytes from other cellular blood elements. This procedure recovers about 80% of the lymphocytes but doesn't differentiate between T cells and B cells. The percentage of T cells and B cells is determined by attaching a label or marker and using different identification techniques.

Null cells possess Fc receptors but no other detectable surface markers and have no diagnostic significance. The number of null cells is usually determined by subtracting the sum of T cells and B cells from total lymphocytes.

Purpose
• To aid diagnosis of primary and secondary immunodeficiency diseases
• To distinguish benign from malignant lymphocytic proliferative diseases
• To monitor response to therapy

Patient preparation
• Explain to the patient that this test measures certain white blood cells.
• Tell him that the test requires a blood sample and who will perform the venipuncture and when.
• Reassure him that although he may experience transient discomfort from

the needle puncture and the pressure of the tourniquet, collecting the sample takes less than 3 minutes.

Procedure and posttest care
• Perform a venipuncture, and collect the sample in a 7-ml *green-top* tube.
• Because many patients with T-cell and B-cell changes have a compromised immune system, keep the venipuncture site clean and dry.
• If a hematoma develops at the venipuncture site, apply warm soaks.

Precautions
• Completely fill the collection tube, and invert it gently several times to adequately mix the sample and anticoagulant.
• Send the sample to the laboratory immediately to ensure viable lymphocytes.
• If antilymphocyte antibodies are suspected, as in autoimmune disease, notify the laboratory.

Reference values
T-cell and B-cell assays are being standardized, and values may differ from one laboratory to another, depending on test technique.
• Percentage of total lymphocytes:
– T cells: 53% to 88%
– B cells: 5% to 20%.
• Total lymphocyte count: 1,500 to 3,000/µl
• T-cell count: 812 to 2,318 cells/µl
• B-cell count: 99 to 426 cells/µl
These counts are higher in children.

Normal T-cell and B-cell counts don't necessarily ensure a competent immune system. In autoimmune diseases, such as systemic lupus erythematosus and rheumatoid arthritis, T cells and B cells, although present in normal numbers, may not be functionally competent.

Abnormal findings

An abnormal T-cell or B-cell count suggests but doesn't confirm specific diseases. The B-cell count is elevated in chronic lymphocytic leukemia, multiple myeloma, Waldenström's macroglobulinemia, and DiGeorge's syndrome.

B cells decrease in acute lymphocytic leukemia and in certain congenital or acquired immunoglobulin deficiency diseases. In other immunoglobulin deficiency diseases, especially if only one immunoglobulin class is deficient, the B-cell count remains normal.

The T-cell count rises occasionally in infectious mononucleosis; it rises more often in multiple myeloma and acute lymphocytic leukemia.

The T-cell count decreases in congenital T-cell deficiency diseases, such as DiGeorge's, Nezelof's, and Wiskott-Aldrich syndromes, and in certain B-cell proliferative disorders, such as chronic lymphocytic leukemia, Waldenström's macroglobulinemia, and acquired immunodeficiency syndrome.

Interfering factors

• Failure to use the proper collection tube
• Failure to adequately mix the sample and the anticoagulant
• Failure to send the sample to the laboratory immediately
• Changes in health status, such as from stress, surgery, chemotherapy, steroid or immunosuppressive therapy, or X-rays (possible rapid change in T- and B-cell counts)
• Immunoglobulins, such as autologous antilymphocyte antibodies that sometimes occur in autoimmune disease (possible change in results)

LYMPHOCYTE TRANSFORMATION TESTS

Transformation tests evaluate lymphocyte competency without injection of antigens into the patient's skin. These in vitro tests eliminate the risk of adverse effects but can still accurately assess the ability of lymphocytes to proliferate and to recognize and respond to antigens.

The mitogen assay evaluates the mitotic response of T lymphocytes and B lymphocytes to a foreign antigen. The antigen assay uses specific substances, such as purified protein derivative, *Candida*, mumps, tetanus toxoid, and streptokinase, to stimulate lymphocyte transformation. The mixed lymphocyte culture (MLC) assay is useful in matching transplant recipients and donors and in testing immunocompetence. (See *Lymphocyte marker assays,* page 266.)

Purpose

• To assess and monitor genetic and acquired immunodeficiency states
• To provide histocompatibility typing of both tissue transplant recipients and donors
• To detect if a patient has been exposed to various pathogens, such as those that cause malaria, hepatitis, and mycoplasmal pneumonia

Patient preparation

• Explain to the patient that this test evaluates lymphocyte function, which is crucial to the immune system.
• If appropriate, inform him that the test monitors his response to therapy.

LYMPHOCYTE MARKER ASSAYS

A normal immune response requires a balance between the regulatory activities of several interacting cell types, most notably T-helper and T-suppressor cells. By using highly specific monoclonal antibodies, levels of lymphocyte differentiation can be defined and both normal and malignant cell populations can be analyzed. Direct and indirect immunofluorescence, microcytotoxicity, and immunoperoxidase immunoassay techniques are used most frequently: They use an anticoagulated blood sample combined with monoclonal antibodies that react with specific T- and B-cell markers. The chart below lists some commonly ordered lymphocyte marker assays and their indications.

LYMPHOCYTE MARKER ASSAY	PURPOSE
Pan T-cell marker (CD3)	• To measure mature T cells in immune dysfunction
T-helper/inducer subset marker (CD4)	• To identify and characterize the proportion of T-helper cells in autoimmune or immunoregulatory disorders • To detect immunodeficiency disorders, such as acquired immunodeficiency syndrome • To differentiate T-cell acute lymphoblastic leukemia from T-cell lymphomas and other lymphoproliferative disorders
T-suppressor/cytotoxic subset marker (CD8)	• To identify and characterize the proportion of T-suppressor cells in autoimmune and immunoregulatory disorders
T-cell/E-Rosette receptor (CD2)	• To differentiate lymphoproliferative disorders of T-cell origin, such as T-cell lymphocytic leukemia and lymphoblastic lymphoma, from those of non-T-cell origin
Pan-B (B-1) marker (CD20)	• To differentiate lymphoproliferative disorders of B-cell origin, such as B-cell chronic lymphocytic leukemia, from those of T-cell origin
Pan-B (BA-1) marker (CD19)	• To identify B-cell lymphoproliferative disorders, such as B-cell chronic lymphocytic leukemia
CALLA (common acute lymphocytic leukemia antigen) marker	• To identify bone marrow regeneration • To identify non-T-cell acute lymphocytic leukemia
Lymphocyte subset panel (B, pan-T, T-helper/inducer, T-suppressor/cytotoxic, and T-helper/T-suppressor ratio)	• To evaluate immunodeficiencies • To identify immunoregulation associated with autoimmune disorders • To characterize lymphoid neoplasms
Lymphocytic leukemia marker panel (T-cell markers [E-Rosette receptor and Leu-9], B-cell markers [B-1 and BA-1], and CALLA)	• To characterize lymphocytic leukemias as T, B, non-T, or non-B, regardless of the stage of differentiation of the malignant cells

• For histocompatibility typing, explain that this test helps determine the best match for a transplant.

• Advise the patient that he needn't restrict food or fluids.

• Tell the patient that the test requires a blood sample and who will perform the venipuncture and when.

• Reassure the patient that although he may experience transient discomfort from the needle puncture and the tourniquet, collecting the sample takes less than 3 minutes.

• If a radioisotope scan is scheduled, be sure the serum sample for this test is drawn first.

Procedure and posttest care

• Perform a venipuncture. If the patient is an adult, collect the sample in a 7-ml *green-top* (heparinized) tube; for a child, use a 5-ml *green-top* tube.

• Because many of these patients may have a compromised immune system, take special care to keep the venipuncture site clean and dry.

• If a hematoma develops at the venipuncture site, apply warm soaks.

Precautions

• Completely fill the collection tube, and invert it gently several times to mix the sample and anticoagulant.

• Send the sample to the laboratory immediately.

Reference values

Results depend on the mitogens used. Reference ranges accompany test results.

Abnormal findings

In the mitogen and antigen assays, a low stimulation index or unresponsiveness indicates a depressed or defective immune system. Serial testing can be performed to monitor the effectiveness

of therapy in a patient with an immunodeficiency disease.

In the MLC test, the stimulation index is a measure of compatibility. A high index indicates poor compatibility. Conversely, a low stimulation index indicates good compatibility.

A high stimulation index, in response to the relevant pathogen, can also demonstrate exposure to malaria, hepatitis, mycoplasmal pneumonia, periodontal disease, and certain viral infections in patients who no longer have detectable serum antibodies.

Interfering factors

• Pregnancy or use of oral contraceptives, depressing lymphocyte response to phytohemagglutinin (low stimulation index)

• Chemotherapy (unless pretherapy baseline values are available for comparison)

• Radioisotope scan within 1 week before the test

• Failure to send the sample to the laboratory immediately

TERMINAL DEOXYNUCLEOTIDYL TRANSFERASE TEST

Using indirect immunofluorescence, this test measures levels of terminal deoxynucleotidyl transferase (TdT). The TdT test differentiates certain types of leukemias and lymphomas marked by primitive cells that can't be identified by histology alone.

Purpose

• To help differentiate acute lymphocytic leukemia (ALL) from acute nonlymphocytic leukemia

• To help differentiate lymphoblastic lymphomas from malignant lymphomas

• To monitor response to therapy, help determine the patient's prognosis, or obtain early diagnosis of a relapse

Patient preparation

• Explain to the patient that this test detects an enzyme that can help classify tissue origin.

If the patient is scheduled for a blood test, prepare him in the following way:

• Tell him to fast for 12 to 14 hours before the test.

• Tell him that the test requires a blood sample and who will perform the venipuncture and when.

• Reassure the patient that although he may experience transient discomfort from the needle puncture and the tourniquet, collecting the sample takes less than 3 minutes.

If the patient is scheduled for bone marrow aspiration, prepare him in the following way:

• Describe the procedure to him and answer any questions.

• Inform the patient that he needn't restrict food or fluids before the test.

• Tell him who will perform the biopsy and where and that it usually takes only 5 to 10 minutes.

• Make sure the patient or a responsible family member has signed an informed consent form.

• Administer a mild sedative 1 hour before the test.

• Check the patient's history for hypersensitivity to the local anesthetic.

• After checking with the doctor, tell the patient which bone will be the biopsy site.

• Inform him that he'll receive a local anesthetic but will feel pressure on insertion of the biopsy needle and a brief, pulling pain when the marrow is withdrawn.

Procedure and posttest care

• If a blood test is scheduled, perform a venipuncture, and collect the sample in one 10-ml heparinized blood tube and one *lavender-top* tube.

• If assisting with bone marrow aspiration, inject 1 ml of bone marrow into a 7-ml *green-top* tube and dilute it with 5 ml of normal saline solution, or submit four air-dried marrow smears.

• Send the sample to the laboratory immediately.

• Because patients with leukemia may bleed excessively, apply pressure to the venipuncture site until bleeding stops.

• If a hematoma develops at the venipuncture site, apply warm soaks.

• Check the bone marrow aspiration site for bleeding and inflammation, and observe the patient for signs of hemorrhage and infection.

Precautions

• Before performing the venipuncture, contact the laboratory to ensure that it can process the sample and to find out how much blood to draw.

• Because patients with leukemia are more susceptible to infection, clean the skin thoroughly before performing the venipuncture.

Reference values

TdT is present in less than 2% of marrow cells and is undetectable in normal peripheral blood.

Abnormal findings

Positive cells are present in more than 90% of patients with ALL, in 33% of patients with chronic myelogenous leukemia in blast crisis, and in 5% of patients with nonlymphocytic leukemias. TdT-positive cells are absent in patients with ALL who are in remission.

Interfering factors

- Failure to obtain a representative sample during bone marrow aspiration
- Performing bone marrow aspiration on a child because of presence of TdT-positive bone marrow in children during proliferation of prelymphocytes (possible false-positive)
- Bone marrow regeneration, idiopathic thrombocytopenic purpura, and neuroblastoma, causing TdT-positive bone marrow (possible false-positive)
- Failure to send the sample to the laboratory immediately

GENERAL HUMORAL FUNCTION

QUANTITATIVE IMMUNOGLOBULINS G, A, AND M

Immunoglobulins, proteins that can function as specific antibodies in response to antigen stimulation, are responsible for the humoral aspects of immunity. Deviations from normal immunoglobulin percentages are characteristic in many immune disorders, including cancer, hepatic disorders, rheumatoid arthritis, and systemic lupus erythematosus.

Immunoelectrophoresis identifies immunoglobulin G (IgG), immunoglobulin A (IgA), and immunoglobulin M (IgM) in a serum sample; the level of each is measured by radial immunodiffusion or nephelometry. Some laboratories detect immunoglobulin by indirect immunofluorescence and radioimmunoassay.

Purpose

- To diagnose paraproteinemias, such as multiple myeloma and Waldenström's macroglobulinemia
- To detect hypogammaglobulinemia and hypergammaglobulinemia as well as nonimmunologic diseases, such as cirrhosis and hepatitis, that are associated with abnormally high immunoglobulin levels
- To assess the effectiveness of chemotherapy and radiation therapy

Patient preparation

- Explain to the patient that this test measures antibody levels.
- If appropriate, tell the patient that the test evaluates the effectiveness of treatment.
- Instruct him to restrict food and fluids, except for water, for 12 to 14 hours before the test.
- Tell him that the test requires a blood sample and who will perform the venipuncture and when.
- Reassure him that although he may experience transient discomfort from the needle puncture and the tourniquet, collecting the sample takes less than 3 minutes.
- Check the patient's medication history, and withhold drugs that may affect test results, including phenytoin and other anticonvulsants, asparaginase, hydralazine, hydantoin derivatives, oral contraceptives, phenylbutazone, dextran, methotrexate, methylprednisolone, prednisolone, and methadone. If these medications must be continued, note this on the laboratory slip.
- Be aware that alcohol or narcotic abuse may affect results.
- Note that patients with severe hypersensitivity to bacille Calmette-Guérin (BCG) vaccine may have altered test results.

Serum Immunoglobulin Levels in Various Disorders

DISORDER	IgG	IgA	IgM
Immunoglobulin disorders			
Lymphoid aplasia	D	D	D
Agammaglobulinemia	D	D	D
Type I dysgammaglobulinemia (selective IgG and IgA deficiency)	D	D	N or I
Type II dysgammaglobulinemia (absent IgA and IgM)	N	D	D
IgA globulinemia	N	D	N
Ataxia-telangiectasia	N	D	N
Multiple myeloma, macroglobulinemia, lymphomas			
Heavy chain disease (Franklin's disease)	D	D	D
IgG myeloma	I	D	D
IgA myeloma	D	I	D
Macroglobulinemia	D	D	I
Acute lymphocytic leukemia	N	D	N
Chronic lymphocytic leukemia	D	D	D
Acute myelocytic leukemia	N	N	N
Chronic myelocytic leukemia	N	D	N
Hodgkin's disease	N	N	N
Hepatic disorders			
Hepatitis	I	I	I
Laënnec's cirrhosis	I	I	N
Biliary cirrhosis	N	N	I
Hepatoma	N	N	D
Other disorders			
Rheumatoid arthritis	I	I	I
Systemic lupus erythematosus	I	I	I
Nephrotic syndrome	D	D	N
Trypanosomiasis	N	N	I
Pulmonary tuberculosis	I	N	N

KEY: N = normal; I = increased; D = decreased.

Procedure and posttest care

• Perform a venipuncture, and collect the sample in a 7-ml *red-top* tube.

• Advise the patient with abnormally low immunoglobulin levels (especially of IgG or IgM) to protect himself against bacterial infection. When caring for such a patient, watch for signs of infection, such as fever, chills, rash, and skin ulcers.

• Instruct the patient with abnormally high immunoglobulin levels and symptoms of monoclonal gammopathies to report bone pain and tenderness. Such a patient has numerous antibody-producing malignant plasma cells in bone marrow, which hamper production of other blood components. Watch for signs of hypercalcemia, renal failure, and spontaneous pathologic fractures.

• If a hematoma develops at the venipuncture site, apply warm soaks.

• Inform the patient that he may resume his normal diet.

• Resume administration of medications withheld before the test.

Precautions

• Send the sample to the laboratory immediately to prevent deterioration of immunoglobulins.

Reference values

When using nephelometry, serum immunoglobulin levels for adults range as follows:

• IgG: 700 to 1,500 mg/dl
• IgA: 60 to 400 mg/dl
• IgM: 60 to 300 mg/dl.

Abnormal findings

The accompanying chart (*Serum immunoglobulin levels in various disorders*) shows IgG, IgA, and IgM levels in various disorders. In congenital and acquired hypogammaglobulinemias, myelomas, and macroglobulinemia, the findings confirm the diagnosis. In he-

patic and autoimmune diseases, leukemias, and lymphomas, such findings are less important, but they can support the diagnosis based on other tests, such as biopsies and white blood cell differential, and on the physical examination.

Interfering factors

• Radiation therapy or chemotherapy (possible decrease due to suppressive effects on bone marrow)

• Anticonvulsants, asparaginase, hydralazine, hydantoin derivatives, oral contraceptives, and phenylbutazone (possible increase)

• Methotrexate and severe hypersensitivity to BCG vaccine (possible decrease)

• Dextrans and methylprednisolone (decrease in all levels)

• Phenytoin (decrease in IgG and IgA levels)

• Methadone (increase in IgA levels)

• Narcotic abuse (possible increase in IgM levels)

• Failure to send the sample to the laboratory immediately

IMMUNE COMPLEX ASSAYS

When immune complexes are produced faster than they can be cleared by the lymphoreticular system, immune complex disease, such as postinfectious syndromes, serum sickness, drug sensitivity, rheumatoid arthritis, and systemic lupus erythematosus (SLE), may occur.

Histologic examination of tissue obtained by biopsy and the use of fluorescence or peroxidase staining with antibodies specific for immunologic types generally detect immune complexes. However, tissue biopsies can't provide information about titers of complexes still in circulation; therefore, serum assays, which detect circulating immune complexes indirectly, may be required. Because of the inherent variability of these complexes, several serum test methods may be appropriate.

Most immune complex assays haven't been standardized, so more than one test may be required to achieve accurate results.

Purpose
- To demonstrate circulating immune complexes in serum
- To monitor response to therapy
- To estimate severity of disease

Patient preparation
- Explain to the patient that these tests help evaluate his immune system.
- If appropriate, inform him that the test will be repeated to monitor his response to therapy.
- Advise him that he needn't restrict food or fluids before the test.
- Tell him that the test requires a blood sample and who will perform the venipuncture and when.
- Reassure him that although he may experience transient discomfort from the needle puncture and the tourniquet, collecting the sample takes less than 3 minutes.
- If the patient is scheduled for C1q assays, check his history for recent heparin therapy and report such therapy to the laboratory.

Procedure and posttest care
- Perform a venipuncture, and collect the sample in a 7-ml *red-top* tube.
- Because many patients with immune complexes have a compromised immune system, keep the venipuncture site clean and dry.
- If a hematoma develops at the site, apply warm soaks.

Precautions
- Send the sample to the laboratory immediately to prevent deterioration of immune complexes.

Normal findings
Normally, immune complexes aren't detectable in serum.

Abnormal findings
The presence of detectable immune complexes in serum has etiologic importance in many autoimmune diseases, such as SLE and rheumatoid arthritis. For definitive diagnosis, the presence of these complexes must be considered with the results of other studies. For example, in SLE, immune complexes are associated with high titers of antinuclear antibodies and circulating antinative deoxyribonucleic acid antibodies.

Because of their filtering function, renal glomeruli seem most vulnerable to immune complex deposition, although blood vessel walls and choroid plexuses (vascular folds in the ventricles of the brain) can be affected. Renal biopsy to detect immune complexes can provide conclusive evidence for immune complex (type III) glomerulonephritis, differentiating it from other types of glomerulonephritis.

Interfering factors
- Failure to send the sample to the laboratory immediately
- Presence of cryoglobulins in the serum
- Inability to standardize rheumatoid factor inhibition tests and platelet aggregation assays

RAJI CELL ASSAY

This assay, which is performed to detect the presence of circulating immune complexes, studies the Raji lymphoblastoid cell line. Identifying these cells, which have receptors for immunoglobulin G complement, helps to evaluate autoimmune disease.

Purpose
- To detect circulating immune complexes
- To aid the study of autoimmune disease

Patient preparation
- As appropriate, explain to the patient the purpose of the test.
- Tell him that the test requires a blood sample and who will perform the venipuncture and when.
- Reassure him that although he may experience transient discomfort from the needle puncture and the tourniquet, collecting the sample takes less than 3 minutes.

Procedure and posttest care
- Perform a venipuncture, and collect a sample in a *red-top, red-marble-top,* or *green-top* tube. Place the sample on ice and send it to the laboratory for assay.
- If a hematoma develops at the venipuncture site, apply warm soaks.

Precautions
- Handle the sample gently to prevent hemolysis.

Reference values
Normal value is less than 13 mg AHG (antihemophilic globulin) Eq/ml.

Abnormal findings
A positive Raji cell assay can detect immune complexes, including those found in viral, microbial, and parasitic infections; metastasis; autoimmune disorders; and drug reactions. This test may also detect immune complexes associated with celiac disease, cirrhosis, Crohn's disease, cryoglobulinemia, dermatitis herpetiformis, sickle cell anemia, and ulcerative colitis.

Interfering factors
- Hemolysis due to rough handling of the sample
- Recent injection of radioactive contrast medium
- Failure to place the sample on ice

COMPLEMENT ASSAYS

Complement is a collective term for a system of at least 15 serum proteins designed to destroy foreign cells and help remove foreign materials. Complement deficiency can increase susceptibility to infection and predispose to other diseases. Complement assays are indicated in patients with known or suspected immunomediated disease or repeatedly abnormal response to infection. Various laboratory methods are used to evaluate and measure total complement and its components; hemolytic assay, laser nephelometry, and radial immunodiffusion are the most common.

Although complement assays provide valuable information about the patient's immune system, the results must be considered in light of serum immunoglobulin and autoantibody tests for a definitive diagnosis of immunomediated disease or abnormal response to infection.

Purpose
• To help detect immunomediated disease and genetic complement deficiency
• To monitor effectiveness of therapy

Patient preparation
• Explain to the patient that this test measures a group of proteins that fight infection.
• Advise him that he needn't restrict food or fluids.
• Tell him that the test requires a blood sample and who will perform the venipuncture and when.
• Reassure him that although he may experience transient discomfort from the needle puncture and the tourniquet, collecting the sample usually takes less than 3 minutes.
• If the patient is scheduled for C1q assay, check his history for recent heparin therapy. Report such therapy to the laboratory.

Procedure and posttest care
• Perform a venipuncture, and collect the sample in a 7-ml *red-top* tube.
• Because many patients with complement defects have a compromised immune system, keep the venipuncture site clean and dry.
• If a hematoma develops at the venipuncture site, apply warm soaks.

Precautions
• Handle the sample gently to prevent hemolysis.
• Send it to the laboratory immediately because complement is heat labile and deteriorates rapidly.

Reference values
Normal values for complement range as follows:
• total complement: 25 to 110 units
• C1 esterase inhibitor: 8 to 24 mg/dl
• C3: 70 to 150 mg/dl
• C4: 14 to 40 mg/dl

Abnormal findings
Complement abnormalities may be genetic or acquired; acquired abnormalities are most common. Depressed total complement levels (which are clinically more significant than elevations) may result from excessive formation of antigen-antibody complexes, insufficient synthesis of complement, inhibitor formation, or increased complement catabolism and are characteristic in such conditions as systemic lupus erythematosus (SLE), acute poststreptococcal glomerulonephritis, and acute serum sickness. Low levels may also occur in some patients with advanced cirrhosis of the liver, multiple myeloma, hypogammaglobulinemia, or rapidly rejecting allografts.

Elevated total complement may occur in obstructive jaundice, thyroiditis, acute rheumatic fever, rheumatoid arthritis, acute myocardial infarction, ulcerative colitis, and diabetes.

C1 esterase inhibitor deficiency is characteristic in hereditary angioedema, the most common genetic abnormality associated with complement; C3 deficiency is characteristic in recurrent pyogenic infection and disease activation in SLE; C4 deficiency is characteristic in SLE and rheumatoid arthritis. C4 is increased in autoimmune hemolytic anemia.

Interfering factors
• Hemolysis due to rough handling of the sample

• Failure to send the sample to the laboratory immediately

• Recent heparin therapy

RADIOALLERGOSORBENT TEST

The radioallergosorbent test (RAST) measures immunoglobulin E (IgE) antibodies in serum by radioimmunoassay and identifies specific allergens that cause rash, asthma, hay fever, drug reactions, and other atopic complaints. RAST is easier to perform and more specific than skin testing; it's also less painful for and less dangerous to the patient. Careful selection of specific allergens, based on the patient's clinical history, is crucial for effective testing.

Although skin testing is still the preferred means of diagnosing IgE-mediated hypersensitivities, RAST may be more useful when a skin disorder makes accurate reading of skin tests difficult, when a patient requires continual antihistamine therapy, or when skin tests are negative but the patient's clinical history supports IgE-mediated hypersensitivity.

Purpose
• To identify allergens to which the patient has an immediate (IgE-mediated) hypersensitivity
• To monitor the patient's response to therapy

Patient preparation
• Explain to the patient that this test may detect the cause of allergy or monitor the effectiveness of allergy treatment.

• Inform him that he needn't restrict food or fluids.

• Tell him that the test requires a blood sample and who will perform the venipuncture and when.

• Reassure him that although he may experience transient discomfort from the needle puncture and the tourniquet, collecting the sample takes less than 3 minutes.

• If the patient is scheduled for a radioactive scan, make sure the sample is collected before the scan.

Procedure and posttest care
• Perform a venipuncture, and collect the sample in a 7-ml *red-top* tube. Generally, 1 ml of serum is sufficient for five allergen assays.

• Note on the laboratory slip the specific allergens to be tested.

• If a hematoma develops at the venipuncture site, apply warm soaks.

Reference values
RAST results are interpreted in relation to a control or reference serum that differs among laboratories.

Abnormal findings
Elevated serum IgE levels suggest hypersensitivity to the specific allergen or allergens used.

Interfering factor
• Radioactive scan within 1 week before sample collection

HAM TEST

The Ham test, or acidified serum lysis test, is performed to determine the cause of undiagnosed hemolytic anemia, hemoglobinuria, and bone marrow aplasia. This test determines the stability of the red blood cell (RBC) membrane. It helps establish a diagnosis of paroxysmal nocturnal hemoglobinuria (PNH), a rare hematologic disease.

Purpose
• To help establish a diagnosis of PNH
• To determine the cause of undiagnosed hemolytic anemia and bone marrow aplasia

Patient preparation
• Explain to the patient that this test helps determine the cause of his anemia or other signs.
• Advise him that he needn't restrict food or fluids.
• Tell him that the test requires a blood sample and who will perform the venipuncture and when.
• Reassure him that although he may experience transient discomfort from the needle puncture and the tourniquet, collecting the sample takes less than 3 minutes.

Procedure and posttest care
• Because the blood sample must be defibrinated immediately, laboratory personnel perform the venipuncture and collect the sample.
• If a hematoma develops at the venipuncture site, apply warm soaks.

Normal findings
Normally, RBCs don't undergo hemolysis. Test results should be negative.

Abnormal findings
Hemolysis of RBCs indicates PNH.

Interfering factors
• Blood containing large numbers of spherocytes (possible false-positive)
• Blood from patients with congenital dyserythropoietic anemia (false-positive)

HUMAN LEUKOCYTE ANTIGEN TEST

The human leukocyte antigen (HLA) test identifies a group of antigens present on the surface of all nucleated cells but most easily detected on lymphocytes. There are four types of HLA: HLA-A, HLA-B, HLA-C, and HLA-D. These antigens are essential to immunity and to determine the degree of histocompatibility between transplant recipients and donors. Numerous antigenic determinants (more than 60, for instance, at the HLA-B locus) are present for each site; one set of each antigen is inherited from each parent.

A high incidence of specific HLA types has been linked to specific diseases, such as rheumatoid arthritis and multiple sclerosis, but these findings have little diagnostic significance.

Purpose
• To provide histocompatibility typing of transplant recipients and donors
• To aid genetic counseling
• To aid paternity testing

Patient preparation
• Explain to the patient that this test detects antigens on white blood cells.
• Advise him that he needn't restrict food or fluids before the test.
• Tell the patient that this test requires a blood sample and who will perform the venipuncture and when.
• Reassure him that although he may experience transient discomfort from the needle puncture and the tourniquet, collecting the blood sample usually takes less than 3 minutes.
• Check the patient's history for recent blood transfusions. HLA testing may need to be postponed if he has recently undergone a transfusion.

Procedure and posttest care
- Perform a venipuncture, and collect the sample in a tube containing anticoagulant acid citrate dextrose solution.
- If a hematoma develops at the venipuncture site, apply warm soaks.

Precautions
- Handle the sample gently to prevent hemolysis.

Normal findings
In HLA-A, HLA-B, and HLA-C testing, lymphocytes that react with the test antiserum undergo lysis; they're detected by phase microscopy. In HLA-D testing, leukocyte incompatibility is marked by blast formation, deoxyribonucleic acid synthesis, and proliferation.

Abnormal findings
Incompatible HLA-A, HLA-B, HLA-C, and HLA-D groups may cause unsuccessful tissue transplantation.

Many diseases have a strong association with certain types of HLAs. For example, HLA-DR5 is associated with Hashimoto's thyroiditis. B8 and Dw3 are associated with Graves' disease, whereas B8 alone is associated with chronic autoimmune hepatitis, celiac disease, and myasthenia gravis. Dw3 alone is associated with Addison's disease, Sjögren's syndrome, dermatitis herpetiformis, and systemic lupus erythematosus.

In paternity testing, a putative father who presents a phenotype (two haplotypes: one from the father and one from the mother) with no haplotype or antigen pair identical to one of the child's is excluded as the father. A putative father with one haplotype identical to one of the child's may be the father; the probability varies with the incidence of the haplotype in the population.

Interfering factors
- Hemolysis due to rough handling of the sample
- HLA from blood transfusion within 72 hours before sample collection

AUTOANTIBODIES

ANTINUCLEAR ANTIBODIES

In conditions such as systemic lupus erythematosus (SLE), scleroderma, and certain infections, the body's immune system may perceive portions of its own cell nuclei as foreign and may produce antinuclear antibodies (ANAs). Specific ANAs include antibodies to deoxyribonucleic acid (DNA), nucleoprotein, histones, nuclear ribonucleoprotein, and other nuclear constituents.

Because they don't penetrate living cells, ANAs are harmless in themselves but sometimes form antigen-antibody complexes that cause tissue damage (as in SLE). Because of multiorgan involvement, test results aren't diagnostic and can only partially confirm clinical evidence. (See *Comparative incidence of antinuclear antibodies*, page 278.)

Purpose
- To screen for SLE (failure to detect ANAs essentially rules out active SLE)
- To monitor the effectiveness of immunosuppressive therapy for SLE

Patient preparation
- Explain to the patient that this test evaluates the immune system and that

COMPARATIVE INCIDENCE OF ANTINUCLEAR ANTIBODIES

CONDITION	INCIDENCE OF POSITIVE A.N.A. (%)
Systemic lupus erythematosus	95 to 100
Lupoid hepatitis	95 to 100
Progressive systemic sclerosis (scleroderma)	60 to 70
Sjögren's syndrome	50 to 60
Rheumatoid arthritis	25 to 30
Polyarteritis nodosa	10
Dermatomyositis, polymyositis	10 to 50

further testing is usually required for diagnosis.

- If appropriate, inform the patient that the test will be repeated to monitor his response to therapy.
- Advise him that he needn't restrict food or fluids.
- Tell him that the test requires a blood sample and who will perform the venipuncture and when.
- Reassure him that although he may experience discomfort from the puncture and the tourniquet, collecting the sample takes less than 3 minutes.
- Check the patient's history for drugs that may affect test results, such as isoniazid, hydralazine, and procainamide. Note findings on the laboratory slip.

Procedure and posttest care
- Perform a venipuncture, and collect the sample in a 7-ml *red-top* tube.
- Because a patient with an autoimmune disease has a compromised immune system, observe the venipuncture site for signs of infection, and report any changes to the doctor immediately.
- Keep a clean, dry bandage over the site for at least 24 hours.

- If a hematoma develops at the venipuncture site, apply warm soaks.

Reference values
Test results are reported as positive (with pattern and serum titer noted) or negative.

Abnormal findings
Although this test is a sensitive indicator of ANAs, it isn't specific for SLE. Low titers may occur in patients with viral diseases, chronic hepatic disease, collagen vascular disease, and autoimmune diseases and in some healthy adults; the incidence increases with age. The higher the titer, the more specific the test is for SLE (titer often exceeds 1:256).

The pattern of nuclear fluorescence helps identify the type of immune disease present. A peripheral pattern is almost exclusively associated with SLE because it indicates the presence of anti-DNA antibodies; sometimes anti-DNA antibodies are measured by radioimmunoassay if ANA titers are high or a peripheral pattern is observed. A homogeneous, or diffuse, pattern is also associated with SLE as well as with related connective tissue disorders; a nucleolar pattern, with scleroderma; and a speckled, irregular pattern, with infectious mononucleosis and mixed connective tissue disorders (for example, SLE and scleroderma).

A single serum sample, especially one collected from a patient with collagen vascular disease, may contain antibodies to several parts of the cell's nucleus. In addition, as serum dilution increases, the fluorescent pattern may change because different antibodies are reactive at different titers.

Interfering factor

• Most commonly isoniazid, hydralazine, and procainamide but also paraaminosalicylic acid, chlorpromazine, clofibrate, phenytoin, griseofulvin, ethosuximide, gold salts, methyldopa, oral contraceptives, penicillin, propylthiouracil, phenylbutazone, methysergide, streptomycin, sulfonamides, tetracyclines, mephenytoin, quinidine, primidone, reserpine, and trimethadione (possible production of a syndrome resembling SLE)

EXTRACTABLE NUCLEAR ANTIGEN ANTIBODIES

Extractable nuclear antigen (ENA) is a complex of at least four antigens. One of them — ribonucleoprotein (RNP) — is susceptible to degradation by ribonuclease. The second — Smith (Sm) antigen — is an acidic nuclear protein that resists ribonuclease degradation. The third and fourth antigens that are sometimes included in this group — Sjögren's syndrome (SS-A) antigen

and Sjögren's syndrome B (SS-B) antigen — form a precipitate when an antibody is present.

Antibodies to these antigens are associated with certain autoimmune disorders. Tests to detect ENA antibodies help differentiate autoimmune disorders with similar signs and symptoms.

Purpose

• To aid differential diagnosis of autoimmune disease

• To distinguish between anti-RNP and anti-Sm antibodies

• To screen for anti-RNP antibodies (common in systemic lupus erythematosus [SLE], progressive systemic sclerosis, and other rheumatic disorders)

• To screen for anti-Sm antibodies (a specific marker for SLE)

• To detect the SS-A and SS-B antibodies produced in Sjögren's syndrome

• To monitor response to therapy in patients with autoimmune disease

Patient preparation

• Explain to the patient that this test detects certain antibodies and that test results help determine diagnosis and treatment.

• When appropriate, explain that the test assesses the effectiveness of treatment.

• Advise the patient that he needn't restrict food or fluids.

• Tell him that the test requires a blood sample and who will perform the venipuncture and when.

• Reassure him that although he may experience transient discomfort from the needle puncture and the pressure of the tourniquet, collecting the sample takes less than 3 minutes.

Procedure and posttest care

• Perform a venipuncture, and collect the sample in a 7-ml *red-top* tube.

• Because a patient with an autoimmune disease has a compromised immune system, check the venipuncture site for infection, and report any change promptly.

• Keep a clean, dry bandage over the site for at least 24 hours.

• If a hematoma develops at the venipuncture site, apply warm soaks.

Precautions
• Send the sample to the laboratory immediately.

Reference values
Expected values range as follows:
• < 20 units (negative)
• 20 to 25 units (borderline)
• ≥ 26 units (positive).

Abnormal findings
Anti-RNP antibodies are elevated in SLE (35% to 40% of patients) and mixed connective tissue disease. Anti-Sm antibodies are specific for SLE. Anti-SS-A and anti-SS-B antibodies are elevated in Sjögren's syndrome (40% to 45% of patients). Anti-SS-B antibodies are also elevated in SLE.

Interfering factor
• Failure to send the sample to the laboratory immediately

ANTIMITOCHONDRIAL ANTIBODIES

Usually performed with the test for anti-smooth-muscle antibodies, this test detects antimitochondrial antibodies in serum by indirect immunofluorescence. These autoantibodies are present in several hepatic diseases.

Their role in disease pathogenesis is unknown, and there's no evidence that they cause hepatic damage. Most commonly, they're associated with primary biliary cirrhosis and, sometimes, chronic active hepatitis and drug-induced jaundice. Antimitochondrial antibodies are also associated with autoimmune diseases, such as systemic lupus erythematosus, rheumatoid arthritis, pernicious anemia, and idiopathic Addison's disease.

Purpose
• To aid diagnosis of primary biliary cirrhosis
• To distinguish between extrahepatic jaundice and biliary cirrhosis

Patient preparation
• Explain to the patient that this test evaluates liver function.

• Advise the patient that he needn't restrict food or fluids.

• Tell him that the test requires a blood sample and who will perform the venipuncture and when.

• Reassure him that although he may experience transient discomfort from the needle puncture and the tourniquet, collecting the sample takes less than 3 minutes.

• Check the patient's medication history for oxyphenisatin use, and report it to the laboratory because it may produce antimitochondrial antibodies.

Procedure and posttest care
• Perform a venipuncture, and collect the sample in a 7-ml *red-top* tube.

• Because patients with hepatic disease may bleed excessively, apply pressure to the venipuncture site until bleeding stops.

• If a hematoma develops at the venipuncture site, apply warm soaks.

Normal findings

Serum is normally negative for antimitochondrial antibodies. Positive results are titered.

Abnormal findings

Although antimitochondrial antibodies appear in 79% to 94% of patients with primary biliary cirrhosis, this test alone doesn't confirm the diagnosis. Further tests, such as serum alkaline phosphatase, serum bilirubin, aspartate aminotransferase, alanine aminotransferase and, possibly, liver biopsy or cholangiography, may also be necessary. The autoantibodies also appear in some patients with chronic active hepatitis, drug-induced jaundice, and cryptogenic cirrhosis. Antimitochondrial antibodies seldom appear in patients with extrahepatic biliary obstruction, and a positive test helps rule out this condition.

Interfering factors

- Confusion of antimitochondrial antibodies with heterophil antibodies, cardiolipin antibodies to syphilis, ribosomal antibodies, and microsomal hepatic or renal autoantibodies
- Oxyphenisatin (possible false-positive results)

ANTI-SMOOTH-MUSCLE ANTIBODIES

Using indirect immunofluorescence, this test measures the relative concentration of anti-smooth-muscle antibodies in serum; it's usually performed with the test for antimitochondrial antibodies.

Anti-smooth-muscle antibodies appear in several hepatic diseases, especially chronic active hepatitis and, less often, primary biliary cirrhosis. Although anti-smooth-muscle antibodies are most commonly associated with hepatic diseases, their etiologic role is unknown, and there's no evidence that they cause hepatic damage.

Purpose

- To aid diagnosis of active chronic hepatitis and primary biliary cirrhosis

Patient preparation

- Explain to the patient that this test helps evaluate liver function.
- Inform him that he needn't restrict food or fluids.
- Tell him that this test requires a blood sample and who will perform the venipuncture and when.
- Reassure him that although he may experience transient discomfort from the needle puncture and the tourniquet, collecting the blood sample usually takes less than 3 minutes.

Procedure and posttest care

- Perform a venipuncture, and collect the sample in a 7-ml *red-top* tube.
- Because patients with hepatic disease may bleed excessively, apply pressure to the venipuncture site until bleeding stops.
- If a hematoma develops at the venipuncture site, apply warm soaks.

Reference values

A normal titer of anti-smooth-muscle antibodies is negative. Positive results are titered.

Abnormal findings

The test for anti-smooth-muscle antibodies isn't specific; these antibodies appear in a number of patients with chronic active hepatitis and in fewer patients with primary biliary cirrhosis.

Anti-smooth-muscle antibodies may also be present in patients with infectious mononucleosis, acute viral hepatitis, malignant tumor of the liver, and intrinsic asthma.

Interfering factors
• None significant

ANTITHYROID ANTIBODIES

In autoimmune disorders such as Hashimoto's thyroiditis and Graves' disease (hyperthyroidism), thyroglobulin, the major colloidal storage compound, is released into the blood. Antithyroglobulin antibodies are produced to attack this foreign substance; the ensuing autoimmune response damages the thyroid gland.

Purpose
• To detect circulating antithyroglobulin antibodies when clinical evidence indicates Hashimoto's thyroiditis, Graves' disease, or other thyroid diseases

Patient preparation
• Explain to the patient that this test evaluates thyroid function.
• Advise him that he needn't restrict food or fluids.
• Tell him that the test requires a blood sample and who will perform the venipuncture and when.
• Reassure him that although he may experience transient discomfort from the needle puncture and the tourniquet,

collecting the sample takes less than 3 minutes.

Procedure and posttest care
• Perform a venipuncture, and collect the sample in a 7-ml *red-top* tube.
• If a hematoma develops at the venipuncture site, apply warm soaks.

Reference values
The normal titer is less than 1:100 for both antithyroglobulin and antimicrosomal antibodies.

Abnormal findings
The presence of antithyroglobulin or antimicrosomal antibodies in serum can indicate subclinical autoimmune thyroid disease, Graves' disease, or idiopathic myxedema. Titers of 1:400 or more strongly suggest Hashimoto's thyroiditis. Antithyroglobulin antibodies may also occur in some patients with other autoimmune disorders, such as systemic lupus erythematosus, rheumatoid arthritis, and autoimmune hemolytic anemia.

Interfering factors
• None significant

THYROID-STIMULATING IMMUNOGLOBULIN

Thyroid-stimulating immunoglobulin (TSI), formerly called long-acting thyroid stimulator, appears in the blood of most patients with Graves' disease. It stimulates the thyroid gland to produce and excrete excessive amounts of thyroid hormone.

Reportedly, 90% of people with Graves' disease have elevated TSI levels. Positive results of this test strongly suggest Graves' disease, despite normal routine thyroid tests in patients still suspected of having Graves' disease or progressive exophthalmos.

Purpose
- To aid evaluation of suspected thyroid disease
- To aid diagnosis of suspected thyrotoxicosis, especially in patients with exophthalmos
- To monitor treatment of thyrotoxicosis

Patient preparation
- As appropriate, explain to the patient that this test evaluates thyroid function.
- Tell him that the test requires a blood sample and who will perform the venipuncture and when.
- Reassure him that although he may experience transient discomfort from the needle puncture and the pressure of the tourniquet, collecting the sample takes less than 3 minutes.

Procedure and posttest care
- Perform a venipuncture, and collect a 5-ml sample in a *red-top* tube.
- If a hematoma develops at the venipuncture site, apply warm soaks.
- If the patient had a radioactive iodine scan with 48 hours of the test, note this on the laboratory slip.

Precautions
- Handle the sample gently to prevent hemolysis.
- Send it to the laboratory promptly.

Reference values
TSI doesn't normally appear in serum. However, it's considered normal at levels equal to or greater than 1.3 index.

Abnormal findings
Increased TSI levels are associated with exophthalmos, Graves' disease (thyrotoxicosis), and recurrence of hyperthyroidism.

Interfering factors
- Hemolysis due to rough handling of the sample
- Failure to send the sample to the laboratory immediately

CARDIOLIPIN ANTIBODIES

This test measures serum concentrations of immunoglobulin G and immunoglobulin M antibodies in relation to the phospholipid cardiolipin. These antibodies appear in some lupus erythematosus (LE) patients whose serum also contains a coagulation inhibitor (lupus anticoagulant). They also appear in some patients who don't fulfill all the diagnostic criteria for LE but who experience recurrent episodes of spontaneous thrombosis, fetal loss, or thrombocytopenia. Serum concentrations of cardiolipin antibodies are measured by enzyme-linked immunosorbent assay.

Purpose
- To aid diagnosis of cardiolipin antibody syndrome in patients with or without LE who experience recurrent episodes of spontaneous thrombosis, fetal loss, or thrombocytopenia

Patient preparation
- Tell the patient that this test helps diagnose cardiolipin antibody syndrome and lupus erythematosus.
- Tell him that he needn't restrict food or fluids before the test.

• Tell him that the test requires a blood sample and who will perform the venipuncture and when.

• Reassure him that although he may experience transient discomfort from the needle puncture and the tourniquet, collecting the sample takes less than 3 minutes.

Procedure and posttest care

• Perform a venipuncture, and collect the sample in a 5-ml *red-top* tube.

• If a hematoma develops at the venipuncture site, apply warm soaks.

Precautions

• Handle the sample gently to prevent hemolysis, and send it to the laboratory immediately.

Reference values

Cardiolipin antibody results are reported as negative or positive. A positive result is titered.

Abnormal findings

A positive result along with a history of recurrent spontaneous thrombosis, fetal loss, or thrombocytopenia suggests cardiolipin antibody syndrome. Treatment may involve anticoagulant or platelet inhibitor therapy.

Interfering factors

• Hemolysis due to rough handling of the sample

• Failure to send the sample to the laboratory immediately

RHEUMATOID FACTOR

The rheumatoid factor (RF) test is the most useful immunologic test for confirming rheumatoid arthritis (RA). In this disease, "renegade" immunoglobulin G (IgG) antibodies, produced by lymphocytes in the synovial joints, react with IgM antibody to produce immune complexes, complement activation, and tissue destruction. How IgG molecules become antigenic is still unknown, but they may be altered by aggregating with viruses or other antigens. Techniques for detecting RF include the sheep cell agglutination test and the latex fixation test. Although the presence of this autoantibody is diagnostically useful, it may not be etiologically related to RA.

Purpose

• To confirm RA, especially when clinical diagnosis is doubtful

Patient preparation

• Explain to the patient that this test helps confirm RA.

• Advise him that he needn't restrict food or fluids before the test.

• Tell him that the test requires a blood sample and who will perform the venipuncture and when.

• Reassure him that although he may experience transient discomfort from the needle puncture and the tourniquet, collecting the blood sample usually takes less than 3 minutes.

Procedure and posttest care

• Perform a venipuncture, and collect the sample in a 7-ml *red-top* tube.

• Because a patient with RA may be immunologically compromised, keep the venipuncture site clean and dry for 24 hours.

• Check regularly for signs of infection.

• If a hematoma develops at the venipuncture site, apply warm soaks.

Reference values

A normal RF titer is nonreactive if it's less than 39 IU/ml, weakly reactive if it's 40 to 79 IU/ml, and reactive if it's equal to or greater than 80 IU/ml.

Abnormal findings

Non-RA and RA populations aren't clearly separated with regard to the presence of RF: 25% of RA patients have a nonreactive titer, 8% of non-RA patients are reactive at greater than 39 IU/ml, and only 3% of non-RA patients are reactive at greater than 80 IU/ml.

Patients with various non-RA diseases characterized by chronic inflammation may test positive for RF. These diseases include systemic lupus erythematosus, polymyositis, tuberculosis, infectious mononucleosis, syphilis, viral hepatic disease, and influenza.

Interfering factors

● Inadequately activated complement (possible false-positive)
● Serum with high lipid or cryoglobulin levels (possible false-positive, requiring repetition of the test after restricting fat intake)
● Serum with high IgG levels (possible false-negative due to competition with IgG on the surface of latex particles or sheep red blood cells used as substrate)

COLD AGGLUTININS

Cold agglutinins are antibodies, usually of the immunoglobulin M (IgM) type, that cause red blood cells (RBCs) to aggregate at low temperatures. They may occur in small amounts in healthy people. Transient elevations of these antibodies develop during certain infectious diseases, notably primary atypical pneumonia. This test reliably detects such pneumonia within 1 to 2 weeks after onset.

Patients with high cold agglutinin titers, such as those with primary atypical pneumonia, may develop acute transient hemolytic anemia after repeated exposure to cold; patients with persistently high titers may develop chronic hemolytic anemia.

Purpose

● To help confirm primary atypical pneumonia
● To provide additional diagnostic evidence for cold agglutinin disease associated with many viral infections and lymphoreticular cancer
● To detect cold agglutinins in patients with suspected cold agglutinin disease

Patient preparation

● Explain to the patient that this test detects antibodies in the blood that attack RBCs after exposure to low temperatures.
● If appropriate, inform him that the test will be repeated to monitor his response to therapy.
● Advise him that he needn't restrict food or fluids.
● Tell him that the test requires a blood sample and who will perform the venipuncture and when.
● Reassure him that although he may experience transient discomfort from the needle puncture and the tourniquet, collecting the sample takes less than 3 minutes.
● If the patient is receiving antimicrobial drugs, note this on the laboratory slip because the use of such drugs may interfere with the development of cold agglutinins.

Procedure and posttest care
• Perform a venipuncture, and collect the sample in a 7-ml *red-top* tube that has been prewarmed to 98.6° F (37° C).
• If cold agglutinin disease is suspected, keep the patient warm. If the patient is exposed to low temperatures, agglutination may occur within peripheral vessels, possibly leading to frostbite, anemia, Raynaud's phenomenon and, rarely, focal gangrene.
• Watch for signs of vascular abnormalities, such as mottled skin, purpura, jaundice, pallor, pain in or swelling of extremities, and cramping of fingers and toes. Hemoglobinuria may result from severe intravascular hemolysis on exposure to severe cold.
• If a hematoma develops at the venipuncture site, apply warm soaks.

Precautions
• Handle the sample gently to prevent hemolysis, and send it to the laboratory immediately.
• Don't refrigerate the sample; cold agglutinins will coat the RBCs, leaving none in the serum for testing.

Reference values
Cold agglutinin screening results are reported as negative or positive. A positive result, indicating the presence of cold agglutinin, is titered. A normal titer is less than 1:64.

Abnormal findings
High titers may occur as primary phenomena or secondary to infections or lymphoreticular cancer. They may be present in infectious mononucleosis, cytomegalovirus infection, hemolytic anemia, multiple myeloma, scleroderma, malaria, cirrhosis, congenital syphilis, peripheral vascular disease, pulmonary embolism, trypanosomiasis, tonsillitis, staphylococcemia, scar-

latina, influenza and, occasionally, pregnancy. Chronically elevated titers are most commonly associated with pneumonia and lymphoreticular cancer; an acute transient elevation commonly accompanies many viral infections.

Extremely high titers (> 1:2,000) can occur with idiopathic cold agglutinin disease that precedes development of lymphoma. Patients with titers this high are susceptible to intravascular agglutination, which causes significant clinical problems.

Interfering factors
• Hemolysis due to rough handling of the sample (possible false-low titer)
• Refrigeration of the sample before serum is separated from RBCs (possible false-low titer)
• Antimicrobial drugs

CRYOGLOBULINS

Cryoglobulins are abnormal serum proteins that precipitate at low laboratory temperatures (39.2° F [4° C]) and redissolve after being warmed. Their presence in the blood (cryoglobulinemia) is usually associated with immunologic disease but can also occur without known immunopathology. If patients with cryoglobulinemia are subjected to cold, they may experience Raynaud-like symptoms (pain, cyanosis, and coldness of fingers and toes), which generally result from precipitation of cryoglobulins in cooler parts of the body. In some patients, for example, cryoglobulins may precipitate at temperatures as high as 86° F (30° C); such temperatures are possible in some peripheral blood vessels.

The cryoglobulin test involves refrigerating a serum sample at 1° C for 24 hours and observing for formation of a heat-reversible precipitate. Such a precipitate requires further study by immunoelectrophoresis or double diffusion to identify cryoglobulin components.

Purpose
• To detect cryoglobulinemia in patients with Raynaud-like vascular symptoms

Patient preparation
• Explain to the patient that this test detects antibodies in blood that may cause sensitivity to low temperatures.
• Instruct him to fast for 4 to 6 hours before the test.
• Tell him that the test requires a blood sample and who will perform the venipuncture and when.
• Reassure him that although he may experience transient discomfort from the needle puncture and the tourniquet, collecting the blood sample usually takes less than 3 minutes.

Procedure and posttest care
• Perform a venipuncture, and collect the sample in a prewarmed 10-ml *red-top* tube.
• Tell the patient that he may resume his usual diet.
• Tell the patient to avoid cold temperatures or contact with cold objects, if the test is positive for cryoglobulins.
• If a hematoma develops at the venipuncture site, apply warm soaks.
• Observe for signs of intravascular coagulation, such as decreased color and temperature in distal extremities, and increased pain.

Precautions
• Warm the syringe and collection tube to 98.6° F (37° C) before venipuncture

and keep the tube at that temperature to prevent loss of cryoglobulins.
• Send the sample to the laboratory immediately.

Normal findings
Normally, serum is negative for cryoglobulins. Positive results are reported as a percentage based on the amount of sample cryoprecipitation.

Abnormal findings
The presence of cryoglobulins in the blood confirms cryoglobulinemia. This finding doesn't always indicate the presence of clinical disease.

Interfering factors
• Failure to adhere to pretest restrictions
• Failure to keep the sample at 98.6° F (37° C) before centrifugation (possible loss of cryoglobulins)
• Reading the sample before the 72-hour precipitation period ends (possible incorrect analysis of results because some cryoglobulins take several days to precipitate)

ACETYLCHOLINE RECEPTOR ANTIBODIES

The acetylcholine receptor (AChR) antibodies test is the most useful immunologic test for confirming acquired (autoimmune) myasthenia gravis (MG), a disorder of neuromuscular transmission. In MG, antibodies block and destroy AChR sites, causing muscle weakness that can be either generalized or localized to the ocular muscles.

Two test methods — a binding assay and a blocking assay — are now available to determine the relative concentration of AChR antibodies in serum. The blocking assay is relatively new, and its clinical significance isn't fully known. However, it's specific for the autoimmune form of MG and useful for research. Determination of AChR antibodies by either method also helps monitor immunosuppressive therapy for MG, although antibody levels don't usually parallel the severity of disease.

Purpose
• To confirm diagnosis of MG
• To monitor the effectiveness of immunosuppressive therapy for MG

Patient preparation
• Explain to the patient that this test helps confirm MG.
• If appropriate, tell him that the test assesses the effectiveness of treatment.
• Advise him that he needn't restrict food or fluids.
• Tell him that the test requires a blood sample and who will perform the venipuncture and when.
• Reassure him that although he may experience transient discomfort from the needle puncture and the tourniquet, collecting the sample takes less than 3 minutes.
• Check the patient's medication history for immunosuppressive drugs that may affect test results, and note such use on the laboratory slip.

Procedure and posttest care
• Perform a venipuncture, and collect the sample in a 7-ml *red-top* tube.
• Because a patient with an autoimmune disease has a compromised immune system, check the venipuncture site for infection, and promptly report any change.
• Keep a clean, dry bandage over the site for at least 24 hours.

• If a hematoma develops at the venipuncture site, apply warm soaks.

Precautions
• Keep the sample at room temperature, and send it to the laboratory immediately.

Normal findings
Normal serum is negative for AChR-binding antibodies and AChR-blocking antibodies.

Abnormal findings
Positive AChR antibodies in symptomatic adults confirm the diagnosis of MG. Patients who have only ocular symptoms have lower antibody titers than those who have generalized symptoms.

Interfering factors
• Failure to maintain the sample at room temperature
• Failure to send the sample to the laboratory immediately
• Thymectomy, thoracic duct drainage, immunosuppressive therapy, and plasmapheresis (possible decrease)
• Amyotrophic lateral sclerosis (possible false-positive)

ANTI-INSULIN ANTIBODIES

Some diabetic patients form antibodies to the insulin they take. These antibodies bind with some of the insulin, making less insulin available for glucose metabolism and necessitating increased insulin dosages. This phenomenon is known as insulin resistance.

Performed on the blood of a diabetic patient receiving insulin, the anti-insulin antibody test detects insulin antibodies. Insulin antibodies are immunoglobulins, called anti-insulin Ab. The most common type of anti-insulin Ab is immunoglobulin G (IgG), but anti-insulin Ab is also found in the other four classes of immunoglobulins — IgA, IgD, IgE, and IgM. IgM may cause insulin resistance, and IgE has been associated with allergic reactions.

Purpose
• To determine insulin allergy
• To confirm insulin resistance
• To determine if hypoglycemia is caused by insulin overuse

Patient preparation
• Tell the patient that this test is used to determine the most appropriate treatment for his diabetes and to determine if he has insulin resistance or an allergy to insulin.
• Tell the patient that the test requires a blood sample and who will perform the venipuncture and when.
• Tell the patient that although he may experience transient discomfort from the needle puncture and the tourniquet, collecting the sample takes only a few minutes.
• Tell him that he needn't fast before the test.
• Ask the patient if he has had a radioactive test recently; if so, note this on the laboratory slip.

Procedure and posttest care
• Perform a venipuncture, and collect the sample in a 7-ml *red-top* tube.
• If a hematoma develops at the venipuncture site, apply warm soaks.

Precautions
• Handle the sample gently to prevent hemolysis.

Normal findings
There should be less than 3% binding of the patient's serum with labeled beef, human, and pork insulin.

Abnormal findings
Elevated levels may occur in insulin allergy or resistance and in factitious hypoglycemia.

Interfering factor
• Radioactive test performed within 1 week before the test

ANTI-DOUBLE-STRANDED DNA ANTIBODIES

About two-thirds of patients with active systemic lupus erythematosus (SLE) have measurable levels of autoantibodies to double-stranded (native) deoxyribonucleic acid (known as anti-ds-DNA). These antibodies are rarely detected in patients with other connective tissue diseases.

The anti-ds-DNA antibody test measures and differentiates these antibody levels in a serum sample, using radioimmunoassay, agglutination, complement fixation, or immunoelectrophoresis. If anti-ds-DNA antibodies are present, they combine with native DNA and form complexes that are too large to pass through a membrane filter. The test counts these oversized complexes.

Purpose
• To confirm a diagnosis of SLE
• To monitor the SLE patient's response to therapy and determine his prognosis

Patient preparation

- Explain to the patient that this test helps diagnose and determine the appropriate therapy for SLE.
- Advise the patient that he needn't restrict food or fluids.
- Tell him that the test requires a blood sample and who will perform the venipuncture and when.
- Reassure him that although he may experience transient discomfort from the needle puncture and the tourniquet, collecting the sample usually takes less than 3 minutes.
- Ask the patient if he has had a recent radioactive test; if so, note this on the laboratory slip.

Procedure and posttest care

- Perform a venipuncture, and collect the sample in a 7-ml *red-top* tube. (Some laboratories may specify a *lavender-* or *gray-top* tube.)
- If a hematoma develops at the venipuncture site, apply warm soaks.

Precautions

- Handle the sample gently to prevent hemolysis.

Reference values

An anti-ds-DNA antibody level less than 25 IU is considered negative for SLE.

Abnormal findings

Elevated anti-ds-DNA antibody levels may indicate SLE. Values of 25 to 30 IU are considered borderline positive. Values of 31 to 200 IU are positive, and those greater than 200 IU are strongly positive.

Depressed anti-ds-DNA antibody levels may follow immunosuppressive therapy, demonstrating effective treatment of SLE.

Interfering factors

- A radioactive scan performed within 1 week before collection of a sample
- Hemolysis due to rough handling of the sample

VIRUSES

RUBELLA ANTIBODIES

Although rubella (German measles) is generally a mild viral infection in children and young adults, it can produce severe infection in the fetus, resulting in spontaneous abortion, stillbirth, or congenital rubella syndrome. Because rubella infection normally induces immunoglobulin G (IgG) and IgM antibody production, measuring rubella antibodies can determine present infection as well as immunity resulting from past infection. The hemagglutination inhibition test is the most commonly used serologic test for rubella antibodies.

Purpose

- To diagnose rubella infection, especially congenital infection
- To determine susceptibility to rubella in children and in women of childbearing age

Patient preparation

- Explain to the patient that this test diagnoses or evaluates susceptibility to rubella.
- Inform her that she needn't restrict food or fluids before the test.
- Tell her that this test requires a blood sample and that if a current infection is suspected, a second blood sample will

be needed in 2 to 3 weeks to identify a rise in the titer.

• Inform her who will perform the venipuncture and when.

• Reassure her that although she may experience transient discomfort from the needle puncture and the tourniquet, collecting the sample takes less than 3 minutes.

Procedure and posttest care

• Perform a venipuncture, and collect the sample in a 7-ml *red-top* tube.

• If a hematoma develops at the venipuncture site, apply warm soaks.

• When appropriate, instruct the patient to return for an additional blood test.

• If a woman of childbearing age is found to be susceptible to rubella (titer of 1:8 or less), explain that vaccination can prevent rubella and that she must wait at least 3 months after the vaccination to become pregnant or risk permanent damage or death to the fetus.

• If the pregnant patient is found to be susceptible to rubella, instruct her to return for follow-up rubella antibody tests to detect possible subsequent infection.

• If the test confirms rubella in a pregnant patient, provide emotional support. As needed, refer her for appropriate counseling.

Precautions

• Handle the specimen gently to prevent hemolysis.

Reference values

An IgG titer less than 10 IU/ml indicates susceptibility to rubella; a titer greater than 10 IU/ml indicates adequate protection against rubella.

IgM results are reported as positive or negative. The presence of IgM class

antibody indicates congenital or recent infection.

Abnormal findings

Hemagglutination inhibition antibodies normally appear 2 to 4 days after the onset of the rash, peak in 2 to 3 weeks, and then slowly decline but remain detectable for life. A fourfold or greater rise from the acute to the convalescent titer indicates a recent rubella infection.

Because maternal antibodies cross the placenta and persist in the infant's serum for up to 6 months, congenital rubella can be detected only after this period. An elevated antibody titer in an infant age 6 months or older who has not been exposed to rubella postnatally confirms congenital rubella.

Interfering factor

• Hemolysis due to rough handling of the sample

HEPATITIS B SURFACE ANTIGEN

Hepatitis B surface antigen (HBsAg), also called hepatitis-associated antigen or Australia antigen, appears in the sera of patients with hepatitis B virus. It can be detected by radioimmunoassay or, less commonly, reverse passive hemagglutination during the extended incubation period and usually during the first 3 weeks of acute infection or if the patient is a carrier.

Because transmission of hepatitis is one of the gravest complications associated with blood transfusion, all donors must be screened for hepatitis B before their blood is stored. This screening, required by the Food and

Drug Administration's Bureau of Biologics, has helped reduce the incidence of hepatitis. This test doesn't screen for hepatitis A virus (infectious hepatitis).

Purpose
• To screen blood donors for hepatitis B
• To screen people at high risk for contracting hepatitis B, such as hemodialysis nurses
• To aid differential diagnosis of viral hepatitis

Patient preparation
• Explain to the patient that this test helps identify a type of viral hepatitis.
• Inform him that he needn't restrict food or fluids before the test.
• Tell him that the test requires a blood sample and who will perform the venipuncture and when.
• Reassure him that although he may experience transient discomfort from the needle puncture and the tourniquet, collecting the sample takes less than 3 minutes.
• Check the patient's history for administration of hepatitis B vaccine.
• If the patient is giving blood, explain the donation procedure to him.

Procedure and posttest care
• Perform a venipuncture, and collect the sample in a 10-ml *red-top* tube.
• Notify the blood donor if test results are positive for HBsAg.
• Report confirmed viral hepatitis to public health authorities. This is a reportable disease in most states.

Precautions
• Wash your hands carefully after the procedure.
• Remember to wear gloves when drawing blood.
• Dispose of the needle properly.

Normal findings
Normal serum is negative for HBsAg.

Abnormal findings
The presence of HBsAg in a patient with hepatitis confirms hepatitis B. In chronic carriers and people with chronic active hepatitis, HBsAg may be present in the serum several months after the onset of acute infection. It may also occur in more than 5% of patients with certain diseases other than hepatitis, such as hemophilia, Hodgkin's disease, and leukemia. If HbsAg is found in donor blood, that blood must be discarded because it carries a risk of transmitting hepatitis. Blood samples that test positive should be retested because inaccurate results do occur.

Interfering factor
• Hepatitis B vaccine (possible positive)

HETEROPHIL ANTIBODY TESTS

Heterophil antibody tests detect and identify two immunoglobulin M (IgM) antibodies in human serum that react against foreign red blood cells (RBCs): Epstein-Barr virus (EBV) antibodies and Forssman antibodies.

In the Paul-Bunnell test — also called the presumptive test — EBV antibodies, found in the sera of patients with infectious mononucleosis, agglutinate with sheep RBCs in a test tube. Forssman antibodies, present in the sera of some normal persons as well as in the sera of patients with conditions such as serum sickness, also agglutinate with sheep RBCs, thus rendering test results inconclusive for infectious mononucleosis.

If the Paul-Bunnell test establishes a presumptive titer, Davidsohn's differential absorption test can then distinguish between EBV antibodies and Forssman antibodies. (See *Monospot test for infectious mononucleosis.*)

Purpose
• To aid differential diagnosis of infectious mononucleosis

Patient preparation
• Explain to the patient that this test helps detect infectious mononucleosis.
• Tell him that the test requires a blood sample and who will perform the venipuncture and when.
• Reassure him that although he may experience transient discomfort from the needle puncture and the tourniquet, collecting the sample takes less than 3 minutes.

Procedure and posttest care
• Perform a venipuncture, and collect the sample in a 7-ml *red-top* tube.
• If a hematoma develops at the venipuncture site, apply warm soaks.
• If the titer is positive and infectious mononucleosis is confirmed, instruct the patient in the treatment plan.
• If the titer is positive but infectious mononucleosis isn't confirmed, or if the titer is negative but symptoms persist, explain that additional testing will be necessary in a few days or weeks to confirm the diagnosis and plan effective treatment.

Precautions
• Handle the sample gently to prevent hemolysis.

Reference values
Normally, the titer is less than 1:56 but may be higher in elderly people. Some

---

MONOSPOT TEST FOR INFECTIOUS MONONUCLEOSIS

Several screening tests can detect the heterophil infectious mononucleosis (IM) antibody. One of these tests — the monospot — converts the Paul-Bunnell and the Davidsohn's differential absorption tests into one rapid slide test without titration. Monospot relies on agglutination of horse red blood cells (RBCs) by heterophil antibodies.

Distinguishing antibodies
Because horse RBCs contain both Forssman and IM antigens, differential absorption of the patient's serum is necessary to distinguish between them. This is done by mixing the serum sample with guinea pig kidney antigen (containing only Forssman antigen) on one end of a slide and with beef RBC stroma (containing only IM antigen) on the other end of the slide. Each absorbs only the heterophil antibody specific to it. After addition of horse RBCs to each spot, agglutination on the beef cell end of the slide indicates the presence of the IM heterophil antibody and confirms IM.

Monospot rivals the classic heterophil agglutination test for sensitivity. False-positives may occur in the presence of lymphoma, hepatitis A and hepatitis B, leukemia, and pancreatic cancer.

---

laboratories refer to a normal titer as "negative" or as having "no reaction."

Abnormal findings
Although heterophil antibodies are present in the sera of about 80% of pa-

tients with infectious mononucleosis 1 month after onset, a positive finding — a titer higher than 1:56 — doesn't confirm this disorder; a high titer can also result from systemic lupus erythematosus, syphilis, cryoglobulinemia, or the presence of antibodies to nonsyphilitic treponemata (yaws, pinta, bejel). A gradual increase in titer during week 3 or 4 followed by a gradual decrease during weeks 4 to 8 proves most conclusive for infectious mononucleosis. A negative titer doesn't always rule out this disorder; occasionally, the titer becomes reactive 2 weeks later. Therefore, if symptoms persist, the test should be repeated in 2 weeks.

Confirmation of infectious mononucleosis depends on heterophil agglutination tests and hematologic tests that show absolute lymphocytosis, with 10% or more atypical lymphocytes.

Interfering factors
• Hemolysis due to handling of the sample
• Narcotic use, lymphomas, hepatitis, leukemia, and phenytoin therapy (false-positive)

EPSTEIN-BARR VIRUS ANTIBODIES

Epstein-Barr virus (EBV), a member of the herpesvirus group, is the causative agent of heterophil-positive infectious mononucleosis, Burkitt's lymphoma, and nasopharyngeal carcinoma. Although the virus doesn't replicate in standard cell cultures, most EBV infections can be recognized by testing the patient's serum for heterophil antibodies (monospot test), which usually appear within the first 3 weeks of illness and then decline rapidly within a few weeks.

In about 10% of adults and a larger percentage of children, the monospot test is negative, despite primary infection with EBV. Further, EBV has been associated with lymphoproliferative processes in immunosuppressed patients. These disorders occur with reactivated, rather than primary, EBV infections and therefore are also monospot-negative.

Alternatively, EBV-specific antibodies, which develop to several antigens of the virus during active infection, can be measured with a high level of sensitivity and specificity by indirect immunofluorescence.

Purpose
• To provide a laboratory diagnosis of heterophil- (or monospot-) negative cases of infectious mononucleosis
• To determine the antibody status to EBV of immunosuppressed patients with lymphoproliferative processes

Patient preparation
• Explain to the patient the purpose of the test.
• Inform him that the test requires a blood sample and who will perform the venipuncture and when.
• Reassure him that although he may experience transient discomfort from the needle puncture and the tourniquet, collecting the sample takes less than 3 minutes.

Procedure and posttest care
• Perform a venipuncture, and collect 5 ml of sterile blood in a *red-top* tube.
• Allow the blood to clot for at least 1 hour at room temperature.
• If a hematoma develops at the venipuncture site, apply warm soaks.

CLINICAL IMPLICATIONS OF ANTIBODY RESPONSE

ANTIGEN	ACUTE INFECTIOUS MONONUCLEOSIS	REMOTE EPSTEIN-BARR VIRUS INFECTION	BURKITT'S LYMPHOMA	NASO-PHARYNGEAL CARCINOMA
Viral capsid antigen *Antibody class*				
IgM	+++	–	–	–
IgG	+++	++	++++	+++
IgA				++
Epstein-Barr nuclear antigen	–	++	++	++
Heterophil antibody (monospot)	++++	–	–	–

KEY: + antibody titer; – negative for antibody titer

Precautions
• Handle the sample gently to prevent hemolysis.
• Transfer the serum to a sterile tube or vial and send it to the laboratory immediately.
• If transfer must be delayed, store the serum at 39.2° F (4° C) for 1 to 2 days or at −4° F (−20° C) for longer periods to prevent contamination.

Reference values
Sera from patients who have never been infected with EBV have no detectable antibodies to the virus as measured by either the monospot test or the indirect immunofluorescence test. The monospot test is positive only during the acute phase of infection with EBV; the indirect immunofluorescence test detects and discriminates between acute and past infection with the virus.

(For a profile of test results and their clinical implications, see *Clinical implications of antibody response*.)

Abnormal findings
EBV infection can be ruled out if no antibodies to EBV antigens are detected in the indirect immunofluorescence test. A positive monospot test or an indirect immunofluorescence test that is either immunoglobulin M (IgM)-positive or Epstein-Barr nuclear antigen (EBNA)-negative indicates acute EBV infection.

A monospot-negative result doesn't necessarily rule out acute or past infection with EBV. Conversely, IgG class antibody to viral capsid antigen (VCA) and EBNA antigens (IgM-negative) indicates remote (more than 2 months) infection with EBV. Recognize that most cases of monospot-negative infectious mononucleosis are caused by cytomegalovirus infections.

Interfering factors
• Hemolysis due to rough handling of the sample
• Failure to store serum at proper temperature

RESPIRATORY SYNCYTIAL VIRUS ANTIBODIES

Respiratory syncytial virus (RSV), a member of the paramyxovirus group, is the major viral cause of severe lower respiratory tract disease in infants but may cause infections in people of any age. RSV infections are most common and produce the most severe disease during the first 6 months of life. Initial infection involves viral replication in epithelial cells of the upper respiratory tract, but in younger children especially, the infection spreads to the bronchi, the bronchioles, and even the parenchyma of the lungs.

In this test, immunoglobulin G (IgG) and IgM class antibodies are quantified using indirect immunofluorescence.

Purpose
• To diagnose infections caused by RSV

Patient preparation
• Explain to the patient (or, to the patient's parents) the purpose of the test.
• Tell the patient or parents that the test requires a blood sample and who will perform the venipuncture and when.

• Reassure the patient that although he may experience transient discomfort from the needle puncture and the tourniquet, collecting the sample takes less than 3 minutes.

Procedure and posttest care
• Perform a venipuncture, and collect 5 ml of sterile blood in a *red-top* tube.
• Allow the blood to clot for at least 1 hour at room temperature.
• If a hematoma develops at the venipuncture site, apply warm soaks.

Precautions
• Handle the sample gently to prevent hemolysis.
• Transfer the serum to a sterile tube or vial, and send it to the laboratory promptly.
• If transfer must be delayed, store the serum at 39.2° F (4° C) for 1 to 2 days or at −4° F (−20° C) for longer periods to avoid contamination.

Reference values
Sera from patients who have never been infected with RSV have no detectable antibodies to the virus (less than 1:10).

Abnormal findings
The qualitative presence of IgM or a fourfold or greater increase in IgG antibodies indicates active RSV infection. Note that, in infants, serologic diagnosis of RSV infections is difficult because of the presence of maternal IgG antibodies. Thus, the presence of IgM antibodies is most significant.

Interfering factors
• Hemolysis due to rough handling of the sample
• Failure to store serum at the proper temperature

HERPES SIMPLEX ANTIBODIES

Herpes simplex virus (HSV), a member of the herpesvirus group, causes various clinically severe manifestations, including genital lesions, keratitis or conjunctivitis, generalized dermal lesions, and pneumonia. Severe involvement is associated with intrauterine or neonatal infections and encephalitis; such infections are most severe in immunosuppressed patients. Of the two closely related antigenic types, Type 1 usually causes infections above the waistline; Type 2 infections predominantly involve the external genitalia. Primary contact with this virus occurs in early childhood as acute stomatitis or, more commonly, as an inapparent infection.

Sensitive assays, such as indirect immunofluorescence and enzyme immunoassay, are used to demonstrate immunoglobulin M (IgM) class antibodies to HSV or to detect a fourfold or greater increase in IgG class antibodies between acute- and convalescent-phase sera.

Purpose
- To confirm systemic infections caused by HSV
- To detect recent or past HSV infection

Patient preparation
- Explain to the patient the purpose of the test.
- Tell him that the test requires a blood sample and who will perform the venipuncture and when.
- Reassure him that although he may experience transient discomfort from the needle puncture and the tourniquet, collecting the sample takes less than 3 minutes.

Procedure and posttest care
- Perform a venipuncture, and collect 5 ml of sterile blood in a *red-top* tube.
- Allow the blood to clot for at least 1 hour at room temperature.
- If a hematoma develops at the venipuncture site, apply warm soaks.

Precautions
- Handle the sample gently to prevent hemolysis.
- Transfer the serum to a sterile tube or vial, and send it to the laboratory promptly.
- If transfer must be delayed, store the serum at 39.2° F (4° C) for 1 to 2 days or at −4° F (−20° C) for longer periods to avoid contamination.

Reference values
Sera from patients who have never been infected with HSV have no detectable antibodies (less than 1:5).

Abnormal findings
Normal serum values indicating the absence of infection are IgG less than 1:5 and IgM less than 1:10; higher levels are considered positive. The presence of IgM or a fourfold or greater increase in IgG antibodies indicates active HSV infection. Reactivated infections caused by HSV can be recognized serologically only by an increase in IgG class antibodies between acute- and convalescent-phase sera.

Interfering factors
- Hemolysis due to rough handling of the sample
- Failure to store serum at proper temperature

CYTOMEGALOVIRUS ANTIBODY SCREEN

After primary infection, cytomegalovirus (CMV) remains latent in white blood cells. The presence of CMV antibodies indicates past infection with this virus. In an immunocompromised patient, CMV can be reactivated to cause active infection. Administration of blood or tissue from a seropositive donor may cause active CMV infection in CMV-seronegative organ transplant recipients or neonates, especially those born prematurely.

Antibodies to CMV can be detected by several methods, including passive hemagglutination, latex agglutination, enzyme immunoassay, and indirect immunofluorescence. The complement fixation test is only 60% sensitive compared with other assays and should not be used to screen for CMV antibodies. Screening tests for CMV antibodies are qualitative; they detect the presence of antibody at a single low dilution. In quantitative methods, several dilutions of the serum sample are tested to indicate acute infection with CMV.

Purpose
• To detect past CMV infection in donors and recipients of organs and blood
• To screen for CMV infection in infants who require blood transfusions or tissue transplants
• To detect past CMV infection in immunocompromised patients

Patient preparation
• As appropriate, explain the purpose of the test to the patient or the parents of an infant.

• Tell the patient that the test requires a blood sample and who will perform the venipuncture and when.
• Reassure him that although he may experience transient discomfort from the needle puncture and the tourniquet, collecting the sample takes less than 3 minutes.

Procedure and posttest care
• Perform a venipuncture, and collect the sample in a 5-ml *red-top* tube.
• Allow the blood to clot for at least 1 hour at room temperature.

Precautions
• Handle the sample gently to prevent hemolysis.
• Transfer the serum to a sterile tube or vial, and send it to the laboratory.
• If transfer must be delayed, store the serum at 39.2° F (4° C) for 1 to 2 days or at −4° F (−20° C) for longer periods to avoid contamination.

Reference values
Patients who have never been infected with CMV have no detectable antibodies to the virus. Immunoglobulin G (IgG) and IgM are normally negative.

Abnormal findings
A serum sample collected early during the acute phase or late in the convalescent stage may not contain detectable IgG or IgM antibodies to CMV. Therefore, a negative result doesn't preclude recent infection. More than a single sample is needed to ensure accurate results.

A serum sample that tests positive for antibodies at this single dilution indicates that the patient has been infected with CMV and that his white blood cells contain latent virus capable of being reactivated in an immunocompromised host. Immunosuppressed patients who lack antibodies to CMV should receive blood products or organ transplants from donors who are also seronegative. Patients with CMV antibodies don't require seronegative blood products.

Interfering factors
● Hemolysis due to rough handling of the sample
● Failure to store serum at the proper temperature

HUMAN IMMUNODEFICIENCY VIRUS ANTIBODIES

This test detects antibodies to human immunodeficiency virus (HIV) in serum. HIV is the virus that causes acquired immunodeficiency syndrome (AIDS). Transmission occurs by direct exposure of a person's blood to body fluids containing the virus. The virus may be transmitted from one person to another through exchange of contaminated blood and blood products; during sexual intercourse with an infected partner; when I.V. drugs are shared; and from an infected mother to her child during pregnancy or breast-feeding.

Initial identification of HIV is usually achieved through enzyme-linked immunosorbent assay. Positive findings are confirmed by Western blot test and immunofluorescence.

Purpose
● To screen for HIV in high-risk patients
● To screen donated blood for HIV

Patient preparation
● Explain to the patient that this test detects HIV infection.
● Provide adequate counseling about the reasons for performing the test, which is usually requested by the patient's doctor.
● If the patient has questions about his condition, be sure to provide full and accurate information.
● Tell the patient that the test requires a blood sample and who will perform the venipuncture and when.
● Reassure him that although he may experience transient discomfort from the needle puncture and the tourniquet, collecting the sample takes less than 3 minutes.

Procedure and posttest care
● Perform a venipuncture, and collect the sample in a 10-ml *red-top* barrier tube. Barrier tubes help prevent contamination when pouring the serum in the laboratory.
● If a hematoma develops at the venipuncture site, apply warm soaks.
● Keep test results confidential.
● When the patient receives the results, give him another opportunity to ask questions.
● Encourage the patient with positive screening tests to seek medical follow-up care, even if he's asymptomatic.
● Tell him to report early signs of AIDS, such as fever, weight loss, axillary or inguinal lymphadenopathy, rash, and persistent cough or diarrhea. Women should also report gynecologic symptoms.
● Tell the patient to assume that he can transmit AIDS to others until conclusively proved otherwise. To prevent possible contagion, advise him about safe sex precautions.
● Instruct him not to share razors, toothbrushes, or utensils (which may be contaminated with blood) and to

clean such items with household bleach diluted 1:10 in water.
• Advise against donating blood, tissues, or an organ.
• Warn the patient to inform his doctor and dentist about his condition so that they can take proper precautions.

Precautions
• Observe standard precautions when drawing a blood sample.
• Use gloves, properly dispose of needles, and use blood-fluid precaution labels on tubes, as necessary.

Normal findings
Test results are normally negative. A positive result, indicating the presence of antibodies, necessitates further investigation.

Abnormal findings
The test detects previous exposure to the virus. However, it doesn't identify patients who have been exposed to the virus but haven't yet made antibodies. Most patients with AIDS have antibodies to HIV. A positive test for the HIV antibody can't determine whether a patient harbors actively replicating virus or when the patient will manifest signs and symptoms of AIDS.

Many apparently healthy people have been exposed to HIV and have circulating antibodies. The test results for such people aren't false-positives. Furthermore, patients in the later stages of AIDS may exhibit no detectable antibody in their sera because they can no longer mount an antibody response.

Interfering factor
• Sample taken less than 12 weeks after exposure (possible false-negative because of absence of antibodies)

PARVOVIRUS B-19 ANTIBODIES

Parvovirus B-19, a small, single-stranded deoxyribonucleic acid virus belonging to the family Parvoviridae, destroys red blood cell (RBC) precursors and interferes with normal RBC production. It's also associated with erythema infectiosum (a self-limiting, low-grade fever and rash in young children) and aplastic crisis (in patients with chronic hemolytic anemia and immunodeficient patients with bone marrow failure). Immunoglobulin G (IgG) antibodies and IgM antibodies can be detected by enzyme-linked immunosorbent assay (ELISA) and immunofluorescence.

Purpose
• To detect parvovirus B-19 antibody, especially in prospective organ donors
• To diagnosis erythema infectiosum, parvovirus B-19 aplastic crisis, and related parvovirus B-19 diseases

Patient preparation
• Explain to the patient the test purpose and procedure. To a potential organ donor, explain that the test is part of a panel of tests performed before organ donation to protect the organ recipient from potential infection.
• Tell the patient that the test requires a blood sample and who will perform the venipuncture and when.
• Reassure the patient that although he may experience transient discomfort from the needle puncture and the tourniquet, collection of the sample takes less than 3 minutes.

Procedure and posttest care
• Perform a venipuncture, collect the blood sample in a 5-ml *red-top* tube, and store it on ice.

• If a hematoma develops at the venipuncture site, apply warm soaks.

Precautions
• Handle the sample gently to prevent hemolysis.

Normal findings
Normally, results are negative for IgM- and IgG-specific antibodies to parvovirus B-19.

Abnormal findings
About 50% of all adults lack immunity to parvovirus B-19, with as many as 20% of susceptible adults becoming infected after exposure. Positive results have been associated with joint arthralgia, hydrops fetalis, fetal loss, transient aplastic anemia, chronic anemia in immunocompromised patients, and bone marrow failure.

Abnormal findings for the parvovirus B-19 should be confirmed using the Western blot test.

Interfering factors
• Failure to send the sample on ice
• Hemolysis due to rough handling of the sample

BACTERIA AND FUNGI

ANTISTREPTOLYSIN-O TEST

This test measures the relative serum concentrations of the antibody to streptolysin O (known as ASO). A serum sample is diluted with a commercial preparation of streptolysin O and incubated. After the addition of human red blood cells, the tube is reincubated and examined visually. Failure of hemolysis to develop indicates recent streptococcal infection.

Purpose
• To confirm recent or ongoing streptococcal infection
• To help diagnose rheumatic fever and poststreptococcal glomerulonephritis in the presence of clinical symptoms
• To distinguish between rheumatic fever and rheumatoid arthritis when joint pains are present

Patient preparation
• Explain to the patient that this test detects an immunologic response to certain bacteria (streptococci).
• Inform him that he needn't restrict food or fluids.
• Tell him that the test requires a blood sample and who will perform the venipuncture and when.
• Reassure him that although he may experience transient discomfort from the needle puncture and the pressure of the tourniquet, collecting the sample takes less than 3 minutes.
• If the test is to be repeated at regular intervals to identify active and inactive states of rheumatic fever or to confirm acute glomerulonephritis, tell the patient that measuring changes in antibody levels helps determine the effectiveness of therapy.
• Check the patient's medication history for drugs that may suppress the streptococcal antibody response, such as antibiotics and corticosteroids. If such drugs must be continued, note this on the laboratory slip.

Procedure and posttest care
• Perform a venipuncture, and collect the sample in a 7-ml *red-top* tube.

• If a hematoma develops at the veni-puncture site, apply warm soaks.

Precautions

• Handle the sample gently to prevent hemolysis.

Reference values

Even healthy people have some detectable ASO titers from previous minor streptococcal infections. Normal ASO titers range as follows:

• school-age children: ≤ 170 Todd units

• preschoolers and adults: ≤ 85 Todd units.

Abnormal findings

High ASO titers usually occur only after prolonged or recurrent infections. Generally, a titer higher than 166 Todd units is considered a definite elevation. A low titer is good evidence for the absence of active rheumatic fever. A higher titer doesn't necessarily mean that rheumatic fever or glomerulonephritis is present; however, it does indicate the presence of a streptococcal infection.

Serial titers, determined at 10- to 14-day intervals, provide more reliable information than a single titer.

Interfering factors

• Streptococcal skin infections, seldom producing abnormal ASO titers even with poststreptococcal disease (probable false-negative)

• Antibiotic or corticosteroid therapy (possible suppression of the streptococcal antibody response)

• Hemolysis due to rough handling of the sample

FEBRILE AGGLUTINATION TESTS

Sometimes bacterial infections (such as tularemia, brucellosis, and the disorders caused by *Salmonella*) and rickettsial infections (such as Rocky Mountain spotted fever and typhus) cause puzzling fevers, called fevers of undetermined origin (FUO). In these infections and others in which microorganisms are difficult to isolate from blood or excreta, febrile agglutination tests can provide important diagnostic information.

The Weil-Felix reaction for rickettsial disease, Widal's test for *Salmonella*, and tests for brucellosis and tularemia are essentially the same. In these tests, a serum sample is mixed with a few drops of prepared antigens in normal saline solution on a slide and the reaction is observed.

The Weil-Felix reaction establishes rickettsial antibody titers. This test uses three forms of *Proteus* antigens (OX-19, OX-2, and OX-K) that cross-react with the various strains of rickettsiae. Antibodies to certain rickettsial strains react with more than one *Proteus* antigen, whereas antibodies to other strains fail to react with any *Proteus* antigens.

Widal's test establishes the titers for flagellar (H) and somatic (O) antigens, which may indicate *Salmonella* gastroenteritis and extraintestinal focal infections caused by *S. enteritidis* or enteric (typhoid) fever, caused by *S. typhosa*. A third antigen, the Vi or envelope antigen, may indicate typhoid carrier status, which often tests negative for H and O antigens. Widal's test isn't recommended for diagnosing *Salmonella* gastroenteritis.

Slide agglutination and tube dilution tests, using killed suspensions of the disease organisms as antigens, establish titers for the gram-negative coccobacilli *Brucella* and *Francisella tularensis*, which cause brucellosis and tularemia, respectively.

Purpose
● To support clinical findings in diagnosis of disorders caused by *Salmonella, Rickettsia, Francisella tularensis,* and *Brucella* organisms
● To identify the cause of FUO

Patient preparation
● Explain to the patient that this test detects and quantifies microorganisms that may cause fever and other symptoms.
● Inform him that he needn't restrict food or fluids.
● Tell him that the test requires a blood sample and who will perform the venipuncture and when.
● Reassure him that although he may experience transient discomfort from the needle puncture and the tourniquet, collecting the blood sample takes less than 3 minutes.
● If appropriate, explain to the patient that this test requires a series of blood samples to detect a pattern of titers that is characteristic of the suspected disorder. Reassure him that a positive titer only suggests a disorder.
● Note on the laboratory slip when antimicrobial therapy began, if appropriate.

Procedure and posttest care
● Perform a venipuncture, and collect the sample in a 7-ml *red-top* tube.
● If a hematoma develops at the venipuncture site, apply warm soaks.

● In FUO and suspected infection, contact the hospital infection-control department. Isolation may be necessary.

Precautions
● Use standard hospital isolation procedures when collecting and handling samples.
● Send samples to the laboratory immediately.

Reference values
Results are reported as negative or positive, and positive results are titered. Normal dilutions are as follows:
● *Salmonella* antibody: < 1:80
● brucellosis antibody: < 1:80
● tularemia antibody: < 1:40
● rickettsial antibody: < 1:32.

Abnormal findings
Observed rise and fall of titers is crucial for detecting active infection. If this isn't possible, certain titer levels can suggest the disorder. For all febrile agglutinins, a fourfold increase in titers is strong evidence of infection.

The Weil-Felix reaction is positive for rickettsiae with antibodies to *Proteus* 6 to 12 days after infection; titers peak in 1 month and usually drop to negative in 5 to 6 months. This test can't be used to diagnose rickettsialpox or Q fever because the antibodies of these diseases don't cross-react with *Proteus* antigens; the test shows positive titers in *Proteus* infections and, in such cases, is nonspecific for rickettsiae.

In *Salmonella* infection, H and O agglutinins usually appear in serum after 1 week, and titers rise for 3 to 6 weeks. O agglutinins usually fall to insignificant levels in 6 to 12 months. H agglutinin titers may remain elevated for years.

In brucellosis, titers usually rise after 2 to 3 weeks and reach their highest levels between 4 and 8 weeks. The absence of *Brucella* agglutinins doesn't rule out brucellosis. In tularemia, titers usually become positive during the second week of infection, exceed 1:320 by the third week, peak within 4 to 7 weeks, and usually decline gradually 1 year after recovery.

Interfering factors
• Failure to immediately send the sample to the laboratory
• Vaccination or continuous exposure to bacterial or rickettsial infection, resulting in immunity (high titers)
• Antibody cross-reaction with bacteria causing other infectious diseases, such as tularemia antibodies cross-reacting with *Brucella* antigens
• Immunodeficiency (negative titers even during symptomatic infection due to inability to form antibodies)
• Antibiotics (low titers early in the course of infection)
• Elevated immunoglobulin levels due to hepatic disease or excessive drug use (high *Salmonella* titers)
• Skin tests with *Brucella* antigen (possible high *Brucella* titers)
• *Proteus* infections (possible positive Weil-Felix titers for rickettsial disease)

FUNGAL SEROLOGY

Most fungal organisms enter the body as spores inhaled into the lungs or infiltrated through wounds in the skin or mucosa. If the body's defenses can't destroy the organisms initially, the fungi multiply to form lesions; blood and lymph vessels may then spread the mycoses throughout the body. Most healthy people easily overcome initial mycotic infection, but elderly people and others with a deficient immune system are more susceptible to acute or chronic mycotic infection and to disorders secondary to such infection. Mycosis may be deep-seated or superficial: Deep-seated mycosis occurs primarily in the lungs; superficial mycosis, in the skin or mucosal linings.

Although cultures are usually performed to diagnose mycoses by identifying the causative organism, serologic tests occasionally provide the sole evidence for mycosis. Such serologic tests use immunodiffusion, complement fixation, precipitin, latex agglutination, or agglutination methods to demonstrate the presence of specific mycotic antibodies. (See *Serum test methods for fungal infections*.)

Purpose
• To rapidly detect the presence of antifungal antibodies, aiding in the diagnosis of mycoses
• To monitor effectiveness of therapy for mycoses

Patient preparation
• Explain to the patient that this test aids diagnosis of certain fungal infections. If appropriate, tell him that this test monitors his response to antimycotic therapy and that it may be necessary to repeat the test.
• Tell him that the test requires a blood sample and who will perform the venipuncture and when.
• Reassure him that although he may experience brief discomfort from the needle puncture and the tourniquet, collecting the sample takes less than 3 minutes.

Procedure and posttest care
• Perform a venipuncture, and collect the sample in a 10-ml sterile *red-top* tube.

SERUM TEST METHODS FOR FUNGAL INFECTIONS

DISEASE AND NORMAL VALUES	CLINICAL SIGNIFICANCE OF ABNORMAL RESULTS
Blastomycosis Complement fixation: titers <1:8	Titers ranging from 1:8 to 1:16 suggest infection; titers > 1:32 denote active disease. A rising titer in serial samples taken every 3 to 4 weeks indicates disease progression; a falling titer indicates regression. This test has limited diagnostic value because of a high percentage of false-negatives.
Immunodiffusion: negative	A more sensitive test for blastomycosis; detects 70% to 85% of infected people.
Coccidioidomycosis Complement fixation: titers <1:2	Most sensitive test for this fungus. Titers > than 1:2 suggest active disease.
Immunodiffusion: negative	Most useful for screening, followed by complement fixation test for confirmation.
Histoplasmosis Complement fixation (histoplasmin): titers <1:8	Titers ranging from 1:8 to 1:16 suggest infection; titers > 1:32 indicate active disease. Antibodies generally appear 10 to 21 days after initial infection. Test is positive in 10% to 15% of cases.
Complement fixation: titers <1:18	More sensitive than histoplasmin complement fixation test; gives positive results in 75% to 80% of cases. (Both histoplasmin and yeast antigens are positive in 10% of cases.) A rising titer in serial samples taken every 2 to 3 weeks indicates progressive infection; a decreasing titer indicates regression. Titers ranging from 1:8 to 1:16 suggest infection; titers > 1:32 indicate active disease.
Immunodiffusion (histoplasmin): negative	Appearance of both H and M bands indicates active infection. If the M band appears first and lasts longer than the H band, the infection may be regressing. The M band alone may indicate early infection, chronic disease, or a recent skin test.
Aspergillosis Complement fixation: titer <1:8	Titers > 1:8 suggest infection; 70% to 90% of patients with known pulmonary aspergillosis or aspergillus allergy present antibodies. This test cannot detect invasive aspergillosis because patients with this disease do not present antibodies; biopsy is required.
Immunodiffusion: negative	One or more precipitin bands suggests infection. The number of bands is related to complement fixation titers; the more precipitin bands, the higher the titer.
Sporotrichosis Agglutination: titers <1:40	Titers of > 1:80 usually indicate active infection. The test usually is negative in cutaneous infections and positive in extracutaneous infections.

(continued)

SᴇRUM TᴇST MᴇTHODS FOR FUNGAL INFᴇCTIONS *(continued)*

DISEASE AND NORMAL VALUES	CLINICAL SIGNIFICANCE OF ABNORMAL RESULTS
Cryptococcosis Latex agglutination for cryptococcal antigen: negative	About 95% of patients with cryptococcal meningitis exhibit positive latex agglutination in cerebrospinal fluid (CSF). (Serum is less frequently positive than CSF.) Culturing is definitive because false-positives do occur. (Presence of rheumatoid factor may cause a positive reaction.) Serum antigen tests are positive in 33% of patients with pulmonary cryptococcosis; biopsy is usually required.

• If a hematoma develops at the venipuncture site, apply warm soaks.

Precautions
• Send the sample to the laboratory immediately.
• If transport to the laboratory is delayed, store the sample at 39.2° F (4° C).

Findings
Depending on the test method, a negative finding, or normal titer, usually indicates the absence of mycosis. The accompanying chart explains the significance of findings for specific organisms.

Interfering factors
• Failure to observe pretest restrictions
• Failure to send a sterile sample to the laboratory immediately or to properly store the sample in case of delay in transportation
• Cross-reaction of antibodies with other antigens, such as blastomycosis and histoplasmosis antigens (possible false-positive or high titers)
• Recent skin testing with fungal antigens (possible high titers)
• Mycosis-caused immunosuppression (low titers or false-negative)

CANDIDA ANTIBODIES

Commonly present in the body, *Candida albicans* is a saprophytic yeast that can become pathogenic when the environment favors proliferation or the host's defenses have been significantly weakened.

Candidiasis is usually limited to the skin and mucous membranes but may cause life-threatening systemic infection. Susceptibility to candidiasis is associated with antibacterial, antimetabolic, and corticosteroid therapy as well as with immunologic defects, pregnancy, obesity, diabetes, and debilitating diseases. Oral candidiasis is common and benign in children; in adults, it may be an early indication of acquired immunodeficiency syndrome.

Diagnosis of candidiasis is usually made by culture or histologic study. When such diagnosis can't be made, identifying *Candida* antibodies may be helpful in diagnosing systemic candidiasis. Be cautioned that serologic testing to detect antibodies in candidiasis isn't reliable, and investigators continue to disagree about its usefulness.

Purpose
• To aid diagnosis of candidiasis when culture or histologic study can't confirm the diagnosis

Patient preparation
• As appropriate, explain the purpose of the test to the patient.
• Inform him that he needn't restrict food or fluids.
• Tell him that the test requires a blood sample and who will perform the venipuncture and when.
• Reassure him that although he may experience transient discomfort from the needle puncture and the tourniquet, collecting the sample takes less than 3 minutes.

Procedure and posttest care
• Perform a venipuncture, and collect the sample in a 5-ml sterile *red-top* tube.
• If a hematoma develops at the venipuncture site, apply warm soaks.

Precautions
• Handle the sample gently to prevent hemolysis.
• Send the sample to the laboratory promptly.
• Note any recent antimicrobial therapy on the laboratory request form.

Normal findings
A normal test result is negative for *Candida* antibodies.

Abnormal findings
A positive test for *C. albicans* antibodies is common in patients with disseminated candidiasis. However, this test yields a significant percentage of false-positive results.

Interfering factor
• Hemolysis due to rough handling of the sample

BACTERIAL MENINGITIS ANTIGEN

This test can detect specific antigens of *Streptococcus pneumoniae, Neisseria meningitidis,* and *Haemophilus influenzae* type B, the principal etiologic agents in meningitis. It can be performed on samples of serum, cerebrospinal fluid (CSF), urine, pleural fluid, and joint fluid, but CSF and urine are preferred.

Purpose
• To identify the etiologic agent in meningitis
• To aid diagnosis of bacterial meningitis
• To aid diagnosis of meningitis when the Gram-stained smear and culture are negative

Patient preparation
• As appropriate, explain the purpose of the test to the patient.
• Inform the patient that this test requires a specimen of urine or CSF.
• If a CSF specimen is required, describe how it will be obtained.
• Tell him who will perform the procedure and when and that he may experience transient discomfort from the needle puncture.
• Advise the patient that a headache is the most common complication of lumbar puncture but that his cooperation during the test minimizes such an effect.
• Make sure the patient or a family member has signed an informed consent form.

Procedure and posttest care
• Collect a 10-ml clean-catch specimen of urine or a 1-ml specimen of

CSF in a sterile container. (For detailed instructions on collecting a CSF specimen, see "Cerebrospinal fluid analysis" in Chapter 7.)

Precautions
• Maintain specimen sterility during collection.
• Wear gloves when obtaining or handling the specimen.
• Make sure the cap is tightly fastened on the specimen container.
• Place the specimen on a refrigerated coolant and send it to the laboratory promptly.

Normal findings
Normally, results are negative for bacterial antigens.

Abnormal findings
Positive results identify the specific bacterial antigen: *S. pneumoniae, N. meningitidis, H. influenzae* type B, or group B streptococci.

Interfering factors
• Previous antimicrobial therapy
• Failure to maintain sterility during specimen collection
• Failure to keep specimen cool
• Failure to send the specimen to the laboratory immediately

LYME DISEASE SEROLOGY

Lyme disease is a multisystem disorder characterized by dermatologic, neurologic, cardiac, and rheumatic manifestations in various stages. Epidemiologic and serologic studies implicate a common tickborne spirochete, *Borrelia burgdorferi*, as the causative agent.

Serologic tests are able to identify 50% of patients with early-stage Lyme disease and all patients with later complications of carditis, neuritis, and arthritis or who are in remission. The test uses one of three methods: Western blot test, enzyme-linked immunosorbent assay (ELISA), or indirect immunofluorescent assay.

ELISA is used as a screening test for identification of infection or past exposure. The Western blot test for immunoglobulin (IgG) antibody and the indirect immunofluorescent assay for IgM antibodies to *B. burgdorferi* are automatically performed to confirm reactive ELISA results greater than 1.0 index.

Purpose
• To confirm a diagnosis of Lyme disease

Patient preparation
• Explain to the patient that this test helps determine whether his symptoms are caused by Lyme disease.
• Instruct the patient to fast for 12 hours before the sample is drawn but to drink fluids as usual.
• Tell the patient that the test requires a blood sample and who will perform the venipuncture and when.
• Reassure him that although he may experience transient discomfort from the needle puncture and the tourniquet, collecting the sample takes less than 3 minutes.

Procedure and posttest care
• Perform a venipuncture, and collect the sample in a 7-ml *red-top* tube.
• If a hematoma develops at the venipuncture site, apply warm soaks.

Precautions
• Handle the specimen carefully to prevent hemolysis.

- Send the specimen to the laboratory immediately.

Reference values
Normal serum values are nonreactive for the ELISA method; the index is less than 1.0. Normal results for the Western blot test are negative for IgM; IgG of less than or equal to 4 bands is nonconfirmatory. Normal titer for the indirect immunofluorescent assay is less than 1:256.

Abnormal findings
A positive Lyme serology can help confirm diagnosis but isn't definitive. Other treponemal diseases and high rheumatoid factor titers can cause false-positive results. More than 15% of patients with Lyme disease fail to develop antibodies.

Interfering factors
- High serum lipid levels (possible in-accurate results, requiring repetition of the test after a period of restricted fat intake)
- Samples contaminated with other bacteria (possible false-positive)
- Hemolysis due to rough handling of the sample
- Failure to observe pretest restrictions

H. PYLORI ANTIBODIES

Helicobacter pylori is a spiral, gram-negative bacterium associated with chronic gastritis and idiopathic chronic duodenal ulceration. Although a gastric specimen can be obtained by endoscopy and cultured for *H. pylori*, the *H. pylori* antibody blood test is a more useful noninvasive screening procedure and

may be performed using the enzyme-linked immunosorbent assay (ELISA) test.

Purpose
- To help diagnose *H. pylori* infection in patients with GI symptoms

Patient preparation
- Inform the patient that this test is used to diagnose the infection that may cause ulcers.
- Tell him that he needn't restrict food or fluids.
- Explain that a blood sample will be taken and who will perform the venipuncture and when.
- Explain to him that, although he may experience slight discomfort from the tourniquet and the needle puncture, the test takes less than 3 minutes.

Procedure and posttest care
- Perform a venipuncture and collect the sample in a 7-ml *red-top* tube.
- Send the sample to the laboratory immediately.
- If a hematoma develops at the veni-puncture site, apply warm soaks.

Precautions
- This test should be performed only on patients with GI symptoms because of the large number of healthy people who have *H. pylori* antibodies.

Normal findings
Normally, no antibodies to *H. pylori* are revealed. Test results are reported as negative or positive.

Abnormal findings
A positive *H. pylori* test result indicates that the patient has antibodies to the bacterium. The serologic results should be interpreted in light of the clinical findings.

Interfering factors
- None significant

MISCELLANEOUS TESTS

VDRL TEST

The Venereal Disease Research Laboratory (VDRL) test is widely used to screen for primary and secondary syphilis. Usually, a serum sample is used in the VDRL test, but this test may also be performed on a specimen of cerebrospinal fluid (CSF) obtained by lumbar puncture to test for tertiary syphilis. The VDRL test of CSF is less sensitive than the fluorescent treponemal antibody absorption test.

Purpose
- To screen for primary and secondary syphilis
- To confirm primary or secondary syphilis in the presence of syphilitic lesions
- To monitor response to treatment

Patient preparation
- Explain to the patient that this test detects syphilis.
- Inform him that the disease often goes undetected in the general population because infected people remain untreated.
- Tell the patient that he needn't restrict food, fluids, or medications but should abstain from alcohol for 24 hours before the test.
- Tell him that the test requires a blood sample and who will perform the venipuncture and when.

- Reassure him that although he may experience transient discomfort from the needle puncture and the tourniquet, collecting the sample takes less than 3 minutes.

Procedure and posttest care
- Perform a venipuncture, and collect the sample in a 7-ml *red-top* tube.
- If a hematoma develops at the venipuncture site, apply warm soaks.
- If the test is nonreactive or borderline but syphilis hasn't been ruled out, instruct the patient to return for follow-up testing. Explain that borderline test results don't necessarily mean that he is free of the disease.
- If the test is reactive, explain the importance of proper treatment. Provide the patient with further information about sexually transmitted diseases and how they're spread, and stress the need for antibiotic therapy. Report the results to state public health authorities, and prepare the patient for mandatory inquiries.
- If the test is reactive but the patient shows no clinical signs of syphilis, explain that many uninfected people show false-positive reactions. Stress the need for further specific tests to rule out syphilis.

Precautions
- Handle the specimen carefully to prevent hemolysis.

Normal findings
Normal serum shows no flocculation and is reported as a nonreactive test.

Abnormal findings
Definite flocculation is reported as a reactive test; slight flocculation is reported as a weakly reactive test. A reactive VDRL test occurs in about 50% of patients with primary syphilis and in nearly all patients with secondary syphilis.

If syphilitic lesions exist, a reactive VDRL test is diagnostic. If no lesions are evident, a reactive VDRL test necessitates repeated testing. Biological false-positive reactions can be caused by conditions unrelated to syphilis, for example, infectious mononucleosis, malaria, leprosy, hepatitis, systemic lupus erythematosus, rheumatoid arthritis, and nonsyphilitic treponemal diseases, such as pinta and yaws.

A nonreactive test doesn't rule out syphilis because *Treponema pallidum* causes no detectable immunologic changes in the serum for 14 to 21 days after infection. Darkfield microscopy of exudate from suspicious lesions can provide early diagnosis by identifying the causative spirochetes.

A reactive VDRL test using a CSF specimen indicates neurosyphilis, which can follow the primary and secondary stages in patients who remain untreated.

Interfering factors
• Ingestion of alcohol within 24 hours of the test (possible transient nonreactive results)
• Immunosuppression (possible nonreactive results)
• Hemolysis due to rough handling of the sample

FLUORESCENT TREPONEMAL ANTIBODY ABSORPTION TEST

The fluorescent treponemal antibody absorption (FTA-ABS or simply FTA) test uses indirect immunofluorescence to detect antibodies to the spirochete *Treponema pallidum* in serum. This spirochete causes syphilis.

Although the FTA-ABS test is generally performed on a serum sample to detect primary or secondary syphilis, a cerebrospinal fluid (CSF) specimen is required to detect tertiary syphilis. Because antibody levels remain constant for long periods, the FTA-ABS test is not recommended for monitoring response to therapy. (See *Two tests for* Treponema pallidum, page 312.)

Purpose
• To confirm primary and secondary syphilis
• To screen for suspected false-positive results of Venereal Disease Research Laboratories (VDRL) tests

Patient preparation
• Explain to the patient that this test can confirm or rule out syphilis.
• Inform him that he needn't restrict food or fluids.
• Tell him that the test requires a blood sample and who will perform the venipuncture and when.
• Reassure him that although he may experience transient discomfort from the needle puncture and the tourniquet, collecting the blood sample usually takes less than 3 minutes.

Procedure and posttest care
• Perform a venipuncture, and collect the sample in a 7-ml *red-top* tube.
• If a hematoma develops at the venipuncture site, apply warm soaks.
• If the test is reactive, explain the nature of syphilis, and stress the importance of proper treatment and the need to find and treat the patient's sexual contacts.
• If appropriate, provide the patient with additional information about syphilis and how it's spread; emphasize the need for antibiotic therapy. Report positive results to state public health

TWO TESTS FOR *TREPONEMA PALLIDUM*

The microhemagglutination assay for the *Treponema pallidum* antibody increases the specificity of syphilis testing by eliminating methodologic interference. In this assay, tanned sheep red blood cells are coated with *T. pallidum* antigen and combined with absorbed test serum. Hemagglutination occurs in the presence of specific anti-*T. pallidum* antibodies in the serum.

In the enzyme-linked immunosorbent assay, tubes coated with *T. pallidum* are washed and then treated with enzyme-labeled antihuman globulin. After the substrate for the enzymes is added to the tubes, the enzymatic activity is measured by quantitating the reaction product formed.

authorities and prepare the patient for mandatory inquiries.

• If the test is nonreactive or findings are borderline but syphilis hasn't been ruled out, instruct the patient to return for follow-up testing; explain that inconclusive results don't necessarily indicate that he's free of the disease.

Precautions

• Handle the sample gently to prevent hemolysis.

Normal findings

Normally, results of the FTA-ABS test are nonreactive.

Abnormal findings

The presence of treponemal antibodies in the serum — a reactive test result — does not indicate the stage or severity of infection. (The presence of these antibodies in CSF is strong evidence of tertiary neurosyphilis.) Elevated antibody levels appear in most patients with primary syphilis and in almost all patients with secondary syphilis. Higher antibody levels persist for several years, with or without treatment.

The absence of treponemal antibodies — a nonreactive test result— does not necessarily rule out syphilis. *T. pallidum* causes no detectable immunologic changes in the blood for 14 to 21 days after initial infection. Organisms may be detected earlier by examining suspicious lesions with a darkfield microscope. Low antibody levels and other nonspecific factors produce borderline findings. In such cases, repeated testing and a thorough review of patient history may be productive.

Although the FTA-ABS test is specific, some patients with nonsyphilitic conditions, such as systemic lupus erythematosus, genital herpes, and increased or abnormal globulins, or those who are pregnant may show minimally reactive levels. In addition, the FTA-ABS test doesn't always distinguish between *T. pallidum* and certain other treponemas, such as those that cause pinta, yaws, and bejel.

Interfering factor

• Hemolysis due to rough handling of the sample

Two cancer tests

Two tests for certain cancers may soon be part of the diagnostic arsenal.

CA19-9 antigen test
The CA19-9 carbohydrate antigen test has proven to be a valuable tool in the early detection of pancreatic cancer. Found in the blood, the antigen is a tumor marker that will help in differentiating benign pancreatic tumors from malignant tumors. High blood levels of the antigen may indicate cancer of the pancreas or other GI sites, such as the liver or colon.

Hercep test
The Food and Drug Administration recently approved the Hercep test as a method of detecting breast cancer. This immunohistochemical assay detects breast tumors that produce excessive amounts of the HER2 protein. It may also be helpful in diagnosing a relapse of breast cancer.

Carcinoembryonic Antigen

Carcinoembryonic antigen (CEA) is a protein normally found in embryonic entodermal epithelium and fetal GI tissue. Production of CEA stops before birth, but it may begin again later if a neoplasm develops. Because CEA levels are also raised by biliary obstruction, alcoholic hepatitis, chronic heavy smoking, and other conditions, this test can't be used as a general indicator of cancer. The measurement of enzyme CEA levels by immunoassay is useful for staging and monitoring treatment of certain cancers.

Other tests are used to diagnose certain types of cancer. (See *Two cancer tests*.)

Purpose
● To monitor the effectiveness of cancer therapy
● To assist in preoperative staging of colorectal cancers, assess adequacy of surgical resection, and test for recurrence of colorectal cancers

Patient preparation
● Explain to the patient that this test detects and measures a special protein that isn't normally present in adults.
● If appropriate, inform him that the test will be repeated to monitor the effectiveness of therapy.
● Advise him that he needn't restrict food, fluids, or medications before the test.
● Tell him that the test requires a blood sample and who will perform the venipuncture and when.
● Reassure him that although he may experience discomfort from the needle puncture and the tourniquet, collecting the sample takes less than 3 minutes.

Procedure and posttest care
● Perform a venipuncture, and collect the sample in a 7-ml *red-top* tube.
● If a hematoma develops at the venipuncture site, apply warm soaks.

Precautions

• Handle the sample gently to prevent hemolysis, and send it to the laboratory immediately.

Reference values

Normal serum CEA values are less than 5 ng/ml.

Abnormal findings

Persistent elevation of CEA levels suggests residual or recurrent tumor. If levels exceed normal before surgical resection, chemotherapy, or radiation therapy, their return to normal within 6 weeks suggests successful treatment.

High CEA levels are characteristic in various malignant conditions, particularly entodermally derived neoplasms of the GI organs and the lungs, and in certain nonmalignant conditions, such as benign hepatic disease, hepatic cirrhosis, alcoholic pancreatitis, and inflammatory bowel disease.

Elevated CEA concentrations may occur in nonendodermal carcinomas, such as breast cancer and ovarian cancer.

Interfering factors

• Chronic cigarette smoking (possible increase)
• Hemolysis due to rough handling of the sample

ALPHA-FETOPROTEIN

Alpha-fetoprotein (AFP) is a glycoprotein produced by fetal tissue and tumors that differentiate from midline embryonic structures. During fetal development, AFP levels in serum and amniotic fluid rise. AFP crosses the placenta and appears in maternal serum.

High maternal serum AFP levels may suggest fetal neural tube defects, such as spina bifida and anencephaly, but positive confirmation requires amniocentesis and ultrasonography. Other congenital anomalies, such as Down syndrome and other chromosomal disorders, may be associated with low maternal serum AFP concentrations.

Elevated AFP levels in patients who aren't pregnant may occur in cancers, such as hepatocellular carcinoma, or certain nonmalignant conditions, such as ataxia-telangiectasia. In these conditions, AFP assays are more useful for monitoring response to therapy than for diagnosis. AFP levels are best determined by enzyme immunoassay on amniotic fluid or serum.

Purpose

• To monitor the effectiveness of therapy in malignant conditions, such as hepatomas and germ cell tumors, and certain nonmalignant conditions, such as ataxia-telangiectasia
• To screen for the need for amniocentesis or high-resolution ultrasonography in a pregnant woman

Patient preparation

• Explain to the patient that this test monitors her response to therapy by measuring a specific blood protein. Advise her that further testing may be necessary.
• Tell her that she needn't restrict food, fluids, or medications before the test.
• Tell her that this test requires a blood sample and who will perform the venipuncture and when.
• Reassure her that although she may experience transient discomfort from the needle puncture and the tourniquet, collecting the sample takes less than 3 minutes.

Procedure and posttest care

• Perform a venipuncture, and collect the sample in a 7-ml *red-top* tube.

• Record the patient's age, race, weight, and gestational period on the laboratory slip.

• If a hematoma develops at the venipuncture site, apply warm soaks.

Precautions

• Handle the sample gently to prevent hemolysis.

Reference values

When testing by immunoassay, AFP values are less than 15 ng/ml in men and nonpregnant women. Values in maternal serum are less than 2.5 multiples of median (Mom) for fetal gestational age.

Abnormal findings

Elevated maternal serum AFP levels may suggest neural tube defects or other tube anomalies. Maternal AFP levels rise sharply in the maternal blood of about 90% of women carrying a fetus with anencephaly and in 50% of those carrying a fetus with spina bifida. Definitive diagnosis requires ultrasonography and amniocentesis. High AFP levels may indicate intrauterine death. Sometimes high levels indicate other anomalies, such as duodenal atresia, omphalocele, tetralogy of Fallot, and Turner's syndrome.

Elevated serum AFP levels occur in 70% of nonpregnant patients with hepatocellular carcinoma. Elevated levels are also related to germ cell tumor of gonadal, retroperitoneal, or mediastinal origin. Serum AFP levels rise in ataxia-telangiectasia and sometimes in cancer of the pancreas, stomach, or biliary system and in nonseminiferous testicular tumor. Transient modest elevations can occur in nonneoplastic hepatocellular disease, such as alcoholic cirrhosis and acute or chronic hepatitis. Elevation of AFP levels after remission suggests tumor recurrence.

In hepatocellular carcinoma, a gradual decrease in serum AFP levels indicates a favorable response to therapy. In germ cell tumors, serum AFP levels and serum human chorionic gonadotropin levels should be measured concurrently.

Low serum AFP values correlate with chromosomal disorders but require further investigation. Failure of the AFP value to return to normal by about 1 month after cancer therapy suggests the presence of residual tumor.

Interfering factors

• Hemolysis due to rough handling of the sample

• Multiple pregnancies (possible false-positive)

TORCH TEST

This test helps detect exposure to pathogens involved in congenital and neonatal infections. TORCH is an acronym for toxoplasmosis, rubella, cytomegalovirus, and herpes simplex antibodies. These pathogens are commonly associated with congenital and neonatal infections that aren't clinically apparent and may cause severe central nervous system impairment. This test detects specific immunoglobulin M-associated antibodies in infant blood.

Purpose

• To aid diagnosis of acute, congenital, and intrapartum infections

Patient preparation
• Explain to the infant's parents the purpose of the test and mention that the test requires a blood sample.
• Tell them who will perform the venipuncture and when. Reassure them that although their child may experience transient discomfort, collecting the sample takes less than 3 minutes.

Procedure and posttest care
• Obtain a 3-ml sample of venous or cord blood.
• If a hematoma develops at the venipuncture site, apply warm soaks.

Precautions
• Handle the sample gently to prevent hemolysis.
• Send the sample to the laboratory immediately.
• Don't freeze the sample.

Normal findings
Normal test result is negative for TORCH agents.

Abnormal findings
Toxoplasmosis is diagnosed by sequential examination that shows rising antibody titers, changing titers, and serologic conversion from negative to positive; a titer of 1:256 suggests recent *Toxoplasma* infection.

In infants less than 6 months old, rubella infection is associated with a marked and persistent rise in complement-fixing antibody titer over time. Persistence of rubella antibody in an infant after age 6 months strongly suggests congenital infection. Congenital rubella is associated with cardiac anomalies, neurosensory deafness, growth retardation, and encephalitic symptoms.

Detection of herpes antibodies in cerebrospinal fluid with signs of herpetic encephalitis and persistent herpes simplex virus type 2 antibody levels confirms herpes simplex infection in a neonate without obvious herpetic lesions.

Interfering factors
• Hemolysis due to rough handling of the sample
• Failure to send the sample to the laboratory immediately

TUBERCULIN SKIN TESTS

Tuberculin skin tests are used to screen for previous infection by the tubercle bacillus. They're routinely performed in children, young adults, and patients with radiographic findings that suggest this infection. In both the old tuberculin (OT) and purified protein derivative (PPD) tests, intradermal injection of the tuberculin antigen causes a delayed hypersensitivity reaction in patients with active or dormant tuberculosis.

The Mantoux test uses a single-needle intradermal injection of PPD, permitting precise measurement of the dose. Multipuncture tests, such as the tine test, MonoVacc tests, and Aplitest, use intradermal injections with tines impregnated with OT or PPD. Because they require less skill and are more rapidly administered, multipuncture tests are generally used for screening. A positive multipuncture test usually requires a Mantoux test for confirmation.

Purpose
• To distinguish tuberculosis from blastomycosis, coccidioidomycosis, and histoplasmosis

• To identify people who need diagnostic investigation for tuberculosis because of possible exposure

Patient preparation
• Explain to the patient that this test helps detect tuberculosis.
• Tell him that the test requires an intradermal injection, which may cause him transient discomfort.
• Check the patient's history for active tuberculosis, the results of previous skin tests, and hypersensitivities.
• If the patient has had tuberculosis, don't perform a skin test.
• If he's had a positive reaction to previous skin tests, consult the doctor or follow hospital policy.
• If he's had an allergic reaction to acacia, don't perform an OT test because this product contains acacia.
• If you're performing a tuberculin test on an outpatient, instruct him to return at the specified time so that test results can be read.
• Inform the patient that a positive reaction to a skin test appears as a red, hard, raised area at the injection site. Although the area may itch, instruct him not to scratch it.
• Stress that a positive reaction doesn't always indicate active tuberculosis.

Procedure and posttest care
• Ask the patient to sit and support his extended arm on a flat surface.
• Clean the volar surface of the upper forearm with alcohol, and allow the area to dry completely.
Mantoux test
• Perform an intradermal injection.
Multipuncture test
• Remove the protective cap on the injection device to expose the four tines.
• Hold the patient's forearm in one hand, stretching the skin of the forearm tightly. Then, with your other hand,

firmly depress the device into the patient's skin, without twisting it.
• Hold the device in place for at least 1 second before removing it.
• If you've applied sufficient pressure, you'll see four puncture sites and a circular depression made by the device on the patient's skin.
Both tests
• Record where the test was given, the date and time, and when the results are to be read. Tuberculin skin tests are generally read 48 to 72 hours after injection; the MonoVacc test can be read 48 to 96 hours after the test.
• If ulceration or necrosis develops at the injection site, apply cold soaks or a topical steroid.

Precautions
• Tuberculin skin tests are contraindicated in patients with current reactions to smallpox vaccinations, a rash, a skin disorder, or active tuberculosis.
• Don't perform a skin test in areas with excessive hair, acne, or insufficient subcutaneous tissue, such as over a tendon or bone.
• If the patient is known to be hypersensitive to skin tests, use a first-strength dose in the Mantoux test to avoid necrosis at the puncture site.
• Have epinephrine available to treat a possible anaphylactoid or acute hypersensitivity reaction.

Normal findings
In tuberculin skin tests, normal findings show negative or minimal reactions. In the Mantoux test, no induration may appear or the patient may develop induration less than 5 mm in diameter.
   In the tine and Aplitest tests, no vesiculation or induration may appear or the patient may develop induration less than 2 mm in diameter. In the MonoVacc tests, no induration appears.

Abnormal findings

A positive tuberculin reaction indicates previous infection by tubercle bacilli. It doesn't distinguish between an active and a dormant infection or provide a definitive diagnosis. If a positive reaction occurs, sputum smear and culture and chest radiography are necessary for further information.

In the Mantoux test, induration 5 to 9 mm in diameter indicates a borderline reaction; larger induration, a positive reaction. Because patients infected with atypical mycobacteria other than tubercle bacilli may have borderline reactions, repeat testing is necessary.

In the tine or Aplitest tests, vesiculation indicates a positive reaction; induration 2 mm in diameter without vesiculation requires confirmation by the Mantoux test. Any induration in the MonoVacc test indicates a positive reaction; however, it requires confirmation by the Mantoux test.

Interfering factors

● Subcutaneous injection, usually indicated by erythema > 10 mm in diameter without induration

● Corticosteroids, other immunosuppressants, and live vaccine viruses, such as measles, mumps, rubella, and polio, within 4 to 6 weeks before the test (possible suppression of skin reaction)

● In elderly people and patients with viral infection, malnutrition, febrile illness, uremia, immunosuppressive disorders, or miliary tuberculosis (possible suppression of skin reaction)

● Less than 10-week period since infection (possible suppression of skin reaction)

● Improper dilution, dosage, or storage of the tuberculin

CHAPTER 6

Urine Tests

URINALYSIS 321

321 Routine urinalysis
324 Urinary calculi
325 Phenolsulfonphthalein
    excretion

327 Concentration and dilution tests
328 Tubular reabsorption of
    phosphate

ENZYMES 329

329 Amylase
330 Arylsulfatase A
331 Lysozyme

332 Cyclic adenosine mono-
    phosphate

HORMONES 334

334 Aldosterone
335 Free cortisol
336 Catecholamines

337 Total urine estrogens
339 Placental estriol
340 Human chorionic gonadotropin

METABOLITES 341

341 Pregnanetriol
342 17-Hydroxycorticosteroids
343 17-Ketosteroids
346 17-Ketogenic steroids

347 Vanillylmandelic acid
348 Homovanillic acid
349 5-Hydroxyindoleacetic acid
350 Pregnanediol

PROTEINS AND PROTEIN METABOLITES 351

351 Proteins
353 Bence Jones protein
353 Amino acid screening
357 Hydroxyproline

358 Creatinine
359 Creatinine clearance
360 Uric acid

PIGMENTS 361

361 Hemoglobin
362 Myoglobin
363 Porphyrins

365 δ-aminolevulinic acid
366 Bilirubin
368 Urobilinogen

SUGARS, KETONES, AND MUCOPOLYSACCHARIDES 369

369 Copper reduction test
370 Glucose oxidase test

372 Ketone test
373 Acid mucopolysaccharides

VITAMINS 374

374 Tryptophan challenge test   375 Vitamin C

MINERALS 376

376 Sodium and chloride   380 Copper
377 Potassium   381 Hemosiderin
378 Calcium and phosphates   382 Oxalate
379 Magnesium

URINALYSIS

ROUTINE URINALYSIS

Routine urinalysis tests screen for urinary and systemic disorders. These tests evaluate physical characteristics (color, odor, and opacity) of urine; determine specific gravity and pH; detect and measure protein, glucose, and ketone bodies; and examine sediment for blood cells, casts, and crystals.

Diagnostic laboratory methods include visual examination, reagent strip screening, refractometry for specific gravity, and microscopic inspection of centrifuged sediment.

Purpose
• To screen patient's urine for renal or urinary tract disease
• To help detect metabolic or systemic disease unrelated to renal disorders

Patient preparation
• Explain to the patient that this test aids diagnosis of renal or urinary tract disease and helps evaluate overall body function.
• Inform him that food or fluids need not be restricted before the test.
• Check his medication history; many drugs may affect test results.

Procedure and posttest care
• Collect a random urine specimen of at least 10 ml.
• Obtain a first-voided morning specimen if possible.

Precautions
• Strain the specimen to catch stones or stone fragments if the patient is being evaluated for renal colic.

• Carefully pour the urine through an unfolded 4″ × 4″ gauze pad or a fine-mesh sieve placed over the specimen container.
• Send the specimen to the laboratory immediately.
• Refrigerate the specimen if analysis will be delayed longer than 1 hour.

Normal findings
See *Normal findings in routine urinalysis*, page 322.

Abnormal findings
Nonpathologic variations in normal values may result from diet, nonpathologic conditions, specimen collection time, and other factors.

Urine pH, which is greatly affected by diet and medications, influences the appearance of urine and the composition of crystals. An alkaline pH (above 7.0) — characteristic of a vegetarian diet — causes turbidity and the formation of phosphate, carbonate, and amorphous crystals. An acid pH (below 7.0) — typical of a high-protein diet — produces turbidity and the formation of oxalate, cystine, leucine, tyrosine, amorphous urate, and uric acid crystals.

Protein, normally absent from the urine, may be present in a benign condition known as orthostatic (postural) proteinuria. Most common in patients ages 10 to 20, this condition is intermittent, appears after prolonged standing, and disappears after recumbency. Transient benign proteinuria can also occur with fever, exposure to cold, emotional stress, or strenuous exercise.

Sugars, usually absent from the urine, may appear under normal conditions. The most common sugar in urine is glucose. Transient nonpathologic glycosuria may result from emotional stress or pregnancy and may follow ingestion of a high-carbohydrate meal.

NORMAL FINDINGS IN ROUTINE URINALYSIS

ELEMENT	FINDINGS
Macroscopic	
Color	Pale yellow to amber
Odor	Slightly aromatic
Appearance	Clear
Specific gravity	1.005 to 1.035
pH	4.5 to 8
Protein	None
Glucose	None
Ketone bodies	None
Bilirubin	None
Urobilinogen	Normal
Hemoglobin	None
Erythrocytes (RBCs)	None
Nitrite (bacteria)	None
Leukocytes (WBCs)	None
Microscopic	
RBCs	0 to 3/high-power field
WBCs	0 to 4/high-power field
Epithelial cells	0 to 5/high-power field
Casts	None, except 1 to 2 hyaline casts/low-power field
Crystals	Present
Bacteria	None
Yeast cells	None
Parasites	None

Centrifuged urine sediment contains cells, casts, crystals, bacteria, yeast, and parasites. Red blood cells (RBCs) don't often appear in urine without pathologic significance, but hard exercise can cause hematuria.

The following abnormal findings generally suggest pathologic conditions:

- *Color:* Color change can result from diet, drugs, and many diseases.
- *Odor:* In diabetes mellitus, starvation, and dehydration, a fruity odor accompanies formation of ketone bodies. In urinary tract infections, a fetid odor commonly is associated with *Escherichia coli.* Maple syrup urine disease and phenylketonuria also cause distinctive odors.
- *Turbidity:* Turbid urine may contain red or white cells, bacteria, fat, or chyle and may reflect renal infection.
- *Specific gravity:* Low specific gravity (< 1.005) is characteristic of diabetes insipidus, nephrogenic diabetes insipidus, acute tubular necrosis, and pyelonephritis. Fixed specific gravity, in which values remain 1.010 regardless of fluid intake, occurs in chronic glomerulonephritis with severe renal damage. High specific gravity (> 1.035) occurs in nephrotic syndrome, dehydration, acute glomerulonephritis, heart failure, liver failure, and shock.
- *pH:* Alkaline urine pH may result from Fanconi's syndrome, urinary tract infection, and metabolic or respiratory alkalosis. Acid urine pH is associated with renal tuberculosis, pyrexia, phenylketonuria, alkaptonuria, and acidosis.
- *Protein:* Proteinuria suggests renal failure or disease (including nephrosis, glomerulosclerosis, glomerulonephritis, nephrolithiasis, and polycystic kidney disease), or possibly multiple myeloma.
- *Sugars:* Glycosuria usually indicates diabetes mellitus but may result from pheochromocytoma, Cushing's syndrome, impaired tubular reabsorption, advanced renal disease, and increased intracranial pressure. Fructosuria, galactosuria, and pentosuria generally suggest rare hereditary metabolic disorders (except for lactosuria during pregnancy and lactation). However, an alimentary form of pentosuria and fructosuria may follow excessive ingestion of pentose or fructose. When the liver fails to metabolize these sugars, they spill into the urine because the renal tubules don't reabsorb them.

- *Ketone bodies:* Ketonuria occurs in diabetes mellitus when cellular energy needs exceed available cellular glucose. In the absence of glucose, cells metabolize fat for energy. Ketone bodies — the end products of incomplete fat metabolism — accumulate in plasma and are excreted in the urine. Ketonuria may also occur in starvation states and following diarrhea or vomiting.
- *Bilirubin:* Bilirubin in urine may occur in liver disease resulting from obstructive jaundice or hepatotoxic drugs or toxins, or from fibrosis of the biliary canaliculi (which may occur in cirrhosis).
- *Urobilinogen:* Intestinal bacteria in the duodenum change bilirubin into urobilinogen. The liver reprocesses the remainder into bile. Increased urobilinogen in the urine may indicate liver damage, hemolytic disease, or severe infection. Decreased levels may occur with biliary obstruction, inflammatory disease, antimicrobial therapy, severe diarrhea, or renal insufficiency.
- *Cells:* Hematuria indicates bleeding within the genitourinary tract and may result from infection, obstruction, inflammation, trauma, tumors, glomerulonephritis, renal hypertension, lupus nephritis, renal tuberculosis, renal vein thrombosis, renal calculi, hydronephrosis, pyelonephritis, scurvy, malaria, parasitic infection of the bladder, subacute bacterial endocarditis, polyarteritis nodosa, and hemorrhagic disorders. Strenuous exercise or exposure to toxic chemicals may also cause hematuria. An excess of white blood cells (WBCs)

in urine usually implies urinary tract inflammation, especially cystitis or pyelonephritis. WBC and WBC casts in urine suggest renal infection. Numerous epithelial cells suggest renal tubular degeneration.

● *Casts (plugs of gelled proteinaceous material [high-molecular-weight mucoprotein]):* Casts form in the renal tubules and collecting ducts by agglutination of protein cells or cellular debris and are flushed loose by urine flow. Excessive numbers of casts indicate renal disease. Hyaline casts are associated with renal parenchymal disease, inflammation, trauma to the glomerular capillary membrane, and some physiologic states (such as after exercise); epithelial casts, with renal tubular damage, nephrosis, eclampsia, amyloidosis, and heavy metal poisoning; coarse and fine granular casts, with acute or chronic renal failure, pyelonephritis, and chronic lead intoxication; fatty and waxy casts, with nephrotic syndrome, chronic renal disease, and diabetes mellitus; RBC casts, with renal parenchymal disease (especially glomerulonephritis), renal infarction, subacute bacterial endocarditis, vascular disorders, sickle cell anemia, scurvy, blood dyscrasias, malignant hypertension, collagen disease, and acute inflammation; and white blood cell casts, with acute pyelonephritis and glomerulonephritis, nephrotic syndrome, pyogenic infection, and lupus nephritis.

● *Crystals:* Some crystals normally appear in urine, but numerous calcium oxalate crystals suggest hypercalcemia or ethylene glycol ingestion. Cystine crystals (cystinuria) reflect an inborn error of metabolism.

● *Other components:* Bacteria, yeast cells, and parasites in urine sediment reflect genitourinary tract infection or contamination of external genitalia. Yeast cells, which may be mistaken for red blood cells, are identifiable by their ovoid shape, lack of color, variable size and, frequently, signs of budding. The most common parasite in sediment is *Trichomonas vaginalis,* which causes vaginitis, urethritis, and prostatovesiculitis.

Interfering factors
● Insufficient urinary volume, < 2 ml (possible limitation of the range of procedures)
● Failure to send specimen to the laboratory immediately (false-low urobilinogen)
● High dietary vitamin C intake (false-negative for presence of glucose; possible false-negative nitrate test)
● Foods, such as beets and rhubarb (false change in color)
● Drugs, such as phenytoin, phenazopyridine and oral anticoagulants (possible false change in color)

URINARY CALCULI

Urinary calculi (urinary stones) are insoluble substances most commonly formed of the mineral salts — calcium oxalate, calcium phosphate, magnesium ammonium phosphate, urate, or cystine. They may appear anywhere in the urinary tract and range in size from microscopic to several centimeters.

Formation of calculi can result from reduced urinary volume, increased excretion of mineral salts, urinary stasis, pH changes, and decreased protective substances. Calculi commonly form in the kidney, pass into the ureter, and are excreted in the urine. Because not all calculi pass spontaneously, they may require surgical extraction. Calculi don't always cause symptoms, but when they do, hematuria is most common. If calculi obstruct the ureter, they may cause severe flank pain, dysuria, and urinary retention, frequency, and urgency.

Purpose
• To detect and identify calculi in the urine

Patient preparation
• Explain to the patient that this test detects urinary stones and that laboratory analysis will reveal their composition.
• Tell him that his urine will be collected and strained.
• Advise him that no prior restriction of food or fluids is required.
• Reassure him that symptoms will subside immediately after excretion of any stones.
• Inform him that medication to control pain will be administered.

Equipment
Strainer (an unfolded 4″ × 4″ dressing or a fine-mesh sieve), specimen container

Procedure and posttest care
• Have the patient void into the strainer.
• Inspect the strainer carefully because calculi may be minute, looking like gravel or sand.
• Document the appearance of the calculi and the number if possible.
• Place the calculi in a properly labeled container.
• Send the container to the laboratory immediately for prompt analysis.
• Observe for severe flank pain, dysuria, and urinary retention, frequency, or urgency. Hematuria should subside.

Precautions
• Keep the strainer and urinal or bedpan within the patient's reach if he has received analgesics because he may be drowsy and unable to get out of bed to void.

Normal findings
Normally, calculi aren't present in urine.

Abnormal findings
More than half of all calculi in urine are of mixed composition, containing two or more mineral salts; calcium oxalate is the most common component. Determination of the composition of calculi helps identify various metabolic disorders, guiding proper treatment and prevention measures.

Interfering factor
• Improper collection technique

PHENOLSULFONPHTHA-LEIN EXCRETION

The phenolsulfonphthalein (PSP) excretion test evaluates kidney function. This test is indicated in patients with abnormal results in the urine concentration test, one of the earliest signs of renal dysfunction.

Purpose
• To determine renal plasma flow
• To evaluate tubular function

Patient preparation
• Explain to the patient that this test evaluates kidney function.
• Inform him that he needn't restrict food before the test. Encourage him to drink fluids before and during the test to maintain adequate urine flow.
• Tell him the test requires an I.V. injection and collection of urine specimens 15 minutes, 30 minutes, 1 hour

and, if ordered, 2 hours after the I.V. injection.

• Inform him who will administer the I.V. injection and when.

• Advise him that he may feel transient discomfort from the needle puncture and the pressure of the tourniquet, and that the dye temporarily turns the urine red.

• If the patient is unable to void and requires catheterization, tell him that he may have the urge to void when the catheter is in place.

• Withhold drugs that may affect test results, such as chlorothiazide, aspirin, phenylbutazone, sulfonamides, penicillin, and probenecid. If they must be continued, note this on the laboratory slip.

Equipment

6 mg of PSP dye in 1 ml of solution, equipment for indwelling urinary catheterization, four urine specimen containers

Procedure and posttest care

• Instruct the patient to empty his bladder, and discard the urine.

• The doctor will administer 1 ml of PSP, which equals 6 mg of dye, I.V.

• Collect a urine specimen at 15 minutes, 30 minutes, 1 hour and, if ordered, 2 hours after the injection.

• Because 40 ml of urine is required for each specimen, encourage fluid intake.

• If the patient is catheterized, make sure to clamp the catheter between collections.

• Record the PSP dosage on the laboratory slip.

• Properly label each specimen, and include the collection time.

• Elevate the arm and apply warm soaks if phlebitis develops at the I.V. site.

• If the patient is catheterized, make sure he voids within 8 to 10 hours after the catheter is removed.

• Resume administration of medications withheld during the test.

Precautions

• Use this test cautiously in a patient with cardiac dysfunction or renal insufficiency because the increased fluid intake necessary for proper hydration may precipitate heart failure.

• Keep epinephrine available because allergic reactions to PSP occasionally occur.

• Don't use the urine in the drainage bag if the patient already has a catheter in place.

• Empty the bag, and clamp the catheter for 1 hour before the test.

• Send specimen to the laboratory immediately after each collection.

• Refrigerate the specimen if more than 10 minutes will elapse before transport.

Reference values

Normally, 25% of the PSP dose is excreted in 15 minutes, 50% to 60% in 30 minutes, 60% to 70% in 1 hour, and 70% to 80% in 2 hours. Normal excretion for children (excluding infants) is 5% to 10% higher than for adults.

Abnormal findings

The 15-minute value is the most sensitive indicator of both tubular function and renal plasma flow because depressed excretion at this interval but normal excretion later suggests relatively mild or early-stage bilateral renal disease. However, a depressed 2-hour value may reveal moderate-to-severe renal impairment. Depressed PSP excretion is also characteristic in renal vascular disease, urinary tract obstruction, heart failure, and gout.

Elevated PSP excretion is characteristic in hypoalbuminemia, hepatic disease, and multiple myeloma.

Interfering factors
- Failure to collect an adequate specimen at required times
- Radiographic contrast agents, chlorothiazide, salicylates, sulfonamides, penicillin, cascara sagrada, ethanol, indomethacin, nitrofurantoin, phenylbutazone, probenecid, and vitamins (possible increase or decrease)
- Beets, carrots, and rhubarb (possible increase or decrease)
- Incorrect PSP dosage (possible increase or decrease)
- High serum protein levels (decrease)
- Severe hypoalbuminemia, excessive albuminuria, or severe liver disease (possible effect on excretion)

CONCENTRATION AND DILUTION TESTS

The kidneys normally concentrate or dilute urine according to fluid intake. When such intake is excessive, the kidneys excrete more water in the urine; when intake is limited, they excrete less. This test evaluates renal capacity to concentrate urine in response to fluid deprivation, or to dilute it in response to fluid overload.

Purpose
- To evaluate renal tubular function
- To detect renal impairment

Patient preparation
- Explain to the patient that this test evaluates kidney function.
- Tell him the test requires multiple urine specimens. Explain how many specimens will be collected and at what intervals.
- Instruct him to discard any urine voided during the night.
- Withhold diuretics as needed.
Concentration test
- Provide a high-protein meal and only 200 ml of fluid the night before the test.
- Instruct the patient to restrict food and fluids for at least 14 hours before the test. (Some concentration tests require that water be withheld for 24 hours but permit relatively normal food intake.)
- Limit salt intake at the evening meal to prevent excessive thirst.
- Emphasize to the patient that his cooperation is necessary to obtain accurate results.
Dilution test
- Generally, this test directly follows the concentration test and necessitates no additional patient preparation. If it's performed alone, simply withhold breakfast.

Procedure and posttest care
Concentration test
- Collect urine specimens at 6 a.m., 8 a.m., and 10 a.m.
Dilution test
- Instruct the patient to void and discard the urine.
- Give him 1,500 ml of water to drink within 30 minutes.
- Collect urine specimens every half hour or every hour for 4 hours thereafter.
Both tests
- Provide a balanced meal or a snack after collecting the final specimen.
- Make sure the patient voids within 8 to 10 hours after the catheter is removed.

Precautions
- May be contraindicated in patients with advanced renal disease or cardiac

dysfunction because fluid overload can precipitate water intoxication, sodium diuresis, or heart failure.
- Send each specimen to the laboratory immediately after collection.
- Provide the patient with a clean bedpan, urinal, or toilet specimen pan if he is unable to urinate into the specimen containers.
- Rinse the collection device after each use.
- If the patient is catheterized, empty the drainage bag before the test. Obtain the specimens from the catheter, and clamp the catheter between collections.

Reference values
Normal specific gravity ranges from 1.005 to 1.035; osmolality normally ranges from 300 to 900 mOsm/kg.
  Concentration test: Specific gravity ranges from 1.025 to 1.032 and osmolality rises above 800 mOsm/kg of water in patients with normal renal function.
  Dilution test: Normally, specific gravity falls below 1.003 and osmolality below 100 mOsm/kg for at least one specimen; 80% or more of the ingested water is eliminated in 4 hours. In elderly persons, depressed values can be associated with normal renal function.

Abnormal findings
Decreased renal capacity to concentrate urine in response to fluid deprivation, or to dilute urine in response to fluid overload, may indicate tubular epithelial damage, decreased renal blood flow, loss of functional nephrons, or pituitary or cardiac dysfunction.

Interfering factors
- Failure to observe pretest restrictions
- Use of radiographic contrast agents within 7 days of test (possible increase in osmolality)

- Diuretics and nephrotoxic drugs (possible increase or decrease in specific gravity and osmolality)
- Glycosuria

TUBULAR REABSORPTION OF PHOSPHATE

The test for tubular reabsorption of phosphate is an indirect measure of parathyroid hormone (PTH) levels. PTH helps maintain optimum blood levels of ionized calcium and controls renal excretion of calcium and phosphate. In this test, urine and serum phosphate and creatinine are measured, and these values are used to calculate the tubular reabsorption of phosphate.

Purpose
- To evaluate parathyroid function
- To aid diagnosis of primary hyperparathyroidism
- To distinguish between hypercalcemia due to hyperparathyroidism and hypercalcemia due to other causes

Patient preparation
- Explain to the patient that this test evaluates the function of the parathyroid glands.
- Advise him that the test requires a blood sample and urine collection over a 24-hour period.
- Tell the patient who'll perform the venipuncture and when.
- Advise the patient that he may experience transient discomfort from the needle puncture and the pressure of the tourniquet.
- Reassure him that collecting the blood sample generally takes less than 3 minutes.

• Instruct the patient to maintain a normal phosphate diet for 3 days before the test because low phosphate intake (< 500 mg/day) may elevate tubular reabsorption values and a high-phosphate diet (3,000 mg/day) may lower them. Common nutritional sources of phosphorus include legumes, nuts, milk, egg yolks, meat, poultry, fish, cereals, and cheese. These foods should be eaten in moderate amounts.

• Instruct the patient to fast after midnight the night before the test.

• As necessary, withhold drugs that may influence test results, such as amphotericin B, chlorothiazide diuretics, furosemide, and gentamicin. If these medications must be continued throughout the test period, note this on the laboratory slip.

Procedure and posttest care

• Perform a venipuncture, and collect the sample in a 10-ml *red-top* tube.

• Instruct the patient to empty his bladder, and discard the urine; record this as time zero.

• Collect the patient's urine over a 24-hour period; occasionally, a 4-hour collection or a random collection is ordered instead.

• Allow the patient to eat, and encourage fluid intake to maintain adequate urine flow after the venipuncture.

• Apply warm soaks if a hematoma develops at the venipuncture site.

• Resume administration of medications withheld during the test.

• Tell the patient that he may resume his usual diet.

Precautions

• Handle the collection tube gently to prevent hemolysis.

• Keep the urine specimen container refrigerated or on ice during the collection period.

• Tell the patient to avoid contaminating the specimen with toilet paper or stool.

• Label the specimen and send it to the laboratory as soon as the collection period has ended.

Normal findings

Renal tubules normally reabsorb 80% or more of phosphate.

Abnormal findings

Reabsorption of less than 74% of phosphate strongly suggests primary hyperparathyroidism. Hypercalcemia is the most common manifestation of primary hyperparathyroidism. However, a patient with hypercalcemia may still require additional testing to confirm primary hyperparathyroidism as the cause.

Interfering factors

• Uremia, renal tubular disease, osteomalacia, and sarcoidosis (possible decrease)

• Renal calculi in patients not having parathyroid tumor (possible decrease)

• Contamination of the specimen with toilet tissue or stool

• Hemolysis due to rough handling of the sample

• Failure to keep the specimen on ice or to send it to the laboratory immediately

ENZYMES

AMYLASE

Amylase is a starch-splitting enzyme produced primarily in the pancreas and salivary glands, which is usually secreted into the alimentary tract and absorbed into the blood; small amounts of amylase are also absorbed into the blood directly from these organs. Following glomerular filtration, amylase is excreted in the urine.

In the presence of adequate renal function, serum and urine levels usually rise in tandem. However, within 2 or 3 days of onset of acute pancreatitis, serum amylase levels fall to normal, but elevated urine amylase persists for 7 to 10 days. One method for determining urine amylase levels is the dye-coupled starch method.

Purpose
• To diagnose acute pancreatitis when serum amylase levels are normal or borderline
• To aid diagnosis of chronic pancreatitis and salivary gland disorders

Patient preparation
• Explain to the patient that this test evaluates the function of the pancreas and the salivary glands.
• Inform him that he needn't restrict food or fluids.
• Tell him the test requires urine collection for 2, 6, 8, or 24 hours, and teach him how to collect a timed specimen.

Procedure and posttest care
• Collect the patient's urine over a 2-, 6-, 8-, or 24-hour period.

Precautions
• If a female patient is menstruating, the test may have to be rescheduled.
• Cover and refrigerate the specimen during the collection period.
• If the patient is catheterized, keep the collection bag on ice.
• Instruct the patient not to contaminate the specimen with toilet tissue or stool.
• Send the specimen to the laboratory as soon as the test is complete.

Reference values
Because urine amylase is reported in various units of measure, values differ from laboratory to laboratory. The Mayo Clinic reports urinary excretion of 10 to 80 amylase units/hour as normal.

Abnormal findings
Elevated amylase levels occur in acute pancreatitis; obstruction of the pancreatic duct, intestines, or salivary duct; carcinoma of the head of the pancreas; mumps; acute injury of the spleen; renal disease, with impaired absorption; perforated peptic or duodenal ulcers; and gallbladder disease.

Depressed levels occur in pancreatitis, cachexia, alcoholism, cancer of the liver, cirrhosis, hepatitis, and hepatic abscess.

Interfering factors
• Hematuria or heavy bacteriuria
• Salivary amylase in the urine due to coughing or talking over the sample (possible increase)
• Failure to collect all urine during the test period, to properly store the specimen, or to send the complete specimen to the laboratory immediately
• Contamination of the specimen with toilet tissue, stool, or menstrual blood
• Morphine, meperidine, codeine, pentazocine, bethanechol, thiazide diuretics, indomethacin, or alcohol within 24 hours of the test (possible increase)
• Fluorides (possible decrease)

ARYLSULFATASE A

Arylsulfatase A (ARSA), a lysosomal enzyme found in every cell except the mature erythrocyte, is principally active in the liver, pancreas, and kidneys, where exogenous substances are detoxified into ester sulfates.

Urine ARSA levels rise in transitional bladder cancer, colorectal cancer, and leukemia. However, research hasn't resolved whether elevated ARSA levels provoke malignant growths or are simply an enzymatic response to them. This test measures urine ARSA levels by colorimetric or kinetic techniques.

Purpose

• To aid diagnosis of bladder, colon, or rectal cancer; myeloid (granulocytic) leukemia; and metachromatic leukodystrophy (an inherited lipid storage disease)

Patient preparation

• Tell the patient that this test measures an enzyme that's present throughout the body.
• Advise him that he needn't restrict food or fluids before the test.
• Tell him the test requires urine collection over a 24-hour period, and teach him how to collect a timed specimen.

Procedure and posttest care

• Collect the patient's urine over a 24-hour period.

Precautions

• If a female patient is menstruating, the test may have to be rescheduled.
• Tell the patient not to contaminate the urine specimen with toilet tissue or stool.
• Keep the collection container refrigerated or on ice during the collection period.
• Send the specimen to the laboratory as soon as the collection period has ended.
• If the patient has an indwelling urinary catheter in place, keep the collection bag on ice for the duration of the test.
• Change the continuous urinary drainage apparatus before beginning the test.

Reference values

Normally, ARSA values are greater than 1 U/L.

Abnormal findings

Elevated ARSA levels may result from cancer of the bladder, colon, or rectum or from myeloid leukemia.

Depressed ARSA levels can result from metachromatic leukodystrophy. In patients with this condition, urine studies show metachromatic granules in the urinary sediment.

Interfering factors

• Failure to collect all urine during the test period, to properly store the specimen, or to send the complete specimen to the laboratory immediately
• Contamination of the specimen with toilet tissue, stool, or menstrual blood
• Surgery within 1 week before the test (possible increase)

LYSOZYME

Lysozyme (or muramidase), a low-molecular-weight enzyme, is present in mucus, saliva, tears, skin secretions, and various internal body cells and fluids. This enzyme splits, or lyses, the cell walls of gram-positive bacteria and, with complement and other blood factors, acts to destroy them. Lysozyme seems to be synthesized in granulocytes and monocytes, and it first appears in serum after destruction of such cells. When the serum lysozyme level exceeds three times the normal level, the enzyme appears in the urine.

However, since renal tissue also contains lysozyme, renal injury alone can cause measurable excretion of this enzyme.

This test measures urine lysozyme levels with a turbidimeter. Serum lysozyme determinations, using the same method, confirm the results of urine testing.

Purpose
• To aid diagnosis of acute monocytic or granulocytic leukemia and to monitor the progression of these diseases
• To evaluate proximal tubular function and to diagnose renal impairment
• To detect rejection or infarction of kidney transplantation

Patient preparation
• Explain to the patient that this test evaluates renal function and the immune system.
• Advise him that he needn't restrict food or fluids before the test.
• Tell him the test requires collection of urine over a 24-hour period, and teach him how to collect the specimen correctly.

Procedure and posttest care
• Collect the patient's urine over a 24-hour period.

Precautions
• If a female patient is menstruating, the test may have to be rescheduled for a later date.
• Tell the patient to avoid contaminating the urine specimen with toilet tissue or stool.
• Cover and refrigerate the specimen throughout the collection period.
• Keep the collection bag on ice if the patient has an indwelling urinary catheter in place.
• Send the specimen to the laboratory as soon as the test is complete.

Reference values
Normally, urine lysozyme values are 0 to 3 mg/24 hours.

Abnormal findings
Elevated urine lysozyme levels are characteristic of impaired renal proximal tubular reabsorption, acute pyelonephritis, nephrotic syndrome, tuberculosis of the kidney, severe extrarenal infection, rejection or infarction of kidney transplantation (levels normally increase during the first few days after transplantation), and polycythemia vera.

Urine levels rise markedly after acute onset or relapse of monocytic or myelomonocytic leukemia and rise moderately after acute onset or relapse of granulocytic (myeloid) leukemia.

Urine lysozyme levels remain normal or decrease in lymphocytic leukemia and remain normal in myeloblastic and myelocytic leukemias.

Interfering factors
• Failure to collect all urine
• Bacteriuria (decrease)
• Blood or saliva in the specimen (increase)
• Specimen contamination with toilet tissue, stool, or menstrual blood

CYCLIC ADENOSINE MONOPHOSPHATE

Formed from adenosine triphosphate by the action of the enzyme adenylate cyclase, the nucleotide cyclic adenosine monophosphate (cAMP) influences the protein synthesis rate within cells. Measurement of urinary excretion of cAMP after I.V. infusion of a standard dose of parathyroid hormone (PTH) can show renal tubular resistance in a patient with hypoparathyroid symptoms and high levels of PTH. Such findings suggest type I pseudohypoparathyroidism, a rare inherited disorder. (Urinary cAMP levels respond normally with type II pseudohypoparathyroidism because the defect is beyond the level of cAMP generation.)

Purpose
• To aid differential diagnosis of pseudohypoparathyroidism

Patient preparation
• Explain to the patient that this test evaluates parathyroid function.
• Tell him the test requires a 15-minute I.V. infusion of PTH and a 3- to 4-hour urine specimen collection.

    CLINICAL ALERT Perform a skin test to detect an allergy to PTH; keep epinephrine readily available in case of an adverse reaction.

• Just before the procedure is performed, instruct the patient not to touch the I.V. line or exert pressure on the arm receiving the infusion.
• Tell him he may experience transient discomfort from the needle puncture. Ask him to notify you if he feels severe burning or if the site becomes inflamed or swollen.

Equipment
PTH (300 units, in refrigerated ampules), vial of sterile water (saline solution causes precipitate to form), urine collection container with hydrochloric acid added as a preservative

Procedure and posttest care
• Instruct the patient to empty his bladder.
• If the patient has an indwelling urinary catheter in place, change the collection bag.
• Send this specimen to the laboratory, if ordered; otherwise, discard it.

• Prepare the PTH for infusion as directed, using sterile water for dilution.
• Start the infusion with dextrose 5% in water, and infuse the PTH over 15 minutes. Record the start of the infusion as time zero.
• Collect a urine specimen 3 to 4 hours after infusion.
• Discontinue the I.V. infusion.
• Observe the patient for symptoms of hypercalcemia, including lethargy, anorexia, nausea, vomiting, vertigo, and abdominal cramps.
• Apply warm soaks if a hematoma or irritation develops at the venipuncture site.

Precautions
• Measurement of cAMP should be performed cautiously in patients receiving a digitalis glycoside and in those with sarcoidosis or renal or cardiac disease.
• Tell the patient to avoid contaminating the urine specimen with toilet tissue or stool.
• Send the specimen to the laboratory immediately; if transport is delayed, refrigerate the specimen.
• Keep the collection bag on ice if the patient has a catheter in place.

Reference values
Levels of cAMP are normally 1.3 to 3.7 nmol/dl of glomerular filtrate.

Abnormal findings
Failure to respond to PTH, indicated by normal urinary excretion of cAMP, suggests type I pseudohypoparathyroidism.

Interfering factors
• Isotopes administered up to 8 hours before specimen collection
• Contamination or improper storage of the specimen or failure to acidify the urine with hydrochloric acid

• Failure to send the specimen to the laboratory immediately

HORMONES

ALDOSTERONE

The aldosterone test measures urine levels of aldosterone, the principal mineralocorticoid secreted by the adrenal cortex. Aldosterone promotes retention of sodium and excretion of potassium by the renal tubules, thereby helping to regulate blood pressure and fluid and electrolyte balance. In turn, aldosterone secretion is controlled by the renin-angiotensin system. This feedback mechanism is vital to maintaining fluid and electrolyte balance.

Urine aldosterone levels, measured through radioimmunoassay, are usually evaluated after measurement of serum electrolyte and renin levels.

Purpose
• To aid diagnosis of primary and secondary aldosteronism

Patient preparation
• Explain to the patient that this test evaluates hormonal balance.
• Instruct him to maintain a normal sodium diet (3 g/day) before the test and to avoid sodium-rich foods, such as bacon, barbecue sauce, corned beef, bouillon cubes or powder, and olives.
• Advise him to avoid strenuous physical exercise and stressful situations during the collection period.
• Tell him the test requires collection of urine during a 24-hour period, and teach him the proper collection technique.

Procedure and posttest care
• Collect the patient's urine over a 24-hour period. Use a bottle containing a preservative to keep the specimen at a pH of 4.0 to 4.5.
• Tell the patient he may resume normal physical activity that was restricted before the test.

Precautions
• Refrigerate the specimen or place it on ice during the collection period.
• Send the specimen to the laboratory as soon as the collection is completed.

Reference values
Normally, urine aldosterone levels in individuals ages 1 year and older range from 2 to 16 µg/24 hours; for neonates (ages 0 to 30 days), 0.7 to 11 µg/24 hours; and for infants ages 1 to 11 months, 0.7 to 22 µg/24 hours.

Abnormal findings
Elevated urine aldosterone levels suggest primary or secondary aldosteronism. The primary form usually arises from an aldosterone-secreting adenoma of the adrenal cortex but may also result from adrenocortical hyperplasia. Secondary aldosteronism, the more common form, results from external stimulation of the adrenal cortex, such as that produced when the renin-angiotensin system is activated by hypertensive and edematous disorders.

Disorders that may result in secondary aldosteronism are malignant hypertension, heart failure, cirrhosis of the liver, nephrotic syndrome, and idiopathic cyclic edema.

Low urine aldosterone levels may result from Addison's disease, salt-losing syndrome, and toxemia of pregnancy. These levels normally rise during pregnancy but rapidly decline following parturition.

Interfering factors

- Failure to maintain normal dietary sodium intake
- Failure to avoid strenuous physical exercise and emotional stress before the test (possible increase due to stimulation of adrenocortical secretions)
- Radioactive scan performed within 1 week before the test
- Failure to collect all urine during the collection period, to properly store the specimen, or to send it to the laboratory immediately
- Antihypertensive drugs (possible decrease due to sodium and water retention)
- Diuretics and most steroids (possible increase due to sodium excretion)
- Some corticosteroids, such as fludrocortisone, which mimic mineralocorticoid activity (possible decrease)

FREE CORTISOL

Used as a screen for adrenocortical hyperfunction, the free cortisol test measures urine levels of the portion of cortisol not bound to the corticosteroid-binding globulin transcortin. It's one of the best diagnostic tools for detecting Cushing's syndrome.

Unlike a single measurement of plasma cortisol, radioimmunoassay determinations of free cortisol levels in a 24-hour urine specimen reflect overall secretion levels instead of diurnal variations. Concurrent measurements of plasma cortisol and corticotropin, with urine 17-hydroxycorticosteroids and the dexamethasone suppression test, may be used to confirm the diagnosis.

Purpose

- To aid diagnosis of Cushing's syndrome

Patient preparation

- Explain to the patient that this test helps evaluate adrenal gland function.
- Inform him that he needn't restrict food or fluids before the test but should avoid stressful situations and excessive physical exercise during the collection period.
- Tell him the test requires collection of urine over a 24-hour period.
- Teach him the proper collection technique for a 24-hour urine specimen.
- Check the patient's recent drug history for medications that may interfere with test results, including steroids, reserpine, phenothiazines, and amphetamines. Review your findings with the laboratory; then notify the doctor.

Procedure and posttest care

- Collect the patient's urine over a 24-hour period. Use a bottle containing a preservative to keep the specimen at a pH of 4.0 to 4.5.
- Tell the patient he may resume normal activity restricted during the test.
- Resume administration of medications withheld during the test.

Precautions

- Refrigerate the specimen or place it on ice during the collection period.

Reference values

Normal free cortisol values range as follows:

- ages 0 to 10: 2 to 27 µg/24 hours
- ages 11 to 17: 1 to 55 µg/24 hours
- ages 18 and older: 5 to 55 µg/24 hours.

Abnormal findings

Elevated free cortisol levels may indicate Cushing's syndrome resulting from adrenal hyperplasia, adrenal or pituitary tumor, or ectopic corticotropin production. Hepatic disease and obesity, which can raise plasma cortisol levels, generally don't appreciably raise urine levels of free cortisol. Low levels have little diagnostic significance and don't necessarily indicate adrenocortical hypofunction.

Interfering factors
• Failure to collect all urine during the test period or to properly store the specimen
• Acute stress, alcoholism, depression, and many drugs, such as exogenous corticosteroids and anticonvulsants (may erase normal diurnal variation, affect response to suppression and stimulation tests, and increase baseline levels)
• Pregnancy (possible increase)
• Reserpine, phenothiazines, morphine, amphetamines, and prolonged steroid therapy (possible increase)

CATECHOLAMINES

The test for catecholamines uses spectrophotofluorometry to measure urine levels of the major catecholamines — epinephrine, norepinephrine, and dopamine. Epinephrine is secreted by the adrenal medulla; dopamine, by the central nervous system; and norepinephrine, by both. Catecholamines help regulate metabolism and prepare the body for the fight-or-flight response to stress. Certain tumors can also secrete catecholamines.

The specimen of choice for this test is a 24-hour urine specimen because catecholamine secretion fluctuates diurnally and in response to pain, heat, cold, emotional stress, physical exercise, hypoglycemia, injury, hemorrhage, asphyxia, and drugs. However, a random specimen may be useful for evaluating catecholamine levels after a hypertensive episode.

For a complete diagnostic workup of catecholamine secretion, urine levels of catecholamine metabolites are also measured. These metabolites — metanephrine, normetanephrine, homovanillic acid (HVA), and vanillylmandelic acid (VMA) — normally appear in the urine in greater quantities than the catecholamines.

Purpose
• To aid diagnosis of pheochromocytoma in a patient with unexplained hypertension
• To aid diagnosis of neuroblastoma, ganglioneuroma, and dysautonomia

Patient preparation
• Explain to the patient that this test evaluates adrenal function.
• Inform him that he needn't restrict food or fluids before the test but should avoid stressful situations and excessive physical activity during the collection period.
• Tell him that the test requires either a specimen collected over 24 hours or a random specimen, and explain the collection procedure.

Procedure and posttest care
• Collect the patient's urine over a 24-hour period. Use a bottle containing a preservative to keep the specimen acidified to a pH of 3.0 or less. (If a random specimen is ordered, collect it immediately after a hypertensive episode.)
• Tell the patient that he may resume activity restricted during the test.

Precautions
• Refrigerate a 24-hour specimen or place it on ice during the collection period.
• Send the specimen to the laboratory as soon as the collection is complete.

Reference values
Values for catecholamine fractionaliza-
tion range as follows.
Epinephrine
- Younger than age 1: 0 to 2.5 μg/
24 hours
- age 1: 0 to 3.5 μg/24 hours
- ages 2 to 3: 0 to 6 μg/24 hours
- ages 4 to 9: 0.2 to 10 μg/24 hours
- ages 10 to 15: 0.5 to 20 μg/24 hours
- ages 16 and older: 0 to 20 μg/
24 hours
Norepinephrine
- Younger than age 1: 0 to 10 μg/
24 hours
- age 1: 1 to 17 μg/24 hours
- ages 2 to 3: 4 to 29 μg/24 hours
- ages 4 to 6: 8 to 45 μg/24 hours
- ages 7 to 9: 13 to 65 μg/24 hours
- ages 10 and older: 15 to 80 μg/
24 hours
Dopamine
- Younger than age 1: 0 to 85 μg/
24 hours
- age 1: 10 to 140 μg/24 hours
- ages 2 to 3: 40 to 260 μg/24 hours
- ages 4 and older: 65 to 400 μg/
24 hours.

Abnormal findings
In a patient with undiagnosed hypertension, elevated urine catecholamine
levels following a hypertensive episode
usually indicate a pheochromocytoma.
If tests indicate a pheochromocytoma,
the patient may also be tested for multiple endocrine neoplasia. With the exception of HVA — a metabolite of
dopamine — catecholamine metabolites may also be elevated. Abnormally
high HVA levels rule out a pheochromocytoma, because this tumor mainly
secretes epinephrine, whose primary
metabolite is VMA, not HVA.

Elevated catecholamine levels, without marked hypertension, may be due
to a neuroblastoma or a ganglioneuroma, although HVA levels reflect
these conditions more accurately.

Myasthenia gravis and progressive
muscular dystrophy commonly cause
urine catecholamine levels to rise
above normal, but this test is rarely
performed to diagnose these disorders.
Consistently low-normal catecholamine levels may indicate dysautonomia marked by orthostatic hypotension.

Interfering factors
- Failure to comply with drug restrictions, to collect all urine during the
collection period, or to properly store
the specimen
- Excessive physical exercise or emotional stress (increase)
- Caffeine, insulin, nitroglycerin,
aminophylline, ethanol, sympathomimetics, methyldopa, tricyclic antidepressants, chloral hydrate, quinidine,
quinine, tetracycline, B-complex vitamins, isoproterenol, levodopa, and
monoamine oxidase inhibitors (possible increase)
- Clonidine, guanethidine, reserpine,
and iodine-containing contrast media
(possible decrease)
- Phenothiazines, erythromycin, and
methenamine compounds (possible increase or decrease)

TOTAL URINE ESTROGENS

The total urine estrogens test is a quantitative analysis of total urine levels of
estradiol, estrone, and estriol — the
major estrogens present in significant
amounts in urine. A common method
for measuring total urine estrogen levels involves purification by gel filtration, followed by spectrophotofluorometry. Supplementary tests that may provide further information about ovarian

function include cytologic examination of vaginal smears, measurement of urine levels of pregnanediol and follicle-stimulating hormone, and evaluation of response to an injection of progesterone.

Purpose
• To evaluate ovarian activity and to help determine the cause of amenorrhea and female hyperestrogenism
• To aid diagnosis of tumors of ovarian, adrenocortical, or testicular origin
• To assess fetoplacental status

Patient preparation
• Explain to the female patient that this test helps evaluate ovarian function; to the pregnant patient that this test helps evaluate fetal development and placental function; and to the male patient that this test helps evaluate testicular function.
• Inform the patient that the test requires collection of urine over a 24-hour period.
• Advise her that no pretest restrictions of food or fluids are necessary.
• If the 24-hour specimen is to be collected at home, teach the patient the proper collection technique.

Procedure and posttest care
• Collect the patient's urine over a 24-hour period. Use a bottle containing a preservative to keep the specimen at a pH of 3.0 to 5.0.
• If the patient is pregnant, note the approximate week of gestation on the laboratory slip.
• If the patient is a nonpregnant female, note the stage of her menstrual cycle.

Precautions
• Refrigerate the specimen or keep it on ice during the collection period.

Reference values
In nonpregnant females, total urine estrogen levels rise and fall during the menstrual cycle, peaking shortly before midcycle, decreasing immediately after ovulation, increasing through the life of the corpus luteum, and decreasing greatly as the corpus luteum degenerates and menstruation begins.

Total estrogen levels range as follows.

Nonpregnant females
• 4 to 60 µg/24 hours
Pregnant females
• First trimester: 0 to 800 µg/24 hours
• Second trimester: 800 to 5,000 µg/24 hours
• Third trimester: 5,000 to 50,000 µg/24 hours

In postmenopausal females, values are less than 10 µg/24 hours. In males, total estrogen levels range from 4 to 25 µg/24 hours.

Abnormal findings
Decreased total urine estrogen levels may reflect ovarian agenesis, primary ovarian insufficiency (due to Stein-Leventhal syndrome, for example), or secondary ovarian insufficiency (due to pituitary or adrenal hypofunction or metabolic disturbances).

Elevated total estrogen levels in nonpregnant females may indicate tumors of ovarian or adrenocortical origin, adrenocortical hyperplasia, or a metabolic or hepatic disorder. In males, elevated total estrogen levels are associated with testicular tumors.

Elevated total urine estrogen levels are normal during pregnancy; serial determinations should show a rising titer.

Interfering factors
• Steroid hormones, methenamine mandelate, phenazopyridine hydrochloride, phenothiazines, tetracyclines, phenolphthalein, ampicillin, meproba-

mate, senna, cascara sagrada, and hydrochlorothiazide (possible increase or decrease)

PLACENTAL ESTRIOL

The placental estriol test monitors fetal viability by measuring urine levels of placental estriol, the predominant estrogen excreted in urine during pregnancy. A steady rise in estriol reflects a properly functioning placenta and, in most cases, a healthy, growing fetus. Normally, estriol is secreted in much smaller amounts by the ovaries in nonpregnant females, by the testes in males, and by the adrenal cortex in both sexes.

The usual clinical indication for this test is high-risk pregnancy. Serial testing is necessary to plot the expected rise in estriol levels, or to show the absence of such a rise. The specimen of choice for this test is a 24-hour urine specimen because estriol levels fluctuate diurnally. Radioimmunoassay is the usual test method. Generally, serum estriol levels are considered more reliable than urine levels.

Purpose
● To assess fetoplacental status, especially in high-risk pregnancy, such as one complicated by maternal hypertension, diabetes mellitus, preeclampsia, toxemia, or a history of stillbirth

Patient preparation
● Explain to the patient that this test helps determine if the placenta is functioning properly, which is essential to the health of the fetus.
● Tell her that she needn't restrict food or fluids.

● Advise her that this test requires urine collection over a 24-hour period, and instruct her how to collect the specimen. Emphasize that proper collection technique is necessary for results to be valid.

Procedure and posttest care
● Collect the patient's urine over a 24-hour period. Use a bottle containing a preservative to keep the specimen at a pH of 3.0 to 5.0.
● Send the specimen to the laboratory. If the patient is pregnant, note the week of gestation on the laboratory slip.
● Resume administration of medications withheld during the test.

Precautions
● Refrigerate the specimen or keep it on ice during the collection period.

Reference values
Normal urine estriol values range as follows.
Nonpregnant females
● Follicular phase: 0 to 14 μg/24 hours
● Ovulatory phase: 13 to 54 μg/24 hours
● Luteal phase: 8 to 60 μg/24 hours
Pregnant females
● First trimester: 0 to 800 μg/24 hours
● Second trimester: 800 to 12,000 μg/24 hours
● Third trimester: 5,000 to 50,000 μg/24 hours

Urine estriol values in postmenopausal females range from 0 to 11 μg/24 hours. In males, urine estriol values range from 1 to 11 μg/24 hours.

Abnormal findings
A 40% drop from baseline values that occurs on 2 consecutive days strongly suggests placental insufficiency and impending fetal distress. A 20% drop over 2 weeks or failure of consecutive estriol levels to rise in a normal curve

similarly indicates inadequate placental function and undesirable fetal status. These developments may necessitate cesarean section, depending on the patient's condition and other apparent signs of fetal distress.

A chronically low urine estriol curve may result from fetal adrenal insufficiency, congenital anomalies (such as anencephaly), Rh isoimmunization, or placental sulfatase deficiency.

A high-risk pregnancy in which maternal glomerular filtration rate decreases may cause a low-normal estriol curve. Such a pregnancy may occur in a patient with hypertension or diabetes mellitus, for example. The pregnancy may continue, as long as no complications develop and estriol levels continue to rise. However, falling estriol levels or a sudden drop from baseline values indicates severe fetal distress.

High urine estriol levels may occur in multiple pregnancy.

Interfering factors

● Failure to properly store the specimen during the collection period
● Steroid hormones, methenamine mandelate, phenothiazines, phenazopyridine hydrochloride, tetracyclines, phenolphthalein, ampicillin, meprobamate, senna, cascara sagrada, and hydrochlorothiazide

HUMAN CHORIONIC GONADOTROPIN

Qualitative analysis of urine levels of human chorionic gonadotropin (hCG) allows for detection of pregnancy as early as 10 days after a missed menstrual period. Production of hCG, a glycoprotein, which prevents degeneration of the corpus luteum at the end of the normal menstrual cycle, begins after conception. During the first trimester, hCG levels rise steadily and rapidly, peaking around the 10th week of gestation, subsequently tapering off to less than 10% of peak levels.

The most common method of evaluating hCG in urine is hemagglutination inhibition. This laboratory procedure can provide both qualitative and quantitative information. The qualitative urine test is easier and less expensive than the serum hCG test (beta-subunit assay); therefore, it's used more frequently to detect pregnancy.

Purpose

● To detect and confirm pregnancy
● To aid diagnosis of hydatidiform mole or hCG-secreting tumors

Patient preparation

● If appropriate, explain to the patient that this test determines whether she is pregnant or the status of her pregnancy. Alternatively, explain how the test functions as a screen for some types of cancer.
● Tell her she needn't restrict food or fluids before the test.
● Inform her that the test requires a first-voided morning specimen or urine collection over a 24-hour period, depending on whether the test is qualitative or quantitative.

Procedure and posttest care

● For verification of pregnancy (qualitative analysis), collect a first-voided morning specimen. If this isn't possible, collect a random specimen.
● For quantitative analysis of hCG, collect the patient's urine over a 24-hour period.
● Specify the date of the patient's last menstrual period on the laboratory slip.

• Resume administration of medications withheld during the test.

Precautions
• Refrigerate the 24-hour specimen or keep it on ice during the collection period.

Reference values
In quantitative analysis, urine hCG levels in the first trimester of a normal pregnancy may be as high as 500,000 IU/24 hours; in the second trimester, they range from 10,000 to 25,000 IU/24 hours; and in the third trimester, from 5,000 to 15,000 IU/24 hours.

Measurable hCG levels don't normally appear in the urine of men or nonpregnant women.

Abnormal findings
During pregnancy, elevated urine hCG levels may indicate multiple pregnancy or erythroblastosis fetalis; depressed urine hCG levels may indicate threatened abortion or ectopic pregnancy.

Measurable levels of hCG in males and nonpregnant females may indicate choriocarcinoma, ovarian or testicular tumors, melanoma, multiple myeloma, or gastric, hepatic, pancreatic, or breast cancer.

Interfering factors
• Failure to properly store the specimen during the collection period
• Gross proteinuria (> 1 g/24 hours), hematuria, or an elevated erythrocyte sedimentation rate (possible false-positive, depending on the laboratory method)
• Early pregnancy, ectopic pregnancy, or threatened abortion (possible false-negative)
• Phenothiazine (possible false-negative or false-positive)
• Injection of hCG to treat infertility (possible false-positive)

METABOLITES

PREGNANETRIOL

Using spectrophotometry, the pregnanetriol test determines urine levels of pregnanetriol, the metabolite of the cortisol precursor 17-hydroxyprogesterone. Pregnanetriol is normally excreted in the urine in minute amounts. However, when cortisol biosynthesis is impaired at the point of 17-hydroxyprogesterone conversion, urinary excretion of pregnanetriol rises significantly.

Elevated urine pregnanetriol levels suggest adrenogenital syndrome. Urine 17-ketosteroids and urine 17-ketogenic steroids may be measured concurrently to assess androgen levels. Elevated androgen levels are characteristic of adrenogenital syndrome (congenital adrenal hyperplasia).

Purpose
• To aid diagnosis of adrenogenital syndrome
• To monitor cortisol replacement

Patient preparation
• Explain to the patient (or to the parents if the patient is a child) that this test evaluates hormonal secretion.
• Inform him that he needn't restrict food or fluids before the test.
• Tell him the test requires collection of urine over a 24-hour period, and teach him the proper collection technique.

Procedure and posttest care
• Collect the patient's urine over a 24-hour period. Use a bottle containing a preservative to keep the specimen at a pH of 4.0 to 4.5.

Precautions
• Refrigerate the specimen or keep it on ice during the collection period.
• Send the specimen to the laboratory as soon as the collection is complete.

Reference values
The normal rate of pregnanetriol excretion ranges as follows.
Males
• ages 0 to 5: < 0.1 mg/24 hours
• ages 6 to 9: < 0.3 mg/24 hours
• ages 10 to 15: 0.2 to 0.6 mg/24 hours
• ages 16 and older: 0.2 to 2 mg/24 hours
Females
• ages 0 to 5: < 0.1 mg/24 hours
• ages 6 to 9: < 0.3 mg/24 hours
• ages 10 to 15: 0.1 to 0.6 mg/24 hours
• ages 16 and older: 0 to 1.4 mg/24 hours.

Abnormal findings
Elevated urine pregnanetriol levels suggest adrenogenital syndrome: excessive adrenal androgen secretion and resulting virilization. Females with this condition fail to develop normal secondary sex characteristics and show marked masculinization of external genitalia at birth. Males usually appear normal at birth but later develop signs of somatic and sexual precocity.

In monitoring treatment with cortisol replacement, elevated urine pregnanetriol levels indicate insufficient dosage of cortisol. When cortisol replacement adequately inhibits hypersecretion of corticotropin and subsequent overproduction of 17-hydroxyprogesterone, pregnanetriol levels fall within the normal range.

Interfering factors
• Failure to store the specimen properly during the collection period or to send the completed sample to the laboratory immediately
• Exercise (possible increase)

17-HYDROXY-CORTICOSTEROIDS

The 17-hydroxycorticosteroids (17-OHCS) test measures urine levels of 17-OHCS — metabolites of the hormones that regulate glyconeogenesis. More than 80% of all urinary 17-OHCS are metabolites of cortisol, the primary adrenocortical steroid. Test findings thus reflect cortisol secretion and, indirectly, adrenocortical function.

Because cortisol secretion varies diurnally and in response to stress and many other factors, urine 17-OHCS levels are most accurately determined from a 24-hour specimen. Column chromatography and spectrophotofluorometry with the Porter-Silber reagent are used to measure 17-OHCS levels.

Levels of plasma cortisol, urine free cortisol, and urine 17-ketosteroids may be measured and corticotropin stimulation and suppression testing performed to confirm results of this test. Of these, urine free cortisol is a more sensitive and specific test for hypercortisolism.

Purpose
• To assess adrenocortical function

Patient preparation
• Explain to the patient that this test evaluates how his adrenal glands are functioning.
• Inform him that he needn't restrict food or fluids but should avoid excessive physical exercise and stressful situations during the collection period.
• Tell him the test requires collection of urine over a 24-hour period, and instruct him in the proper collection technique.

• Check the patient's medication history for drugs that may affect 17-OHCS levels, including meprobamate, phenothiazines, spironolactone, ascorbic acid, chloral hydrate, glutethimide, chlordiazepoxide, penicillin G, hydroxyzine, quinidine, quinine, iodides, and methenamine. Review your findings with the laboratory, and then notify the doctor; he may restrict medications before the test.

Procedure and posttest care

• Collect the patient's urine over a 24-hour period. Use a bottle containing a preservative to prevent deterioration of the specimen.
• Tell the patient that he may resume activity restricted during the test.
• Resume administration of any medications restricted before the test.

Precautions

• Refrigerate the specimen or place it on ice during the collection period.

Reference values

Normally, urine 17-OHCS values range from 3 to 10 mg/24 hours in males, and from 2 to 6 mg/24 hours in females. In children, levels range from 1 to 5 mg/24 hours.

Abnormal findings

Elevated urine 17-OHCS levels may indicate Cushing's syndrome, adrenal carcinoma or adenoma, or pituitary tumor. Increased levels may also occur in patients with virilism, hyperthyroidism, and severe hypertension. Extreme stress induced by conditions such as acute pancreatitis and eclampsia also causes urine 17-OHCS levels to rise above normal.

Low urine 17-OHCS levels may indicate Addison's disease, hypopituitarism, or myxedema.

Interfering factors

• Failure to observe restrictions, to collect all urine during the test period, or to properly store the specimen
• Meprobamate, phenothiazines, spironolactone, ascorbic acid, chloral hydrate, glutethimide, chlordiazepoxide, penicillin G, hydroxyzine, quinidine, quinine, iodides, and methenamine (possible increase)
• Hydralazine, phenytoin, thiazide diuretics, ethinamate, nalidixic acid, and reserpine (possible decrease)

17-KETOSTEROIDS

The 17-ketosteroids (17-KS) test uses the spectrophotofluorometric technique to measure urine levels of 17-KS. Steroids and steroid metabolites characterized by a ketone group on carbon 17 in the steroid nucleus, 17-KS originate primarily in the adrenal glands but also in the testes and ovaries.

Although not all 17-KS are androgens, they cause androgenic effects. For example, excessive secretion of 17-KS may result in hirsutism and may increase clitoral or phallic size; in utero, elevated 17-KS levels may cause a female fetus to develop a male urogenital tract. Because 17-KS don't include all the androgens (testosterone, for example, the most potent androgen, isn't a 17-KS), these levels provide only a rough estimate of androgenic activity. To provide additional information about androgen secretion, plasma testosterone levels may be measured concurrently.

Purpose

• To aid diagnosis of adrenal and gonadal dysfunction

Normal Values for the 17-Ketosteroid Fractionation Test

Through gas-liquid chromatography, this fractionation test shows which specific steroids in the 17-ketosteroid (17-KS) group are elevated or suppressed and thus aids differential diagnosis of conditions suggested by abnormal 17-KS levels. Note that 17-KS levels are measured in milligrams per 24 hours.

STEROID	ADULT MALE	ADULT FEMALE	MALE AGES 10 TO 15	FEMALE AGES 10 TO 15	BOTH SEXES AGES 6 TO 9
Androsterone	0.9 to 6.1	0 to 3.1	0.2 to 2	0.5 to 2.5	0.1 to 1
Dehydroepian-drosterone	0 to 3.1	0 to 1.5	< 0.4	< 0.4	< 0.2
Etiocholanolone	0.9 to 5.2	0.1 to 3.5	0.1 to 1.6	0.7 to 3.1	0.3 to 1
11-Hydroxy-androsterone	0.2 to 1.6	0 to 1.1	0.1 to 1.1	0.2 to 1	0.4 to 1
11-Hydroxy-etiocholanolone	0.1 to 0.9	0.1 to 0.8	< 0.3	0.1 to 0.5	0.1 to 0.5
11-Ketoandro-sterone	0 to 0.5	0 to 0.3	< 0.1	< 0.1	< 0.1
11-Ketoetiocho-lanolone	0 to 1.6	0 to 1	< 0.3	0.1 to 0.5	0.1 to 0.5
Pregnanetriol	0.2 to 2	0 to 1.4	0.2 to 0.6	0.1 to 0.6	< 0.3

• To aid diagnosis of adrenogenital syndrome (congenital adrenal hyperplasia)
• To monitor cortisol therapy in the treatment of adrenogenital syndrome

Patient preparation
• Explain to the patient that this test evaluates hormonal balance.
• Inform him that he needn't restrict food or fluids before the test but should avoid excessive physical exercise and stressful situations during the collection period.
• Tell him the test requires urine collection over a 24-hour period, and in-struct him in the proper collection technique.

Procedure and posttest care
• Collect the patient's urine over a 24-hour period. Use a bottle containing a preservative to keep the specimen at a pH of 4.0 to 4.5.
• Tell the patient that he may resume activity restricted during the test.
• Resume administration of medications withheld before the test.

Precautions
• If a woman is menstruating, urine collection may have to be postponed

BOTH SEXES AGES 3 TO 5	BOTH SEXES AGES 1 TO 2	BOTH SEXES BIRTH TO AGE 1
< 0.3	< 0.3	< 0.1
< 0.1	< 0.1	< 0.1
< 0.7	< 0.4	< 0.1
< 0.4	< 0.3	< 0.3
< 0.4	< 0.1	< 0.1
< 0.1	< 0.1	< 0.1
< 0.4	< 0.1	< 0.1
< 0.1	< 0.1	< 0.1

because presence of blood in the specimen interferes with test findings.
● Refrigerate the specimen or place it on ice during the collection period.
● When the collection is completed, send the specimen to the laboratory immediately.

Reference values
Normally, urine 17-KS values range from 6 to 21 mg/24 hours in men and from 4 to 17 mg/24 hours in women. Children between ages 11 and 14 excrete 2 to 7 mg/24 hours; younger children and infants excrete 0.1 to 3 mg/24 hours.

For more information about specific steroids in the 17-KS group, the 17-KS fractionation test may be performed. (See *Normal values for the 17-ketosteroid fractionation test.*)

Abnormal findings
Elevated urine 17-KS levels may result from adrenal hyperplasia, carcinoma or adenoma, or adrenogenital syndrome. In women, elevated levels may also indicate ovarian dysfunction, such as polycystic ovary disease (Stein-Leventhal syndrome), lutein cell tumor of the ovary, or androgenic arrhenoblastoma. In men, elevated 17-KS levels may indicate interstitial cell tumor of the testis. Characteristically, 17-KS levels also rise during pregnancy, severe stress, chronic illness, or debilitating disease.

Depressed urine 17-KS levels may result from Addison's disease, panhypopituitarism, eunuchoidism, or castration and may occur in cretinism, myxedema, and nephrosis. When this test is used to monitor cortisol therapy for adrenogenital syndrome, 17-KS levels typically return to normal with adequate cortisol administration.

Interfering factors
● Failure to observe restrictions, to collect all urine during the collection period, to properly store the specimen, or to send it to the laboratory immediately
● Presence of menstrual blood in the specimen
● Meprobamate, phenothiazines, spironolactone, and oleandomycin (possible increase)
● Estrogens, penicillin, ethacrynic acid, and phenytoin (possible decrease)
● Nalidixic acid and quinine (possible increase or decrease)

17-Ketogenic Steroids

Using spectrophotofluorometry, the 17-ketogenic steroids (17-KGS) test determines urine levels of 17-KGS, which consist of the 17-hydroxycorticosteroids — cortisol and its metabolites, for example — and other adrenocortical steroids, such as pregnanetriol, that can be oxidized in the laboratory to 17-ketosteroids. Because 17-KGS represent such a large group of steroids, this test provides an excellent overall assessment of adrenocortical function. For accurate diagnosis of a specific disease, 17-KGS levels must be compared with results of other tests, including plasma corticotropin, plasma cortisol, corticotropin stimulation, single-dose metyrapone, and dexamethasone suppression.

Purpose
• To evaluate adrenocortical function
• To aid diagnosis of Cushing's syndrome and Addison's disease

Patient preparation
• Explain to the patient that this test evaluates adrenal function.
• Inform him that he needn't restrict food or fluids before the test but should avoid excessive physical exercise and stressful situations during the collection period.
• Tell him the test requires urine collection over a 24-hour period, and teach him how to collect the specimen correctly.

Procedure and posttest care
• Collect the patient's urine over a 24-hour period. Use a bottle containing a preservative to keep the specimen at a pH of 4.0 to 4.5.

• Tell the patient he may resume activity restricted during the test.
• Resume administration of drugs withheld before the test.

Precautions
• Refrigerate the specimen or keep it on ice during the collection period.
• Send the specimen to the laboratory as soon as the collection is complete.

Reference values
Normally, urine 17-KGS levels range from 4 to 14 mg/24 hours in men and from 2 to 12 mg/24 hours in women. Children ages 11 to 14 excrete 2 to 9 mg/24 hours; younger children and infants excrete 0.1 to 4 mg/24 hours.

Abnormal findings
Elevated urine 17-KGS levels indicate hyperadrenalism, which may occur in Cushing's syndrome, adrenogenital syndrome (congenital adrenal hyperplasia), and adrenal carcinoma or adenoma. Levels also rise with severe physical stress (burns, infections, or surgery, for example) or emotional stress.

Low levels may reflect hypoadrenalism, which may occur in Addison's disease and may also be associated with panhypopituitarism, cretinism, and general wasting.

Interfering factors
• Failure to observe restrictions, to collect all urine during the collection period, to properly store the specimen, or to send it to the laboratory immediately
• Corticotropin, meprobamate, phenothiazines, spironolactone, penicillin, oleandomycin, and hydralazine (possible increase)
• Estrogens, quinine, reserpine, thiazide diuretics, and long-term corticosteroid therapy (possible decrease)
• Nalidixic acid and dexamethasone (possible increase or decrease)

Vanillylmandelic Acid

Using spectrophotofluorometry, the vanillylmandelic acid (VMA) test determines urine levels of VMA, a phenolic acid. VMA is the catecholamine metabolite that is normally most prevalent in the urine and is the product of hepatic conversion of epinephrine and norepinephrine; urine VMA levels reflect endogenous production of these major catecholamines. Like the test for urine total catecholamines, this test helps to detect catecholamine-secreting tumors — especially pheochromocytoma — and helps evaluate the function of the adrenal medulla, the primary site of catecholamine production.

The VMA test ideally should be performed on a 24-hour urine specimen (not a random specimen) to overcome the effects of diurnal variations in catecholamine secretion. Other catecholamine metabolites — metanephrine, normetanephrine, and homovanillic acid (HVA) — may be measured at the same time.

Purpose
- To help detect pheochromocytoma, neuroblastoma, and ganglioneuroma
- To evaluate the function of the adrenal medulla

Patient preparation
- Explain to the patient that this test evaluates hormonal secretion.
- Instruct him to restrict foods and beverages containing phenolic acid, such as coffee, tea, bananas, citrus fruits, chocolate, and vanilla, for 3 days before the test.
- Advise him to avoid stressful situations and excessive physical activity during the urine collection period.

- Tell him the test requires collection of urine over a 24-hour period, and teach him the proper collection technique.

Procedure and posttest care
- Collect the patient's urine over a 24-hour period. Use a bottle containing a preservative to keep the specimen at a pH of 3.0.
- Resume administration of medications withheld before the test.
- Tell the patient he may resume normal diet and activity.

Precautions
- Refrigerate the specimen or keep it on ice during the collection period.
- Send the specimen to the laboratory immediately after the collection period.

Reference values
Normally, VMA levels in adults are less than 8 mg/24 hours. In children, reference values are as follows:
- younger than age 1: < 27 µg/mg creatinine
- age 1: < 18 µg/mg creatinine
- ages 2 to 4: < 13 µg/mg creatinine
- ages 5 to 9: < 8.5 µg/mg creatinine
- ages 10 to 14: < 7 µg/mg creatinine.

Abnormal findings
Elevated urine VMA levels may result from a catecholamine-secreting tumor. Further testing, such as measurement of urine HVA levels to rule out pheochromocytoma, is necessary for precise diagnosis. If pheochromocytoma is confirmed, the patient may be tested for multiple endocrine neoplasia, an inherited condition commonly associated with pheochromocytoma. (Family members of a patient with confirmed pheochromocytoma should also be carefully evaluated for multiple endocrine neoplasia.)

Interfering factors
• Failure to observe restrictions, to properly store the specimen during the collection period, or to send the completed sample to the laboratory immediately
• Epinephrine, norepinephrine, lithium carbonate, methocarbamol, chlorpromazine, guanethidine, reserpine, monoamine oxidase inhibitors, levodopa, and salicylates

HOMOVANILLIC ACID

The homovanillic acid test (HVA) is a quantitative analysis of urine levels of HVA, which is a metabolite of dopamine, one of the three major catecholamines. Synthesized primarily in the brain, dopamine is a precursor to epinephrine and norepinephrine, the other principal catecholamines. The liver breaks down most dopamine into HVA for eventual excretion; a minimal amount of dopamine appears in the urine.

Using two-dimensional chromatography, urine HVA levels are usually measured simultaneously with the major catecholamines and other catecholamine metabolites — metanephrine, normetanephrine, and vanillylmandelic acid.

Purpose
• To aid diagnosis of neuroblastoma and ganglioneuroma
• To rule out pheochromocytoma

Patient preparation
• Explain to the patient that this test assesses hormone secretion.
• Inform him that he needn't restrict food or fluids before the test but should avoid stressful situations and excessive physical exercise during the collection period.
• Tell him the test requires collection of urine over a 24-hour period, and teach him the proper collection technique.

Procedure and posttest care
• Collect the patient's urine over a 24-hour period. Use a bottle containing a preservative to keep the specimen at a pH of 2.0 to 4.0.
• Resume administration of medications withheld before the test.
• Tell the patient that he may resume activity restricted during the test.

Precautions
• Refrigerate the specimen or keep it on ice during the collection period.
• Send the specimen to the laboratory immediately after the collection is completed.

Reference values
The normal urine HVA value for adults is less than 8 mg/24 hours. The normal range for children varies with age, as follows:
• younger than age 1: < 35 µg/mg creatinine
• age 1: < 23 µg/mg creatinine
• ages 2 to 4: < 13.5 µg/mg creatinine
• ages 5 to 9: < 9 µg/mg creatinine
• ages 10 to 14: < 12 µg/mg creatinine

Abnormal findings
Elevated urine HVA levels suggest neuroblastoma, a malignant soft-tissue tumor that develops in infants and young children, or ganglioneuroma, a tumor of the sympathetic nervous system that develops in older children and adolescents and rarely metastasizes. HVA levels don't usually rise in patients with pheochromocytoma because this tumor secretes mainly epinephrine, which metabolizes primarily

into vanillylmandelic acid. Thus, an abnormally high urine HVA level generally rules out pheochromocytoma.

Interfering factors
• Failure to observe restrictions, to collect all urine during the test period, to store the specimen properly, or to send the completed sample to the laboratory immediately
• Excessive physical exercise or emotional stress during the collection period (possible increase)
• Monoamine oxidase inhibitors (decrease due to inhibition of dopamine metabolism)
• Aspirin, methocarbamol, and levodopa (possible increase or decrease)

5-HYDROXYINDOLE-ACETIC ACID

The quantitative analysis of urine levels of 5-hydroxyindoleacetic acid (5-HIAA) is used mainly to screen for carcinoid tumors (argentaffinomas). Such tumors, found generally in the intestine or appendix, secrete an excessive amount of serotonin, which is reflected by high 5-HIAA levels. This test measures 5-HIAA levels by the colorimetric technique and is most accurate when performed with a 24-hour urine specimen, which can detect small or intermittently secreting carcinoid tumors.

Purpose
• To aid diagnosis of carcinoid tumors (argentaffinomas)

Patient preparation
• Explain to the patient what serotonin is and why this test is important.

• Instruct him not to eat foods containing serotonin, such as bananas, plums, pineapples, avocados, eggplants, tomatoes, or walnuts, for 4 days before the test.
• Tell him the test requires collection of urine over a 24-hour period, and teach him the proper collection technique.

Procedure and posttest care
• Collect the patient's urine over a 24-hour period. Use a bottle containing a preservative to keep the specimen at a pH of 2.0 to 4.0
• Resume administration of medications withheld before the test.
• Tell the patient that he may resume his normal diet.

Precautions
• Refrigerate the specimen or keep it on ice during the collection period.
• Send the specimen to the laboratory as soon as the collection is complete.

Reference values
Normally, urine 5-HIAA values are less than or equal to 6 mg/24 hours.

Abnormal findings
Marked elevation of urine 5-HIAA levels, possibly as high as 200 to 600 mg/24 hours, indicates a carcinoid tumor. However, because these tumors vary in their capacity to store and secrete serotonin, some patients with carcinoid syndrome (metastatic carcinoid tumors) may not show elevated levels. Repeated testing is often necessary.

Interfering factors
• Failure to observe pretest restrictions, to collect all urine during the test period, to properly store the specimen, or to send the completed sample to the laboratory immediately
• Severe GI disturbance or diarrhea

● Melphalan, reserpine, and fluoro-uracil (increase)
● Ethanol, tricyclic antidepressants, monoamine oxidase inhibitors, methyldopa, and isoniazid (decrease in most cases)
● Methenamine compounds, phenothiazines, salicylates, guaifenesin, mephenesin, methocarbamol, and acetaminophen (possible increase or decrease)

PREGNANEDIOL

Using gas chromatography or radioimmunoassay, this test measures urine levels of pregnanediol, the chief metabolite of progesterone. Although biologically inert, pregnanediol has diagnostic significance because it reflects about 10% of the endogenous production of its parent hormone.

Progesterone is produced in nonpregnant females by the corpus luteum during the latter half of each menstrual cycle, preparing the uterus for implantation of a fertilized ovum. If implantation doesn't occur, progesterone secretion drops sharply; if implantation does occur, the corpus luteum secretes more progesterone to further prepare the uterus for pregnancy and to begin development of the placenta. Toward the end of the first trimester, the placenta becomes the primary source of progesterone secretion, producing the progressively larger amounts needed to maintain pregnancy.

Normally, urine levels of pregnanediol reflect variations in progesterone secretion during the menstrual cycle and during pregnancy. Direct measurement of plasma progesterone levels by radioimmunoassay may also be done.

Purpose
● To evaluate placental function in pregnant females
● To evaluate ovarian function in non-pregnant females

Patient preparation
● Explain to the patient that this test evaluates placental or ovarian function.
● Inform her that she needn't restrict food or fluids.
● Tell her the test requires collection of urine over a 24-hour period, and teach her the proper collection technique.
● Advise the pregnant patient that this test may be repeated several times to obtain serial measurements.

Procedure and posttest care
● Collect the patient's urine over a 24-hour period.
● Resume administration of drugs withheld before the test.

Precautions
● Refrigerate the specimen or keep it on ice during the collection period.
● If the patient is pregnant, note the approximate week of gestation on the laboratory slip.
● For premenopausal women who aren't pregnant, note the stage of the menstrual cycle on the laboratory slip.

Reference values
In nonpregnant females, urine pregnanediol values normally range from 0.5 to 1.5 mg/24 hours during the follicular phase of the menstrual cycle. In pregnant females, the values range as follows:
● first trimester: 10 to 30 mg/24 hours
● second trimester: 35 to 70 mg/ 24 hours
● third trimester: 70 to 100 mg/ 24 hours.
    Normal postmenopausal values range from 0.2 to 1 mg/24 hours. In

males, urine pregnanediol levels are 0 to 1 mg/24 hours.

Abnormal findings

During pregnancy, a marked decrease in urine pregnanediol levels based on a single 24-hour urine specimen or a steady decrease in pregnanediol levels in serial measurements may indicate placental insufficiency and requires immediate investigation. A precipitous drop in pregnanediol values may suggest fetal distress — for example, threatened abortion or preeclampsia — or fetal death. However, pregnanediol measurements are not reliable indicators of fetal viability because levels can remain normal even after fetal death, as long as maternal circulation to the placenta remains adequate.

In nonpregnant females, abnormally low urine pregnanediol levels may occur with anovulation, amenorrhea, or other menstrual abnormalities. Low to normal pregnanediol levels may be associated with hydatidiform mole. Elevations may indicate luteinized granulosa or theca cell tumors, diffuse thecal luteinization, or metastatic ovarian cancer.

Adrenal hyperplasia or biliary tract obstruction may elevate urine pregnanediol values in males or females. Some forms of primary hepatic disease produce abnormally low levels in both sexes.

Interfering factors

● Failure to properly store the specimen during the collection period
● Methenamine mandelate, methenamine hippurate, progestogens, combination oral contraceptives, and drugs containing corticotropin (possible increase or decrease)

PROTEINS AND PROTEIN METABOLITES

PROTEINS

A protein test is a quantitative test for proteinuria. Normally, the glomerular membrane allows only proteins of low molecular weight to enter the filtrate. The renal tubules then reabsorb most of these proteins, normally excreting a small amount that's undetectable by a screening test. A damaged glomerular capillary membrane and impaired tubular reabsorption allow excretion of proteins in the urine.

A qualitative screening often precedes this test. A positive result requires quantitative analysis of a 24-hour urine specimen by acid precipitation tests. Electrophoresis can detect Bence Jones protein, hemoglobins, myoglobins, or albumin.

Purpose

● To aid diagnosis of pathologic states characterized by proteinuria, primarily renal disease

Patient preparation

● Explain to the patient that this test detects proteins in the urine.
● Inform him that he needn't restrict food or fluids.
● Tell him that the test usually requires urine collection over a 24-hour period.

Procedure and posttest care

● Collect the patient's urine over a 24-hour period. A special specimen container can be obtained from the laboratory.

• Resume administration of medications withheld before the test.

Precautions
• Tell the patient not to contaminate the urine with toilet tissue or stool.
• Refrigerate the specimen or place it on ice during the collection period.

Reference values
In males, normal urine protein values range from 0 to 150 mg/24 hours; in females, from 27 to 93 mg/24 hours.

Abnormal findings
Proteinuria is a chief characteristic of renal disease. When proteinuria is present in a single specimen, a 24-hour urine collection is required to identify specific renal abnormalities.

Proteinuria can result from glomerular leakage of plasma proteins (a major cause of protein excretion), from overflow of filtered proteins of low molecular weight (when these are present in excessive concentrations), from impaired tubular reabsorption of filtered proteins, and from the presence of renal proteins derived from the breakdown of kidney tissue.

Persistent proteinuria indicates renal disease resulting from increased glomerular permeability. *Minimal proteinuria* (< 0.5 g/24 hours), however, is most often associated with renal diseases in which glomerular involvement isn't a major factor, as in chronic pyelonephritis.

Moderate proteinuria (0.5 to 4 g/24 hours) occurs in several types of renal disease — acute or chronic glomerulonephritis, amyloidosis, toxic nephropathies — or in diseases in which renal failure often develops as a late complication (diabetes or heart failure, for example). *Heavy protein-uria* (> 4 g/24 hours) is commonly associated with nephrotic syndrome.

When accompanied by an elevated white blood cell (WBC) count, proteinuria indicates urinary tract infection. When accompanied by hematuria, proteinuria indicates local or diffuse urinary tract disorders. Other pathologic states (infections and lesions of the central nervous system, for example) can also result in detectable amounts of proteins in the urine.

Many drugs (such as amphotericin B, gold preparations, aminoglycosides, polymyxins, and trimethadione) inflict renal damage, causing true proteinuria. This makes the routine evaluation of urine proteins essential during such treatment. In all forms of proteinuria, fractionation results obtained by electrophoresis provide more precise information than the screening test. For example, excessive hemoglobin in the urine indicates intravascular hemolysis; elevated myoglobin suggests muscle damage; albumin, increased glomerular permeability; and Bence Jones protein, multiple myeloma.

Not all forms of proteinuria have pathologic significance. *Benign proteinuria* can result from changes in body position. *Functional proteinuria* is associated with exercise as well as emotional or physiologic stress, and is usually transient.

Interfering factors
• Contamination of the specimen with toilet tissue or stool
• Failure to properly store the specimen during the collection period
• Tolbutamide, para-aminosalicylic acid, acetazolamide, sodium bicarbonate, penicillin, sulfonamides, cephalosporins, and iodine-containing contrast media (possible false-positive or false-negative)

BENCE JONES PROTEIN

Bence Jones proteins are abnormal light-chain immunoglobulins of low molecular weight that are derived from the clone of a single plasma cell. This globulin appears in the urine of 50% to 80% of patients with multiple myeloma and in most patients with Waldenström's macroglobulinemia.

Screening tests, such as thermal coagulation and Bradshaw's test, can detect Bence Jones proteins, but urine immunoelectrophoresis is usually the method of choice for quantitative studies. Serum immunoelectrophoresis, which is sometimes used, is less sensitive than other tests. Nevertheless, both urine and serum studies are frequently used when multiple myeloma is suspected.

Purpose
• To confirm the presence of multiple myeloma in patients with characteristic clinical signs, such as bone pain (especially in the back and the thorax) and persistent anemia and fatigue

Patient preparation
• Tell the patient that this test can detect an abnormal protein in the urine.
• Tell him the test requires an early-morning urine specimen; teach him how to collect a clean-catch specimen.

Procedure and posttest care
• Collect an early-morning urine specimen of at least 50 ml.

Precautions
• Instruct the patient not to contaminate the urine specimen with toilet tissue or stool.
• Send the specimen to the laboratory immediately, or refrigerate it if transport is delayed.

Normal findings
Normal urine should contain no Bence Jones proteins.

Abnormal findings
The presence of Bence Jones proteins in urine suggests multiple myeloma or Waldenström's macroglobulinemia. Very low levels, in the absence of other symptoms, may result from benign monoclonal gammopathy. However, clinical evidence figures prominently in diagnosis of multiple myeloma.

Interfering factors
• Connective tissue disease, renal insufficiency, and certain cancers (possible false-positive)
• Contamination of the specimen with menstrual blood, prostatic secretions, or semen (possible false-positive)
• Contamination of the specimen with toilet tissue or stool
• Failure to properly store the specimen during the collection period or to send the completed sample to the laboratory immediately (possible false-positive from deterioration of protein)

AMINO ACID SCREENING

Amino acid screening tests screen for aminoaciduria — elevated urine amino acid levels — a condition that may result from inborn errors of metabolism due to the absence of specific enzymatic activities. Abnormal metabolism causes an excess of one or more amino acids to appear in plasma and, as the renal threshold is exceeded, in urine. (See *Chromatographic identification of amino acid disorders*, pages 354 and 355.)

(Text continues on page 356.)

CHROMATOGRAPHIC IDENTIFICATION OF AMINO ACID DISORDERS

In chromatography — the preferred method for screening aminoacidurias — amino acids migrate into multicolored bands. The sequence of amino acids and their corresponding band numbers, as listed below, reflect these standard migratory patterns. When congenital enzyme deficiencies and subsequent metabolic disorders increase plasma and urine amino acid levels, these bands intensify.

| Chromatographic band number | Amino acids | METABOLIC AMINO ACID DISORDERS | | | | | | |
| | | Phenylketonuria | | Maple syrup urine disease | | Cystinuria | | |
		Plasma	Urine	Plasma	Urine	Plasma	Urine	
1	Leucine, isoleucine			+	+			
2	Phenylalanine	+	+					
3	Valine, methionine			+	+			
4	Tryptophan, beta-amino isobutyric acid							
5	Tyrosine							
6	Proline			+				
7	Alanine, ethanolamine							
8	Threonine, glutamic acid							
9	Homocitrulline, glycine, serine, hydroxyproline, aspartic acid, glutamine, citrulline			+				
10	Homocystine, asparagine							
11	Argininosuccinic acid, histidine, arginine, lysine, ornithine, cystathionine, cystine, cysteine, hydroxylysine						+	

KEY: + = increased amino acids in plasma or urine

	Homocystinuria		Hartnup disease		Argininosuccinicaciduria		Histidinemia		Hyperprolinemia type A		Citrullinuria	
	Plasma	Urine	Plasma	Urine	Plasma	Urine	Plasma	Urine	Plasma	Urine	Plasma	Urine
				+								
				+								
	+			+							+	
				+								
				+								
									+	+		
				+				+				+
								+				+
				+		+				+	+	+
		+										
				+		+	+	+				+

Aminoacidurias may be classified as either primary (overflow) aminoacidopathies or as secondary (renal) aminoacidopathies. The latter type is associated with conditions marked by defective tubular reabsorption from congenital disorders. A more specific defect, such as cystinuria, may cause one or more amino acids to appear in urine.

To screen newborns, children, and adults for congenital aminoacidurias, plasma or urine specimens may be used. The plasma test is the better indicator of overflow aminoacidurias; urine testing is used to confirm or monitor certain amino acid disorders and to screen for renal aminoacidurias.

Various laboratory techniques are available to screen for aminoacidurias, but chromatography is the preferred method. Positive findings on chromatography can be elaborated by fractionation, showing specific amino acid levels. Testing for specific amino acid levels is also necessary for infants or young children with acidosis, severe vomiting and diarrhea, and abnormal urine odor. Such testing is especially important in newborns because early diagnosis and prompt treatment of aminoacidurias may prevent mental retardation.

Purpose
• To screen for renal aminoacidurias
• To follow up on plasma test findings when results of these tests suggest overflow aminoacidurias

Patient preparation
• Explain to the patient (or to parents if the patient is an infant or a child) that this test helps detect amino acid disorders. Advise him that additional tests may be necessary.
• Inform him that he needn't restrict food or fluids before the test.

• Tell him the test requires a urine specimen.
• Check the patient's medication history for drugs that may interfere with test results. If such drugs must be continued, note this on the laboratory slip. (If the patient is a breast-fed infant, record any drugs the mother is receiving.)

Procedure and posttest care
• If the patient is an infant, clean and dry the genital area, attach the collection device, and observe for voiding. Transfer urine — at least 20 ml — to a specimen container. Remove the collection device carefully to prevent skin irritation.
• If the patient is an adult or a child, collect a fresh random specimen.

Precautions
• For an infant, apply the adhesive flanges of the collection device securely to the skin to prevent leakage.
• Send the specimen to the laboratory immediately.

Normal findings
Patterns on thin-layer chromatography are reported as normal.

Abnormal findings
If thin-layer chromatography shows gross changes or abnormal patterns, blood and 24-hour urine quantitative column chromatography are performed to identify specific amino acid abnormalities and to differentiate overflow and renal aminoacidurias.

Interfering factors
• Failure to send the urine specimen to the laboratory immediately
• In newborns, failure to ingest dietary protein during the 48 hours preceding the test
• Amphetamines, norepinephrine, levodopa, and all antibiotics (possible increase or decrease)

HYDROXYPROLINE

Total urine levels of hydroxyproline, an amino acid found mainly in collagen (a component of skin and bone), are a good index of bone matrix turnover because levels increase when collagen breaks down during bone resorption. Bone matrix turnover and hydroxyproline levels normally rise in children during periods of rapid skeletal growth. However, they also rise in disorders that increase bone resorption, such as Paget's disease, metastatic bone tumors, and certain endocrine disorders.

Hydroxyproline levels are most often determined colorimetrically on a timed urine sample; they may also be determined by ion-exchange or gas-liquid chromatography. A collagen-restricted diet is essential for this test because hydroxyproline levels reflect collagen intake. Free hydroxyproline, a small component of total hydroxyproline and a sensitive indicator of dietary collagen intake, may be measured to validate results.

Purpose

- To monitor treatment for disorders characterized by bone resorption, including Paget's disease, metastatic bone tumors, and certain endocrine disorders
- To aid diagnosis of disorders characterized by bone resorption

Patient preparation

- Explain to the patient that this test helps monitor treatment or detect an amino acid disorder related to bone formation.
- Inform him that he must follow a collagen-free diet and avoid eating ice cream, candy, meat, fish, poultry, jelly, and any foods containing gelatin for 24 hours before the test and during the test period itself.
- Tell him the test requires urine collection over a 2-hour or 24-hour period, and teach him the correct collection technique.
- Note the patient's age and sex on the laboratory slip.

Procedure and posttest care

- Collect the patient's urine over a 2-hour or 24-hour period. Use a container that has a preservative to prevent degradation of hydroxyproline.
- Tell the patient he may resume foods and drugs withheld before the test.

Precautions

- Refrigerate the specimen or keep it on ice during the collection period.
- Send the specimen to the laboratory immediately.

Reference values

For adults, normal values typically range from 14 to 45 mg/24 hours or 0.4 to 5 mg/2-hour specimen (males) and 0.4 to 2.9 mg/2-hour specimen (females). Normal values for children are much higher and peak between ages 11 and 18. Values also rise during the third trimester of pregnancy, reflecting fetal skeletal growth.

Abnormal findings

Hydroxyproline levels should decrease slowly during therapy for bone resorption disorders. Elevated levels may indicate bone disease, metastatic bone tumors, or endocrine disorders that stimulate hormonal secretion.

Interfering factors

- Failure to observe restrictions, to collect all urine during the collection period, to properly store the specimen, or to send the completed specimen to the laboratory immediately

- Ascorbic acid, vitamin D, aspirin, glucocorticoids, calcitonin, and mithramycin used to treat Paget's disease (possible decrease)
- Psoriasis and burns (possible increase due to collagen turnover)

CREATININE

The creatinine test measures urine levels of creatinine, the chief metabolite of creatine. Produced in amounts proportional to total body muscle mass, creatinine is removed from the plasma primarily by glomerular filtration and is excreted in the urine. Because the body doesn't recycle it, creatinine has a relatively high, constant clearance rate, making it an efficient indicator of renal function. However, the creatinine clearance test, which measures both urine and plasma creatinine clearance, is a more precise index than this test. A standard method for determining urine creatinine levels is based on Jaffé's reaction, in which creatinine treated with an alkaline picrate solution yields a bright orange-red complex.

Purpose
- To help assess glomerular filtration
- To check the accuracy of 24-hour urine collection, based on the relatively constant levels of creatinine excretion

Patient preparation
- Explain to the patient that this test helps evaluate kidney function.
- Inform him that he needn't restrict fluids but shouldn't eat an excessive amount of meat before the test.
- Advise him that he should avoid strenuous physical exercise during the collection period.
- Tell him the test usually requires urine collection over a 24-hour period,

and teach him the proper collection technique.

Procedure and posttest care
- Collect the patient's urine over a 24-hour period. Use a specimen bottle that contains a preservative to prevent the degradation of creatinine.
- Resume administration of medications withheld during the test.
- Tell the patient he may resume normal diet and activity.

Precautions
- Refrigerate the specimen or keep it on ice during the collection period.
- Once the collection is completed, send the specimen to the laboratory immediately.

Reference values
Normally, urine creatinine levels range from less than 0.8 to 1.8 g/24 hours in males and from 0.6 to 1.6 g/24 hours in females.

Abnormal findings
Decreased urine creatinine levels may result from impaired renal perfusion (associated with shock, for example) or from renal disease due to urinary tract obstruction. Chronic bilateral pyelonephritis, acute or chronic glomerulonephritis, and polycystic kidney disease may also depress creatinine levels. Increased levels generally have little diagnostic significance.

Interfering factors
- Failure to observe restrictions, to collect all urine during the test period, to properly store the specimen, or to send the completed specimen to the laboratory immediately
- Corticosteroids, gentamycin, tetracyclines, diuretics, and amphotericin B (possible decrease)

CREATININE CLEARANCE

An anhydride of creatine, creatinine is formed and excreted in constant amounts by an irreversible reaction and functions solely as the main end product of creatine. Creatinine production is proportional to total muscle mass and is relatively unaffected by urine volume or normal physical activity or diet.

An excellent diagnostic indicator of renal function, the creatinine clearance test determines how efficiently the kidneys are clearing creatinine from the blood. The rate of clearance is expressed in terms of the volume of blood (in milliliters) that can be cleared of creatinine in 1 minute. Creatinine levels become abnormal when more than 50% of the nephrons have been damaged.

Purpose
• To assess renal function (primarily glomerular filtration)
• To monitor progression of renal insufficiency

Patient preparation
• Explain to the patient that this test assesses kidney function.
• Inform him that he needn't restrict fluids but shouldn't eat an excessive amount of meat before the test.
• Advise him that he should avoid strenuous physical exercise during the collection period.
• Tell him the test requires a timed urine specimen and at least one blood sample.
• Tell him how the urine specimen will be collected. Also inform him who'll perform the venipuncture and when and that he may feel some discomfort from the needle puncture. Reassure

him that collecting the blood sample takes less than 3 minutes.
• Explain that more than one venipuncture may be necessary.

Procedure and posttest care
• Collect a timed urine specimen at 2, 6, 12, or 24 hours in a bottle containing a preservative to prevent degradation of creatinine.
• Perform a venipuncture anytime during the collection period, and collect the sample in a 7-ml *red-top* tube.
• Apply warm soaks to ease discomfort if a hematoma develops at the venipuncture site.
• Resume administration of medications withheld before the test.
• Tell the patient that he may resume normal diet and activity.

Precautions
• Refrigerate the urine specimen or keep it on ice during the collection period.
• Send the specimen to the laboratory as soon as the collection is complete.

Reference values
Normal creatinine clearance varies with age; in males, it ranges from 55 to 146 ml/minute/1.73 m^2; in females, from 52 to 134 ml/minute/1.73m^2. For older patients, creatinine clearance normally decreases by 6 ml/minute for each decade.

Abnormal findings
Low creatinine clearance may result from reduced renal blood flow (associated with shock or renal artery obstruction), acute tubular necrosis, acute or chronic glomerulonephritis, advanced bilateral chronic pyelonephritis, advanced bilateral renal lesions (which may occur in polycystic kidney disease, renal tuberculosis, and cancer), nephrosclerosis, heart failure, or severe dehydration.

High creatinine clearance rates generally have little diagnostic significance.

Interfering factors
• Failure to observe restrictions, to collect all urine during the test period, to properly store the specimen, or to send the completed sample to the laboratory immediately
• Amphotericin B, thiazide diuretics, furosemide, and aminoglycosides (possible decrease)

URIC ACID

A quantitative analysis of urine uric acid levels may supplement serum uric acid testing when seeking to identify disorders that alter production or excretion of uric acid (such as leukemia, gout, and renal dysfunction).

The most specific laboratory method for detecting uric acid is spectrophotometric absorption after treatment of the specimen with the enzyme uricase.

Purpose
• To detect enzyme deficiencies and metabolic disturbances that affect uric acid production, such as gout
• To help measure the efficiency of renal clearance and to determine the risk of stone formation

Patient preparation
• Explain to the patient that this test measures the body's production and excretion of a waste product known as uric acid.
• Inform him that he needn't restrict food or fluids before the test.

• Tell him the test requires urine collection over a 24-hour period, and teach him the proper collection technique.

Procedure and posttest care
• Collect the patient's urine over a 24-hour period.
• Resume administration of medications withheld before the test.

Precautions
• Send the specimen to the laboratory immediately after the collection period.

Reference values
Normal urine uric acid values vary with diet but generally are less than 750 mg/24 hours.

Abnormal findings
Elevated urine uric acid levels may result from chronic myeloid leukemia, polycythemia vera, multiple myeloma, early remission in pernicious anemia, lymphosarcoma and lymphatic leukemia during radiotherapy, or tubular reabsorption defects, such as Fanconi's syndrome and hepatolenticular degeneration (Wilson's disease).

Low urine uric acid levels occur in gout (when associated with normal uric acid production but inadequate excretion) and in severe renal damage, such as that resulting from chronic glomerulonephritis, diabetic glomerulosclerosis, and collagen disorders.

Interfering factors
• Failure to send the sample to the laboratory immediately
• Diuretics, pyrazinamide, salicylates, phenylbutazone, probenecid, and allopurinol (possible increase or decrease)

PIGMENTS

HEMOGLOBIN

An abnormal finding, free hemoglobin in the urine may occur in hemolytic anemias, infection, strenuous exercise, or severe intravascular hemolysis from a transfusion reaction. Contained in red blood cells (RBCs), hemoglobin consists of an iron-protoporphyrin complex (heme) and a polypeptide (globin). Usually, RBC destruction occurs within the reticuloendothelial system. However, when RBC destruction occurs within the circulation, free hemoglobin enters the plasma and binds with haptoglobin. If the plasma level of hemoglobin exceeds that of haptoglobin, the excess of unbound hemoglobin is excreted in the urine (hemoglobinuria).

Heme proteins act like enzymes that catalyze oxidation of organic substances. This reaction produces a blue coloration; the intensity of color varies with the amount of hemoglobin present. Microscopic examination is required to identify intact RBCs in urine (hematuria), which can occur in the presence of unbound hemoglobin.

Purpose
• To aid diagnosis of hemolytic anemias, infection, or severe intravascular hemolysis from a transfusion reaction

Patient preparation
• Explain to the patient that this test detects excessive RBC destruction.
• Inform him that he needn't restrict food or fluid.

• Tell him the test requires a random urine specimen, and teach him the proper collection technique.

Procedure and posttest care
• Collect a random urine specimen. (See *Bedside testing for urine blood pigments,* page 362.)
• Resume administration of medications withheld during the test.

Precautions
• Because contamination of the specimen with menstrual blood alters results, a female patient who is menstruating should reschedule her test.
• Send the specimen to the laboratory immediately.

Normal findings
Normally, hemoglobin isn't present in the urine.

Abnormal findings
Hemoglobinuria may result from severe intravascular hemolysis due to a blood transfusion reaction, burns, or a crushing injury. It may result from acquired hemolytic anemias caused by chemical or drug intoxication or malaria; congenital hemolytic anemias, such as hemoglobinopathies or enzyme defects; or paroxysmal nocturnal hemoglobinuria (another type of hemolytic anemia). Less commonly, it may signal cystitis, ureteral calculi, or urethritis.

Hemoglobinuria and hematuria occur in renal epithelial damage (which may result from acute glomerulonephritis or pyelonephritis), renal tumor, and tuberculosis.

Interfering factors
• Failure to send the specimen to the laboratory immediately
• Nephrotoxic drugs, anticoagulants, and drugs that contain vitamin C as a preservative

---

BEDSIDE TESTING FOR URINE BLOOD PIGMENTS
═══════════════════════════════════════

To test a patient's urine for blood pigments at bedside, use one of the methods that follow.

Dipstick, Multistix, or Chemstrip
• Collect a urine specimen.
• Dip the stick into the specimen and withdraw it.
• After 30 seconds, compare the stick to the color chart. Blue indicates a positive reaction; the intensity of color indicates pigment concentration.

Occult tablet
• Collect a urine specimen.
• Put one drop of urine on the filter paper. Place the tablet on the urine, and then put two drops of water on the tablet.
• After 2 minutes, inspect the filter paper around the tablet. Blue indi-

cates a positive reaction; the intensity of color indicates pigment concentration.

Occult solution
• Collect a urine specimen.
• After placing one drop of urine on the filter paper, close the package and turn it over. Open the opposite ends, and place two drops of solution on the filter paper.
• After 30 seconds, inspect the filter paper. Blue indicates a positive reaction; the intensity of color indicates pigment concentration.

Distinguishing hemoglobin
Because these methods detect only blood pigments, immunochemical studies are necessary to differentiate hemoglobin from other blood pigments such as myoglobin.

• Contamination of the specimen by menstrual blood

MYOGLOBIN
═══════════════════════════════════════

The myoglobin test detects the presence of myoglobin — a red pigment found in the cytoplasm of cardiac and skeletal muscle cells — in the urine. When muscle cells are extensively damaged, as by disease or severe crushing trauma, myoglobin is released into the blood, quickly cleared by renal glomerular filtration, and eliminated in the urine (myoglobinuria). For example, myoglobin appears in the urine within 24 hours after myocardial infarction.

Because of marked structural similarities, urine myoglobin must be differentiated from urine hemoglobin. The most commonly used test method is the differential precipitation test. Hemoglobin — bound to haptoglobin — precipitates when urine is mixed with ammonium sulfate. Myoglobin, however, remains soluble and can be measured.

Purpose
• To aid diagnosis of muscular disease
• To detect extensive infarction of muscle tissue
• To assess the extent of muscular damage from crushing trauma

Patient preparation
• Explain to the patient that this test detects a red pigment found in muscle

cells and helps evaluate muscle injury or disease.

• Inform him that he needn't restrict food or fluids before the test.

• Tell him that this test requires a random urine specimen, and teach him the proper collection technique.

Procedure and posttest care
• Collect a random urine specimen.

Precautions
• Send the specimen to the laboratory immediately.

Normal findings
Normally, myoglobin doesn't appear in urine.

Abnormal findings
Myoglobinuria occurs in acute or chronic muscular disease, alcoholic polymyopathy, familial myoglobinuria, extensive myocardial infarction, and in severe trauma to the skeletal muscles (which may result from a crushing injury, extreme hyperthermia, or severe burns). It also occurs in strenuous or prolonged exercise, but disappears after rest.

Interfering factor
• Failure to send the specimen to the laboratory immediately

PORPHYRINS

The test for porphyrins is a quantitative analysis of urine porphyrins (most notably, uroporphyrins and coproporphyrins) and their precursors (porphyrinogens, such as porphobilinogen [PBG]). Porphyrins are red-orange fluorescent compounds, consisting of four pyrrole rings that are produced during heme biosynthesis. They're present in all protoplasm, figure in energy storage and utilization, and are normally excreted in urine in small amounts. Elevated urine levels of porphyrins or porphyrinogens, therefore, reflect impaired heme biosynthesis. Such impairment may result from inherited enzyme deficiencies (congenital porphyrias) or from defects due to disorders such as hemolytic anemias and hepatic disease (acquired porphyrias).

Determination of the specific porphyrins and porphyrinogens found in a urine specimen can help identify the impaired metabolic step in hemebiosynthesis. Occasionally, a preliminary qualitative screening is performed on a random specimen; a positive finding on the screening test must be confirmed by the quantitative analysis of a 24-hour specimen. For correct diagnosis of a specific porphyria, urine porphyrin levels should be correlated with plasma and fecal porphyrin levels.

Purpose
• To aid diagnosis of congenital or acquired porphyrias

Patient preparation
• Explain to the patient that this test detects abnormal hemoglobin formation.

• Inform him that he needn't restrict food or fluids before the test.

• Tell him the test requires urine collection over a 24-hour period, and teach him the proper collection technique.

• Note whether the patient is taking any drugs that may interfere with test results, such as oral contraceptives, griseofulvin, or rifampin. Inform the laboratory and the doctor, who may reschedule the test or restrict drugs before the test.

URINE PORPHYRIN LEVELS IN PORPHYRIA

In porphyria, defective heme biosynthesis increases urinary porphyrins and their corresponding precursors.

PORPHYRIA	PORPHYRINS		PORPHYRIN PRECURSORS	
	Uroporphy-rins	Coproporphy-rins	δ-amino-levulinic acid	Porphobilin-ogen
Erythropoietic porphyria	Highly increased	Increased	Normal	Normal
Erythropoietic protoporphyria	Normal	Normal	Normal	Normal
Acute intermittent porphyria	Variable	Variable	Highly increased	Highly increased
Variegate porphyria	Normal or slightly increased; may be high-ly increased during acute attack	Normal or slightly increased; may be highly increased during acute attack	Highly increased during acute attack	Normal or slightly increased; highly increased during acute attack
Coproporphyria	Not applicable	May be highly increased during acute attack	Increased during acute attack	Increased during acute attack
Porphyria cutanea tarda	Highly increased	Increased	Variable	Variable

Procedure and posttest care

• Collect the patient's urine over a 24-hour period. Use a light-resistant specimen bottle containing a preservative to prevent degradation of the light-sensitive porphyrins and their precursors.

• Resume administration of medications withheld during the test.

Precautions

• Be aware that pregnancy or menstruation may affect the accuracy of test results.

• Refrigerate the specimen or keep it on ice during the collection period.

• Send it to the laboratory as soon as the collection is completed.

• Protect the specimen from light exposure if a light-resistant container is not available.

• Put the collection bag in a dark plastic bag if an indwelling urinary catheter is in place.

Reference values

Normal urine porphyrin and precursor values fall in the following ranges:
- uroporphyrins: in women, ≤ 22 μg/ 24 hours; in men, ≤ 46 μg/24 hours
- coproporphyrins: in women, ≤ 60 μg/ 24 hours; in men, ≤ 96 μg/24 hours
- PBG: in both sexes, up to 1.5 mg/ 24 hours.

Abnormal findings

Increased urine levels of porphyrins and porphyrin precursors are characteristic of porphyria. (See *Urine porphyrin levels in porphyria.*) Infectious hepatitis, Hodgkin's disease, central nervous system disorders, cirrhosis, and heavy metal, benzene, or carbon tetrachloride toxicity may also increase porphyrin levels.

Interfering factors

- Failure to properly store the specimen during the collection period, to protect it from exposure to light, or to send the completed specimen to the laboratory immediately
- Phenazopyridine, procaine, sulfamethoxazole, tetracyclines, griseofulvin, rifampin, oral contraceptives, and diazepam (possible increase or decrease)
- Pregnancy or menstruation (possible increase or decrease)

δ-AMINOLEVULINIC ACID

Using the colorimetric technique, the quantitative analysis of urine δ-aminolevulinic acid (ALA) levels helps diagnose porphyrias, hepatic disease, and lead poisoning. In an emergency, a simple qualitative screening test may be performed.

ALA, the basic precursor of the porphyrins, normally converts to porphobilinogen during heme synthesis. Impaired conversion, which occurs in porphyrias and lead poisoning, causes urine ALA levels to rise before other chemical or hematologic changes occur.

Purpose

- To screen for lead poisoning
- To aid diagnosis of porphyrias and certain hepatic disorders, such as hepatitis and hepatic carcinoma

Patient preparation

- Explain to the patient that this test detects abnormal hemoglobin formation.
- If lead poisoning is suspected, tell the patient (or parents, because the patient is usually a child) that the test helps detect the presence of excessive lead in the body.
- Inform the patient or his parents that he needn't restrict food or fluids.
- Tell him that the test requires urine collection over a 24-hour period, and teach him or his parents the proper collection technique.

Procedure and posttest care

- Collect the patient's urine over a 24-hour period. Use a light-resistant bottle containing a preservative (usually glacial acetic acid) to prevent degradation of ALA.
- Resume administration of medications withheld during the test.

Precautions

- Refrigerate the specimen or keep it on ice during the collection period.
- Send the specimen to the laboratory as soon as the collection is complete.

- Protect the specimen from direct sunlight.
- Insert the drainage bag in a dark plastic bag if the patient has an indwelling urinary catheter in place.

Reference values

Normally, urine ALA values range from 1.5 to 7.5 mg/dl/24 hours in persons ages 6 and older, and 0 to 0.66 mg/dl/24 hours in persons ages 9 months to 5 years. ALA values are not established for neonates and infants up to age 8 months.

Abnormal findings

Elevated urine ALA levels may occur in lead poisoning, acute porphyria, hepatic carcinoma, or hepatitis.

Interfering factors

- Failure to collect all urine during the test period, to properly store the specimen and protect it from light, or to send the completed specimen to the laboratory immediately
- Barbiturates and griseofulvin (increase due to accumulation of porphyrins in the liver)
- Vitamin E in pharmacologic doses (possible decrease)

BILIRUBIN

The bilirubin screening test, based on a color reaction with a specific reagent, detects water-soluble direct (conjugated) bilirubin in the urine. Detectable amounts of bilirubin in the urine may indicate liver disease caused by infections, biliary disease, or hepatotoxicity.

When combined with urobilinogen measurements, the bilirubin test helps identify disorders that can cause jaundice. The analysis can be performed at the bedside, using a bilirubin reagent strip, or in the laboratory.

Purpose

- To help identify the cause of jaundice

Patient preparation

- Explain to the patient that this test helps determine the cause of jaundice.
- Inform him that he needn't restrict food or fluids before the test.
- Tell him the test requires a random urine specimen.
- Advise him that the specimen will be tested at bedside or in the laboratory.

Procedure and posttest care

- Collect a random urine specimen in the container provided.

Bedside analysis using the dipstrip procedure

- Dip the reagent strip into the specimen and remove it immediately.
- Compare the strip color with the color standards after 20 seconds.
- Record the test results on the patient's chart.

Bedside analysis using the ictotest procedure

- Place five drops of urine on the asbestos-cellulose test mat. If bilirubin is present, it'll be absorbed into the mat.
- Put a reagent tablet on the wet area of the mat, and place two drops of water on the tablet. If bilirubin is present, a blue to purple coloration will develop on the mat. Pink or red indicates absence of bilirubin.

Precautions

- Use only a freshly voided specimen. Bilirubin disintegrates after 30 minutes of exposure to room temperature or light.
- If the specimen is to be analyzed in the laboratory, send it there at once.

COMPARATIVE VALUES OF BILIRUBIN AND UROBILINOGEN

CAUSES OF JAUNDICE	Indirect bilirubin	Direct bilirubin	Bilirubin	Urobilinogen	Urobilinogen
	SERUM		URINE		STOOL
Unconjugated hyperbilirubinemia					
Hemolytic disorders: hemolytic anemia, erythroblastosis fetalis	↑	N	O	N↑	↑
Gilbert's disease: constitutional hepatic dysfunction	↑↑	N	O	N↓	N↓
Crigler-Najjar syndrome: congenital hyper-bilirubinemia	↑↑↑	N	O	N↓	N↓
Conjugated hyperbilirubinemia					
Extrahepatic obstruction: calculi, tumor, scar tissue in common bile duct or hepatic excretory duct	N	↑	+	↓O	↓O
Hepatocellular disorders: viral, toxic, or alcoholic hepatitis; cirrhosis; parenchymal injury	↑	↑	+	↓N↑	N↑
Hepatocanalicular disorders or intrahepatic obstruction: drug-induced cholestasis; some familial defects, such as Dubin-Johnson and Rotor's syndromes; viral hepatitis; and primary biliary cirrhosis	↑	↑	+	↓N↑	N↑

KEY:

↑	Increased	O	Absent
N↑	May be increased	+	Present
↑↑	Moderately increased	N↓	Normal or reduced
↑↑↑	Markedly increased	↓O	Decreased or absent
N	Normal	↓N↑	Variable

● If the specimen is tested at the bedside, make sure 20 seconds elapse before interpreting the color change on the dipstrip.

● Be sure lighting is adequate to make this color determination.

Normal findings

Normally, bilirubin isn't found in urine in a routine screening test.

Abnormal findings

High concentrations of direct bilirubin in urine may be evident from the specimen's appearance (dark, with a yellow foam). To diagnose jaundice, however, the presence or absence of direct bilirubin in urine must be correlated with serum test results and with urine and fecal urobilinogen levels. (See *Comparative values of bilirubin and urobilinogen.*)

Interfering factors
• Failure to test the specimen promptly or to send it to the laboratory immediately

UROBILINOGEN

The urobilinogen test detects impaired liver function by measuring urine levels of urobilinogen, the colorless, water-soluble product that results from the reduction of bilirubin by intestinal bacteria. Absent or altered urobilinogen levels can indicate hepatic damage or dysfunction. Increased urine urobilinogen levels may indicate hemolysis of red blood cells.

Quantitative analysis of urine urobilinogen involves addition of Ehrlich's reagent to a 2-hour urine specimen. The resulting color reaction is read promptly by spectrophotometry.

Purpose
• To aid diagnosis of extrahepatic obstruction, such as blockage of the common bile duct
• To aid differential diagnosis of hepatic and hematologic disorders

Patient preparation
• Explain to the patient that this test helps assess liver and biliary tract function.
• Inform him that he needn't restrict fluids or food, except for bananas, which he should avoid for 48 hours before the test.
• Tell him that the test requires a 2-hour urine specimen, and teach him how to collect it.

Procedure and posttest care
• Most laboratories request a random urine specimen; others prefer a 2-hour specimen, usually during the afternoon (ideally, between 1 p.m. and 3 p.m.), when urobilinogen levels peak.
• Tell the patient he may resume his normal diet.
• Resume administration of drugs withheld during the test.

Precautions
• Send the specimen to the laboratory immediately. This test must be performed within 30 minutes of collection because urobilinogen quickly oxidizes to an orange compound called urobilin.

Reference values
Normally, urine urobilinogen values are less than 4 mg/24 hours.

Abnormal findings
Absence of urine urobilinogen may result from complete obstructive jaundice or treatment with broad-spectrum antibiotics, which destroy the intestinal bacterial flora. Low urine urobilinogen levels may result from congenital enzymatic jaundice (hyperbilirubinemia syndromes) or from treatment with drugs that acidify urine, such as ammonium chloride or ascorbic acid.

Elevated levels may indicate hemolytic jaundice, hepatitis, or cirrhosis.

Interfering factors
• Failure to observe pretest restrictions or to immediately send the specimen to the laboratory
• Para-aminosalicylic acid, phenazopyridine, procaine, phenothiazines, and sulfonamides (possible decrease)

SUGARS, KETONES, AND MUCOPOLY-SACCHARIDES

COPPER REDUCTION TEST

The copper reduction test measures the concentration of reducing substances in the urine through the reaction of these substances with a commercially prepared tablet called Clinitest. Clinitest, which reacts to glucose and to other reducing substances (mostly sugars), has almost replaced Benedict's test.

This test is most valuable for providing the patient with overt or latent diabetes a simple, at-home method of monitoring urine sugar levels. It's sometimes used as a rapid laboratory screening tool.

Purpose
● To detect mellituria
● To monitor urine glucose levels during insulin therapy, after determination that the sugar in the urine is glucose

Patient preparation
● Explain to the patient that this test determines urine sugar level.
● If the patient has been recently diagnosed as diabetic, teach him how to perform the Clinitest tablet test.
● Provide written guidelines and a flow sheet to help him record Clinitest results at home, if appropriate.

Equipment
Specimen container, 10-ml test tube, medicine dropper, Clinitest tablets, Clinitest color chart

Procedure and posttest care
● Have the patient void; then give him a drink of water.
● Collect a second-voided urine specimen after 30 to 45 minutes.

Five-drop Clinitest tablet test
● Hold the medicine dropper vertically, and instill five drops of urine from the specimen container into the test tube.
● Rinse the dropper with water, and add 10 drops of water to the test tube.
● Add one Clinitest tablet, and observe the color change, especially during effervescence (the pass-through phase).
● Wait 15 seconds after effervescence subsides, and gently agitate the test tube.
● If color develops at the 15-second interval, read the color against the Clinitest color chart, and record the results.
● Ignore any changes that develop after 15 seconds.
● Rapid color changes (bright orange to dark brown or green-brown) in the pass-through phase in a five-drop Clinitest reaction indicate glycosuria of 2% or more. Record the results as over 2% without comparison to the color chart.

Two-drop Clinitest tablet test
● Hold the medicine dropper vertically, and instill two drops of urine into the test tube.
● Flush urine residue from the dropper with water; then add 10 drops of water to the test tube.
● Add one Clinitest tablet, and observe the color change during the pass-through phase.
● Wait 15 seconds after effervescence stops; compare the color with the appropriate color reference chart, and record results.
● In a two-drop Clinitest reaction, rapid color changes (bright orange to dark brown or green-brown) in the pass-through phase indicate glycosuria of 5% or more.

Precautions

• Instruct the patient not to contaminate the specimen with toilet tissue or stool.

• Make sure hands are dry when handling Clinitest tablets, and avoid contact with eyes, mucous membranes, GI tract, and clothing because sodium hydroxide and moisture produce caustic burns.

• Store tablets in a well-marked, child-proof bottle to prevent accidental ingestion.

• Don't use discolored tablets (dark blue). The normal color of fresh tablets is light blue, with darker blue flecks.

• During effervescence, hold the test tube near the top to avoid burning your hand; it becomes boiling hot.

Normal findings

Normally, no glucose is present in urine.

Abnormal findings

Glycosuria occurs in diabetes mellitus, adrenal and thyroid disorders, hepatic and central nervous system diseases, conditions involving low renal threshold (such as Fanconi's syndrome), toxic renal tubular disease, heavy metal poisoning, glomerulonephritis, and nephrosis; in pregnant women; and in those receiving total parenteral nutrition. It also occurs with administration of large amounts of glucose and some drugs, such as asparaginase, corticosteroids, carbamazepine, ammonium chloride, thiazide diuretics, dextrothyroxine, large amounts of nicotinic acid, lithium carbonate, and long-term phenothiazines.

Interfering factors

• Failure to use freshly voided urine or to flush urine residue from the medicine dropper

• Contamination of the specimen with toilet tissue or stool

• Failure to use whole or fresh Clinitest tablets or to keep the tablet container tightly closed to protect specimen from exposure to light or moisture

• Failure to detect the pass-through phenomenon or to use the correct reference chart for color comparison of the specimen

• Cephalosporins, nalidixic acid, and large doses of probenecid (possible false-positive)

• Tetracycline and ascorbic acid (possible false-positive or false-negative, depending on test method)

• Low renal threshold for glucose

• Presence of reducing substances other than glucose

GLUCOSE OXIDASE TEST

The glucose oxidase test — which involves the use of commercial, plastic-coated reagent strips (Clinistix, Diastix) or Tes-Tape — is a specific, qualitative test for glycosuria. The test is used primarily to monitor urine glucose in patients with diabetes. Because of this test's simplicity and convenience, patients can perform it at home.

Purpose

• To detect glycosuria

• To monitor urine glucose levels during insulin therapy

Patient preparation

• Explain to the patient that this test determines urine glucose concentration.

- If he's a newly diagnosed patient with diabetes, teach him how to perform a reagent strip test.
- Check his drug history. If he's receiving levodopa, ascorbic acid, phenazopyridine, salicylates, peroxides, or hypochlorites, use Clinitest tablets instead.

Equipment
Specimen container, glucose test strips, reference color blocks

Procedure and posttest care
- Have the patient void; then give him a drink of water.
- Collect a second-voided specimen after 30 to 45 minutes.

Clinistix test
- Dip the test area of the reagent strip in the specimen for 2 seconds.
- Remove excess urine by tapping the strip against a clean surface or the side of the container, and begin timing.
- Hold the strip in the air, and "read" the color *exactly 10 seconds* after taking the strip out of the urine by comparing it with the reference color blocks on the label of the container.
- Record the results.
- Ignore color changes that develop after 10 seconds.

Diastix test
- Dip the reagent strip in the specimen for 2 seconds.
- Remove excess urine by tapping the strip against the container, and begin timing.
- Hold the strip in the air, and compare the color to the color chart *exactly 30 seconds* after taking the strip out of the urine.
- Record the results.
- Ignore color changes that develop after 30 seconds.

Tes-Tape
- Withdraw about 1″ (3.8 cm) of the reagent tape from the dispenser; dip ¼″ (0.6 cm) in the specimen for 2 seconds.

- Remove excess urine by tapping the strip against the side of the container, and begin timing.
- Hold the tape in the air, and compare the color of the darkest part of the tape to the color chart *exactly 60 seconds* after taking the strip out of the urine.
- If the tape indicates 0.5% or higher, wait an additional 60 seconds to make the final color comparison.
- Record the results.

Precautions
- Instruct the patient not to contaminate the urine specimen with toilet tissue or stool.
- Keep the test strip container tightly closed to prevent deterioration of strips by exposure to light or moisture.
- Store it in a cool place (under 86° F [30° C]) to avoid heat degradation.
- Don't use discolored or darkened Clinistix or Diastix or dark yellow or yellow-brown Tes-Tape.

Normal findings
Normally, no glucose is present in urine.

Abnormal findings
Glycosuria occurs in diabetes mellitus, adrenal and thyroid disorders, hepatic and central nervous system diseases, conditions involving low renal threshold (such as Fanconi's syndrome), toxic renal tubular disease, heavy metal poisoning, glomerulonephritis, and nephrosis; in pregnant women; and in those receiving total parenteral nutrition. It also occurs with administration of large amounts of glucose and of certain drugs, such as asparaginase, corticosteroids, carbamazepine, ammonium chloride, thiazide diuretics, dextrothyroxine, large doses of nicotinic acid, lithium carbonate, and prolonged use of phenothiazines.

Interfering factors
- Dilute, stale urine or contamination of the specimen due to toilet tissue, stool, or bacteria
- Use of reagent strips after the expiration date, failure to keep the reagent strip container tightly closed, or failure to record the reagent strip method used
- Presence of reducing substances, such as levodopa, ascorbic acid, phenazopyridine, methyldopa, and salicylates (possible false-negative)
- Tetracyclines (false-negative)

KETONE TEST

In the ketone test, a routine, semiquantitative screening test, a commercially prepared product is used to measure the urine level of ketone bodies. Ketone bodies are the by-products of fat metabolism; they include acetoacetic acid, acetone, and beta-hydroxybutyric acid. Excessive amounts may appear in patients with carbohydrate dehydration, which may occur in starvation or diabetic ketoacidosis (DKA).

Commercially available tests include the Acetest tablet, Chemstrip K, Ketostix, or Keto-Diastix. Each product measures a specific ketone body. For example, Acetest measures acetone and Ketostix measures acetoacetic acid.

Purpose
- To screen for ketonuria
- To identify DKA and carbohydrate deprivation
- To distinguish between a diabetic and a nondiabetic coma
- To monitor control of diabetes mellitus, ketogenic weight reduction, and treatment of DKA

Patient preparation
- Explain to the patient that this test evaluates fat metabolism.
- If the patient is newly diagnosed with diabetes, tell him how to perform the test.

Procedure and posttest care
- Instruct the patient to void; then give him a drink of water.
- Collect a second-voided midstream specimen about 30 minutes later.

Acetest
- Lay the tablet on a piece of white paper, and place one drop of urine on the tablet.
- Compare the tablet color (white, lavender, or purple) with the color chart after 30 seconds.

Ketostix
- Dip the reagent stick into the specimen and remove it immediately.
- Compare the stick color (buff or purple) with the color chart after 15 seconds.
- Record the results as negative, small, moderate, or large amounts of ketones.

Keto-Diastix
- Dip the reagent strip into the specimen, and remove it immediately.
- Tap the edge of the strip against the container or a clean, dry surface to remove excess urine.
- Hold the strip horizontally to prevent mixing the chemicals from the two areas.
- Interpret each area of the strip separately. Compare the color of the ketone section (buff or purple) with the appropriate color chart after exactly 15 seconds; compare the color of the glucose section after 30 seconds.
- Ignore color changes that occur after the specified waiting periods.
- Record the results as negative or positive for small, moderate, or large amounts of ketones.

Precautions
- Test the specimen within 60 minutes after it is obtained, or you must refrigerate it.
- Allow refrigerated specimens to return to room temperature before testing.
- Don't use tablets or strips that have become discolored or darkened.

Normal findings
Normally, no ketones are present in urine.

Abnormal findings
Ketonuria may occur in uncontrolled diabetes mellitus or starvation. It also occurs as a metabolic complication of total parenteral nutrition.

Interfering factors
- Failure to keep the reagent container tightly closed to prevent absorption of light or moisture or bacterial contamination of the specimen (false-negative)
- Failure to test the specimen within 1 hour or to refrigerate it
- Levodopa, phenazopyridine, and sulfobromophthalein (false-positive results when Ketostix or Keto-Diastix is used instead of Acetest)

ACID MUCOPOLY-SACCHARIDES

The acid mucopolysaccharides test is a quantitative test that helps detect mucopolysaccharidosis, a rare disorder that may affect the skeleton, joints, liver, spleen, eye, ear, skin, teeth, and the cardiovascular, respiratory, and central nervous systems. This test measures the urine level of acid mucopolysaccharides (AMPs), a group of polysaccharides or carbohydrates.

Purpose
- To diagnose mucopolysaccharidosis in infants with a family history of the disease

Patient preparation
- Explain to the parents of the infant that this test helps determine the efficiency of carbohydrate metabolism.
- Inform them that they needn't restrict the child's food or fluids.
- Tell the parents that the test requires urine collection for 24 hours, and instruct them on the proper way to collect the specimen at home.

Equipment
Pediatric urine collectors, 24-hour collection container, 20 ml toluene (usually obtained from the laboratory)

Procedure and posttest care
- Collect the patient's urine over a 24-hour period.
- Add 20 ml toluene as a preservative at the start of the collection.
- Indicate the patient's age on the laboratory slip.
- Send the specimen to the laboratory immediately after the 24-hour collection period.
- Be sure to remove all adhesive from the urine collector from the infant's perineum.
- Wash the area gently with soap and water, and watch for irritation.

Precautions
- Refrigerate the specimen or place it on ice during the collection period.

Reference values
The AMP value is expressed as milligrams of glucuronic acid divided by the amount of creatinine in the same

specimen (which reflects glomerular filtration rate) to overcome irregularities in the 24-hour urine collection.

Normal AMP values for infants are as follows:

- ages 0 to 2 months: < 40 mg/mmol creatinine
- ages 3 to 4 months: < 25 mg/mmol creatinine
- ages 5 to 6 months: < 20 mg/mmol creatinine
- ages 7 to 11 months: < 17.5 mg/mmol creatinine.

Abnormal findings
Elevated AMP levels reliably indicate mucopolysaccharidosis. Supplementary quantitative analysis and detailed blood studies can identify the defective enzyme.

Interfering factors
- Failure to collect all urine during the test period, to properly store the specimen, or to send the completed specimen to the laboratory immediately
- Heparin (increase)

VITAMINS

TRYPTOPHAN CHALLENGE TEST

Measurement of urine xanthurenic acid after a challenge dose of tryptophan confirms deficiency of vitamin B_6 long before symptoms appear.

Although vitamin B_6 isn't directly involved in energy metabolism, it's essential for reactions that occur in protein metabolism and for amino acid synthesis. Vitamin B_6 deficiency can cause hypochromic microcytic anemia without iron deficiency and central nervous system disturbances. When normal magnesium levels accompany a vitamin B_6 deficiency, urinary citrate and oxalate solubility may decrease, causing formation of urinary calculi.

Purpose
- To detect vitamin B_6 deficiency

Patient preparation
- Explain to the patient that this test determines the body's stores of vitamin B_6.
- Tell him he'll receive an oral dose of medication.
- Explain that this test requires urine collection over a 24-hour period.

Procedure and posttest care
- Administer L-tryptophan by mouth (usually, 50 mg/kg for children and up to 2 g/kg for adults).
- Have the patient void and discard the urine. Immediately begin collection of a 24-hour urine specimen.
- Inform the patient with vitamin B_6 deficiency that yeast, wheat, corn, liver, and kidneys are good sources of pyridoxine.

Precautions
- Make sure the specimen bottle contains a crystal of thymol, a preservative.
- Tell the patient not to contaminate the urine specimen with toilet tissue or stool.
- Refrigerate the specimen, or place it on ice during the collection period.

Reference values
Normal excretion of xanthurenic acid after a tryptophan challenge dose is less than 50 mg/24 hours.

Abnormal findings

Urine levels of xanthurenic acid exceeding 100 mg/24 hours indicate vitamin B_6 deficiency. This rare disorder may result from malnutrition, malignancy, pregnancy, familial xanthurenic aciduria, or use of oral contraceptives, hydralazine, D-penicillamine, or isoniazid.

Interfering factors

• Contamination of the specimen with toilet tissue or stool
• Failure to properly handle the specimen
• Oral contraceptives, hydralazine, D-penicillamine, and isoniazid (decrease)

VITAMIN C

Through colorimetric measurement of urinary levels, the vitamin C test determines body stores of vitamin C (ascorbic acid). This water-soluble vitamin, which is easily absorbed by the intestine, acts as a reversible reducing agent in metabolic processes, aids collagen formation, and helps maintain connective and osteoid tissues.

This analysis is particularly useful in diagnosing scurvy, an extreme deficiency of vitamin C characterized by the degeneration of connective and osteoid tissues, dentin, and endothelial membranes. Although now uncommon in North America, scurvy may occur in alcoholics, people on low-residue or low-citrus diets, and infants who have been weaned to cow's milk that does not contain a vitamin C supplement.

Purpose

• To aid diagnosis of scurvy, scurvy-like conditions, and metabolic disorders, such as malnutrition, that interfere with oxidative processes

Patient preparation

• Explain to the patient that this test detects vitamin C deficiency.
• Inform the patient that he should maintain a normal diet.
• Tell him the test requires urine collection over a 24-hour period.
• If the specimen is to be collected at home, instruct the patient on proper collection technique.

Procedure and posttest care

• Collect the patient's urine over a 24-hour period.
• Advise the patient with vitamin C deficiency that citrus fruits, tomatoes, potatoes, cabbage, and strawberries are good dietary sources of vitamin C.

Precautions

• Tell the patient not to contaminate the specimen with toilet tissue or stool.
• Refrigerate the specimen, or place it on ice during the collection period.

Reference values

Normal urine vitamin C excretion is 30 mg/24 hours.

Abnormal findings

Depressed urine vitamin C levels are common in patients with infection, cancer, burns, or other stress-producing conditions. Decreased vitamin C levels may also indicate malnutrition, malabsorption, renal deficiencies, or prolonged I.V. therapy without vitamin C replacement. Severe vitamin C deficiency causes scurvy.

Interfering factors

• Improper specimen collection or storage or exposure to light
• Contamination of the specimen with toilet tissue or stool

MINERALS

SODIUM AND CHLORIDE

The sodium and chloride test determines urine levels of sodium, the major extracellular cation, and of chloride, the major extracellular anion. Less significant than serum levels (and, consequently, performed less frequently), measurement of urine sodium and urine chloride concentrations is used to evaluate renal conservation of these two electrolytes and to confirm serum sodium and chloride values.

In the body, sodium and chloride help maintain osmotic pressure and water and acid-base balance. Normal ranges of sodium and chloride in the urine vary greatly with dietary salt intake and perspiration.

Purpose
● To help evaluate fluid and electrolyte imbalance
● To monitor the effects of a low-salt diet
● To help evaluate renal and adrenal disorders

Patient preparation
● Explain to the patient that this test helps determine the balance of salt and water in the body.
● Advise him that no special restrictions are necessary.
● Tell him the test requires urine collection over a 24-hour period.
● If the specimen is to be collected at home, instruct the patient on proper collection technique.

Procedure and posttest care
● Collect the patient's urine over a 24-hour period.

Precautions
● Tell the patient not to contaminate the specimen with toilet tissue or stool.

Reference values
Normal urine sodium excretion ranges from 40 to 220 mEq/L/24 hours or 40 to 220 mmol/day in an adult; in a child, from 41 to 115 mEq/L/24 hours. Normal urine chloride excretion ranges from 140 to 250 mEq/L/24 hours in an adult; in children ages 6 to 10, from 15 to 40 mEq/L/24 hours; and in children ages 10 to 14, from 64 to 176 mEq/L/24 hours.

Abnormal findings
Usually, urine sodium and urine chloride levels are parallel, rising and falling in tandem. Abnormal levels of both minerals may indicate the need for more specific testing.

Elevated urine sodium levels may reflect increased salt intake, adrenal failure, salicylate toxicity, diabetic acidosis, salt-losing nephritis, and water-deficient dehydration.

Decreased urine sodium levels suggest decreased salt intake, primary aldosteronism, acute renal failure, and heart failure.

Elevated urine chloride levels may result from water-deficient dehydration, salicylate toxicity, diabetic ketoacidosis, adrenocortical insufficiency (Addison's disease), or salt-losing renal disease. Decreased levels may result from excessive diaphoresis, heart failure, hypochloremic metabolic alkalosis, or prolonged vomiting or gastric suctioning.

To evaluate fluid-electrolyte imbalance, results must be correlated with findings of serum electrolyte studies.

Interfering factors

• Contamination of the specimen with toilet tissue or stool

• Caffeine, diuretics, dopamine, postmenopausal diuresis, and increased sodium intake (possible increase in sodium)

• Corticosteroids, epinephrines, propranolol, low sodium intake, premenstrual sodium and water retention, and stress diuresis (possible decrease in sodium)

• Carbenicillin therapy, reduced chloride intake, ingestion of large amounts of licorice, alkali ingestion (possible decrease in chloride)

• Ammonium chloride administration, excessive infusion of normal saline solution, sulfides, cyanides, halogens, and bromides (possible increase in chloride)

POTASSIUM

The potassium test is a quantitative test that measures urine levels of potassium, a major intracellular cation that helps regulate acid-base balance and neuromuscular function. Potassium imbalance may cause such signs and symptoms as muscle weakness, nausea, diarrhea, confusion, hypotension, and electrocardiogram changes; severe imbalance may lead to cardiac arrest.

Most commonly, a serum potassium test is performed to detect hyperkalemia (abnormally high levels) or hypokalemia (abnormally low levels). A urine potassium test may be performed to evaluate hypokalemia when a history and physical examination fail to uncover the cause. If results suggest a renal disorder, additional renal function tests may be ordered.

Purpose

• To determine whether hypokalemia is caused by renal or extrarenal disorders

Patient preparation

• Explain to the patient that this test evaluates his kidney function.

• Advise him that no special dietary restrictions are necessary.

• Tell him that the test requires urine collection over a 24-hour period.

• If the specimen is to be collected at home, teach him the correct collection technique.

Procedure and posttest care

• Collect the patient's urine over a 24-hour period.

• Administer potassium supplements and monitor serum levels as appropriate.

• Provide dietary supplements and nutritional counseling as necessary.

• Replace volume loss with I.V. or oral fluids as necessary.

• Resume administration of drugs withheld during the test.

Precautions

• Tell the patient not to contaminate the specimen with toilet tissue or stool.

• Refrigerate the specimen or place it on ice during the collection period.

• Send the specimen to the laboratory immediately after collection or refrigerate it.

Reference values

Normal potassium excretion in adults is 25 to 125 mEq/24 hours, or 25 to 125 mmol/24 hours. In children, normal excretion is 22 to 57 mmol/24 hours.

Abnormal findings

In a patient with hypokalemia, potassium concentration less than 10 mEq/L suggests normal renal function, indicating that potassium loss is most likely the result of a GI disorder such as malabsorption syndrome.

In a patient with hypokalemia lasting more than 3 days, urine potassium concentration above 10 mEq/L indicates renal loss of potassium. These losses may result from such disorders as aldosteronism, renal tubular acidosis, or chronic renal failure. However, extrarenal disorders, such as dehydration, starvation, Cushing's disease, or salicylate intoxication, may also elevate urine potassium levels.

Interfering factors
• Contamination of the specimen with toilet tissue or stool
• Failure to send the specimen to the laboratory immediately or to refrigerate it
• Ammonium chloride, thiazide diuretics, and acetazolamide

CALCIUM AND PHOSPHATES

The calcium and phosphates test measures the urine levels of calcium and phosphates, elements essential for the formation and resorption of bone. Urine calcium and phosphate levels generally parallel serum levels.

Normally absorbed in the upper intestine and excreted in stool and urine, calcium and phosphates help maintain tissue and fluid pH, electrolyte balance in cells and extracellular fluids, and permeability of cell membranes. Calcium promotes enzymatic processes, aids blood coagulation, and lowers neuromuscular irritability; phosphates aid carbohydrate metabolism.

Purpose
• To evaluate calcium and phosphate metabolism and excretion
• To monitor treatment of calcium or phosphate deficiency

Patient preparation
• Explain to the patient that this test measures the amount of calcium and phosphates in the urine.
• Encourage him to be as active as possible before the test.
• Tell him the test requires urine collection over a 24-hour period.
• If the patient is to collect the specimen, teach him the proper technique.
• Provide the Albright-Reifenstein diet (which contains about 130 mg of calcium/24 hours) for 3 days before the test or provide a copy of the diet for the patient to follow at home.

Procedure and posttest care
• Collect the patient's urine over a 24-hour period.
• Observe a patient with low urine calcium levels for tetany.

Precautions
• Tell the patient not to contaminate the specimen with toilet tissue or stool.

Reference values
Normal values depend on dietary intake. For a normal diet, urine calcium levels for a 24-hour period range from 25 to 300 mg/24 hours in males and 20 to 275 mg/24 hours in females. Normal excretion of phosphate is less than 1,000 mg/24 hours.

Abnormal findings
A variety of disorders may affect calcium and phosphorus levels. (See *Disorders that affect urine calcium and urine phosphorus levels.*)

Disorders That Affect Urine Calcium and Urine Phosphorus Levels

DISORDER	URINE CALCIUM LEVEL	URINE PHOSPHATE LEVEL
Hyperparathyroidism	Elevated	Elevated
Vitamin D intoxication	Elevated	Suppressed
Metastatic carcinoma	Elevated	Normal
Sarcoidosis	Elevated	Suppressed
Renal tubular acidosis	Elevated	Elevated
Multiple myeloma	Elevated or normal	Elevated or normal
Paget's disease	Normal	Normal
Milk-alkali syndrome	Suppressed or normal	Suppressed or normal
Hypoparathyroidism	Suppressed	Suppressed
Acute nephrosis	Suppressed	Suppressed or normal
Chronic nephrosis	Suppressed	Suppressed
Acute nephritis	Suppressed	Suppressed
Renal insufficiency	Suppressed	Suppressed
Osteomalacia	Suppressed	Suppressed
Steatorrhea	Suppressed	Suppressed

Interfering factors
- Contamination of the specimen with toilet tissue or stool
- Thiazide diuretics, sodium phosphate, and glucocorticoids

MAGNESIUM

Measurement of urine magnesium is especially useful because magnesium deficiency is detectable in urine before it changes serum magnesium levels. This test may be used to rule out magnesium deficiency as the cause of neurologic symptoms and to help evaluate glomerular function in suspected renal disease.

Magnesium is a cation found primarily in the bones and in intracellular fluid; a small amount is present in extracellular fluid. This element activates many enzyme systems, helps transport sodium and potassium across cell membranes, affects nucleic acid and protein metabolism, and influences intracellular calcium levels through its effect on secretion of parathyroid hormone.

Purpose
• To rule out magnesium deficiency in patients with symptoms of central nervous system irritation
• To detect excessive urinary excretion of magnesium
• To help evaluate glomerular function in renal disease

Patient preparation
• Explain to the patient that this test determines urine magnesium levels.
• Tell him that this test requires urine collection over a 24-hour period.

Procedure and posttest care
• Collect the patient's urine over a 24-hour period.

Precautions
• Tell the patient to be careful not to contaminate the urine specimen with toilet tissue or stool.

Reference values
Normal urinary excretion of magnesium is 6 to 10 mEq/24 hours or 3 to 5 mmol/24 hours.

Abnormal findings
Low urine magnesium levels may result from malabsorption, acute or chronic diarrhea, diabetic ketoacidosis, dehydration, pancreatitis, advanced renal failure, and primary aldosteronism. They may also result from decreased dietary intake of magnesium.
    Elevated urine magnesium levels may result from early chronic renal disease, adrenocortical insufficiency (Addison's disease), chronic alcoholism, or chronic ingestion of magnesium-containing antacids.

Interfering factors
• Contamination of the specimen with toilet tissue or stool

• Magnesium-containing antacids, ethacrynic acid, thiazide diuretics, and aldosterone (possible increase)

COPPER

The copper test measures the urine level of copper, an essential trace element and a component of several metalloenzymes and proteins necessary for hemoglobin synthesis and oxidation reduction. Most copper in plasma is bound to and transported by an alpha$_2$-globulin (plasma protein) called ceruloplasmin. When copper is unbound, the ions can inhibit many enzyme reactions, resulting in copper toxicity. Urine normally contains only a small amount of free copper.
    Determination of urine copper levels is frequently used to detect Wilson's disease, a rare, inborn metabolic error that is most common among people of eastern European Jewish, southern Italian, or Sicilian ancestry.

Purpose
• To help detect Wilson's disease
• To screen infants with family histories of Wilson's disease

Patient preparation
• Explain to the patient that this test determines the amount of copper in urine.
• Inform him that no special restrictions are necessary.
• Tell him the test requires urine collection over a 24-hour period. If the specimen is to be collected at home, describe the proper collection technique.

Procedure and posttest care
• Collect the patient's urine over a 24-hour period.

- Refrigerate the specimen during the collection period.

Precautions
- Tell the patient not to contaminate the urine specimen with toilet tissue or stool.

Reference values
Normal urinary excretion of copper is 15 to 60 μg/24 hours.

Abnormal findings
Elevated urine copper levels usually indicate Wilson's disease (a liver biopsy helps establish this diagnosis). Wilson's disease is marked by decreased ceruloplasmin, increased urinary excretion of copper, and accumulation of copper in the interstitial tissues of the liver and brain. Early detection and treatment (low-copper diet and D-penicillamine) are vital to prevent irreversible changes, such as nerve tissue degeneration and cirrhosis of the liver.

Elevated copper levels may also occur in nephrotic syndromes, chronic active hepatitis, biliary cirrhosis, rheumatoid arthritis, chelation therapy, and estrogen therapy.

Interfering factors
- Contamination of the specimen with toilet tissue or stool
- Failure to refrigerate specimen

HEMOSIDERIN

The test for hemosiderin measures the urine level of hemosiderin — a colloidal iron oxide and one of the two forms of iron that are stored and deposited in body tissue.

When iron storage mechanisms fail to manage iron overload, excess iron may escape to cells unaccustomed to high iron concentrations and may produce toxic effects. Toxicity may affect the liver, myocardium, bone marrow, pancreas, kidneys, and skin. Subsequent tissue damage is referred to as hemochromatosis. Hemochromatosis may occur in a rare hereditary form (primary hemochromatosis) and in exogenous forms.

Purpose
- To aid diagnosis of hemochromatosis

Patient preparation
- Explain to the patient that this test helps determine if the body is accumulating excessive amounts of iron.
- Inform him that no restrictions are necessary and that the test requires a urine specimen.

Procedure and posttest care
- Collect a random urine specimen of approximately 30 ml.

Precautions
- Seal the container securely, and send the specimen to the laboratory immediately.

Normal findings
Normally, hemosiderin is not found in urine.

Abnormal findings
The presence of hemosiderin, appearing as yellow-brown granules in urinary sediment, indicates hemochromatosis; liver or bone marrow biopsy is necessary for confirmation of primary hemochromatosis. Hemosiderin may also suggest pernicious anemia, chronic hemolytic anemia, multiple blood transfusions, and paroxysmal nocturnal hemoglobinuria, the result of excessive iron injections or dietary intake of iron.

Interfering factor
• Failure to send the specimen to the laboratory immediately

OXALATE

Oxalate, a salt of oxalic acid, is an end product of metabolism and is excreted almost exclusively in the urine. Measuring urine levels of oxalate detects hyperoxaluria, a disorder in which oxalate accumulates in the soft and connective tissue, especially in the kidneys and bladder, causing chronic inflammation and fibrosis. Calcium oxalate deposits are the most common cause of renal calculi, which may produce kidney damage.

Purpose
• To detect primary hyperoxaluria in infants
• To rule out hyperoxaluria in renal insufficiency

Patient preparation
• Explain to the patient (or to the parents if the patient is a child) that this test determines if the urine contains excess oxalate.
• Tell the patient or parents that the test requires urine collection over a 24-hour period.
• Tell the patient to avoid foods high in oxalate — such as tomatoes, strawberries, rhubarb, and spinach — for 1 week before the test.

Procedure and posttest care
• Collect the patient's urine over a 24-hour period. Use a light-protected container with hydrochloric acid.

Precautions
• Tell the patient not to urinate directly into the 24-hour specimen container, but to use an appropriate container.
• Advise him not to contaminate the urine specimen with toilet tissue or stool.

Reference values
Urine oxalate levels of 0.11 to 0.46 mmol/24 hours are considered normal.

Abnormal findings
Elevated urine oxalate levels (hyperoxaluria) may result from excessive metabolic production of oxalate or increased oxalate intake. Levels as high as 100 to 400 mg/24 hours can occur.

Primary hyperoxaluria, a rare inborn metabolic disorder, causes excessive production and urinary excretion of oxalate. In this type of hyperoxaluria, urine oxalate levels become elevated before serum levels become elevated.

Secondary hyperoxaluria can result from pancreatic insufficiency, diabetes mellitus, cirrhosis, pyridoxine deficiency, Crohn's disease, ileal resection, or ingestion of antifreeze (ethylene glycol) or stain-remover, or it can occur as a reaction to a methoxyflurane anesthetic.

Interfering factors
• Tomatoes, strawberries, rhubarb, and spinach (possible false increase)
• Contamination of the specimen with toilet tissue or stool

CHAPTER 7

Additional Specimen Tests

RESPIRATORY SYSTEM   384

384   Examination of sputum for ova   385   Pleural fluid analysis
      and parasites

GASTROINTESTINAL SYSTEM   387

387   Basal gastric secretion test   398   Fecal urobilinogen
389   Gastric acid stimulation test   399   Examination of stool for ova
390   Peritoneal fluid analysis   and parasites
393   Test for duodenal parasites   401   Examination of stool for
395   Fecal occult blood test   rotavirus antigen
397   Fecal lipids

REPRODUCTIVE SYSTEM   402

402   Sex chromatin tests   414   Papanicolaou test
403   Chromosome analysis   417   Semen analysis
409   Amniotic fluid analysis   420   Contraction stress test

MISCELLANEOUS TESTS   421

421   Cerebrospinal fluid analysis   429   Pericardial fluid analysis
425   Soluble amyloid beta protein   433   Sweat test
      precursor   435   Examination of urogenital
427   Synovial fluid analysis   secretions for trichomonads

RESPIRATORY SYSTEM

EXAMINATION OF SPUTUM FOR OVA AND PARASITES

Parasitic infestation is rare in North America but may result from exposure to *Entamoeba histolytica, Ascaris lumbricoides, Echinococcus granulosus, Strongyloides stercoralis, Paragonimus westermani,* or *Necator americanus.* A sputum specimen is obtained by expectoration or tracheal suctioning to evaluate for parasites.

Purpose
● To identify pulmonary parasites

Patient preparation
● Explain to the patient that this test helps identify parasitic pulmonary infection.
● Tell him the test requires a sputum specimen or, if necessary, tracheal suctioning.
● Inform him that early morning collection is preferred because secretions accumulate overnight.
● Encourage the patient to help sputum production by drinking fluids the night before collection.
● Teach the patient how to expectorate by taking three deep breaths and forcing a deep cough.
● Tell him that he'll experience some discomfort from the catheter during tracheal suctioning.

Equipment
For expectoration: Sterile, disposable, impermeable container with screw cap

or tight-fitting cap, nebulizer, intermittent positive-pressure breathing ventilator, and 10% sodium chloride, acetylcysteine, or sterile or distilled water aerosols, to induce cough
For tracheal suctioning: #16 or #18 French suction catheter, sterile gloves, sterile specimen container or sputum trap, sterile 0.9% sodium chloride solution

Procedure and posttest care
Expectoration
● Instruct the patient to breathe deeply a few times and then to "deep cough" and expectorate into the container.
● Use chest physiotherapy, or heated aerosol spray (nebulization), if cough is unproductive.
● Take proper precautions in sending the specimen to the laboratory.
Tracheal suctioning
● Administer oxygen before and after the procedure, if necessary.
● Attach a sputum trap to the suction catheter.
● Wearing a sterile glove, lubricate the tip of the catheter; then pass the catheter through the patient's nostril without suction. (The patient will cough when the catheter passes into the larynx.)
● Advance the catheter into the trachea.
● Apply suction for no longer than 15 seconds to obtain the specimen.
● Stop suction, and gently remove the catheter.
● Discard the catheter and glove in a proper receptacle.
● Detach the sputum trap from the suction apparatus and cap the opening.
● Label all specimens carefully.
● Provide proper mouth care. After suctioning, offer water.
● Monitor vital signs every hour until the patient is stable.

Precautions

- Be sure to wear gloves when performing procedures and handling specimens.

CLINICAL ALERT Don't perform tracheal suctioning on patients with esophageal varices.

- If the patient has asthma or chronic bronchitis, watch for aggravated bronchospasms with use of more than 10% concentration of sodium chloride or acetylcysteine in an aerosol.

CLINICAL ALERT Suction for only 5 to 10 seconds at a time during tracheal suctioning. *Never* suction for longer than 15 seconds. If the patient shows signs of hypoxia *or* cyanosis, remove the suctioning catheter immediately and administer oxygen.

- Send the specimen to the laboratory immediately, or place it in preservative.

Normal findings

Normally, no parasites or ova are present.

Abnormal findings

The parasite identified indicates the type of pulmonary infection and the presence of adult-stage intestinal infection.

- *Entamoeba histolytica* trophozoites: pulmonary amebiasis
- *A. lumbricoides* larvae and adults: pneumonitis
- *Echinococcus granulosus* cysts of larval stage: hydatid disease
- *P. westermani* ova: paragonimiasis
- *S. stercoralis* larvae: strongyloidiasis
- *N. americanus* larvae: hookworm disease

Interfering factors

- Improper collection technique or failure to send the specimen to the laboratory immediately
- Recent therapy with antihelmintics or amebicides

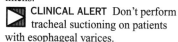

PLEURAL FLUID ANALYSIS

The pleura, a two-layer membrane that covers the lungs and lines the thoracic cavity, maintains a small amount of lubricating fluid between its layers to minimize friction during respiration. Increased fluid in this space may result from diseases such as cancer or tuberculosis, or from blood or lymphatic disorders, and can cause respiratory difficulty.

In pleural fluid aspiration (thoracentesis), the thoracic wall is punctured to obtain a specimen of pleural fluid for analysis or to relieve pulmonary compression and resultant respiratory distress.

Purpose

- To determine the cause and nature of pleural effusion

Patient preparation

- Explain to the patient that the test assesses the space around the lungs for fluid.
- Inform him that he needn't restrict food or fluids.
- Tell him who will perform the test and where.
- Explain that chest X-rays or an ultrasound study may precede the test to help locate the fluid.
- Check the patient's history for hypersensitivity to local anesthetics.
- Warn the patient that he may feel a stinging sensation on injection of the anesthetic and some pressure during withdrawal of the fluid.
- Advise him not to cough, breathe deeply, or move during the test to minimize the risk of injury to the lung.

Equipment

Sterile collection bottles, sterile gloves, adhesive tape, sterile thoracentesis tray (a prepackaged, disposable tray with the following: 70% alcohol or povidone-iodine solution, drapes, local anesthetic [usually 1% lidocaine], 5-ml sterile syringe for local anesthetic, 25G needle, 50-ml syringe for removing fluid, 17G aspiration needle, sterile specimen bottle or tube, three-way stopcock or sterile tubing to prevent air from entering the pleural cavity, small sterile dressing)

Procedure and posttest care

• Record baseline vital signs.
• If necessary, shave the area around the needle insertion site.
• Position the patient to widen intercostal spaces and to allow easier access to the pleural cavity. He must be well-supported and comfortable, preferably seated at the edge of the bed with a chair or stool supporting his feet and his head and arms resting on a padded overbed table. If the patient can't sit up, he may be positioned on his unaffected side, with the arm on the affected side elevated above his head.
• Remind him not to cough, breathe deeply, or move suddenly during the procedure.
• During aspiration, observe the patient for signs of respiratory distress, such as weakness, dyspnea, pallor, cyanosis, changes in heart rate, tachypnea, diaphoresis, blood-tinged frothy mucus, and hypotension.
• After the needle is withdrawn, apply slight pressure and a small adhesive bandage to the puncture site.
• Label the specimen container, and record the date and time of the test and the amount, color, and character of the fluid (clear, frothy, purulent, bloody) on the laboratory slip.
• Note any signs of distress exhibited during the procedure.

• Record the exact location from which fluid was removed to aid diagnosis.
• Reposition the patient comfortably on the affected side. Tell him to remain on this side for at least 1 hour to seal the puncture site. Elevate the head of the bed to facilitate breathing.
• Monitor vital signs every 30 minutes for 2 hours, and then every 4 hours until they are stable.
• Tell the patient to call a nurse immediately if he experiences difficulty breathing.

CLINICAL ALERT Watch for signs of pneumothorax, tension pneumothorax, fluid reaccumulation and, if a large amount of fluid was withdrawn, pulmonary edema or cardiac distress due to mediastinal shift. Usually, a posttest X-ray is ordered to detect these complications before clinical symptoms appear.
• Check the puncture site for any fluid leakage. A large amount of leakage is abnormal. Also check the site and surrounding area for subcutaneous emphysema.

Precautions

• Thoracentesis is contraindicated in patients who have a history of bleeding disorders.
• Use strict aseptic technique.
• Note the patient's temperature and whether he's receiving antimicrobial therapy on the laboratory slip.
• Add a small amount (about 0.5 ml) of sterile heparin to the container to prevent coagulation of the fluid.
• Send the specimen to the laboratory immediately.

Reference values

Normally, the pleural cavity maintains negative pressure and contains less than 20 ml of serous fluid.

Abnormal findings

Pleural effusion results from the abnormal formation or reabsorption of pleural fluid. Certain characteristics classify pleural fluid as either a transudate (a low-protein fluid that has leaked from normal blood vessels) or an exudate (a protein-rich fluid that has leaked from blood vessels with increased permeability).

Pleural fluid may contain blood (hemothorax), chyle (chylothorax), or pus and necrotic tissue. Blood-tinged fluid may indicate a traumatic tap; if so, the fluid should clear as aspiration progresses.

Transudative effusion generally results from diminished colloidal pressure, increased negative pressure within the pleural cavity, ascites, systemic and pulmonary venous hypertension, heart failure, hepatic cirrhosis, and nephritis.

Exudative effusion results from disorders that increase pleural capillary permeability (possibly with changes in hydrostatic or colloid osmotic pressures), lymphatic drainage interference, infections, pulmonary infarctions, and neoplasms. Exudative effusion associated with depressed glucose levels, elevated lactate dehydrogenase (LD) isoenzymes, rheumatoid arthritis cells, and negative smears, cultures, and cytologic examination may indicate pleurisy associated with rheumatoid arthritis.

The most common pathogens that appear in culture studies of pleural fluid are *Mycobacterium tuberculosis, Staphylococcus aureus, Streptococcus pneumoniae* and other streptococci, *Haemophilus influenzae* and, in the case of a ruptured pulmonary abscess, anaerobes such as *Bacteroides*. Cultures are usually positive during the early stages of infection; however, antibiotic therapy may produce a negative culture despite a positive Gram stain and grossly purulent fluid. Empyema may result from complications of pneumonia, pulmonary abscess, perforation of the esophagus, or penetration from mediastinitis. A high percentage of neutrophils suggests septic inflammation; predominating lymphocytes suggest tuberculosis, or fungal or viral effusions.

Serosanguineous fluid may indicate pleural extension of a malignant tumor. Elevated LD in a nonpurulent, nonhemolyzed, nonbloody effusion may also suggest malignancy. Pleural fluid glucose levels that are 30 to 40 mg/dl lower than blood glucose levels may indicate a malignant tumor, a bacterial infection, nonseptic inflammation, or metastasis. Increased amylase levels occur in pleural effusions associated with pancreatitis.

Interfering factors

- Failure to use aseptic technique
- Failure to send the specimen to the laboratory immediately
- Antimicrobial therapy before aspiration of fluid for culture (possible decrease in numbers of bacteria, making it difficult to isolate the infecting organism)

GASTROINTESTINAL SYSTEM

BASAL GASTRIC SECRETION TEST

The basal gastric secretion test measures basal secretion during fasting by aspirating stomach contents through a nasogastric (NG) tube. It's indicated in patients with obscure epigastric pain, anorexia, and weight loss. Because external factors — such as the sight or odor of food — and psychological stress stimulate gastric secretion, accurate testing requires that the patient be relaxed and isolated from all sources of sensory stimulation. Although abnormal basal secretion can suggest various gastric and duodenal disorders, complete evaluation of secretion requires the gastric acid stimulation test.

Purpose
• To determine gastric output while the patient is fasting

Patient preparation
• Explain to the patient that this test measures the stomach's secretion of acid.
• Instruct him to restrict food for 12 hours and fluids and smoking for 8 hours before the test.
• Tell him who will perform the test and that the procedure takes approximately 1½ hours (or 2½ hours, if followed by the gastric acid stimulation test).
• Inform the patient that the test requires insertion of a tube through the nose and into the stomach and that he may initially experience discomfort and may cough or gag.
• Withhold antacids, anticholinergics, cholinergics, alcohol, cimetidine, reserpine, adrenergic blockers, and adrenocorticosteroids for 24 hours before the test. If these medications must be continued, note this on the laboratory slip.
• Check the patient's pulse rate and blood pressure just before the test. Then encourage him to relax.

Procedure and posttest care
• Insert the NG tube after seating the patient comfortably.
• Attach a 20-ml syringe to it, and aspirate the stomach contents.

• To ensure complete emptying of the stomach, ask the patient to assume three positions in sequence — supine and right and left lateral decubitus — while stomach contents are aspirated.
• Label the specimen container "Residual Contents."
• Connect the NG tube to the suction machine. Aspirate gastric contents by continuous low suction for 1½ hours. Aspiration can also be performed manually with a syringe.
• Collect a specimen every 15 minutes, but discard the first two; this eliminates the specimen that could be affected by the stress of the intubation.
• Record the color and odor of each specimen, and note the presence of food, mucus, bile, or blood.
• Label these specimens "Basal Contents," and number them 1 through 4.
• Next, secretion volume and acid concentration are measured.
• If the NG tube is to be left in place, clamp it or attach it to low intermittent suction.
• Watch for complications, such as nausea, vomiting, and abdominal distention or pain, following removal of the NG tube.
• If the patient complains of a sore throat, provide soothing lozenges.
• Tell the patient to resume his usual diet and any medications that were withheld for the test, unless the gastric acid stimulation test will also be performed.

Precautions
• The basal gastric secretion test is contraindicated in patients with conditions that prohibit NG intubation.
• During insertion, make sure the NG tube enters the esophagus, and not the trachea; remove it immediately if the patient develops cyanosis or paroxysmal coughing.

• Monitor vital signs during intubation, and observe carefully for arrhythmias.

• To prevent contamination of the specimens with saliva, instruct the patient to expectorate excess saliva.

• When collection is completed, send the specimens to the laboratory immediately.

Reference values

Normally, basal secretion ranges from 0 to 5 mmol/hour.

Abnormal findings

Abnormal basal secretion findings are nonspecific and must be considered with the results of the gastric acid stimulation test. Elevated secretion may suggest duodenal or jejunal ulcer (after partial gastrectomy); markedly elevated secretion, Zollinger-Ellison syndrome. Depressed secretion may indicate gastric carcinoma or benign gastric ulcer. Absence of secretion may indicate pernicious anemia.

Interfering factors

• Failure to observe pretest restrictions (increase)

• Psychological stress (possible increase)

• Cholinergics, reserpine, alcohol, adrenergic blockers, and adrenocorticosteroids (possible increase)

• Antacids, anticholinergics, and cimetidine (possible decrease)

GASTRIC ACID STIMULATION TEST

The gastric acid stimulation test measures the secretion of gastric acid for 1 hour after subcutaneous injection of pentagastrin or a similar drug that stimulates gastric acid output. This test is indicated when the basal secretion test suggests abnormal gastric secretion and is commonly performed immediately afterward. Although this test detects abnormal gastric secretion, radiographic studies and endoscopy are necessary to determine the cause.

Purpose

• To aid diagnosis of duodenal ulcer, Zollinger-Ellison syndrome, pernicious anemia, and gastric carcinoma

Patient preparation

• Explain to the patient that this test determines if the stomach is secreting acid properly.

• Instruct him to refrain from eating, drinking, and smoking after midnight before the test.

• Tell him who will perform the test, where it will take place, and that it takes 1 hour.

• Explain that the test requires passing a tube through the nose and into the stomach and a subcutaneous injection of pentagastrin.

• Describe the possible adverse effects of the test, such as abdominal pain, nausea, vomiting, flushing, and transitory dizziness, faintness, and numbness of extremities. Instruct him to report such symptoms immediately.

• Check the patient's history for hypersensitivity to pentagastrin.

• Withhold antacids, anticholinergics, adrenergic blockers, cimetidine, and reserpine for 24 hours before the test. If these drugs must be continued, note this on the laboratory slip.

• Record baseline vital signs before beginning the procedure.

Procedure and posttest care

• After basal gastric secretions have been collected, the nasogastric (NG) tube remains in place.

• Pentagastrin is injected subcutaneously. After 15 minutes, collect a specimen every 15 minutes for 1 hour.
• Record the color and odor of each specimen, and note the presence of food, mucus, bile, or blood.
• Label the specimens "Stimulated Contents," and number them 1 through 4.
• If the NG tube is kept in place, it should be clamped or attached to low intermittent suction.
• Watch for nausea, vomiting, and abdominal distention and pain after the NG tube is removed.
• If the patient complains of a sore throat, provide soothing lozenges.
• Tell the patient he may resume his usual diet.
• Resume any medications withheld for the test.

Precautions
• The gastric acid stimulation test is contraindicated in patients with hypersensitivity to pentagastrin or with conditions that prohibit NG intubation.
• Observe for adverse effects of pentagastrin.
• To prevent contamination of the specimens with saliva, instruct the patient to expectorate excess saliva.
• When collection is completed, send the specimens to the laboratory immediately.

Reference values
Following stimulation, gastric acid secretion ranges from 10 to 20 mmol/hour.

Abnormal findings
Elevated gastric secretion may indicate duodenal ulcer; markedly elevated secretion suggests Zollinger-Ellison syndrome. Depressed secretion may indicate gastric carcinoma; achlorhydria may indicate pernicious anemia.

Interfering factors
• Failure to observe pretest restrictions
• Cholinergics, adrenergic blockers, and reserpine (increase)
• Antacids, anticholinergics, and cimetidine (decrease)

PERITONEAL FLUID ANALYSIS

Peritoneal fluid analysis assesses a specimen of peritoneal fluid obtained by paracentesis. This procedure requires inserting a trocar and cannula through the abdominal wall while the patient receives a local anesthetic. If the fluid specimen is removed for therapeutic purposes, the trocar may be connected to a drainage system. However, if only a small amount of fluid is removed for diagnostic purposes, an 18G needle may be used in place of the trocar and cannula. In a four-quadrant tap, fluid is aspirated from each quadrant of the abdomen to verify abdominal trauma and confirm the need for surgery.

Purpose
• To determine the cause of ascites
• To detect abdominal trauma

Patient preparation
• Explain to the patient that this procedure helps determine the cause of ascites or detects abdominal trauma.
• Inform him that he needn't restrict food or fluids before the test.
• Tell him that the test requires a peritoneal fluid specimen, that he'll receive a local anesthetic to minimize discomfort, and that the procedure takes about 45 minutes to perform.

• Provide psychological support to decrease the patient's anxiety, and assure him that complications are rare.

• If the patient has severe ascites, inform him that the procedure will relieve his discomfort and allow him to breathe more easily.

• Tell the patient to void just before the test. This helps prevent accidental bladder injury during needle insertion.

Procedure and posttest care

• Have the patient sit on a bed or in a chair with his feet flat on the floor and his back well supported. If he cannot tolerate being out of bed, place him in high Fowler's position and make him as comfortable as possible.

• Except for the puncture site, keep him covered to prevent chilling.

• Provide a plastic sheet or absorbent pad to collect spillage and to protect the patient and bed linens.

• Shave the puncture site, prepare the skin, and drape the area.

• Inject the local anesthetic.

• Insert the needle or trocar and cannula 1″ to 2″ (2.5 to 5 cm) below the umbilicus. (However, you may also insert them through the flank, the iliac fossa, the border of the rectus, or at each quadrant of the abdomen.)

• If a trocar and cannula are used, make a small incision to facilitate insertion. When the needle pierces the peritoneum, it "gives" with an audible sound. Remove the trocar and aspirate a sample of fluid with a 50-ml luer-lock syringe.

• Apply a gauze dressing to the puncture site. Make sure it's thick enough to absorb all drainage. Check the dressing frequently (for example, whenever you check vital signs); reinforce or apply a pressure dressing, if needed.

• Monitor vital signs until stable. If the patient's recovery is poor, check vital signs every 15 minutes. Weigh the patient and measure abdominal girth;

compare these with baseline measurements.

• Allow the patient to rest and, if possible, withhold treatment or procedures that may cause undue stress, such as linen changes.

• Monitor urine output for at least 24 hours, and watch for hematuria, which may indicate bladder trauma.

• If a large amount of fluid was aspirated, watch for signs of vascular collapse (color change, elevated pulse and respiratory rates, decreased blood pressure and central venous pressure, mental changes, and dizziness). Administer fluids orally if the patient is alert and can accept them.

CLINICAL ALERT Watch for signs of hemorrhage or shock and for increasing pain or abdominal tenderness. These may indicate a perforated intestine or, depending on the site of the tap, puncture of the inferior epigastric artery, hematoma of the anterior cecal wall, or rupture of the iliac vein or bladder.

CLINICAL ALERT Observe the patient with severe hepatic disease for signs of hepatic coma, which may result from loss of sodium and potassium accompanying hypovolemia. Watch for mental changes, drowsiness, and stupor. Such a patient is also prone to uremia, infection, hemorrhage, and protein depletion.

• Administer I.V. infusions and albumin. Check the laboratory report for electrolytes (especially sodium) and serum protein levels.

Precautions

• Peritoneal fluid analysis should be performed cautiously in pregnant patients and in patients with bleeding tendencies or unstable vital signs.

• Check vital signs every 15 minutes during the procedure. Watch for deviations from baseline findings. Observe

PERITONEAL FLUID ANALYSIS

ELEMENT	NORMAL VALUE OR FINDING
Gross appearance	Sterile, odorless, clear to pale yellow color; scant amount (< 50 ml)
Red blood cells	None
White blood cells	< 300/μl (undiluted peritoneal fluid) or < 500/μl (lavage fluid)
Protein	< 4.1 g/dl
Glucose	70 to 100 mg/dl
Amylase	140 to 400 U/L
Ammonia	< 50 μg/dl
Alkaline phosphatase	30 to 110 U/L
Cytology	No abnormal cells present
Bacteria	None
Fungi	None

for dizziness, pallor, perspiration, and increased anxiety.

• If rapid fluid aspiration induces hypovolemia and shock, reduce the vertical distance between the trocar and the collection bag to slow the drainage rate. If necessary, stop drainage by turning off the stopcock or by clamping the tubing.

• Avoid contamination of specimens, which alters their bacterial content. Send them to the laboratory immediately.

Reference values

For normal peritoneal fluid values, see *Peritoneal fluid analysis.*

Abnormal findings

Milk-colored peritoneal fluid may result from chyle or lymph fluid escaping from a thoracic duct that is damaged or blocked by a malignant tumor, lymphoma, tuberculosis, parasitic infestation, adhesion, or hepatic cirrhosis; a pseudochylous condition may result from the presence of leukocytes or tumor cells. Differential diagnosis of true chylous ascites depends on the presence of elevated triglyceride levels (≥ 400 mg/dl) and microscopic fat globules.

Cloudy or turbid fluid may indicate peritonitis due to primary bacterial infection, ruptured bowel (after trauma), pancreatitis, strangulated or infarcted intestine, or appendicitis. Bloody fluid may result from a benign or malignant tumor, hemorrhagic pancreatitis, or a traumatic tap; however, if the fluid fails to clear on continued aspiration, traumatic tap isn't the cause. Bile-stained green fluid may indicate a ruptured gallbladder, acute pancreatitis, or perforated intestine or duodenal ulcer.

A red blood cell count over 100/µl indicates neoplasm or tuberculosis; a count over 100,000/µl indicates intra-abdominal trauma. An elevated white blood cell count with more than 25% neutrophils occurs in 90% of patients with spontaneous bacterial peritonitis and in 50% of those with cirrhosis. A high percentage of lymphocytes suggest tuberculous peritonitis or chylous ascites. Numerous mesothelial cells indicate tuberculous peritonitis.

Protein levels rise above 3 g/dl in malignancy and above 4 g/dl in tuberculosis. Peritoneal fluid glucose levels fall below 60 mg/dl in 30% to 50% of patients with tuberculous peritonitis and peritoneal carcinomatosis.

Amylase levels rise in about 90% of patients with pancreatic trauma, pancreatic pseudocyst, or acute pancreatitis and may also rise in intestinal necrosis or strangulation.

Peritoneal alkaline phosphatase levels rise to more than twice the normal serum levels in about 90% of patients with ruptured or strangulated small intestine. Peritoneal ammonia levels also exceed twice the normal serum levels in ruptured or strangulated large and small intestines, and in ruptured ulcer or appendix.

A protein ascitic fluid to serum ratio of 0.5 or greater may suggest malignant, tuberculous, or pancreatic ascites. The presence of this finding indicates a nonhepatic cause; its absence suggests uncomplicated hepatic disease. An albumin gradient between ascitic fluid and serum over 1 g/dl indicates chronic hepatic disease; a lesser value suggests malignancy.

Cytologic examination of peritoneal fluid accurately detects malignant cells. Microbiological examination can reveal coliforms, anaerobes, and enterococci, which can enter the peritoneum from a ruptured organ, or from infections accompanying appendicitis, pancreatitis, tuberculosis, or ovarian disease. Gram-positive cocci often indicate primary peritonitis; gram-negative organisms, secondary peritonitis. The presence of fungi may indicate histoplasmosis, candidiasis, or coccidioidomycosis.

Interfering factors

• Unsterile collection technique or failure to send the specimen to the laboratory immediately

• Contamination of the specimen with blood, bile, urine, or stool due to injury to underlying structures during paracentesis

TEST FOR DUODENAL PARASITES

This test evaluates duodenal contents for the presence of parasites in a specimen obtained by duodenal intubation and aspiration or by the string test (Entero test). Such parasites include trophozoites of *Giardia lamblia, G. duodenalis,* the ova and larvae of *Strongyloides stercoralis,* and the ova of *Entamoeba histolytica, Necator americanus,* or *Ancylostoma duodenale* in various stages of cleavage. This test can also detect ova of the liver flukes *Clonorchis sinensis* and *Fasciola hepatica* in the biliary tract. However, liver fluke infestations are rare in North America.

Examination of duodenal contents for ova and parasites is performed only in a symptomatic patient with negative stool examinations.

Purpose
● To detect parasitic infestation when stool examinations are negative

Patient preparation
● Explain to the patient that this test detects parasitic infestation of the GI tract.
● Instruct him to restrict food and fluids for 12 hours before the test.
● Tell him who will perform the test and when.
● If the test will be done with a nasoenteric tube, warn him that he may gag during the tube's passage, but assure him that following the examiner's instructions about positioning, breathing, and swallowing will minimize discomfort.
● Instruct the patient to empty his bladder just before the procedure.

Equipment
Gloves, double-lumen tube with olive tip (or weighted gelatin capsule with string attached, for string test), water-soluble jelly, 30-ml sterile syringe, emesis basin, sterile specimen container, adhesive tape ½″ wide

Procedure and posttest care
Nasoenteric tube
● After inserting the tube, place the patient in a left lateral decubitus position, with his feet elevated, to allow peristalsis to move the tube into the duodenum.
● The pH of a small amount of aspirated fluid determines tube position: If the tube is in the stomach, pH is lower than 7.0; if it's in the duodenum, pH is higher than 7.0.
● Fluoroscopy can also determine correct positioning. When position is confirmed, residual duodenal contents are aspirated.
● Transfer the entire specimen to a sterile container, and label the container appropriately.

Entero test capsule with string
● Tape the free end of the string to the patient's cheek.
● Instruct him to swallow the capsule (on the other end of the string) with water.
● Leave the string in place for 4 hours; then pull it out gently and place it in a sterile container.
● Label the container appropriately.
● Dispose of equipment properly.
● Provide oral hygiene and offer the patient water.
● Observe carefully for signs of perforation, such as dysphagia or fever.
● Tell the patient he can resume his normal diet.

Precautions
● Use gloves when performing the procedure and handling specimens.
● Duodenal intubation is contraindicated for pregnant women and for patients with acute cholecystitis; acute pancreatitis; esophageal varices, stenosis, diverticula, or malignant neoplasms; recent severe gastric hemorrhage; aortic aneurysm; or heart failure.
● When possible, obtain the specimen before the start of drug therapy.
● Send the specimen to the laboratory immediately.
● Withdraw the tube slowly (about 6″ to 8″ [15 to 20 cm] every 10 minutes) to the esophagus; then clamp the tube and remove it quickly. *Never* force the tube.

Normal findings
Normally, no ova or parasites appear in duodenal contents.

Abnormal findings
Finding *G. lamblia* or *G. duodenalis* indicates giardiasis, possibly causing malabsorption syndrome; *S. stercoralis* suggests strongyloidiasis; *A. duodenale* and *N. americanus* imply hookworm disease; and *C. sinensis* and

F. hepatica signify histopathologic changes in the bile ducts.

Interfering factors
- Failure to observe pretest restrictions (possible dilution of the specimen)
- Previous drug therapy or delay in transporting the specimen to the laboratory

FECAL OCCULT BLOOD TEST

Fecal occult blood is detected by microscopic analysis or by chemical tests for hemoglobin, such as the guaiac test. Normally, stool contains small amounts of blood (2 to 2.5 ml/day); therefore, tests for occult blood detect quantities larger than this. Testing is indicated when clinical symptoms and preliminary blood studies suggest GI bleeding. Additional tests are required to pinpoint the origin of the bleeding. (See *Common sites and causes of GI blood loss*, page 396.)

Purpose
- To detect GI bleeding
- To aid early diagnosis of colorectal cancer

Patient preparation
- Explain to the patient that this test helps detect abnormal GI bleeding.
- Instruct him to maintain a high-fiber diet and to refrain from eating red meats, turnips, and horseradish for 48 to 72 hours before the test as well as throughout the collection period.
- Tell him the test requires collection of three stool specimens. Occasionally, only a random specimen is collected.
- Withhold iron preparations, bromides, iodides, rauwolfia derivatives, indomethacin, colchicine, salicylates, phenylbutazone, steroids, and ascorbic acid for 48 hours before the test and throughout the collection period. If these medications must be continued, note this on the laboratory slip.

Procedure and posttest care
- Collect three stool specimens or a random specimen. Testing may take place in the laboratory or in a utility room on the nursing unit, depending on hospital policy.
- Place a small amount of stool on a piece of filter paper.
- Add 2 drops each of tap water, glacial acetic acid, 1:60 solution of gum guaiac in 95% ethyl alcohol, and 3% hydrogen peroxide *or* 2 drops each of 0.2% orthotoluidine and 0.3% hydrogen peroxide. (Most solutions are premixed and bottled.) Mix thoroughly with a tongue blade. Note the color immediately, and check it again after 5 minutes.
- Be sure to obtain specimens from two different areas of each stool to allow for variance in distribution of blood.
- Tell the patient to resume his usual diet and medication schedule.

Precautions
- Instruct the patient to avoid contaminating the stool specimen with toilet tissue or urine.
- Send the specimen to the laboratory or perform the test immediately.

Reference values
Normally, stool contains 2 mg or less total hemoglobin/g. A marginal finding is 2 to 3 mg total hemoglobin/g, and an elevated finding is greater than 3 mg total hemoglobin/g.

Abnormal findings
A dark blue reaction that appears within 5 minutes indicates that the test is positive for occult blood; a strongly positive reaction within 3 to 4 minutes

COMMON SITES AND CAUSES OF G.I. BLOOD LOSS

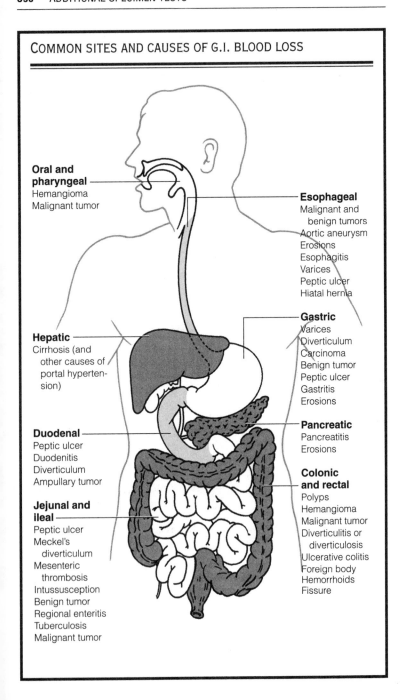

Oral and pharyngeal
Hemangioma
Malignant tumor

Esophageal
Malignant and
  benign tumors
Aortic aneurysm
Erosions
Esophagitis
Varices
Peptic ulcer
Hiatal hernia

Hepatic
Cirrhosis (and
  other causes of
  portal hyperten-
  sion)

Gastric
Varices
Diverticulum
Carcinoma
Benign tumor
Peptic ulcer
Gastritis
Erosions

Duodenal
Peptic ulcer
Duodenitis
Diverticulum
Ampullary tumor

Pancreatic
Pancreatitis
Erosions

Jejunal and ileal
Peptic ulcer
Meckel's
  diverticulum
Mesenteric
  thrombosis
Intussusception
Benign tumor
Regional enteritis
Tuberculosis
Malignant tumor

Colonic and rectal
Polyps
Hemangioma
Malignant tumor
Diverticulitis or
  diverticulosis
Ulcerative colitis
Foreign body
Hemorrhoids
Fissure

is always abnormal. A faint blue reaction is weakly positive and isn't necessarily abnormal. A positive test indicates GI bleeding, which may result from many disorders, such as varices, peptic ulcer, carcinoma, ulcerative colitis, dysentery, or hemorrhagic disease. This test is particularly important for early diagnosis of colorectal cancer. Further tests, such as barium swallow, analyses of gastric contents, and endoscopic procedures, are necessary to define the site and extent of bleeding.

Interfering factors
• Failure to observe pretest restrictions, to test the specimen immediately, or to send it to the laboratory immediately
• Iron preparations, bromides, rauwolfia derivatives, indomethacin, colchicine, phenylbutazone, and steroids (possible increase due to association with GI blood loss)
• Ascorbic acid (false-normal, even with significant bleeding)
• Ingestion of 2 to 5 ml of blood, such as from bleeding gums
• Consumption of food or meat, such as red meat (possible false increase)

FECAL LIPIDS

Lipids excreted in stool include monoglycerides, diglycerides, triglycerides, phospholipids, glycolipids, soaps (fatty acids and fatty acid salts), sterols, and cholesterol esters. When biliary and pancreatic secretions are adequate, emulsified dietary lipids are almost completely absorbed in the small intestine.

Excessive excretion of fecal lipids (steatorrhea) occurs in several malabsorption syndromes. Qualitative and quantitative tests are used to detect excessive excretion of lipids in patients exhibiting signs of malabsorption, such as weight loss, abdominal distention, and scaly skin.

The qualitative test involves staining a specimen of stool with Sudan III dye and then examining it microscopically for evidence of malabsorption, such as undigested muscle fibers and various fats. The quantitative test involves drying and weighing a 72-hour specimen, and then using a solvent to extract the lipids, which are subsequently evaporated and weighed. Only the quantitative test confirms steatorrhea.

Purpose
• To confirm steatorrhea

Patient preparation
• Explain to the patient that this test evaluates digestion of fats.
• Instruct him to abstain from alcohol and to maintain a high-fat diet (100 g/day) for 3 days before the test and during the collection period.
• Tell him the test requires a 72-hour stool collection.
• Withhold azathioprine, bisacodyl, cholestyramine, kanamycin, neomycin, colchicine, aluminum hydroxide, calcium carbonate, alcohol, potassium chloride, and mineral oil because they may affect test results. If these medications must be continued, note this on the laboratory slip.
• Teach the patient how to collect a timed stool specimen, and provide him with the necessary equipment.
• Inform him that the laboratory requires 1 or 2 days to complete the analysis.

Procedure and posttest care
• Collect a 72-hour stool specimen.
• Tell the patient he may resume his usual diet.
• Administer medications withheld before the test.

Precautions

- Don't use a waxed collection container because the wax may become incorporated in the stool and interfere with accurate testing.
- Tell the patient to avoid contaminating the stool specimen with toilet tissue or urine.
- Refrigerate the collection container and keep it tightly covered.

Reference values

Fecal lipids normally comprise less than 20% of excreted solids, with excretion of 2 to 7 g/24 hours.

Abnormal findings

Both digestive and absorptive disorders cause steatorrhea. Digestive disorders may affect the production and release of pancreatic lipase or bile; absorptive disorders may affect the integrity of the intestine.

In pancreatic insufficiency, impaired lipid digestion may result from insufficient production of lipase. Pancreatic resection, cystic fibrosis, chronic pancreatitis, or ductal obstruction by stone or tumor may prevent the normal release or action of lipase.

In impaired hepatic function, faulty lipid digestion may result from inadequate production of bile salts. Biliary obstruction, which may accompany gallbladder disease, may prevent the normal release of bile salts into the duodenum.

Extensive small-bowel resection or bypass may also interrupt normal enterohepatic circulation of bile salts.

Diseases of the intestinal mucosa affect normal absorption of lipids; regional ileitis and atrophy due to malnutrition cause gross structural changes in the intestinal wall, and celiac disease and tropical spruce produce mucosal abnormalities.

Scleroderma, radiation enteritis, fistulas, intestinal tuberculosis, small intestine diverticula, and altered intestinal flora may also cause steatorrhea.

Whipple's disease and lymphomas cause lymphatic obstruction that may inhibit fat absorption.

Interfering factors

- Failure to observe pretest restrictions or use of a waxed collection container
- Contaminated or incomplete stool specimen (total weight less than 300 g)
- Azathioprine, bisacodyl, cholestyramine, kanamycin, neomycin, colchicine, aluminum hydroxide, calcium carbonate, alcohol, potassium chloride, and mineral oil (possible increase or decrease due to inhibited absorption or altered chemical digestion)

FECAL UROBILINOGEN

Urobilinogen, the end product of bilirubin metabolism, is a brown pigment formed by bacterial enzymes in the small intestine. It's excreted in stool or reabsorbed into portal blood, where it's returned to the liver and excreted in bile; a small amount is excreted in urine. Proper bilirubin metabolism depends on normal hepatobiliary system functioning and normal erythrocyte lifespan.

Although measuring fecal urobilinogen is a useful indicator of hepatobiliary and hemolytic disorders, the test is rarely performed because it's easier to measure serum bilirubin and urine urobilinogen.

Purpose

- To aid diagnosis of hepatobiliary and hemolytic disorders

Patient preparation

- Explain to the patient that this test evaluates function of the liver and bile ducts or detects red blood cell disorders.

• Inform him that he needn't restrict food or fluids before the test.

• Tell him the test requires collection of a random stool specimen.

• Withhold broad-spectrum antibiotics, sulfonamides, and salicylates for 2 weeks before the test. If these medications must be continued, note this on the laboratory slip.

Procedure and posttest care

• Collect a random stool specimen.

• Tell the patient that he may resume his usual diet.

• Resume administration of medications withheld for the test.

Precautions

• Tell the patient not to contaminate the stool specimen with toilet tissue or urine.

• Use a light-resistant collection container because urobilinogen breaks down to urobilin when exposed to light.

• Send the specimen to the laboratory immediately.

• Refrigerate the specimen if transport or testing is delayed more than 30 minutes; freeze the specimen if test is to be performed by an outside laboratory.

Reference values

Normally, fecal urobilinogen values range from 50 to 300 mg/24 hours.

Abnormal findings

Absent or low levels of urobilinogen in the stool indicate obstructed bile flow, the result of intrahepatic disorders (such as hepatocellular jaundice due to cirrhosis or hepatitis) or extrahepatic disorders (such as choledocholithiasis or tumor of the head of the pancreas, the ampulla of Vater, or the bile duct). Low fecal urobilinogen levels are also characteristic of depressed erythropoiesis, as in aplastic anemia.

Elevated fecal urobilinogen levels may occur in hemolytic jaundice, thalassemia, and hemolytic, sickle cell, and pernicious anemias.

Interfering factors

• Contamination of the specimen or failure to use a light-resistant collection container

• Broad-spectrum antibiotics (possible decrease due to inhibition of bacterial growth in the colon)

• Sulfonamides, which react with the reagent used by the laboratory in this test, and large doses of salicylates (possible increase)

EXAMINATION OF STOOL FOR OVA AND PARASITES

Examination of a stool specimen can detect several types of intestinal parasites. Some of these parasites live in nonpathogenic symbiosis; others cause intestinal disease. In North America, the most common parasites include the roundworms *Ascaris lumbricoides* and *Necator americanus* (also called hookworms); the tapeworms *Diphyllobothrium latum, Taenia saginata,* and *Taenia solium* (rare); the amoeba *Entamoeba histolytica*; and the flagellate *Giardia lamblia.*

Purpose

• To confirm or rule out intestinal parasitic infection and disease

Patient preparation

• Explain to the patient that this test detects intestinal parasitic infection.

COLLECTION PROCEDURE FOR PINWORMS

The ova of the pinworm *Enterobius vermicularis* seldom appear in stool because the female migrates from the anus during the night and deposits the eggs in the perianal area. To collect them, place a piece of cellophane tape, sticky side out, on the end of a tongue depressor, and press it firmly on the anal area. Then transfer the tape, sticky side down, to a slide (kits with tape and a slide or a sticky paddle are available). If tape is unavailable, use an anal swab technique. Because the female usually deposits her ova at night, collect the specimen early in the morning before the patient bathes or defecates.

• Instruct him to avoid treatments with castor or mineral oil, bismuth, magnesium or antidiarrheal compounds, barium enemas, and antibiotics for 7 to 10 days before the test.
• Tell him the test requires three stool specimens — one every other day or every third day. Up to six specimens may be required to confirm the presence of *E. histolytica.*
• Record recent dietary and travel history if the patient has diarrhea. Check the patient's history for antiparasitic drugs, such as carbarsone, tetracycline, paromomycin, metronidazole, and diiodohydroxyquin, within 2 weeks of the test.

Equipment
Gloves, waterproof container with tight-fitting lid, bedpan (if necessary), tongue blade

Procedure and posttest care
• Put on gloves and collect a stool specimen directly into the container. (See *Collection procedure for pinworms.*)
• Collect the specimen into a clean, dry bedpan if the patient is bedridden; then, using a tongue blade, transfer it into a properly labeled container.
• Note on the laboratory slip the date and time of collection and the specimen's consistency.
• Also record any recent or current antimicrobial therapy and any pertinent travel or dietary history.
• Resume administration of medications discontinued before the test.

Precautions
• Do not contaminate the stool specimen with urine, which can destroy trophozoites.
• Don't collect stool from a toilet bowl because water is toxic to trophozoites and may contain organisms that interfere with test results.
• Send the specimen to the laboratory immediately. If a liquid or soft stool specimen can't be examined within 30 minutes of passage, place some of it in a preservative; if a formed stool specimen can't be examined immediately, refrigerate it or place it in preservative.
• If the entire stool can't be sent to the laboratory, include macroscopic worms or worm segments and bloody and mucoid portions of the specimen.
• Use gloves when performing the procedure and handling the specimen, disposing of equipment, sealing the container, and transporting it. Dispose of gloves after specimen collection.

Normal findings
No parasites or ova appear in stool.

Abnormal findings
The presence of *E. histolytica* confirms amebiasis; *G. lamblia,* giardiasis.

However, the extent of infection depends on the degree of tissue invasion. If amebiasis is suspected but stool examinations are negative, specimen collection after saline cathartic using buffered sodium biphosphate or during sigmoidoscopy may be necessary. If giardiasis or the presence of *Strongyloides stercoralis* is suspected but stool examinations are negative, examination of duodenal contents may be necessary.

Because injury to the host is difficult to detect — even when helminth ova or larvae appear — the number of worms is usually correlated with the patient's clinical symptoms to distinguish between helminth infestation and helminth diseases. Eosinophilia may also indicate parasitic infection.

Helminths may migrate from the intestinal tract, producing pathologic changes in other parts of the body. For example, the roundworm *Ascaris* may perforate the bowel wall, causing peritonitis, or may migrate to the lungs, causing pneumonitis. Hookworms can cause hypochromic microcytic anemia secondary to bloodsucking and hemorrhage, especially in patients with iron-deficient diets. The tapeworm *D. latum* may cause megaloblastic anemia by removing vitamin B_{12}.

Interfering factors
• Caster or mineral oil, bismuth, magnesium or antidiarrheal compounds, and barium enema
• Failure to observe pretest restrictions
• Improper collection technique, collection of too few specimens, or contamination of the sample with urine (possible false-negative)
• Failure to transport the specimen to the laboratory promptly or to refrigerate or preserve it
• Exposure of specimen to excessive heat or cold

• Antibiotic therapy
• Antiparasitic drugs, such as carbarsone, tetracycline, paromomycin, metronidazole, and diiodohydroxyquin

EXAMINATION OF STOOL FOR ROTAVIRUS ANTIGEN

Rotaviruses are the most common cause of infectious diarrhea in infants and young children. They are most prevalent in children ages 3 months to 2 years during the winter months. Clinical features include diarrhea, vomiting, fever, and abdominal pain. Symptoms of infection may range from mild in adults to severe in young children, especially hospitalized infants.

Rotavirus infections are easily transmitted in group settings, such as nursing homes, preschools, and day-care centers. Transmission is presumed to occur from person to person by the fecal-oral route. In a hospital setting, nosocomial spread of this viral infection can cause significant harm.

Because human rotaviruses don't replicate efficiently in laboratory cell cultures, detection typically requires sensitive, specific enzyme immunoassays that provide results within minutes or hours (depending on the assay).

Purpose
• To obtain a laboratory diagnosis of rotavirus gastroenteritis

Patient preparation
• Explain the purpose of the test to the patient or to his parents if the patient is a child.

• Inform him that the test requires a stool specimen.

• Collect the specimens during the prodromal and acute stages of clinical infection to ensure detection of the viral antigens by enzyme immunoassay.

Procedure and posttest care

• Usually, a stool specimen (1 g in a screw-capped tube or vial) is used to detect rotaviruses. If a microbiological transport swab is used, it must be heavily stained with stool to be diagnostically productive for rotavirus.

• Provide fluids to the patient to avoid dehydration caused by vomiting and diarrhea.

Precautions

• Avoid using collection containers with preservatives, metal ions, detergents, and serum, which may interfere with the assay.

• Store stool specimens for up to 24 hours at 35.6° to 46.4° F (2° to 8° C). If a longer period of storage or shipment is necessary, freeze specimens at −4° F (−20° C) or colder. Repeated freezing and thawing will cause the specimen to deteriorate and yield misleading results.

• Don't store the specimen in a self-defrosting freezer.

• Use gloves when obtaining or handling all specimens.

Normal findings

The detection of rotavirus by enzyme immunoassay is laboratory evidence of current infection with the organism.

Interfering factor

• Collection of specimen in containers with preservatives such as metal ions, detergents, or serum (decreased number of pathogens)

REPRODUCTIVE SYSTEM

SEX CHROMATIN TESTS

Although sex chromatin tests can screen for abnormalities in the number of sex chromosomes, the faster, simpler, and more accurate full karyotype (chromosome analysis) has all but replaced them. Sex chromatin tests are usually indicated for abnormal sexual development, ambiguous genitalia, amenorrhea, and suspected chromosomal abnormalities.

Purpose

• To quickly screen for abnormal sexual development (both X and Y chromatin tests)

• To aid assessment of an infant with ambiguous genitalia (X chromatin test only)

• To determine the number of Y chromosomes in an individual (Y chromatin test only)

Patient preparation

• Explain to the patient or to his parents, if appropriate, why the test is being performed.

• Tell him the test requires that the inside of his cheek be scraped to obtain a specimen and who will perform the test.

• Assure the patient the test takes only a few minutes but may require a follow-up chromosome analysis.

• Inform him that the laboratory generally requires as long as 4 weeks to complete the analysis.

Equipment

Wooden or metal spatula, clean glass slide, cell fixative

Procedure and posttest care

• Scrape the buccal mucosa firmly with a wooden or metal spatula at least twice to obtain a specimen of healthy cells (vaginal mucosa is occasionally used in young women).

• Rub the spatula over the glass slide, making sure the cells are evenly distributed.

• Spray the slide with cell fixative, and send the slide to the laboratory with a brief patient history and indications for the test.

Precautions

• Make sure the buccal mucosa is scraped firmly to ensure a sufficient number of cells.

• Check that the specimen isn't saliva, which contains no cells.

Normal findings

A normal female (XX) has only one X chromatin mass (the number of X chromatin masses discernible is one less than the number of X chromosomes in the cells examined). For various reasons, an X chromatin mass is ordinarily discernible in only 20% to 50% of the buccal mucosal cells of a normal woman.

A normal male (XY) has only one Y chromatin mass (the number of Y chromatin masses equals the number of Y chromosomes in the cells examined).

Abnormal findings

In most laboratories, if less than 20% of the cells in a buccal smear contain an X chromatin mass, some cells are presumed to contain only one X chromosome, necessitating full karyotyping. Persons with female phenotypes

and positive Y chromatin masses run a high risk of developing malignancies in their *intra-abdominal* gonads. In such persons, removal of these gonads is indicated and should generally be performed before age 5.

The patient or his parents require genetic counseling after the cause of chromosomal abnormal sexual development has been identified. A medical team comprising of doctors, psychologists, psychiatrists, and educators must decide the child's sex if a child is phenotypically of one sex and genotypically of the other. This careful evaluation should be made early to prevent developmental problems related to incorrect gender identification. (See *Sex chromosome anomalies,* pages 404 and 405.)

Interfering factors

• Obtaining saliva instead of buccal cells (false specimen)

• Cell deterioration due to failure to apply cell fixative to the slide

• Presence of bacteria or wrinkles in the cell membrane, analysis of degenerative cells, or use of an outdated stain

CHROMOSOME ANALYSIS

Chromosome analysis studies the relationship between the microscopic appearance of chromosomes and an individual's phenotype — the expression of the genes in physical, biochemical, or physiologic traits.

Ideally, chromosomes are studied during metaphase, the middle phase of mitosis, when new cell poles appear. During metaphase, colchicine (a cell

SEX CHROMOSOMES ANOMALIES

DISORDER AND CHROMOSOMAL ANEUPLOIDY	CAUSE AND INCIDENCE
Klinefelter's syndrome • 47,XXY • 48,XXXY • 49,XXXXY • 48,XX,YY • 49,XXX,YY • Mosaics: XXY, XXXY, or XXXXY/XX or XY	• Nondisjunction or improper chromatid separation during anaphase I or II of oogenesis or spermatogenesis results in abnormal gamete • 1 per 500 to 600 male births
Polysomy Y • 47,XYY	• Nondisjunction during anaphase II of spermatogenesis causes both Y chromosomes to pass to the same pole and results in a YY sperm • 1 per 1,000 male births
Turner's syndrome • 45,XO • Mosaics: XO/XX or XO/XXX • Aberrations of X chromosomes, including deletion of short arm of one X chromosome, presence of a ring chromosome, or presence of an isochromosome on the long arm of an X chromosome	• Nondisjunction during anaphase I or II of spermatogenesis results in sperm without any sex chromosomes • 1 per 3,500 female births (most common chromosome complement in first-trimester abortions)
Other X polysomes	• Nondisjunction at anaphase I or II of oogenesis
• 47,XXX	• 1 per 1,400 female births
• 48,XXXX	• Rare
• 49,XXXXX	• Rare

PHENOTYPIC FEATURES

- Syndrome usually inapparent until puberty
- Small penis and testes
- Sparse facial and abdominal hair; feminine distribution of pubic hair
- Somewhat enlarged breasts (gynecomastia)
- Sexual dysfunction
- Sterility
- Possible mental retardation

- Above average stature (often over 72″ [1.8 m])
- Normal fertility

- Short stature (usually under 57″ [145 cm])
- Webbed neck
- Low hairline
- Broad chest with widely spaced nipples
- Underdeveloped breasts
- Juvenile external genitalia
- Primary amenorrhea common
- Sterility
- No mental retardation but possible problems with space perception and orientation

- Often, no obvious anatomical abnormalities
- Normal fertility

- Mental retardation
- Ocular hypertelorism
- Reduced fertility

- Severe mental retardation
- Ocular hypertelorism, with uncoordinated eye movement
- Abnormal development of sexual organs
- Various skeletal anomalies

poison) is added to arrest cell division. Cells are harvested, stained, and then examined under a microscope. These cells are then photographed to record the karyotype — the systematic arrangement of chromosomes in groupings according to size and shape.

Only rapidly dividing cells, such as bone marrow or neoplastic cells, permit direct, immediate study. In other cells, mitosis is stimulated by the addition of phytohemagglutinin. Indications for the test determine the specimen required (blood, bone marrow, amniotic fluid, skin, or placental tissue) and the specific analytic procedure.

Purpose
- To identify chromosomal abnormalities, such as hypoploidy or hyperploidy, as the underlying cause of malformation, maldevelopment, or disease

Patient preparation
- Explain to the patient or to his parents, if appropriate, the purpose of this test.
- Tell him who will perform the test and what kind of specimen will be required.
- Inform him when results will be available, according to the specimen required.

Procedure and posttest care
- Collect a blood sample (in a 5- to 10-ml *green-top* heparinized tube), a tissue specimen, 1 ml of bone marrow, or at least 20 ml of amniotic fluid.
- Provide appropriate posttest care, depending on the procedure used to collect the specimen.
- Explain the test results and their implications to the patient or to the parents of a child with a chromosomal abnormality.

• Recommend appropriate genetic or other counseling and follow-up care if necessary, such as an infant stimulation program for a patient with Down syndrome.

Precautions

• Keep all specimens sterile, especially those requiring a tissue culture.

• To facilitate interpretation of test results, send the specimen to the laboratory immediately, with a brief patient history and the indication for the test.

• Refrigerate the specimen if transport is delayed, but *never* freeze it.

• Make sure the povidone-iodine solution is thoroughly removed with alcohol before skin biopsy to prevent cell growth in tissue culture.

Normal findings

The normal cell contains 46 chromosomes: 22 pairs of nonsex chromosomes (autosomes) and 1 pair of sex chromosomes (Y for the male-determining chromosome, X for the female-determining chromosome). On a karyotype, chromosomes are arranged according to size and the location of their primary constrictions, or centromeres.

The centromere may be medial (metacentric), slightly to one end of the chromosome (submetacentric), or entirely to one end (acrocentric). The largest chromosomes are displayed first; the others are arranged in order of decreasing size, with the two sex chromosomes traditionally placed last. By convention, the centromere is always placed at the top in a karyotype. Thus, if the two pairs of chromosomal arms are of unequal length, the arm above the centromere will be shorter. The letter "p" designates the short arm; the letter "q," the long arm.

Special stains identify individual chromosomes and locate and enumerate particular portions of chromosomes. Trypsin, alkali, heat denaturation, and Giemsa stain are used for visible light microscopy; quinacrine stain, for ultraviolet microscopy. These techniques produce nonuniform staining of each chromosome in a repetitive, banded pattern. The mechanism of chromosome banding is unknown, but seems related to primary deoxyribonucleic acid sequence and protein composition of the chromosome.

Abnormal findings

Chromosomal abnormalities may be numerical or structural. Any numerical deviation from the norm of 46 chromosomes is called *aneuploidy*. Less than 46 chromosomes is called *hypoploidy*; more than 46, *hyperploidy*. Special designations exist for whole multiples of the haploid number 23: *diploidy* for the normal somatic number of 46, *triploidy* for 69, *tetraploidy* for 92, and so forth.

When the deviation occurs within a single pair of chromosomes, the suffix "–somy" is used, as in *trisomy* for the presence of three chromosomes instead of the usual pair or *monosomy* for the presence of only one chromosome.

Aneuploidy most commonly follows failure of the chromosomal pair to separate (nondisjunction) during anaphase, the mitotic stage that follows metaphase. It may also result from anaphase lag, in which one of the normally separated chromosomes fails to move to a pole and is left out of the daughter cells.

If nondisjunction or anaphase lag occurs during meiosis, the cells of the zygote will all be the same. Errors in mitotic division after zygote formation will produce more than one cell line (mosaicism).

Structural chromosomal abnormalities result from chromosome breakage. Intrachromosomal rearrangement occurs within a single chromosome in the

CHROMOSOME ANALYSIS FINDINGS

SPECIMEN AND INDICATION	RESULT	IMPLICATION
Blood		
• To evaluate abnormal appearance or development, suggesting chromosomal irregularity	• Abnormal chromosome number (aneuploidy) or arrangement	• Identifies specific chromosomal abnormality
• To evaluate couples with history of miscarriages or to identify balanced translocation carriers having unbalanced offspring	• Normal chromosomes • Parental balanced translocation carrier	• Miscarriage unrelated to parental chromosomal abnormality • Increased risk of repeated abortion or unbalanced offspring indicates need for amniocentesis in future pregnancies
• To detect chromosomal rearrangements in rare genetic diseases predisposing patient to malignant neoplasms	• Chromosomal rearrangements, gaps, and breaks	• Occurs in Bloom's syndrome, Fanconi's syndrome, telangiectasia; patient predisposed to malignant neoplasms
Blood or bone marrow		
• To identify Philadelphia chromosome and confirm chronic myelogenous leukemia	• Translocation of chromosome 22q (long arm) to another chromosome (often chromosome 9)	• Aids diagnosis of chronic myelogenous leukemia
	• Aneuploidy (usually due to abnormalities in chromosomes 8 and 12)	• Occurs in acute myelogenous leukemia
	• Trisomy 21	• Occasionally occurs in chronic lymphocytic leukemia cells
Skin		
• To evaluate abnormal appearance or development, suggesting chromosomal irregularity	• All chromosomal abnormalities possible	• Same as chromosomal abnormality in blood; rarely, mosaic individual has normal blood but abnormal skin chromosomes
Amniotic fluid		
• To evaluate developing fetus with possible chromosomal abnormality	• All chromosomal abnormalities possible	• Same as chromosomal abnormality in blood or fetus

(continued)

CHROMOSOME ANALYSIS FINDINGS *(continued)*

SPECIMEN AND INDICATION	RESULT	IMPLICATION
Placental tissue		
● To evaluate products of conception after a miscarriage to determine if abnormality is fetal or placental in origin	● All chromosomal abnormalities possible	● Over 50% of aborted tissue is chromosomally abnormal
Tumor tissue		
● For research purposes only	● Many chromosomal abnormalities possible	● Although malignant tumors aren't associated with specific chromosomal aberrations, most are aneuploid, usually hyperploid.

---

following forms:
● *deletion:* loss of an end (terminal) or middle (interstitial) portion of a chromosome
● *inversion:* end-to-end reversal of a chromosome segment, which may be pericentric inversion (including the centromere) or paracentric inversion (occurring in only one arm of the chromosome)
● *ring chromosome formation:* breakage of both ends of a chromosome and reunion of the ends
● *isochromosome formation:* abnormal splitting of the centromere in a transverse rather than a longitudinal plane.

Interchromosomal rearrangements (of more than one chromosome, usually two) also occur. The most common rearrangement is translocation, or exchange, of genetic material between two chromosomes. Translocations may be balanced, in which the cell neither loses nor gains genetic material; unbalanced, in which a piece of genetic material is gained or lost from each cell; reciprocal (in children), in which two chromosomes exchange material; or Robertsonian, in which two chromosomes join to form one combined chromosome, with little or no loss of material.

Implications of chromosome analysis results depend on the specimen and indications for the test. (See *Chromosome analysis findings*.)

Interfering factors
● Chemotherapy (possible abnormal results due to chromosome breaks)
● Contamination of tissue with bacteria, fungus, or a virus (possible inhibition of culture growth)
● Inclusion of maternal cells in a specimen obtained by amniocentesis, with subsequent culturing (possible false results)
● Failure to maintain a sterile specimen, to send the specimen to the laboratory immediately, or to refrigerate it

AMNIOTIC FLUID ANALYSIS

Amniocentesis is the transabdominal needle aspiration of 10 to 20 ml of amniotic fluid for laboratory analysis. This analysis may be used to detect certain birth defects, such as Down syndrome or spina bifida; to determine fetal maturity; to detect hemolytic disease of the newborn; or, through karyotyping, to detect gender and chromosomal abnormalities. This test can be performed only when the amniotic fluid level reaches 150 ml, usually after the 16th week of pregnancy.

Amniocentesis is indicated if the mother is over age 35; has a family history of genetic, chromosomal, or neural tube defects; or has had a miscarriage. Although adverse effects are rare, potential complications include spontaneous abortion, trauma to the fetus or placenta, bleeding, premature labor, infection, and Rh sensitization from fetal bleeding into the maternal circulation. Because of the severity of possible complications, amniocentesis is contraindicated as a general screening test. Abnormal test results or failure of the tissue cultures to grow may necessitate repetition of the test.

Another method of detecting fetal chromosomal and biochemical disorders in early pregnancy is chorionic villi sampling. (See *Chorionic villi sampling,* pages 410 and 411.)

Purpose
• To detect fetal abnormalities, particularly chromosomal and neural tube defects
• To detect hemolytic disease of the newborn

• To diagnose metabolic disorders, amino acid disorders, and mucopolysaccharidosis
• To determine fetal age and maturity, especially pulmonary maturity
• To assess fetal health by detecting the presence of meconium or blood, or measuring amniotic levels of estriol and fetal thyroid hormone
• To identify fetal gender when one or both parents are carriers of a sex-linked disorder

Patient preparation
• Describe the procedure to the patient, and explain that this test detects fetal abnormalities.
• Assess her understanding of the test, and answer any questions she may have.
• Inform her that she needn't restrict food or fluids.
• Tell her the test requires a specimen of amniotic fluid and who will perform the test.
• Advise her that normal test results can't guarantee a normal fetus because some fetal disorders are undetectable.
• Make sure the patient has signed a consent form.
• Explain that she'll feel a stinging sensation when the local anesthetic is injected.
• Provide emotional support before and during the test and reassure her that adverse effects are rare.
• Ask her to void just before the test to minimize the risk of puncturing the bladder and aspirating urine instead of amniotic fluid.

Equipment
70% alcohol or povidone-iodine solution, sponge forceps, 2″ × 2″ gauze pads, local anesthetic (1% lidocaine), 25G sterile needle, 3-ml syringe, 20G sterile spinal needle with stylet, 10-ml

CHORIONIC VILLI SAMPLING

Chorionic villi sampling (CVS) is a prenatal test for quick detection of fetal chromosomal and biochemical disorders that's performed during the first trimester of pregnancy. Preliminary results may be available within hours; complete results, within a few days. In contrast, amniocentesis can't be performed before the 16th week of pregnancy, and the results aren't available for at least 2 weeks. Thus, CVS can detect fetal abnormalities as much as 10 weeks sooner than amniocentesis.

The chorionic villi are fingerlike projections that surround the embryonic membrane and eventually give rise to the placenta. Cells obtained from an appropriate sample are of fetal, rather than maternal, origin and thus can be analyzed for fetal abnormalities.

Collection time

Samples are best obtained between the 8th and 10th weeks of pregnancy. Before 7 weeks, the villi cover the embryo and make selective sampling difficult. After 10 weeks, maternal cells begin to grow over the villi, and the amniotic sac begins to fill the uterine cavity, making the procedure difficult and potentially dangerous.

Collection method

To collect a chorionic villi sample, place the patient in the lithotomy position. The doctor checks the placement of the patient's uterus bimanually, and then inserts a Graves speculum and swabs the cervix with an antiseptic solution. If necessary, he may use a tenaculum to straighten an acutely flexed uterus, permitting cannula insertion. Guided by ultrasound and, possibly, endoscopy, he directs the catheter through the cannula to the villi. Suction is applied to the catheter to remove about 30 mg of tissue from the villi. The sample is withdrawn, placed in a Petri dish, and examined with a dissecting microscope. Part of the specimen is then cultured for further testing.

Interpretation

CVS can be used to detect about 200 diseases prenatally. For example, direct analysis of rapidly dividing fetal cells can detect chromosome disorders, deoxyribonucleic acid analysis can detect hemoglobinopathies, and lysosomal enzyme assays can screen for lysosomal storage disorders such as Tay-Sachs disease.

The test appears to provide reliable

---

syringe, amber or foil-covered sterile 10-ml test tube

Procedure and posttest care

• A pool of amniotic fluid is located after determining fetal and placental position, usually through palpation and ultrasonic visualization.
• The skin is prepared with antiseptic and alcohol; then 1 ml of 1% lidocaine is injected with a 25G needle, first intradermally and then subcutaneously.

• Then a 20G spinal needle, with a stylet, is inserted into the amniotic cavity and the stylet is withdrawn.
• A 10-ml syringe is attached to the needle; then the fluid is aspirated and placed in an amber or foil-covered test tube.
• The needle is withdrawn, and an adhesive bandage is placed over the needle insertion site.

results except when the sample contains too few cells or the cells fail to grow in culture. Patient risks for this procedure appear to be similar to those for amniocentesis: a small chance of spontaneous abortion, cramps, infection, and bleeding. However, recent research reports an incidence of limb malformations in neonates when CVS has been performed.

Unlike amniocentesis, CVS can't detect complications in cases of Rh sensitization, uncover neural tube defects, or determine pulmonary maturity. However, it may prove to be the best way to detect other serious fetal abnormalities early in pregnancy.

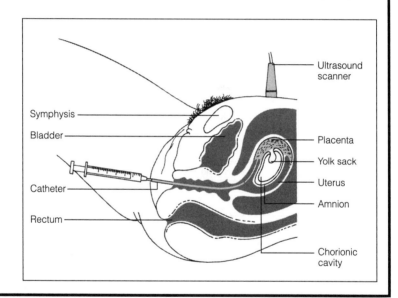

- Ultrasound scanner
- Symphysis
- Bladder
- Placenta
- Yolk sack
- Catheter
- Uterus
- Amnion
- Rectum
- Chorionic cavity

- Monitor fetal heart rate (FHR) and maternal vital signs every 15 minutes for at least 30 minutes.
- Position the patient on her left side if she sweats profusely or feels faint or nauseated to counteract uterine pressure on the vena cava.
- Instruct the patient before she is discharged to report immediately abdominal pain or cramping, chills, fever, vaginal bleeding or leakage of serous vaginal fluid, or fetal hyperactivity or unusual fetal lethargy.

Precautions
- Instruct the patient to fold her hands behind her head to prevent her from accidentally touching the sterile field and causing contamination.
- Send the specimen to the laboratory immediately.

ANALYSIS OF AMNIOTIC FLUID

TEST	NORMAL FINDINGS	FETAL IMPLICATIONS OF ABNORMAL FINDINGS
Color	Clear, with white flecks of vernix caseosa in a mature fetus	Blood of maternal origin is usually harmless. "Port wine'" fluid may indicate abruptio placentae. Fetal blood may indicate damage to the fetal, placental, or umbilical cord vessels.
Bilirubin	• Early: < 0.075 mg/dl or < 1.3 Umol/L • Term: < 0.025 mg/dl or < 0.41 Umol/L	High levels indicate hemolytic disease of the newborn in isoimmunized pregnancy.
Meconium	Absent (except in breech presentation)	Presence indicates fetal hypotension or distress.
Creatinine	• Early: 0.8 to 1 mg/dl or 71 to 97 Umol/L • Term: 1.8 to 4 mg/dl or 159 to 354 Umol/L	Decreased levels may indicate immature fetus (less than 37 weeks).
Lecithin-sphingomyelin ratio	> 3:1 generally indicates fetal pulmonary maturity.	Less than 2:1 indicates pulmonary immaturity and subsequent increased risk of respiratory distress syndrome.
Phosphatidylglycerol	Present at 36 weeks	Absence indicates pulmonary immaturity.
Glucose	< 45 mg/dl	Excessive increases at term or near term indicates hypertrophy of fetal pancreas and subsequent neonatal hypoglycemia.
Alpha-fetoprotein	• Early: 13 to 41 ng/ml • Term: 0.2 to 3 ng/ml (Values vary, depending on gestational age and laboratory technique.)	Inappropriate increases indicate neural tube defects, such as spina bifida or anencephaly, impending fetal death, congenital nephrosis, or contamination by fetal blood.
Chromosome	Normal karyotype	Abnormal karyotype may indicate fetal sex and chromosome disorders.
Acetylcholinesterase	Absent	Presence may indicate neural tube defects, exomphalos, or other serious malformations.

Normal findings

Normal amniotic fluid is clear but may contain white flecks of vernix caseosa when the fetus is near term. For a detailed analysis of the appearance and components of amniotic fluid, see *Analysis of amniotic fluid.*

Abnormal findings

Blood, which is found in about 10% of amniocenteses, results from a faulty tap and doesn't indicate an abnormality. However, it does inhibit cell growth and changes the level of other amniotic fluid constituents. "Port wine" fluid, on the other hand, may be a sign of abruptio placentae, and blood of fetal origin may indicate damage to the fetal, placental, or umbilical cord vessels by the amniocentesis needle.

Large amounts of *bilirubin,* a breakdown product of red blood cells, may indicate hemolytic disease of the newborn. Normally, the bilirubin level increases from the 14th to the 24th week of pregnancy, then declines as the fetus matures, essentially reaching zero at term. Testing for bilirubin usually isn't performed until the 26th week because that's the earliest time successful therapy for Rh sensitization can begin. Bilirubin level is determined by spectrophotometric measurement of the optic density of the amniotic fluid. The deviation of the scan at 450μ from a straight line drawn between 375μ and 525μ represents the bilirubin peak.

Meconium, a semisolid viscous material found in the fetal GI tract, consists of mucopolysaccharides, desquamated cells, vernix, hair, and cholesterol. Meconium passes into the amniotic fluid when hypoxia causes fetal distress and relaxation of the anal sphincter. Meconium is a normal finding in breech presentation. Meconium in the amniotic fluid produces a peak of 410μ on the spectrophotometric analysis. However, serial amniocentesis may show a clearing of meconium over a 2- to 3-week period. If meconium is present during labor, the newborn's nose and throat require thorough cleaning to prevent meconium aspiration.

Creatinine, a product of fetal urine, increases in the amniotic fluid as the fetal kidneys mature. Generally, the creatinine value exceeds 2 mg/dl in a mature fetus.

Alpha-fetoprotein (AFP) is a fetal alpha globulin produced first in the yolk sac and later in the parenchymal cells of the liver and GI tract. Fetal serum AFP levels are about 150 times higher than amniotic fluid levels; maternal serum AFP levels are far lower than amniotic fluid levels. High amniotic fluid levels indicate neural tube defects, but the AFP level may remain normal if the defect is small and closed. Elevated AFP levels may also occur in multiple pregnancy; in disorders such as omphalocele, congenital nephrosis, esophageal or duodenal atresia, cystic fibrosis, exomphalos, Turner's syndrome, and fetal bladder neck obstruction with hydronephrosis; and in impending fetal death.

The amount of *uric acid* in the amniotic fluid increases as the fetus matures, but these levels fluctuate widely and can't accurately predict maturity. Laboratory studies indicate that severe erythroblastosis fetalis, familial hyperuricemia, and Lesch-Nyhan syndrome tend to increase the level of uric acid.

Estrone, estradiol, estriol, and *estriol conjugates* appear in amniotic fluid in varying amounts. Levels of estriol, the most prevalent estrogen, increase from 25.7 ng/ml during the 16th to 20th weeks to almost 1,000 ng/ml at term. Severe erythroblastosis fetalis decreases the estriol level.

The type II cells lining the fetal lung alveoli produce *lecithin* slowly in early pregnancy and then markedly increase production around the 35th week.

The *sphingomyelin* level parallels that of lecithin until the 35th week, when it gradually decreases. Measuring the ratio of lecithin to sphingomyelin (L-S ratio) confirms fetal pulmonary maturity (L-S ratio > 3:1) or suggests a risk of respiratory distress (L-S ratio < 3:1). However, fetal respiratory distress may develop in the fetus of a patient with diabetes, even though the L-S ratio is greater than 3:1, a level that usually indicates pulmonary maturity.

Phosphatidylglycerol (PG) levels are present with pulmonary maturity; *phosphatidylinositol* (PI) levels decrease. The phospholipid content of the amniotic fluid reflects the amount of fetal lung development and degree of risk for neonatal respiratory distress. Testing for both the L-S ratio and for the presence or absence of PG provides a better assessment of neonatal risk than either test done alone. For example, an L-S ratio of 3:1 and the presence of PG indicates minimal risk of respiratory distress; an L-S ratio of less than 3:1 and a lack of PG indicates an increased risk of respiratory distress. Presence of PI and absence of PG indicates that PG should be detectable in 1 to 4 weeks and that the infant is at increased risk during that time.

Measuring *glucose* levels in the fluid can aid in assessing glucose control in the patient with diabetes, but this isn't done routinely. A level greater than 45 mg/dl indicates poor maternal and fetal control. *Insulin* levels normally increase slightly from the 27th to the 40th week but increase sharply (up to 27 times normal) in a poorly controlled patient with diabetes.

Laboratory analysis can identify at least 25 different *enzymes* (usually in low concentrations) in amniotic fluid. The enzymes have few known clinical implications, although elevated acetylcholinesterase levels may occur with neural tube defects, exomphalos, and other serious malformations.

When the mother carries an *X-linked disorder,* determination of fetal sex is important. If chromosome karyotyping identifies a male fetus, there's a 50% chance he'll be affected; a female fetus won't be affected but has a 50% chance of being a carrier.

Interfering factors
● Use of plastic disposable syringes (possible toxicity to amniotic fluid cells)
● Failure to place the specimen in an appropriate amber or foil-covered tube (possible decrease in bilirubin)
● Blood or meconium in the fluid (effect on L-S ratio)
● Maternal blood in the fluid (possible decrease in creatinine)
● Any amount of fetal blood in the fluid specimen (possible doubling of AFP concentrations)
● Several disorders that are not associated with pregnancy, including infectious mononucleosis, cirrhosis, hepatic cancer, teratoma, endodermal sinus tumor, gastric carcinoma, pancreatic carcinoma, and subacute hereditary tyrosinemia (possible increase in AFP levels)

PAPANICOLAOU TEST

The Papanicolaou (Pap) test is a widely known cytologic test for early detection of cervical cancer. A doctor or specially trained nurse scrapes secretions from the patient's cervix and spreads them on a slide, which is sent to the laboratory for cytologic analysis. The test relies on the ready exfoliation of malignant cells from the cervix and shows cell maturity, metabolic activity, and morphology variations.

Although cervical scrapings are the most common test specimen, the test may involve cytologic evaluation of the vaginal pool, prostatic secretions, urine, gastric secretions, cavity fluids, bronchial aspirations, sputum, or solid tumor cells obtained by fine needle aspiration. If a Pap test is positive or suggests malignancy, cervical biopsy can confirm diagnosis.

Purpose
- To detect malignant cells
- To detect inflammatory tissue changes
- To assess response to chemotherapy and radiation therapy
- To detect viral, fungal and, occasionally, parasitic invasion

Patient preparation
- Explain to the patient that the test allows the study of cervical cells.
- Stress its importance as an aid for detection of cancer at a stage when the disease is often asymptomatic and still curable.
- The test should not be scheduled during the menstrual period; the best time is mid-cycle.
- Instruct the patient not to douche or insert vaginal medications for 24 hours before the test because doing so can wash away cellular deposits and change the vaginal pH.
- Tell her the test requires that the cervix be scraped, who will perform the procedure and when, and that she may experience slight discomfort but no pain from the speculum.
- Inform her that the procedure takes 5 to 10 minutes or slightly longer if the

vagina, pelvic cavity, and rectum are examined bimanually.
- Obtain an accurate patient history, and ask the following questions: When did you last have a Pap test? Have you ever had an abnormal Pap test? When was your last menstrual period? Are your periods regular? How many days do they last? Is bleeding heavy or light? Have you taken or are you presently taking hormones or oral contraceptives? Do you use an intrauterine device? Do you have any vaginal discharge, pain, or itching? Which, if any, gynecologic disorders have occurred in your family? Have you ever had gynecologic surgery, chemotherapy, or radiation therapy? If so, describe it fully. Note any pertinent patient history data on the laboratory slip.
- Provide emotional support if the patient is anxious; tell her that test results should be available in a few days.
- Ask the patient to empty her bladder just before the test.

Equipment
Gloves; drape; vaginal speculum; collection device, such as a Pap stick (wooden spatula), cotton-tipped swab, or clean, dry glass pipette with rubber bulb; saline solution; glass microscopic slides; fixative (commercial spray or 95% ethyl alcohol solution in a jar) for slides

Procedure and posttest care
- Instruct the patient to disrobe from the waist down and to drape herself.
- Ask her to lie on the examining table and to place her heels in the stirrups. (She may be more comfortable if she keeps her shoes on.) Tell her to slide her buttocks to the edge of the table. Adjust the drape to minimize exposure.
- To avoid startling the patient, tell her when the examination will begin.

- The examiner puts on gloves and inserts an unlubricated speculum into the vagina. To make insertion easier, the speculum may be moistened with saline solution or warm water.
- After the examiner locates the cervix, he collects secretions from the cervix and material from the endocervical canal with a saline-moistened cotton-tipped swab or wooden spatula.
- He then spreads the specimen on the slide according to laboratory recommendations and immediately immerses the slide in (or sprays it with) a fixative.
- Alternatively, posterior vaginal pool secretions and pancervical material may be collected and smeared on a single slide, which must be fixed immediately according to laboratory instructions.
- Label the specimen appropriately, including the date, the patient's name, age, the date of her last menstrual period, and the collection site and method.
- A bimanual examination may follow removal of the speculum. Help the patient up and instruct her to dress when the examination is completed.
- Supply the patient with a sanitary napkin if cervical bleeding occurs.
- Tell the patient when to return for her next Pap test.

Precautions

- Make sure that the cervical specimen is aspirated and scraped from the cervix. Aspiration of the posterior fornix of the vagina can supplement a cervical specimen but should not replace it.
- Scrapings taken directly from the lesion are preferred if vaginal or vulval lesions are present.
- Use a small pipette, if necessary, in a patient whose uterus is involuting or atrophying from age, to aspirate cells

from the squamocolumnar junction and the cervical canal.
- Preserve the slides immediately.

Normal findings

Normally, no malignant cells or other abnormalities are present.

Abnormal findings

Malignant cells usually have relatively large nuclei and only small amounts of cytoplasm. They show abnormal nuclear chromatin patterns and marked variation in size, shape, and staining properties and may have prominent nucleoli.

A Pap smear may be graded in different ways, so check your laboratory's reporting format. The following list contains the traditional classifications:
- *Class I:* normal pattern; absence of atypical or abnormal cells
- *Class II:* benign abnormality; atypical, but nonmalignant, cells present
- *Class III:* atypical cells consistent with dysplasia
- *Class IV:* suggestive of, but inconclusive for, malignancy
- *Class V:* conclusive for malignancy.

To confirm a suggestive or positive cytology report, the test may be repeated or followed by a biopsy.

Interfering factors

- Douching before the test (can wash away cellular deposits)
- Excessive use of lubricating jelly on the speculum
- Collection of the specimen during menstruation
- Exclusive use of a specimen collected from the vaginal fornix (possible false-negative)
- Delay in fixing the specimen (difficult cytologic interpretation due to dehydration of cells)

SEMEN ANALYSIS

Semen analysis is a simple, inexpensive, and reasonably definitive test that's used in a broad range of applications, including evaluation of a man's fertility. Fertility analysis usually includes measuring the volume of seminal fluid, performing sperm counts, and microscopic examination of spermatozoa. Sperm are counted in much the same way that white blood cells, red blood cells, and platelets are counted on an anticoagulated blood sample. Motility and morphology are studied microscopically after staining a drop of semen.

If analysis detects an abnormality, additional tests (for example, liver, thyroid, pituitary, or adrenal function tests) may be performed to identify the underlying cause and to screen for metabolic abnormalities (such as diabetes mellitus). Significant abnormalities — such as greatly decreased sperm count or motility, or marked increase in morphologically abnormal forms — may require testicular biopsy.

Purpose
● To evaluate male fertility in an infertile couple
● To substantiate the effectiveness of vasectomy
● To detect semen on the body or clothing of a suspected rape victim or elsewhere at the crime scene
● To identify blood group substances to exonerate or incriminate a criminal suspect
● To rule out paternity on grounds of complete sterility

Patient preparation
Evaluation of fertility
● Provide written instructions, and inform the patient that the most desirable specimen requires masturbation, ideally in a doctor's office or a laboratory.
● Tell him to follow the instructions given to him regarding the period of sexual continence before the test because this may increase his sperm count. Some doctors specify a fixed number of days, usually between 2 and 5; others advise a period of continence equal to the usual interval between episodes of sexual intercourse.
● If the patient prefers to collect the specimen at home, emphasize the importance of delivering the specimen to the laboratory within 3 hours after collection. Warn him not to expose the specimen to extreme temperatures or to direct sunlight (which can also increase its temperature). Ideally, the specimen should remain at body temperature until liquefaction is complete (about 20 minutes). To deliver a semen specimen during cold weather, suggest that the patient keep the specimen container in a coat pocket on the way to the laboratory to protect the specimen from exposure to cold.
● Alternatives to collection by masturbation include coitus interruptus or the use of a condom. For collection by coitus interruptus, instruct the patient to withdraw immediately before ejaculation and to deposit the ejaculate in a suitable specimen container. For collection by condom, tell the patient to first wash the condom with soap and water, rinse it thoroughly, and allow it to dry completely. (Powders or lubricants applied to the condom may be spermicidal.) After collection, instruct him to tie the condom, place it in a glass jar, and promptly deliver it to the laboratory.

● Fertility may also be determined by collecting semen from the woman after coitus to assess the ability of the spermatozoa to penetrate the cervical mucus and remain active. For the postcoital cervical mucus test, instruct the patient to report for examination during the ovulatory phase of her menstrual cycle, as determined by basal temperature records, and as soon as possible after sexual intercourse (within 8 hours). Explain to the patient scheduled for this test that the procedure takes only a few minutes. Tell her that she'll be placed in the lithotomy position and that a speculum will be inserted into the vagina to collect the specimen. She may feel some pressure but no pain during this procedure.

Semen collection from rape victim
● Explain to the patient that the examiner will try to obtain a semen specimen from her vagina.
● Prepare her for insertion of the speculum as you would the patient scheduled for postcoital examination.
● Handle the victim's clothes as little as possible. If her clothes are moist, put them in a paper bag — not a plastic bag (which causes seminal stains and secretions to mold). Label the bag properly, and send it to the laboratory immediately.
● Provide emotional support by speaking to the patient calmly and reassuringly. Encourage her to express her fears and anxieties. Listen sympathetically.
● If she's scheduled for vaginal lavage, tell the rape victim to expect a cold sensation when saline solution is instilled to wash out the specimen.
● Help her relax during this procedure by instructing her to breathe deeply and slowly through her mouth.
● Instruct the victim to urinate just before the test, but warn her not to wipe the vulva afterward because this may remove semen.

Equipment
For semen collection by masturbation, coitus interruptus, or condom: clean plastic specimen container (for example, disposable urine or sputum container with lid)

For semen collection from rape victim: clean plastic specimen container, vaginal speculum, rubber gloves, cotton applicator sticks, glass microscopic slides with frosted ends, physiologic (0.85%) saline solution, Pap sticks, jars containing 95% ethanol, large syringe, rubber bulb or other device suitable for vaginal lavage

For a postcoital specimen collection: clean plastic specimen container, vaginal speculum, rubber gloves, cotton applicator sticks, glass microscopic slides with frosted ends, 1-ml tuberculin syringe without a cannula or needle

Procedure and posttest care
● Obtain a semen specimen for a fertility study by asking the patient to collect semen in a clean plastic specimen container.
● A specimen is obtained from the vagina of a rape victim by direct aspiration, saline lavage, or a direct smear of vaginal contents, using a Pap stick or, less desirably, a cotton applicator stick. Dried smears are usually collected from the suspected rape victim's skin by gently washing the skin with a small piece of gauze moistened with physiologic saline solution.
● Prepare direct smears on glass microscopic slides after labeling the frosted end. Immediately place smeared slides in Coplin jars containing 95% ethanol.
● Before postcoital examination, the examiner wipes any excess mucus from the external cervix and collects

the specimen by direct aspiration of the cervical canal, using a 1-ml tuberculin syringe without a cannula or needle.

• Inform a patient who is undergoing infertility studies that test results should be available in 24 hours.

• Refer the suspected rape victim to an appropriate specialist for counseling — a gynecologist, psychiatrist, clinical psychologist, nursing specialist, member of the clergy, or representative of a community support group, such as Women Organized Against Rape (WOAR).

Precautions

• If the patient prefers to collect the specimen during coitus interruptus, tell him he must prevent any loss of semen during ejaculation.

• Deliver all specimens, regardless of source or method of collection, to the laboratory promptly.

• Protect semen specimens for fertility studies from extremes of temperature and direct sunlight during delivery to the laboratory.

• Never lubricate the vaginal speculum. Oil or grease hinders examination of spermatozoa by interfering with smear preparation and staining and by inhibiting sperm motility through toxic ingredients. Instead, moisten the speculum with water or physiologic saline solution.

• Use extreme caution in securing, labeling, and delivering all specimens to be used for medicolegal purposes. You may be asked to testify as to when, where, and from whom the specimen was obtained; the specimen's general appearance and identifying features; steps taken to ensure the specimen's integrity; and when, where, and to whom the specimen was delivered for analysis. If your hospital or clinic uses routing slips for such specimens, fill them out carefully, and place them in the permanent medicolegal file.

Normal findings

Normal semen volume is greater than or equal to 2 ml. Paradoxically, the semen volume of many men in infertile couples is increased. Abstinence for 1 week or more results in progressively increased semen volume. (With abstinence of up to 10 days, sperm counts increase, sperm motility progressively decreases, and sperm morphology stays the same.) Liquefied semen is generally highly viscid, translucent, and gray-white, with a musty or acrid odor. After liquefaction, specimens of normal viscosity can be poured in drops. Normally, semen is slightly alkaline, with a pH of 7.2 to 8.

Other normal characteristics of semen: It coagulates immediately and liquefies within 20 minutes; the normal sperm count is 20 million/ml or more; 30% of spermatozoa have normal morphology; and 50% or more of spermatozoa show progressive motility within 4 hours of collection.

The normal postcoital cervical mucus test shows at least 10 motile spermatozoa per microscopic high-power field and spinnbarkeit (a measurement of the tenacity of the mucus) of at least 4″ (10 cm). These findings indicate adequate spermatozoa and receptivity of the cervical mucus.

Abnormal findings

Abnormal semen is *not* synonymous with infertility. Only one viable spermatozoon is needed to fertilize an ovum. Although a normal sperm count is 20 million/ml or more, many men with sperm counts below 1 million/ml have fathered normal children. Only men who can't deliver *any* viable spermatozoa in their ejaculate during sexual intercourse are absolutely sterile.

Nevertheless, subnormal sperm counts, decreased sperm motility, and abnormal morphology are usually associated with decreased fertility.

Other tests may be necessary to evaluate the patient's general health, metabolic status, or the function of specific endocrine glands (pituitary, thyroid, adrenal, or gonadal).

Interfering factors
- Poor timing of test within the menstrual cycle (abnormal postcoital test results)
- Prior cervical conization or cryotherapy and some medications, such as clomiphene citrate (possible abnormal postcoital test results due to changes in cervical mucus)
- Delayed transport of the specimen, exposure to extreme temperatures or direct sunlight, or the presence of toxic chemicals in the container or the condom (possible decrease in number of viable sperm)
- An incomplete specimen — for example, from coitus interruptus or improper collection technique (decrease in specimen volume)

CONTRACTION STRESS TEST

The contraction stress test (CST), also known as the oxytocin challenge test, measures the fetus's ability to withstand a decreased oxygen supply and the stress of contractions induced before actual labor begins. An infusion of oxytocin is given to stimulate uterine contractions while the fetal heart rate (FHR) is assessed, to evaluate the placenta's ability to provide sufficient oxygen to the fetus.

Purpose
- To determine and evaluate the fetus's in utero risk of hypoxia or ability to withstand uterine contractions before labor begins
- To determine effects of maternal diabetes or hypertension on fetoplacental adequacy and fetal well-being
- To evaluate high-risk pregnancies
- To determine if cesarean delivery will place the fetus at risk
- To determine the need to terminate the pregnancy by labor induction and early birth when performed in conjunction with other diagnostic studies

Patient preparation
- Explain that the procedure takes about 2 hours and is performed within a controlled environment with specially trained nurses and a doctor nearby.
- Inform the patient that food and fluid will be restricted for 4 to 8 hours before the study.
- Review breathing and relaxation techniques the patient may have learned in Lamaze or other childbirth classes, or teach these techniques before the test.
- Inform the patient that she will experience mild contractions and that the fetus and she will be evaluated at all times.
- Vital signs, FHR, assessment, and history will be performed before the test.

Equipment
External monitor for FHR, oxytocin in ordered dosages, I.V. tubing, I.V. access device, dextrose 5% in water, for infusion, ultrasound transducer, tocodynamometer

Procedure and posttest care

• Have the patient empty her bladder.

• Assist her into a semi-Fowler, side-lying position and drape her for privacy.

• Take the patient's blood pressure before and every 10 minutes during the procedure.

• Place the fetal monitor on her abdomen to monitor FHR and the toco-dynamometer on the lower abdomen to monitor contractions. A baseline recording is made and then the FHR is monitored and recorded continuously for 20 minutes.

• An I.V. line is inserted and I.V. oxytocin (Pitocin) is administered via I.V. pump as ordered. The FHR and contractions are monitored and recorded, and the infusion is discontinued to determine the FHR response to the contractions.

• Encourage the patient to use deep-breathing and relaxation skills while the oxytocin is administered and she feels the contractions.

• Continue to monitor FHR for 30 minutes as uterine movements return to normal.

• If premature labor begins, note the frequency, strength, and length of contractions, and prepare for labor or cesarean delivery.

Precautions

• This test is contraindicated in multiple pregnancy, previous cesarean birth or surgical hysterotomy, previous premature labor, premature ruptured membranes, abruptio placentae, placenta previa, and fetus of less than 34 weeks' gestation.

Normal findings

A negative result occurs when the FHR is within normal range, indicating that the fetus can tolerate the stress of labor.

Abnormal findings

Late decelerations in FHR during 2 or more contractions or late decelerations that are inconsistent indicate risk of fetal asphyxia.

Interfering factors

• Maternal hypotension (false-positive results due to diminished placental blood flow)

• Full bladder

MISCELLANEOUS TESTS

CEREBROSPINAL FLUID ANALYSIS

For qualitative analysis, cerebrospinal fluid (CSF) is most commonly obtained by lumbar puncture (usually between the third and fourth lumbar vertebrae) and, rarely, by cisternal or ventricular puncture. A CSF specimen may also be obtained during other neurologic tests such as myelography.

Purpose

• To measure CSF pressure as an aid in detecting obstruction of CSF circulation

• To aid diagnosis of viral or bacterial meningitis, subarachnoid or intracranial hemorrhage, tumors, and brain abscesses

• To aid diagnosis of neurosyphilis and chronic central nervous system infections

Patient preparation
- Describe the procedure to the patient, and explain that this test analyzes the fluid around the spinal cord.
- Inform him that he needn't restrict food or fluids.
- Tell him who will perform the procedure and where.
- Advise the patient that a headache is the most common adverse effect of a lumbar puncture, but reassure him that his cooperation during the test helps minimize this effect.
- Make sure the patient or his legal guardian has signed the appropriate consent form.
- If the patient is unusually anxious, assess and report his vital signs.

Equipment
Lumbar puncture tray, sterile gloves, local anesthetic (usually 1% lidocaine), povidone-iodine solution, small adhesive bandage

Procedure and posttest care
- Position the patient on his side at the edge of the bed, with his knees drawn up to his abdomen and his chin on his chest. Provide pillows to support the spine on a horizontal plane. This position allows full flexion of the spine and easy access to the lumbar subarachnoid space. Help him maintain this position by placing one arm around his knees and the other arm around his neck.
- If the sitting position is preferred, have the patient sit up and bend his chest and head toward his knees. Help him maintain this position throughout the procedure.
- After the skin is prepared for injection, the area is draped. Warn the patient that he'll probably experience a transient burning sensation when the local anesthetic is injected.
- Tell him that when the spinal needle is inserted, he may feel some transient

local pain as the needle transverses the dura mater.
- Ask him to report any pain or sensations that differ from or continue after this expected discomfort because such sensations may indicate irritation or puncture of a nerve root, requiring repositioning of the needle.
- Instruct the patient to remain still and breathe normally; movement and hyperventilation can alter pressure readings or cause injury.
- The anesthetic is injected, and the spinal needle is inserted in the midline, between the spinous processes of the vertebrae (usually between the third and fourth lumbar vertebrae). At this point, initial (or opening) CSF pressure is measured and a specimen is obtained.
- After the specimen is collected, label the containers in the order in which they were filled, and find out if any specific instructions are required for the laboratory.
- Next, a final pressure reading is taken, and the needle is removed.
- Clean the puncture site with a local antiseptic, such as povidone-iodine solution, and apply a small adhesive bandage.
- Check whether the patient must lie flat or if the head of his bed may be slightly elevated. In most cases, you'll be instructed to keep the patient lying flat for 8 hours after lumbar puncture. Some doctors, however, allow a 30-degree elevation at the head of the bed. Remind the patient that although he must not raise his head, he can turn from side to side.
- Encourage the patient to drink fluids. Provide a flexible straw.
- Check the puncture site for redness, swelling, and drainage every hour for the first 4 hours, then every 4 hours for the first 24 hours.

ANALYSIS OF CEREBROSPINAL FLUID

TEST	NORMAL	ABNORMAL	IMPLICATIONS
Pressure	50 to 180 mm H_2O	Increase	Increased intracranial pressure due to hemorrhage, tumor, or edema caused by trauma
		Decrease	Spinal subarachnoid obstruction above puncture site
Appearance	Clear, colorless	Cloudy	Infection (elevated white blood cell [WBC] count and protein levels, or many microorganisms)
		Xanthochromic or bloody	Subarachnoid, intracerebral, or intraventricular hemorrhage; spinal cord obstruction; traumatic tap (usually noted only in initial specimen)
		Brown, orange, or yellow	Elevated protein levels, red blood cell (RBC) breakdown (blood present for at least 3 days)
Protein	*Lumbar:* – neonates: 15 to 100 mg/dl – ages 3 months to 60 years: 15 to 45 mg/dl – Over age 60: 15 to 60 mg/dl *Cisternal:* 15 to 25 mg/dl *Ventricular:* 15 to 16 mg/dl	Marked increase Marked decrease	Tumors, trauma, hemorrhage, diabetes mellitus, polyneuritis, blood in cerebrospinal fluid (CSF) Rapid CSF production
Glucose	40 to 70 mg/dl (two-thirds of blood glucose level)	Increase Decrease	Systemic hyperglycemia Systemic hypoglycemia, bacterial or fungal infection, meningitis, mumps, postsubarachnoid hemorrhage
Cell count	0 to 5 WBCs in adults; 0 to 30 WBCs in neonates	Increase	Active disease: meningitis, acute infection, onset of chronic illness, tumor, abscess, infarction, demyelinating disease (such as multiple sclerosis)
	No RBCs	RBCs	Hemorrhage or traumatic tap

(continued)

ANALYSIS OF CEREBROSPINAL FLUID *(continued)*

TEST	NORMAL	ABNORMAL	IMPLICATIONS
VDRL and other serologic tests	Nonreactive	Positive	Neurosyphilis
Chloride	118 to 132 mEq/L	Decrease	Infected meninges (as in tuberculosis or meningitis)
Gram stain	No organisms	Gram-positive or gram-negative organisms	Bacterial meningitis

• If CSF pressure is elevated, assess neurologic status every 15 minutes for 4 hours. If the patient is stable, assess him every hour for 2 hours, and then every 4 hours or according to pretest schedule.

CLINICAL ALERT Watch for complications of lumbar puncture, such as reaction to the anesthetic, meningitis, bleeding into the spinal canal, and cerebellar tonsillar herniation and medullary compression. Signs of meningitis include fever, neck rigidity, and irritability; signs of herniation include decreased level of consciousness, changes in pupil size and equality, altered vital signs (including widened pulse pressure, decreased pulse rate, and irregular respirations), or respiratory failure.

Precautions
• Infection at the puncture site contraindicates removal of CSF; in a patient with increased intracranial pressure, CSF should be removed with extreme caution because the rapid reduction in pressure that follows withdrawal of fluid can cause cerebellar tonsillar herniation and medullary compression.

• During the procedure, observe closely for adverse reactions, such as elevated pulse rate, pallor, or clammy skin. Report any significant changes immediately.
• Record the collection time on the test request form. Send the form and labeled specimens to the laboratory immediately.

Normal findings
Normally, the CSF pressure is recorded and the appearance of the specimen is checked. Three tubes are collected routinely and are sent to the laboratory for analysis of protein, sugar, and cells as well as for serologic testing, such as the Venereal Disease Research Laboratory (VDRL) test for neurosyphilis. A separate specimen is also sent to the laboratory for culture and sensitivity testing. Electrolyte analysis and Gram stain may be ordered as supplementary tests. CSF electrolyte levels are of special interest in patients with abnormal serum electrolyte levels or CSF infection and in those receiving hyperosmolar agents.

For a summary of normal and abnormal findings in CSF analysis, see *Analysis of cerebrospinal fluid.*

Interfering factors

• Patient position and activity (possible increase or decrease in CSF pressure)

• Crying, coughing, or straining (possible increase in CSF pressure)

• Delay between collection time and laboratory testing (possible invalidation of test results, especially cell counts)

SOLUBLE AMYLOID BETA PROTEIN PRECURSOR

The presence of the amyloid beta protein in the senile plaques of the brain is a hallmark of Alzheimer's disease, leading researchers to believe that this protein may be responsible for the disease's neurotoxic effects. Although amyloid is found in the cerebrospinal fluid (CSF) of healthy people, it's found in smaller amounts in some patients with dementia, making it a useful diagnostic tool.

Purpose

• To assist in the diagnosis of Alzheimer's disease (see *Two new tests for Alzheimer's disease*)

Patient preparation

• Explain to the patient that a specimen of CSF is collected by lumbar puncture, and a small portion is tested using the enzyme-linked immunosorbent assay (ELISA) test.

• Tell the patient who will perform the procedure and where.

• Inform him that he needn't restrict food or fluids.

TWO NEW TESTS FOR ALZHEIMER'S DISEASE

Two new tests were recently introduced for use in patients with symptoms of dementia. One test determines the level of tau protein in conjunction with beta amyloid in the cerebrospinal fluid and requires a lumbar puncture. Elevated levels of tau and reduced levels of beta amyloid are associated with Alzheimer's disease. The manufacturer claims that this test is 95% accurate in ruling out or confirming Alzheimer's disease in about 60% of symptomatic patients over age 60.

The second test determines apolipoprotein E (ApoE) genotype, which is statistically significant in determining the probability of Alzheimer's. The presence of two copies of the ApoE4 allele may increase the probability to over 90%.

Although these tests may prove helpful in diagnosing Alzheimer's disease, experts caution that further studies are necessary to confirm their reliability.

• Advise him that a headache is the most common adverse effect of lumbar puncture, but reassure him that his cooperation during the test helps minimize this effect.

• Make sure that a signed consent form has been obtained.

Equipment

Lumbar puncture tray, sterile gloves, local anesthetic (1% lidocaine), povidone-iodine solution, small adhesive bandage

Procedure and posttest care

• Position the patient on his side at the edge of the bed, with his knees drawn up to his abdomen and his chin on his chest. Provide pillows to support the spine on a horizontal plane. This position allows full flexion of the spine and easy access to the lumbar subarachnoid space. Help the patient maintain this position by placing one arm around his knees and the other arm around his neck.

• If the sitting position is preferred, have the patient sit up and bend his chest and head toward his knees. Help him maintain this position throughout the procedure.

• After the skin is prepared for injection, the area is draped. Warn the patient that he'll probably experience a transient burning sensation when the local anesthetic is injected.

• Tell the patient that when the spinal needle is inserted, he may feel some transient local pain as the needle transverses the dura mater.

• Ask him to report any pain or other sensations that differ from or continue after this expected discomfort because such sensations could indicate irritation or puncture of a nerve root, requiring repositioning of the needle.

• Instruct the patient to remain still and breathe normally during the procedure; movement and hyperventilation can alter pressure readings or cause injury.

• The anesthetic is injected, and the spinal needle is inserted in the midline, between the spinous processes of the vertebrae (usually between the third and fourth lumbar vertebrae). At this point, initial (or opening) CSF pressure is measured and a specimen is obtained.

• After the specimen is collected, label the containers in the order in which they were filled, and determine if there are any specific instructions for the laboratory.

• Next, a final pressure reading is taken, and the needle is removed.

• Clean the puncture site with a local antiseptic, such as povidone-iodine solution, and apply a small adhesive bandage.

• Check whether the patient must lie flat or if the head of his bed may be slightly elevated. In most cases, you'll be instructed to keep the patient lying flat for 8 hours after lumbar puncture. Some doctors, however, allow a 30-degree elevation at the head of the bed. Remind the patient that although he should not raise his head, he can turn from side to side.

• Encourage the patient to drink fluids. Provide a flexible straw.

• Check the puncture site for redness, swelling, and drainage every hour for the first 4 hours, then every 4 hours the first 24 hours.

• If CSF pressure is elevated, assess neurologic status every 15 minutes for 4 hours. If the patient is stable, assess him every hour for 2 hours, and then every 4 hours or according to pretest schedule.

Precautions

• Infection at the puncture site contraindicates removal of CSF; in a patient with increased intracranial pressure, CSF should be removed with extreme caution because the rapid reduction in pressure that follows withdrawal of fluid can cause cerebellar tonsillar herniation and medullary compression.

• During the procedure, observe closely for adverse reactions, such as elevated pulse rate, pallor, or clammy skin. Report any significant changes immediately.

• Record the collection time on the test request form. Send the form and labeled specimens to the laboratory immediately.

Normal findings
Normal amyloid beta protein levels in CSF are greater than 450 units/L, based on age-matched controls using the ELISA test.

Abnormal findings
Soluble amyloid beta protein precursor is found in the CSF of healthy people. Low CSF levels suggest an alteration in the amyloid beta protein precursor processing and amyloid beta protein formation. Low soluble amyloid beta protein precursor levels correlate with clinically diagnosed and autopsy-confirmed Alzheimer's disease.

Interfering factors
• Patient positioning and activity (possible increase or decrease in CSF pressure)
• Crying, coughing, or straining (possible increase in CSF pressure)
• Delay in collection time and laboratory testing

SYNOVIAL FLUID ANALYSIS

In synovial fluid aspiration, or arthrocentesis, a sterile needle is inserted into a joint space — most commonly the knee — to obtain a fluid specimen for analysis. This procedure is indicated for patients with undiagnosed articular disease and symptomatic joint effusion, a condition marked by the excessive accumulation of synovial fluid. Although rare, complications associated with synovial fluid aspiration include joint infection and hemorrhage leading to hemarthrosis (accumulation of blood within the joint).

Purpose
• To aid differential diagnosis of arthritis, particularly septic or crystal-induced arthritis
• To identify the cause and nature of joint effusion
• To relieve the pain and distention resulting from accumulation of fluid within the joint
• To administer a drug locally (usually corticosteroids)

Patient preparation
• Describe the procedure to the patient, and answer any questions he may have.
• Explain that this test helps determine the cause of joint inflammation and swelling and also helps relieve the associated pain.
• Instruct him to fast for 6 to 12 hours before the test if glucose testing of synovial fluid is ordered; otherwise, inform him that he needn't restrict food or fluids before the test.
• Tell him who will perform the test and where.
• Warn him that although he'll receive a local anesthetic, he may still feel transient pain when the needle penetrates the joint capsule.
• Make sure that the patient or his legal guardian has signed a consent form.
• Check the patient's history for hypersensitivity to iodine compounds (such as povidone-iodine), procaine, lidocaine, or other local anesthetics.
• Administer a sedative.

Equipment
Surgical detergent; skin antiseptic (usually tincture of povidone-iodine);

alcohol sponges; local anesthetic (procaine or lidocaine, 1% or 2%); sterile, disposable 1½″ 25G needle; sterile, disposable 1½″ to 2½″ 20G needle; sterile 5-ml syringe for injecting anesthetic; sterile 20-ml syringe for aspiration; 3-ml syringe for administering sedative; sterile dressings; 2″ × 2″ sterile gauze pads; sterile drapes; elastic bandage; tubes for culture, cytologic, clot, and glucose analysis; anticoagulants (heparin, ethylenediaminetetraacetic acid [EDTA], and potassium oxalate); venipuncture equipment

For corticosteroid administration: corticosteroid suspension such as hydrocortisone, 2-ml and 5-ml syringes (or one 10-ml syringe if procaine and steroid are to be injected simultaneously)

Procedure and posttest care
● Position the patient, and explain that he'll need to maintain this position throughout the procedure.
● Tell him that although he'll receive a local anesthetic to minimize pain, he'll probably feel some discomfort when the needle is inserted. (A sedative may be administered to a young child.)
● Clean the skin over the puncture site with surgical detergent and alcohol.
● Paint the site with tincture of povidone-iodine, and allow it to air-dry for 2 minutes.
● After the local anesthetic is administered, the aspirating needle is quickly inserted through the skin, subcutaneous tissue, and synovial membrane into the joint space.
● As much fluid as possible is aspirated into the syringe; at least 15 ml should be obtained, although a smaller amount is usually adequate for analysis.
● The joint (except for the area around the puncture site) may be wrapped with an elastic bandage to compress

the free fluid into this portion of the sac, ensuring maximal collection of fluid.
● If a corticosteroid is being injected, prepare the dose as necessary. For instillation, the syringe is detached, leaving the needle in the joint, and the syringe containing the steroid is attached to the needle instead.
● After the steroid is injected and the needle withdrawn, wipe the puncture site with an alcohol sponge.
● Apply pressure to the puncture site for about 2 minutes to prevent bleeding; then apply a sterile dressing.
● If synovial fluid glucose levels are being measured, perform a venipuncture to obtain a specimen for blood glucose analysis.
● Apply ice or cold packs to the affected joint for 24 to 36 hours after aspiration to decrease pain and swelling. Use pillows for support. If a large quantity of fluid was aspirated, apply an elastic bandage to stabilize the joint.
● If the patient's condition permits, tell him he may resume normal activity immediately after the procedure. However, warn him to avoid excessive use of the affected joint for a few days after the test even if pain and swelling subside.
● Watch for increased pain or fever; these symptoms may indicate joint infection.
● Be careful when handling the dressings and linens of patients with drainage from the joint space, especially if septic arthritis is confirmed or suspected.
● Advise the patient that he may resume his usual diet.

Precautions
● Wear gloves when handling all specimens.
● Use strict sterile technique throughout aspiration to prevent contamination

of joint space or synovial fluid specimen.

• Add an anticoagulant to the specimen, according to the laboratory tests requested. Gently invert the tube several times to mix the specimen and anticoagulant adequately.

• *For cultures,* obtain 2 to 5 ml of synovial fluid and, if possible, inoculate the medium immediately. Otherwise, add one or two drops of heparin to the specimen.

• *For cytologic analysis,* add 5 mg of EDTA or one or two drops of heparin to 2 to 5 ml of synovial fluid.

• *For glucose analysis,* add potassium oxalate, as specified by the laboratory, to 3 to 5 ml of fluid.

• *For crystal examination,* add heparin if specified by the laboratory.

• *For other studies,* such as general appearance and clot evaluation, obtain 2 to 5 ml of synovial fluid, but don't add an anticoagulant.

• Send the properly labeled specimens to the laboratory immediately — gonococci are particularly labile. If a WBC count is being obtained as well, clearly label the specimen "Synovial Fluid" and "Caution: Don't Use Acid Diluents."

Normal findings

Examination of synovial fluid in the laboratory can take many forms. Routine examination includes gross analysis for color, clarity, quantity, viscosity, pH, and the presence of a mucin clot as well as microscopic analysis for WBC count and differential. Special examination includes microbiological analysis for formed elements (including crystals) and bacteria, serologic analysis, and chemical analysis for such components as glucose, protein, and enzymes.

Abnormal findings

Examination of synovial fluid may reveal various joint diseases, including noninflammatory disease (traumatic arthritis and osteoarthritis), inflammatory disease (systemic lupus erythematosus, rheumatic fever, pseudogout, gout, and rheumatoid arthritis), and septic disease (tuberculous and septic arthritis).

Interfering factors

• Failure to observe pretest restrictions
• Specimen contamination
• Acid diluents added to the specimen for WBC count (alteration in cell count)
• Failure to adequately mix the specimen and the anticoagulant or to send the specimen to the laboratory immediately

PERICARDIAL FLUID ANALYSIS

Analysis of the fluid inside the pericardial sac of the heart is usually done for patients with pericardial effusion (an accumulation of excess pericardial fluid), which may result from inflammation (as in pericarditis), rupture, or penetrating trauma.

Obtaining a specimen for analysis requires needle aspiration of pericardial fluid, a procedure called *pericardiocentesis.* This procedure must be performed cautiously because of the risk of potentially fatal complications, such as myocardial or coronary artery laceration, ventricular fibrillation or vasovagal arrest, pleural infection, or accidental puncture of the lung, liver, or stomach. If possible, echocardiography should determine the effusion site

ASPIRATING PERICARDIAL FLUID

In pericardiocentesis, a needle and syringe assembly is inserted through the chest wall into the pericardial sac, as illustrated below. Electrocardiographic monitoring with a leadwire attached to the needle and electrodes placed on the limbs (right arm [RA], right leg [RL], left arm [LA], and left leg [LL]) helps to ensure proper needle placement and to avoid damage to the heart.

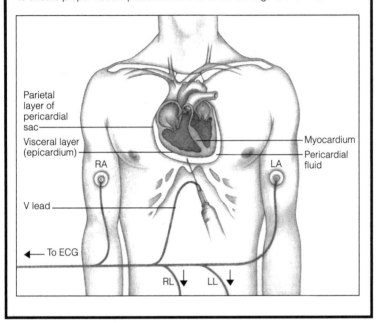

Parietal layer of pericardial sac

Visceral layer (epicardium)

Myocardium

Pericardial fluid

RA

LA

V lead

To ECG

RL

LL

before pericardiocentesis is performed to minimize the risk of complications. (See *Aspirating pericardial fluid.*)

Purpose
• To assist in identifying the cause of pericardial effusion and to help determine appropriate therapy

Patient preparation
• Explain to the patient that this test detects excessive fluid around the heart, determines its cause, and helps determine appropriate therapy.

• Inform him that he needn't restrict food or fluids before the test.
• Tell him who will perform the test and where and that it takes 10 to 20 minutes.
• Inform the patient that a local anesthetic will be injected before the aspiration needle is inserted.
• Warn him that although fluid aspiration isn't painful, he may experience pressure upon insertion of the needle into the pericardial sac.
• Advise him that he may be asked to briefly hold his breath to aid needle insertion and placement.

- Tell the patient that an I.V. line will be started at a slow rate in case medications need to be administered.
- Assure him that someone will remain with him during the test and that his pulse and blood pressure will be monitored after the procedure.
- Check the patient's history for current antimicrobial usage, and record such usage on the test request form.
- Make sure the patient or a responsible member of the family has signed a consent form.
- Explain the test to the family if pericardiocentesis is performed to relieve cardiac tamponade and the patient is in shock.

Equipment

70% alcohol or povidone-iodine solution; local anesthetic (1% procaine or 1% lidocaine); sterile 25G needle for the anesthetic; sterile 14G, 16G, and 18G 4″ or 5″ cardiac needles; 50-ml syringe with luer-lock tip; 7-ml sterile test tubes (one *red-top,* one *green-top* [heparin], and one *lavender-top* [EDTA]); sterile specimen container for culture; vial of heparin 1:1,000; 4″ × 4″ gauze pads; bandage; three-way stopcock. All of these items may be included in a prepackaged pericardiocentesis tray.

Also needed: electrocardiograph (ECG) or bedside monitor, Kelly clamp, alligator clips, defibrillator, and emergency drugs.

Procedure and posttest care

- Place the patient in the supine position with the thorax elevated 60 degrees.
- When the patient is comfortable and well-supported, instruct him to remain still during the procedure.
- A local anesthetic is administered at the insertion site after the skin is prepared with alcohol or povidone-iodine solution from the left costal margin to the xiphoid process.
- With the three-way stopcock open, a 50-ml syringe is aseptically attached to one end and the cardiac needle to the other end.
- The ECG lead wire is attached to the hub of the needle with an alligator clip. The ECG is set to lead V and turned on (or the patient is connected to a bedside monitor).
- The needle is inserted through the chest wall into the pericardial sac, maintaining gentle aspiration until fluid appears in the syringe.
- The needle is angled 35 to 45 degrees toward the tip of the right scapula between the left costal margin and the xiphoid process. A Kelly clamp is attached at the skin surface once the needle is properly positioned so it won't advance further.
- While the fluid is being aspirated, label and number the specimen tubes.
- When the needle is withdrawn, apply pressure to the site *immediately* with sterile gauze pads for 3 to 5 minutes. Then apply a bandage.
- Check blood pressure readings, pulse, respiration, and heart sounds every 15 minutes until stable, then every ½ hour for 2 hours, every hour for 4 hours, and every 4 hours thereafter. Reassure the patient that such monitoring is routine.

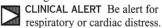 **CLINICAL ALERT** Be alert for respiratory or cardiac distress. Watch especially for signs of cardiac tamponade: muffled and distant heart sounds, distended neck veins, paradoxical pulse, and shock. Cardiac tamponade may result from rapid reaccumulation of pericardial fluid or puncture of a coronary vessel causing bleeding into the pericardial sac.

Precautions
- Carefully observe the ECG tracing during insertion of the cardiac needle; an ST-segment elevation indicates that the needle has reached the epicardial surface and should be retracted slightly; an abnormally shaped QRS complex may indicate perforation of the myocardium. Premature ventricular contractions usually indicate that the needle has touched the ventricular wall.
- Watch for grossly bloody aspirate — a sign of inadvertent puncture of a cardiac chamber.
- Be sure to use specimen tubes with the proper additives. Although fibrin isn't a normal component of pericardial fluid, it does appear in fluid in some pericardial diseases and in carcinoma, and clotting is possible.
- If bacterial culture and sensitivity tests are scheduled, record any antimicrobial therapy the patient is receiving on the laboratory slip.
- If anaerobic organisms are suspected, consult the laboratory concerning the proper collection technique to avoid exposing the aspirate to air. The aspirate may be placed in an anaerobic collection tube or the syringe may be filled completely, displacing all air, and the collection tube capped tightly with a sterile rubber tip.
- Send all specimens to the laboratory immediately.
- Have resuscitation equipment on hand.

Normal findings
Normally, 10 to 50 ml of sterile fluid is present in the pericardium. Pericardial fluid is clear and straw-colored, without evidence of pathogens, blood, or malignant cells. It normally contains fewer than 1,000 white blood cells (WBCs)/ml. Its glucose concentration approximately equals the levels in whole blood.

Abnormal findings
Generally, pericardial effusions are classified as transudates or exudates. Transudates are protein-poor effusions that usually arise from mechanical factors altering fluid formation or resorption, such as increased hydrostatic pressure, decreased plasma oncotic pressure, or obstruction of the pericardial lymphatic drainage system by a tumor.

Most exudates result from inflammation and contain large amounts of protein. In these effusions, inflammation damages the capillary membrane, allowing protein molecules to leak into the pericardial fluid. Exudate effusions may occur in pericarditis, neoplasms, acute myocardial infarction, tuberculosis, rheumatoid disease, and systemic lupus erythematosus.

An elevated WBC count or neutrophil fraction may also accompany inflammatory conditions such as bacterial pericarditis; a high lymphocyte fraction may indicate fungal or tuberculous pericarditis. Turbid or milky effusions may result from the accumulation of lymph or pus in the pericardial sac, or from tuberculosis or rheumatoid disease.

Bloody pericardial fluid may indicate hemopericardium, hemorrhagic pericarditis, or a traumatic tap. Hemopericardium, the accumulation of blood in the pericardium, may result from myocardial rupture after infarction or aortic rupture secondary to dissecting aortic aneurysm or thoracic trauma. In hemopericardium, the fluid has a hematocrit level similar to that of whole blood; in hemorrhagic pericarditis, it has a relatively low hematocrit level and doesn't clot on standing.

Hemorrhagic effusions may indicate a malignant tumor, closed chest trauma, Dressler's syndrome, or postcardiotomy syndrome. A traumatic tap is easily distinguished from hemopericardium or hemorrhagic pericarditis because the fluid becomes progressively clearer.

Glucose concentrations below whole blood levels may reflect increased local metabolism due to malignancy, inflammation, or infection. Possible causes of bacterial pericarditis include *Staphylococcus aureus, Haemophilus influenzae,* and various gram-negative organisms; possible causes of granulomatous pericarditis include *Mycobacterium tuberculosis* or various fungal agents; and possible causes of viral pericarditis include coxsackieviruses, echoviruses, and others.

Interfering factors

• Failure to use aseptic collection technique, allowing skin contaminants to be mistaken for the causative organism
• Failure to use proper additives in test tubes

SWEAT TEST

The sweat test is a quantitative measurement of electrolyte concentrations (primarily sodium and chloride) in sweat, usually performed using pilocarpine iontophoresis (pilocarpine is a sweat inducer). Although this test is primarily used to confirm cystic fibrosis (CF) in children, it's also performed in adults to determine if they're homozygous or heterozygous for CF.

Purpose

• To confirm CF

Patient preparation

• Explain the test to the child (if he's old enough to understand), using clear, simple terms.
• Inform the child and his parents that there are no restrictions on diet, medication, or activity before the test.
• Tell the child who'll perform the test and where and that it takes 20 to 45 minutes (depending on the equipment used).
• Tell him he may feel a slight tickling sensation during the procedure but won't feel any pain.
• Encourage the parents to assist with preparations and to stay with their child during the test. Their presence will minimize the child's anxiety.

Equipment

Analyzer, two skin chloride electrodes (positive and negative), distilled water, two standardizing solutions (chloride concentrations), $2'' \times 2''$ sterile gauze pads (kept in airtight container), pilocarpine pads, forceps (for handling pads), straps (for securing electrodes), gram scale, normal saline solution

Procedure and posttest care

• Wash the area that will undergo iontophoresis with distilled water and dry it. (The flexor surface of the right forearm is commonly used or, when the patient's arm is too small to secure electrodes [as with an infant], the right thigh.)
• Place a gauze pad saturated with premeasured pilocarpine solution on the positive electrode; place the pad saturated with normal saline solution on the negative electrode.
• Apply both electrodes to the area to undergo iontophoresis, and secure them with straps. Lead wires to the analyzer are given a current of 4 milliamperes in 15 to 20 seconds. Ion-

tophoresis will continue at 15- to 20-second intervals for 5 minutes.

• Try to distract the child with a book, television, a toy, or another diversion if he becomes nervous or frightened during the test.

• Remove both electrodes after iontophoresis.

• Discard the pads, clean the skin with distilled water, and then dry it.

• Using forceps, place a dry gauze pad or filter paper (previously weighed on a gram scale) on the area that underwent iontophoresis.

• Cover the pad or filter paper with a slightly larger piece of plastic, and seal the edges of the plastic with waterproof adhesive tape.

• Leave the gauze pad or filter paper in place for about 30 to 40 minutes. (The appearance of droplets on the plastic usually indicates induction of an adequate amount of sweat.)

• Remove the pad or filter paper with the forceps, place it immediately in the weighing bottle, and insert the stopper in the bottle. (The difference between the first and second weights indicates the weight of the sweat specimen collected.)

• Wash the area that underwent iontophoresis with soap and water, and dry it thoroughly. If the area looks red, reassure the patient that this is normal and will disappear within a few hours.

• Tell the patient or his parents that he may resume his usual activities.

Precautions

• Always perform iontophoresis on the right arm (or right thigh) rather than on the left.

• Never perform iontophoresis on the chest, especially in a child, because the current can induce cardiac arrest.

• Use battery-powered equipment to prevent electric shock if possible.

• Stop the test immediately if the patient complains of a burning sensation, which usually indicates that the positive electrode is exposed or positioned improperly. Adjust the electrode and continue the test.

• Make sure at least 100 mg of sweat is collected for analysis.

• Carefully seal the gauze pad or filter paper in the weighing bottle, and send the bottle to the laboratory at once.

Reference values

Normal sodium values in sweat range from 16 to 46 mmol/L or mEq/liter. Normal chloride values from 8 to 43 mmol/L.

Abnormal findings

Sodium levels of 75 mmol/L or more and chloride levels of 79 mmol/L or more are suggestive of CF.

Only a few conditions other than CF result in elevated sweat electrolyte levels — most notably, untreated adrenal insufficiency, as well as type I glycogen storage disease, vasopressin-resistant diabetes insipidus, meconium ileus, and renal failure. In women, sweat electrolyte levels fluctuate cyclically; chloride concentrations usually peak 5 to 10 days before onset of menses, and most women retain fluid before menses. Men also show fluctuations (up to 70 mmol/L). However, CF is the only condition that raises sweat electrolyte levels above 80 mmol/L.

Interfering factors

• Dehydration or edema, especially in the area of collection

• Failure to obtain an adequate amount of sweat, a common problem in neonates

• Presence of pure salt depletion, common during hot weather (possible false-normal)

• Failure to clean the skin thoroughly or to use sterile gauze pads (possible false-high)

• Failure to seal the gauze pad or filter paper carefully (possible false-high electrolyte levels due to evaporation)

EXAMINATION OF UROGENITAL SECRETIONS FOR TRICHOMONADS

Microscopic examination of urine or vaginal, urethral, or prostatic secretions can detect urogenital infection by *Trichomonas vaginalis,* a parasitic, flagellate protozoan that's usually transmitted sexually. This test is more commonly performed on women than on men because women are more likely to exhibit symptoms of trichomoniasis; men may exhibit symptoms of urethritis or prostatitis.

Purpose
• To confirm trichomoniasis

Patient preparation
• Explain that this test can identify the cause of urogenital infection.
• If the patient is a woman, tell her the test requires a specimen of vaginal secretions or urethral discharge, and ask her not to douche before the test.
• If the patient is a man, tell him the test requires a specimen of urethral or prostatic secretions.
• Inform the patient who will perform the procedure and when.

Equipment
Gloves, cotton swab, test tube containing small amount of normal saline solution, vaginal speculum, specimen

cup (if a urine specimen is being collected)

Procedure and posttest care
Vaginal secretions
• With the patient in the lithotomy position, an unlubricated vaginal speculum is inserted, and discharge is collected with a cotton swab. The swab is then placed in the tube containing normal saline solution, and the speculum is removed.
• Another method is to smear the specimen on a glass slide, allow it to air-dry, and then transport it to the laboratory.
Prostatic material
• After prostatic massage, collect secretions with a cotton swab, and place the swab in normal saline solution.
Urethral discharge
• Collect the discharge with a cotton swab, and place the swab in normal saline solution.
Urine
• Include the first portion of a voided random specimen (not midstream).
All procedures
• Label the specimen container appropriately, including the date and time of collection.
• Provide perineal care.

Precautions
• Remember to use gloves when performing procedures and handling specimens.
• If possible, obtain the urogenital specimen before treatment with a trichomonacide begins.
• Send the specimen to the laboratory immediately because trichomonads can be identified only while they're still motile.

Normal findings
Trichomonads are normally absent from the urogenital tract.

Abnormal findings

Trichomonads confirm trichomoniasis. In approximately 25% of women and in most infected men, trichomonads may be present without associated pathology.

Interfering factors

- Improper collection technique
- Failure to send the specimen to the laboratory immediately, causing trichomonads to lose motility
- Collection of the specimen after trichomonacide therapy begins (fewer trichomonads in the specimen)

CHAPTER 8

Cultures

GENERAL CULTURES 438

438 Urine culture
439 Stool culture
441 Throat culture
442 Nasopharyngeal culture
444 Sputum culture

446 Blood culture
447 Wound culture
449 Gastric culture
451 Duodenal contents culture

GENITAL CULTURES 453

453 Culture for gonorrhea
455 Culture for herpes simplex virus

457 Culture for *Chlamydia*

GENERAL CULTURES

Urine culture

Laboratory examination and culture of urine are used to evaluate urinary tract infections (UTIs), especially bladder infections. Urine in the kidneys and bladder is normally sterile, but a urine specimen may contain various organisms due to bacteria in the urethra and on external genitalia. Bacteriuria generally results from one prevalent bacteria type; the presence of more than two bacterial species in a specimen strongly suggests contamination during collection. A single negative culture does not always rule out infection; a quantitative examination of urine culture is needed.

Purpose
• To diagnose UTI
• To monitor microorganism colonization after urinary catheter insertion

Patient preparation
• Explain to the patient that this test is used to detect UTI.
• Inform the patient that the test requires a urine specimen and that no restriction of food or fluids is necessary. Tell him that the first voided specimen of the day is preferred because it will reflect a high colony count after an overnight incubation period.
• Instruct him how to collect a clean-voided midstream specimen; emphasize that external genitalia must be cleaned thoroughly.
• If appropriate, explain catheterization or suprapubic aspiration to the patient, and inform him that he may ex-

perience some discomfort during specimen collection.
• For the patient with suspected tuberculosis, specimen collection may be required on three consecutive mornings.
• Check the patient's history for current antimicrobial therapy.

Equipment
Gloves, sterile specimen cup, towelettes or sterile water, cleansing solution (such as aqueous green soap), and cotton balls or sterile gauze sponges (Note that commercial clean-catch urine kits are available.)

Procedure and posttest care
• Collect a urine specimen.
• Record on the laboratory slip the suspected diagnosis, the collection time and method, current antimicrobial therapy, and fluid- or drug-induced diuresis.

Precautions
• Wear gloves when performing the procedure and handling specimens.
• Collect at least 3 ml of urine, but don't fill the specimen cup more than halfway.
• When obtaining a specimen from an indwelling catheter, clamp the tubing below the collection port to collect a specimen in the tubing. Then use an alcohol pad to clean the port. Next, using a sterile needle and syringe, aspirate a 4-ml specimen from the port and transfer it into a sterile specimen cup.
• Seal the cup with a sterile lid, and send it to the laboratory immediately. If transport is delayed longer than 30 minutes, store the specimen at 39.2° F (4° C) or place it on ice, unless a urine transport tube containing preservative is used.

Normal findings

Culture results that contain 10,000 or fewer organisms per milliliter are considered negative.

Abnormal findings

Bacterial counts of 100,000/ml or more of a single microbe species indicate probable UTI. Counts under 100,000/ml may be significant, depending on the patient's age, sex, history, and other individual factors. Counts under 10,000/ml usually suggest that the organisms are contaminants, except in symptomatic patients, those with urologic disorders, and those whose urine specimens were collected by suprapubic aspiration. A special test for acid-fast bacteria isolates *Mycobacterium tuberculosis,* thus indicating tuberculosis of the urinary tract.

Isolation of more than two species of organisms or of vaginal or skin organisms usually suggests contamination and requires a repeat culture. Prolonged catheterization or urinary diversion may cause polymicrobial infection.

Interfering factors

● Failure to use proper collection technique
● Failure to preserve the specimen properly or to immediately send it to the laboratory
● Fluid- or drug-induced diuresis and antimicrobial therapy (possible decrease)

STOOL CULTURE

Normal bacterial flora in stool include several potentially pathogenic organisms. Bacteriologic examination is valuable for identifying pathogens that cause overt GI disease — such as typhoid and dysentery — and carrier states. A sensitivity test may follow isolation of the pathogen. Stool culture may also be used to detect certain viruses, such as enterovirus, which can cause aseptic meningitis.

Purpose

● To identify pathogenic organisms, especially in a debilitated patient
● To aid treatment of disease, prevent possibly fatal complications, and confine severely infectious diseases

Patient preparation

● Explain to the patient that this test is used to determine the cause of GI distress or to determine if he's a carrier of infectious organisms.
● Advise him that food and fluids needn't be restricted.
● Tell the patient that the test requires the collection of a stool specimen on 3 consecutive days.
● Check the patient's history for dietary patterns, recent antimicrobial therapy, and recent travel that might suggest endemic infections or infestations.

Equipment

Gloves, waterproof container with tight-fitting lid or sterile swab and commercial sterile collection and transport system, tongue blade, bedpan (if needed)

Procedure and posttest care

● Collect a stool specimen directly into the container. If the patient isn't ambulatory, collect the specimen in a clean, dry bedpan and, using a tongue blade, transfer the specimen to the container.
● If you must collect the specimen by rectal swab, insert the swab past the anal sphincter, rotate it gently, and

withdraw it. Then, place the swab in the appropriate container.
• Check with the laboratory for the proper collection procedure before obtaining a specimen for a virus test.
• Label the specimen with the patient's name, doctor's name, facility number, and date and time of collection.
• Indicate the suspected cause of enteritis and current antimicrobial therapy on the laboratory slip.

Precautions
• Wear gloves when performing the procedure and handling the specimen.
• If the patient uses a bedpan or a diaper, avoid contaminating the stool specimen with urine.
• The specimen must represent the first, middle, and last portion of the stool passed. Be sure to include mucoid and bloody portions.
• Put the specimen container in a leakproof bag, and send it to the laboratory immediately. Trophozoites and cysts may be destroyed if exposed to heat, cold, or a delay in delivery to the laboratory.

Normal findings
A large percentage of normal fecal flora consists of anaerobes, including non-spore-forming bacilli, clostridia, and anaerobic streptococci. The remaining percentage consists of aerobes, including gram-negative bacilli (predominantly *Escherichia coli* and other Enterobacteriaceae, plus small amounts of *Pseudomonas*), gram-positive cocci (mostly enterococci), and a few yeasts.

Abnormal findings
The most common pathogenic organisms of the GI tract are *Shigella, Salmonella,* and *Campylobacter jejuni.* Less common pathogenic organisms include *Vibrio cholerae, V. parahae-*
molyticus, Clostridium botulinum, C. difficile, C. perfringens, Staphylococcus aureus, enterotoxigenic *E. coli,* and *Yersinia enterocolitica.* Isolation of some pathogens indicates bacterial infection in patients with acute diarrhea and may require antimicrobial sensitivity tests. Normal fecal flora may include *C. difficile, E. coli,* and other organisms. Therefore, isolation of these organisms may require further tests to demonstrate invasiveness or toxin production.

Isolation of pathogens such as *C. botulinum* indicates food poisoning; the pathogens must also be isolated from the contaminated food. In a patient undergoing long-term antimicrobial therapy, isolation of large numbers of *S. aureus* or yeast may indicate infection. (Asymptomatic carrier states are also indicated by these enteric pathogens.) Isolation of enteroviruses may indicate aseptic meningitis.

If a stool culture shows no unusual growth, detection of viruses by immunoassay or electron microscopy may be used to diagnose nonbacterial gastroenteritis. Highly increased polymorphonuclear leukocytes in fecal material may indicate an invasive pathogen.

Interfering factors
• Failure to use proper collection technique
• Contamination of the specimen by urine (possible injury to or destruction of enteric pathogens)
• Antimicrobial therapy (possible decrease in bacterial growth)
• Failure to transport the specimen promptly or, if delivery is delayed, to use a transport medium, such as buffered glycerol, that stabilizes pH (possible loss of enteric pathogens or overgrowth of nonpathogenic organisms)
• Bismuth-containing toilet tissue placed in the collection container

• Barium and mineral or castor oil when testing for protozoa

THROAT CULTURE

A throat culture is used primarily to isolate and identify pathogens. Culture results are considered in relation to the patient's clinical status, recent antimicrobial therapy, and amount of normal flora.

Purpose

• To isolate and identify group A beta-hemolytic streptococci *(Streptococcus pyogenes)* — allowing early treatment of pharyngitis — and to prevent sequelae, such as rheumatic heart disease and glomerulonephritis
• To screen asymptomatic carriers of pathogens, especially *Neisseria meningitidis*
• Rarely, to identify *Corynebacterium diphtheriae* and *Bordetella pertussis*
• To identify *Candida albicans*, although direct potassium hydroxide preparation usually provides the same information faster

Patient preparation

• Explain to the patient that this test is used to identify microorganisms that may be causing his symptoms or to screen for asymptomatic carriers.
• Inform him that he needn't restrict food or fluids before the test.
• Tell him that a specimen will be collected from his throat and who will collect the specimen and when.
• Describe the procedure, and warn him that he may gag during the swabbing.
• Check the patient's history for recent antimicrobial therapy. Determine im-

munization history if pertinent to preliminary diagnosis.

Equipment

Gloves, sterile swab and culture tube with transport medium or commercial collection and transport system

Procedure and posttest care

• Tell the patient to tilt his head back and close his eyes.
• With the throat well illuminated, check for inflamed areas, using a tongue blade.
• Swab the tonsillar areas from side to side; include inflamed or purulent sites.
• *Do not* touch the tongue, cheeks, or teeth with the swab.
• Immediately place the swab in the culture tube.
• If a commercial sterile collection and transport system is used, crush the ampule and force the swab into the medium to keep the swab moist.
• Note recent antimicrobial therapy on the laboratory slip; label the specimen with the patient's name, the doctor's name, the date and time of collection, and the origin of the specimen; indicate the suspected organism, especially *C. diphtheriae* (requires two swabs and special growth medium), *B. pertussis* (requires a nasopharyngeal culture and a special growth medium), and *N. meningitidis* (requires enriched selective media).
• Nonculture antigen testing methods can be used to detect group A streptococcal antigen in as little as 10 minutes. Cultures are then performed on negative specimens.

Precautions

• Procure the throat specimen before beginning antimicrobial therapy.
• Wear gloves when performing the procedure and handling specimens.

• Send the specimen to the laboratory immediately. Unless a commercial sterile collection and transport system is used, keep the container upright during transport.

• To protect the specimen and prevent its exposure to pathogens, use aseptic technique during the procedure, and observe proper precautions when sending the specimen to the laboratory.

◤ **CLINICAL ALERT** Laryngospasm may occur after the culture is obtained if the patient has epiglottitis or diphtheria. Keep resuscitation equipment nearby.

Normal findings
Normal throat flora include nonhemolytic and alpha-hemolytic streptococci, *Neisseria* species, staphylococci, diphtheroids, some hemophilus, pneumococci, yeasts, and enteric gram-negative rods.

Abnormal findings
Pathogens that may be cultured include group A beta-hemolytic streptococci *(S. pyogenes),* which can cause scarlet fever and pharyngitis; *C. albicans,* which can cause thrush; *C. diphtheriae,* which can cause diphtheria; and *B. pertussis,* which can cause whooping cough. The laboratory report should indicate the prevalent organisms and the quantity of pathogens cultured.

Interfering factors
• Failure to report recent or current antimicrobial therapy on the laboratory slip (possible false-negative)
• Failure to use the proper transport medium
• More than a 15-minute delay in sending the specimen to the laboratory

NASOPHARYNGEAL CULTURE

This test is used to evaluate nasopharyngeal secretions for the presence of pathogenic organisms. It requires direct microscopic examination of a Gram-stained smear of the specimen. Preliminary identification of organisms may be used to guide clinical management and determine the need for additional testing. Cultured pathogens may then require susceptibility testing to determine appropriate antimicrobial therapy.

Purpose
• To identify pathogens causing upper respiratory tract symptoms
• To identify proliferation of normal nasopharyngeal flora, which may be pathogenic in debilitated and other immunocompromised patients
• To identify *Bordetella pertussis* and *Neisseria meningitidis,* especially in very young, elderly, or debilitated patients and asymptomatic carriers
• Infrequently, to isolate viruses, especially to identify carriers of influenza virus A and B

Patient preparation
• Explain to the patient that this test is used to isolate the cause of nasopharyngeal infection.
• Describe the procedure to the patient; tell him that secretions will be obtained from the back of the nose and the throat, using a cotton-tipped swab, and who will collect the specimen.
• Warn him that he may experience slight discomfort and gagging, but reassure him that obtaining the specimen takes less than 15 seconds.

Equipment

Gloves; penlight; sterile, flexible wire swab; small, sterile, open-ended glass Pyrex tube or sterile nasal speculum; tongue blade; culture tube; transport medium (broth)

Procedure and posttest care

- Put on gloves.
- Ask the patient to cough before you begin collecting the specimen.
- Position the patient with his head tilted back.
- Using a penlight and a tongue blade, inspect the nasopharyngeal area.
- Gently pass the swab through the nostril and into the nasopharynx, keeping the swab near the septum and floor of the nose. Rotate the swab quickly and remove it.
- Alternatively, place the Pyrex tube in the patient's nostril, and carefully pass the swab through the tube into the nasopharynx. Rotate the swab for 5 seconds; then place it in the culture tube with transport medium. Remove the Pyrex tube.
- Label the specimen with the patient's name, the doctor's name, the date and time of collection, the origin of the material, and the suspected organism.
- Ideally, specimens for *B. pertussis* should be inoculated to fresh culture medium at the patient's bedside because of the organism's susceptibility to environmental changes.
- If the purpose of specimen collection is to isolate a virus, follow the laboratory's recommended collection technique.

Precautions

- Wear gloves when performing the procedure and handling the specimen.
- *Do not* let the swab touch the sides of the patient's nostril or his tongue to prevent specimen contamination.

⚠ **CLINICAL ALERT** Laryngospasm may occur after the culture is obtained if the patient has epiglottitis or diphtheria. Keep resuscitation equipment nearby.

- Note recent antimicrobial therapy or chemotherapy on the laboratory slip.
- Keep the container upright.
- Tell the laboratory if the suspected organism is *Corynebacterium diphtheriae* or *B. pertussis* because these need special growth media.
- Refrigerate a viral specimen according to your laboratory's procedure.

Normal findings

Flora commonly found in the nasopharynx include nonhemolytic streptococci, alpha-hemolytic streptococci, *Neisseria* species (except *N. meningitidis* and *N. gonorrhoeae*), coagulase-negative staphylococci such as *Staphylococcus epidermidis* and, occasionally, the coagulase-positive *S. aureus*.

Abnormal findings

Pathogens include group A beta-hemolytic streptococci, *B. pertussis, C. diphtheriae, S. aureus, N. gonorrhoeae,* and large amounts of *Haemophilus influenzae,* pneumococci, or *Candida albicans.*

Interfering factors

- Recent antimicrobial therapy (decrease in bacterial growth)
- Failure to use proper collection technique
- Failure to place the specimen in transport medium
- Failure to keep a viral specimen cold
- Failure to send the specimen to the laboratory immediately

SPUTUM CULTURE

Bacteriologic examination of sputum (material raised from the lungs and bronchi) is an important aid to the management of lung disease. The usual method of specimen collection is deep coughing and expectoration, which may require ultrasonic nebulization, hydration, or chest physiotherapy; other methods include tracheal suctioning and bronchoscopy.

Purpose
• To identify the cause of pulmonary infection, thus aiding diagnosis of respiratory diseases (most frequently bronchitis, tuberculosis, lung abscess, and pneumonia)

Patient preparation
• Explain to the patient that this test is used to identify the organism causing respiratory tract infection.
• Tell him that the test requires a sputum specimen and who will collect the specimen.
• If the suspected organism is *Mycobacterium tuberculosis,* tell the patient that as many as three morning specimens may be required.
• If testing is for tuberculosis, explain that cultures for tuberculosis may take some time to develop; therefore, diagnosis of this disorder generally depends on clinical symptoms, a smear for acid-fast bacilli, a chest X-ray, and response to a purified protein derivative skin test.
• If the specimen is to be collected by expectoration, encourage fluid intake the night before collection to help sputum production, unless contraindicated by a fluid restriction. Teach the patient how to expectorate by taking three deep breaths and forcing a deep cough;

emphasize that sputum isn't the same as saliva, which is unacceptable for culturing. Tell him not to brush his teeth or use mouthwash before the specimen collection, although he may rinse his mouth with water.
• If the specimen is to be collected by tracheal suctioning, tell the patient he'll experience discomfort as the catheter passes into the trachea.
• If the specimen is to be collected by bronchoscopy, instruct the patient to fast for 6 hours before the procedure. Make sure he or a responsible family member has signed an informed consent form. Tell him he'll receive a local anesthetic just before the test to minimize discomfort during passage of the tube.

Equipment
For expectoration: sterile, disposable, impermeable container with a tight-fitting cap; 10% sodium chloride, acetylcysteine, propylene glycol, or sterile or distilled water aerosols to induce cough; leakproof bag
For tracheal suctioning: #16 or #18 French suction catheter, water-soluble lubricant, sterile gloves, sterile specimen container or in-line specimen trap, normal saline solution
For bronchoscopy: bronchoscope, local anesthetic, sterile needle and syringe, sterile specimen container, normal saline solution, bronchial brush, sterile gloves

Procedure and posttest care
Expectoration
• Put on gloves.
• Instruct the patient to cough deeply and expectorate into the container. If the cough is nonproductive, use chest physiotherapy or heated aerosol spray (nebulization) to induce sputum. Using aseptic technique, close the container securely.

● Dispose of equipment properly; seal the container in a leakproof bag before sending it to the laboratory.

Tracheal suctioning

● Administer oxygen to the patient before and after the procedure, if necessary.

● Attach the sputum trap to the suction catheter. Using sterile gloves, lubricate the catheter with normal saline solution, and pass it through the patient's nostril without suction. (The patient will cough when the catheter passes through the larynx.) Advance the catheter into the trachea. Apply suction for no longer than 15 seconds to obtain the specimen.

● Stop suction and gently remove the catheter. Discard the catheter and gloves in the proper receptacle. Then detach the in-line sputum trap from the suction apparatus and cap the opening.

● After tracheal suctioning, offer the patient a drink of water.

Bronchoscopy

● After a local anesthetic is sprayed into the patient's throat or the patient gargles with a local anesthetic, the bronchoscope is inserted through the pharynx and trachea into the bronchus.

● Secretions are then collected with a bronchial brush or aspirated through the inner channel of the scope, using an irrigating solution, such as normal saline solution, if necessary.

● After the specimen is obtained, the bronchoscope is removed.

◤ **CLINICAL ALERT** During and after bronchoscopy, observe the patient carefully for signs of hypoxemia (change in mental status), laryngospasm (laryngeal stridor), bronchospasm (paroxysms of coughing or wheezing), pneumothorax (dyspnea, cyanosis, pleural pain, tachycardia), perforation of the trachea or bronchus (subcutaneous crepitus), and trauma to respiratory structures (blood-tinged sputum, coughing up blood). Also,

check for difficulty in breathing or swallowing. *Do not* give liquids until the gag reflex returns.

All collection methods

● A specimen of at least 3 ml is necessary.

● Label the container with the patient's name. Include on the test request form the nature and origin of the specimen, the date and time of collection, the initial diagnosis, and any current antimicrobial therapy.

Precautions

● Tracheal suctioning is contraindicated in patients with esophageal varices.

● In a patient with asthma or chronic bronchitis, watch for aggravated bronchospasms with use of more than 10% concentration of sodium chloride or acetylcysteine in an aerosol.

◤ **CLINICAL ALERT** During tracheal suctioning, suction for only 5 to 10 seconds at a time. *Never* suction longer than 15 seconds. If the patient becomes hypoxic or cyanotic, remove the catheter immediately and administer oxygen.

● Wear gloves when performing the procedure and handling specimens.

● Because the patient may cough violently during suctioning, wear gloves, a mask and, if necessary, a gown to avoid exposure to pathogens.

● *Do not* use more than 20% propylene glycol with water as an inducer for a specimen scheduled for tuberculosis culturing because higher concentrations inhibit the growth of *M. tuberculosis.* (If propylene glycol is not available, use 10% to 20% acetylcysteine with water or saline solution.)

● Send the specimen to the laboratory immediately after collection. Don't refrigerate the specimen.

Normal findings

A Gram stain of expectorated sputum must be examined to ensure that it's a representative specimen of secretions from the lower respiratory tract. Sputum is invariably contaminated with normal oropharyngeal flora, such as alpha-hemolytic streptococci, *Neisseria* species, diphtheroids, some *Haemophilus* species, pneumococci, staphylococci, and yeasts, such as *Candida*. The presence of normal flora does not rule out infection; interpretation of a culture isolate must include consideration of the patient's overall clinical condition.

Abnormal findings

Pathogenic organisms commonly found in sputum include *Streptococcus pneumoniae, M. tuberculosis, Klebsiella pneumoniae (*and other Enterobacteriaceae), *Haemophilus influenzae, Staphylococcus aureus, Pseudomonas aeruginosa, Pneumocystis carinii, Legionella,* and *Mycoplasma pneumoniae.* Isolation of *M. tuberculosis* is a significant finding.

Respiratory viruses usually require serologic or histologic diagnosis rather than diagnosis by sputum culture.

Interfering factors

• Failure to use proper collection technique
• Failure to report current or recent antimicrobial therapy on the laboratory slip (possible false-negative)
• Collection over an extended period, which may cause pathogens to deteriorate or become overgrown by commensals (not accepted as a valid specimen by laboratories)

BLOOD CULTURE

A blood culture is performed to isolate and aid identification of the pathogens in bacteremia (bacterial invasion of the bloodstream) and septicemia (systemic spread of such infection). It requires inoculating a culture medium with a blood sample and incubating it.

Purpose

• To confirm bacteremia
• To identify the causative organism in bacteremia and septicemia

Patient preparation

• Explain to the patient that this procedure is used to help identify the organism causing his symptoms.
• Inform him that he needn't restrict food or fluids before the test.
• Tell him how many samples the test will require and who will perform the venipunctures and when.
• Inform him that he may experience transient discomfort from the needle punctures and the tourniquet. Reassure him that collecting each sample usually takes less than 5 minutes.

Equipment

Gloves; tourniquet; small adhesive bandages; alcohol swabs; povidone-iodine swabs; 10- to 20-ml syringe for an adult, 6-ml syringe for a child; three or four sterile needles; two blood culture bottles, one vented (aerobic) and one unvented (anaerobic), with nutritionally enriched broths and sodium polyethanol sulfonate added, or bottles with resin or a lysis-centrifugation tube

Procedure and posttest care

• Put on gloves.
• Clean the venipuncture site with an alcohol swab and then with an iodine swab, working in a circular motion from the site outward.
• Wait at least 1 minute for the skin to dry, and remove the residual iodine with an alcohol swab. (Or remove the iodine after venipuncture.)
• Apply the tourniquet.

- Perform a venipuncture; draw 10 to 20 ml of blood for an adult, one syringe of 2 to 6 ml for a child, or 0.1 to 1 ml for neonates, infants, and small children.
- Clean the diaphragm tops of the culture bottles with alcohol or iodine, and change the needle on the syringe.
- If broth is used, add blood to each bottle until a 1:5 or 1:10 dilution is obtained. For example, add 10 ml of blood to a 100-ml bottle. (The size of the bottle varies, depending on facility procedure.)
- If a special resin is used, such as Bactec resin medium or Antimicrobial Removal Device, add blood to the resin in the bottles and invert them gently to mix.
- If you're using the lysis-centrifugation technique (Isolator), draw the blood directly into a special collection and processing tube.
- Indicate the tentative diagnosis on the laboratory slip, and note any current or recent antimicrobial therapy.
- If a hematoma develops at the venipuncture site, apply warm soaks.

Precautions
- Wear gloves when performing the procedure and handling specimens.
- Send each specimen to the laboratory immediately after collection.
- Don't draw blood from an existing I.V. catheter. Use a vein below an I.V. catheter or in the opposite arm.

Normal findings
Normally, blood cultures are negative for pathogens.

Abnormal findings
Positive blood cultures don't necessarily confirm pathologic septicemia. Mild, transient bacteremia may occur during the course of many infectious diseases or may complicate other dis-orders. Persistent, continuous, or recurrent bacteremia reliably confirms the presence of serious infection. To detect most causative agents, blood cultures are ideally drawn on 2 consecutive days.

Isolation of most organisms takes about 72 hours; negative cultures are held for 1 or more weeks before being reported negative.

Common blood pathogens include *Streptococcus pneumoniae* and other *Streptococcus* species, *Haemophilus influenzae, Staphylococcus aureus, Pseudomonas aeruginosa,* Bacteroidaceae, *Brucella,* Enterobacteriaceae, coliform bacilli, and *Candida albicans*. Although 2% to 3% of cultured blood samples are contaminated by skin bacteria, such as *Staphylococcus epidermidis,* diphtheroids, and *Propionibacterium,* these organisms may be clinically significant when isolated from multiple cultures or from immunocompromised patients.

Interfering factors
- Failure to report recent or current antimicrobial therapy on the laboratory slip (possible false-negative)
- Failure to use proper collection technique
- Removal of culture bottle caps at the bedside (possible prevention of anaerobic growth)
- Use of incorrect bottle and media (possible prevention of aerobic growth)

WOUND CULTURE

Performed to confirm infection, a wound culture is a microscopic analysis of a specimen from a lesion. Wound cultures may be aerobic, for detection of organisms that usually appear in a

ANAEROBIC SPECIMEN COLLECTOR

Some anaerobes die when exposed to oxygen. To facilitate anaerobic collection and culturing, tubes filled with carbon dioxide (CO_2) or nitrogen are used for oxygen-free transport.

The anaerobic specimen collector shown here consists of a rubber-stoppered tube filled with CO_2, a small inner tube, and a swab attached to a plastic plunger. The drawing on the left shows the tube before specimen collection. The small inner tube containing the swab is held in place by the rubber stopper.

After specimen collection (right), the swab is quickly replaced in the inner tube and the plunger is depressed. This separates the inner tube from the stopper, forcing it into the larger tube and exposing the specimen to the CO_2-rich environment.

The tube should be kept upright.

Before

After

superficial wound, or anaerobic, for organisms that need little or no oxygen and appear in areas of poor tissue perfusion, such as postoperative wounds, ulcers, and compound fractures. Indications for wound culture include fever as well as inflammation and drainage in damaged tissue.

Purpose
• To identify an infectious microbe in a wound

Patient preparation
• Explain to the patient that this test is used to identify infectious microbes.
• Describe the procedure, informing the patient that a drainage specimen from the wound is withdrawn by a syringe or removed on sterile cotton swabs.
• Tell him who will collect the specimen.

Equipment
Sterile cotton swabs and sterile culture tube or commercial sterile collection and transport system (for aerobic culture); sterile cotton swabs or sterile 10-ml syringe with 21G needle, and special culture tube containing carbon dioxide or nitrogen (for anaerobic culture); sterile gloves; alcohol sponges; sterile gauze; povidone-iodine solution

Procedure and posttest care
• Put on gloves, prepare a sterile field, and clean the area around the wound with antiseptic solution.
• For an *aerobic culture,* express the wound and swab as much exudate as possible, or insert the swab deeply into the wound and gently rotate. Immediately place the swab in the aerobic culture tube.
• For an *anaerobic culture,* insert the swab deeply into the wound, gently rotate, and immediately place the swab in the anaerobic culture tube (see *Anaero-*

bic specimen collector). Or insert the needle into the wound, aspirate 1 to 5 ml of exudate into the syringe, and immediately inject the exudate into the anaerobic culture tube. If the needle is covered with a rubber stopper, the aspirate may be sent to the laboratory in the syringe.

• Record on the laboratory slip recent antimicrobial therapy, the source of the specimen, and the suspected organism. Label the specimen container appropriately with the patient's name, the doctor's name, the facility number, the wound site, and the time of specimen collection.

• Dress the wound.

Precautions

• Clean the area around the wound thoroughly to limit contamination of the culture by normal skin flora, such as diphtheroids, *Staphylococcus epidermidis,* and alpha-hemolytic streptococci. *Do not* clean the area around a perineal wound.

• Make sure no antiseptic enters the wound.

• Obtain exudate from the entire wound, using more than one swab if necessary.

• Because some anaerobes die in the presence of even a small amount of oxygen, place the specimen in the culture tube quickly, take care that no air enters the tube, and check that double stoppers are secure.

• Keep the specimen container upright, and send it to the laboratory within 15 minutes to prevent growth or deterioration of microbes.

• Wear gloves during the procedure and when handling the specimen, and take necessary isolation precautions when sending the specimen to the laboratory.

Normal findings

Normally, no pathogenic organisms are present in a clean wound.

Abnormal findings

The most common aerobic pathogens for wound infection include *Staphylococcus aureus,* group A beta-hemolytic streptococci, *Proteus, Escherichia coli* and other Enterobacteriaceae, and some *Pseudomonas* species; the most common anaerobic pathogens include some *Clostridium* and *Bacteroides* species.

Interfering factors

• Failure to report recent or current antimicrobial therapy (possible false-negative)

• Failure to use proper collection technique

• Failure to use the proper transport medium, allowing the specimen to dry and the bacteria to deteriorate

GASTRIC CULTURE

This test requires aspiration of gastric contents and cultivation of any microbes present. Performed in conjunction with a chest X-ray and a purified protein derivative skin test, it's especially useful when a sputum specimen can't be obtained by expectoration or nebulization. Gastric aspiration also provides a specimen for rapid presumptive identification of bacteria (by Gram stain) in neonatal septicemia.

Purpose

• To aid diagnosis of mycobacterial infections

• To identify the infectious bacteria in neonatal septicemia

- To determine if *Helicobacter pylori* is the cause of a patient's gastritis or peptic ulcer disease

Patient preparation
- Explain to the patient (or parents if the patient is a child) that gastric culture is used to diagnose tuberculosis or to identify the infectious organism in neonatal septicemia.
- Instruct him to fast for 8 hours before the test.
- Tell him who will perform the procedure and that the same procedure may be performed on 3 consecutive mornings.
- Instruct him to remain in bed each morning until specimen collection has been completed to prevent premature emptying of stomach contents.
- Describe the procedure to the patient. Tell him that the nasogastric (NG) tube may make him gag but that it passes more easily if he relaxes and follows instructions about breathing and swallowing.
- Just before the procedure, obtain baseline heart rate and rhythm, and place the patient in high Fowler's position.
- Check the patient's history for recent antimicrobial therapy. Inform the doctor of your findings; he may want to discontinue medications before the test.

Equipment
Water-soluble lubricating jelly; sterile water; #16 or #18 French disposable, plastic NG tube; 50-ml sterile syringe; sterile specimen container; sterile gloves; emesis basin; stethoscope; clamp (if necessary)

Procedure and posttest care
- As soon as the patient awakens in the morning, put on gloves, perform NG intubation, and obtain gastric washings.
- Clamp the tube before quickly removing it from the patient.
- Note recent antimicrobial therapy on the laboratory slip, along with the site and time of collection.
- Label the specimen container with the patient's name, the doctor's name, and the facility number.
- Resume administration of medications discontinued before the test.
- Instruct the patient not to blow his nose for 4 to 6 hours to prevent bleeding.
- Tell the patient that he may resume his normal diet.

Precautions
- Gastric intubation is contraindicated in pregnancy, esophageal disorders (varices, stenosis, diverticula), malignant neoplasms, recent severe gastric hemorrhage, aortic aneurysm, heart failure, and myocardial infarction.
- If possible, obtain the specimens before the start of antimicrobial therapy.
- Watch for signs that the tube has entered the trachea, including coughing, cyanosis, and gasping.

CLINICAL ALERT *Never* inject water into an NG tube unless you're sure the tube is correctly placed in the patient's stomach. During lavage, use sterile distilled water to decrease the risk of contamination with saprophytic mycobacteria.
- Check the patient's pulse rate for irregularities during this procedure to detect arrhythmias.
- Wear gloves when performing the procedure and when handling specimens and the NG tube.
- Put the specimen in a tightly capped container, wipe the outside of the container with disinfectant, place it upright

in a plastic bag, and send it to the laboratory immediately.

• Dispose of all equipment carefully to prevent staff contamination.

Normal findings

Normally, the culture specimen is negative for pathogenic mycobacteria.

Abnormal findings

Isolation and identification of the organism *Mycobacterium tuberculosis* indicates the presence of active tuberculosis; other species of *Mycobacterium*, such as *M. bovis, M. kansasii,* and *M. avium-intracellulare* complex, may cause pulmonary disease that is clinically indistinguishable from tuberculosis. Treatment of these mycobacterial infections may be difficult and commonly requires susceptibility studies to determine the most effective antimicrobial therapy. Pathogenic bacteria causing neonatal septicemia may also be identified through culture.

Isolation of *H. pylori* implicates it as a cause of gastritis or peptic ulcer disease.

Interfering factors

• Failure to observe an 8-hour fast before the test (possible decrease)

• Drugs such as tetracycline and aminoglycosides (possible false-negative)

• Presence of saprophytic mycobacteria in gastric contents because these mycobacteria can't be microscopically distinguished from pathogenic mycobacteria (possible false-positive acid-fast smears)

DUODENAL CONTENTS CULTURE

This test requires duodenal intubation, aspiration of duodenal contents, and cultivation of microbes to isolate and identify pathogens that may cause duodenitis, cholecystitis, and cholangitis. Occasionally, a specimen may be obtained during surgery.

Purpose

• To detect bacterial infection of the biliary tract and duodenum

• To differentiate between infection and gallstones

• To rule out bacterial infection as the cause of persistent GI symptoms (epigastric pain, nausea, vomiting, and diarrhea)

Patient preparation

• Explain to the patient that this test is used to determine the cause of his symptoms.

• Instruct him to restrict food and fluids for 12 hours before the test.

• Tell him who will perform the procedure and where.

• Describe the intubation procedure to the patient. Assure him that although this procedure is uncomfortable, it isn't dangerous; tell him that passage of the tube may cause gagging but that following the examiner's instructions about proper positioning, breathing, swallowing, and relaxing will minimize his discomfort.

• Suggest that he empty his bladder before the procedure to increase his general comfort.

Equipment

Gloves, double-lumen nasoenteric tube with olive tip, water-soluble jelly,

30-ml sterile syringe, emesis basin, sterile specimen container, ½" adhesive tape

Procedure and posttest care
● After the nasoenteric tube is inserted, place the patient in a left lateral decubitus position with his feet elevated to allow peristalsis to move the tube into the duodenum.
● Determine the pH of a small amount of aspirated fluid to ascertain tube position. If the tube is in the stomach, pH is lower than 7.0; if the tube is in the duodenum, pH is higher than 7.0.
● The position of the tube can also be confirmed by fluoroscopy.
● Aspirate duodenal contents.
● Occasionally, a specimen for culture of duodenal contents is obtained during duodenoscopy (see "Esophagogastroduodenoscopy" in Chapter 10).
● Transfer the specimen to a sterile container, and label it with the patient's name, doctor's name, and date and time of collection.
● After duodenal intubation or duodenoscopy, observe the patient carefully for signs of perforation, such as dysphagia, epigastric or shoulder pain, dyspnea, and fever, from tube passage.
● After duodenoscopy, monitor vital signs until the patient is stable; keep the side rails up, and enforce bed rest until the patient is fully alert.
● Tell the patient that he may resume his normal diet.

Precautions
● Wear gloves when assisting with this procedure and handling the specimen.
● Duodenal intubation is contraindicated in pregnancy; acute pancreatitis or cholecystitis; esophageal varices, stenosis, and diverticular malignant neoplasms; recent severe gastric hemorrhage; aortic aneurysm; heart failure; and myocardial infarction.

● Collect the specimen for culture before antimicrobial therapy begins.
● Send the specimen to the laboratory immediately.
● Withdraw the tube slowly (6" to 8" [15 to 20 cm] every 10 minutes) until it reaches the esophagus; then clamp the tube and remove it quickly. Report the problem if you can't withdraw the tube easily; *never* force the tube.

Normal findings
Normally, a duodenal contents culture contains small amounts of polymorphonuclear leukocytes and epithelial cells with no pathogens. The bacterial count is usually less than 100,000/ml of body fluid.

Abnormal findings
Duodenal contents (pancreatic and duodenal enzymes as well as bile) are subject to infection by many pathogens. Generally, bacterial counts of 100,000/ml or more or the presence of pathogens in any number indicates infection. Susceptibility testing may be required.

Numerous polymorphonuclear leukocytes, copious mucous debris, and bile-stained epithelial cells in the bile fluid suggest inflammation of the biliary tract; many segmented neutrophils and exfoliated epithelial cells suggest inflammation of the pancreas, duodenum, or bile ducts. The presence of bile sand indicates cholelithiasis or calculi in the biliary tract. Differential diagnosis requires further testing.

Interfering factors
● Failure to observe a 12-hour fast before the test (possible decrease)
● Failure to use proper collection technique

GENITAL CULTURES

CULTURE FOR GONORRHEA

Gonorrhea almost always results from sexual transmission of *Neisseria gonorrhoeae*. A stained smear of genital exudate can confirm gonorrhea in 90% of males with characteristic symptoms, but a culture is often necessary, especially in asymptomatic females. Possible culture sites include the urethra (usual site in males), endocervix (usual site in females), anal canal, and oropharynx.

Purpose
● To confirm gonorrhea

Patient preparation
● Describe the procedure to the patient. Explain that this test is used to confirm gonorrhea.
● Inform the patient who will perform the test and when.
●Instruct the female patient not to douche for 24 hours before the test.
● Tell the male patient not to void during the hour preceding the test. Warn him that males sometimes experience nausea, sweating, weakness, and fainting due to stress or discomfort when the cotton swab or wire loop is introduced into the urethra.

Equipment
Sterile gloves, sterile cotton swabs, tongue blade, wire bacteriologic loop or thin urogenital alginate swabs (for male), vaginal speculum, modified Thayer-Martin medium in plates (or Transgrow medium in specimen bottles if laboratory is not readily available), ring forceps, cotton balls

Procedure and posttest care
Endocervical culture
● Place the patient in the lithotomy position, drape her appropriately, and instruct her to take deep breaths.
● Using gloved hands, insert a vaginal speculum that has been lubricated only with warm water. Clean mucus from the cervix, using cotton balls in ring forceps.
● Insert a dry, sterile cotton swab into the endocervical canal and rotate it from side to side. Leave the swab in place for several seconds for optimum absorption of organisms.
Urethral culture
● Place the patient in a supine position, and drape him appropriately.
● Clean the urethral meatus with sterile gauze or a cotton swab; then insert a thin urogenital alginate swab or a wire bacteriologic loop ⅜″ to ¾″ (1 to 2 cm) into the urethra, and rotate the swab or loop from side to side. Leave it in place for several seconds for optimum absorption of organisms. If permitted, the patient may milk the urethra, bringing urethral secretions to the meatus for collection on a cotton swab.
Rectal culture
● After obtaining an endocervical or a urethral specimen (while the patient is still on the examination table), insert a sterile cotton swab into the anal canal about 1″ (2.5 cm), move the swab from side to side, and leave it in place for several seconds for optimum absorption.
● If the swab is contaminated with stool, discard it and repeat the procedure with a clean swab.
Throat culture
● Position the patient with his head tilted back.
● Check his throat for inflamed areas, using a tongue blade. Rub a sterile

CULTURING FOR *NEISSERIA GONORRHOEAE*

Culturing for *Neisseria gonorrhoeae* requires use of a modified Thayer-Martin (MTM) medium. If a laboratory isn't readily available, you may use Transgrow medium.

Modified Thayer-Martin

MTM medium is a combination of hemoglobin, gonococcal growth-enhancing chemicals, and antimicrobial agents for culturing endocervical, urethral, and rectal specimens. To inoculate a culture plate treated with MTM medium and to spread organisms out of their associated mucus, take the following steps:

● Roll the swab in a Z pattern (1).
● Using the swab or a sterile wire loop, immediately cross-streak the plate (2).
  To demonstrate *N. gonorrhoeae,* incubate within 15 minutes of streaking.

Two-step method of streaking Thayer-Martin plate

Transgrow

A modification of MTM medium, Transgrow is available in a screw-cap bottle containing air and carbon dioxide. Transgrow bottles are used to transport suspect cultures when laboratory facilities aren't available at the site of specimen collection. Use the following procedure:

● To prevent loss of carbon dioxide, inoculate the specimen bottle while it's upright.
● After uncapping the bottle, immediately insert the swab and soak up all excess moisture.
● Starting at the bottom of the bottle, roll the swab from side to side across the medium.
● Recap the bottle, and send it to the laboratory immediately. Subculturing should begin within 24 to 48 hours.

One-step method of streaking Transgrow medium

swab from side to side over the tonsillar areas, including any inflamed or purulent sites. Be careful not to touch the teeth, cheeks, or tongue with the swab.

After specimen collection
• Roll the swab in a Z pattern in a plate containing modified Thayer-Martin medium. Then, cross-streak the medium with a sterile wire loop or the tip of the swab, and cover the plate. (See *Culturing for* Neisseria gonorrhoeae.)
• Label the specimen with the patient's name and room number (if applicable), the doctor's name, and the date and time of collection.
• If laboratory facilities are not readily available, do the following: Uncap the Transgrow medium specimen bottle just before inserting the swab of test material into the bottle. Keep the bottle upright to minimize loss of carbon dioxide. With the swab, absorb the excess moisture within the bottle; then roll the swab across the Transgrow medium. Discard the swab. Place the lid on the bottle, and label the bottle appropriately.
• Advise the patient to avoid all sexual contact until test results are available.
• Explain that treatment usually begins after confirmation of a positive culture, except in a person who has symptoms of gonorrhea or who has had intercourse with someone known to have gonorrhea.
• Advise the patient that a repeat culture is required 1 week after completion of treatment to evaluate the effectiveness of therapy.
• Inform the patient that positive culture findings must be reported to the local health department.

Precautions
• Wear gloves when performing the procedures and handling the specimens.

• Place the male patient in the supine position to prevent falling if vasovagal syncope occurs when the cotton swab or wire loop is introduced into the urethra. Observe for profound hypotension, bradycardia, pallor, and sweating.
• Collect a urethral specimen at least 1 hour after the patient has voided to prevent loss of urethral secretions.
• After collecting the specimens, carefully dispose of gloves, swabs, and speculum to prevent staff exposure.
• Send the specimens to the laboratory immediately, or arrange for transport of the Transgrow bottle because the specimen must be subcultured within 24 to 48 hours.

Normal findings
Normally, no *N. gonorrhoeae* appears in the culture.

Abnormal findings
A positive culture confirms gonorrhea.

Interfering factors
• Pretest antimicrobial therapy
• Contamination due to fecal material in a rectal culture or improper collection technique
• In males, voiding within 1 hour of specimen collection; in females, douching within 24 hours of specimen collection (fewer organisms available for culture)

CULTURE FOR HERPES SIMPLEX VIRUS

Herpes simplex virus (HSV) produces a wide spectrum of clinical manifestations, including keratitis, gingivostomatitis, and encephalitis. In immunocompromised individuals, it may lead to disseminated illness. The herpes-

RAPID MONOCLONAL TEST FOR CYTOMEGALOVIRUS

Cytomegalovirus (CMV), a member of the herpesvirus group, can cause systemic infection in congenitally infected infants and immunocompromised patients, such as transplant recipients, patients receiving chemotherapy, and patients with acquired immunodeficiency syndrome.

Laboratory detection of CMV
In the past, CMV infections were detected in the laboratory by recognizing the distinctive cytopathic effects (CPE) produced by the virus in conventional tube cell cultures. In this slow method of detecting CMV, CPE cultures grow in 9 days on average.

The faster rapid monoclonal test (shell vial assay) is based on centrifugal inoculation of specimens onto cell monolayers grown on round cover slips in 1-dram shell vials. The immunologic detection of early products of viral replication with specific monoclonal antibodies usually occurs after 16 hours of incubation. This assay is based on the availability of a monoclonal antibody specific for the 72-kd protein of CMV synthesized during the immediate early stage of viral replication.

Through indirect immunofluorescence, CMV-infected fibroblasts are recognized by their dense, homogeneous staining confined to the nucleus of these cells. Because of the smooth, regular shape of the nucleus and the surrounding nuclear membrane, infected cells are readily differentiated from nonspecific background fluorescence, which may be present in some specimens.

This test is used to obtain rapid laboratory diagnosis of CMV infection, especially in immunocompromised patients who have or are at risk for developing systemic infections caused by this virus.

Specimen collection
Specimens should be collected during the prodromal and acute stages of clinical infection to ensure the best chance of detecting CMV. As required by the laboratory, collect a specimen for culture. Each type of specimen requires a specific collection device, as listed below:
• *Throat:* microbiologic transport swab
• *Urine, cerebrospinal fluid:* sterile screw-capped tube or vial
• *Bronchoalveolar lavage tissue:* sterile screw-capped jar
• *Blood:* sterile tube with anticoagulant (heparin).

CMV can be detected in urine and throat specimens from asymptomatic patients. The detection of CMV from these sites indicates active, asymptomatic infection, which may herald symptomatic involvement, especially in immunocompromised patients. Detection of CMV in specimens of blood, tissue, or bronchoalveolar lavage generally indicates systemic infection and disease.

virus group includes Epstein-Barr virus, cytomegalovirus (CMV), varicella-zoster virus (VZV), human herpesvirus-6, and HSV Types 1 and 2. Only CMV, VZV, and HSV replicate in the standard cell cultures used in diagnostic laboratories.

About 50% of the strains of HSV can be detected by characteristic cytopathic effects (CPE) within 24 hours after the laboratory receives the specimen; 5 to 7 days are required to detect the remaining HSV strains. (See *Rapid monoclonal test for cytomegalovirus.*)

Purpose
• To confirm diagnosis of HSV infection by culturing the virus from specimens

Patient preparation
• Explain to the patient that this test is performed to detect infection by HSV.
• Explain to the patient that specimens will be collected from suspected lesions during the prodromal and acute stages of clinical infection.

Procedure and posttest care
• Collect a specimen for culture into the appropriate collection device.
• For the throat, skin, eye, or genital area, use a microbiologic transport swab.
• For body fluids or other respiratory specimens (washings, lavage), use a sterile screw-capped jar.
• Store or transport the specimen to the laboratory as soon as possible after collection. If the anticipated time between collection and inoculation of cell cultures is more than 2 hours, the specimen should be stored and transported at 39.2° F (4° C).

Precautions
• Wear gloves when obtaining and handling all specimens.
• Don't freeze the specimen or allow it to dry up.

Normal findings
HSV is seldom recovered from immunocompetent patients who show no overt signs of disease.

Abnormal findings
HSV detected in specimens taken from dermal lesions, the eye, or cerebrospinal fluid is highly significant. Specimens from the upper respiratory tract may be associated with intermittent shedding of the virus, particularly in an immunocompromised patient.

Like other herpesviruses, HSV can be shed from immunocompromised patients intermittently in the absence of apparent disease. For epidemiologic purposes, HSV detected by CPE in standard tube cell cultures is confirmed and identified as Type 1 or 2.

Interfering factor
• Administration of antiviral drugs before specimen collection

CULTURE FOR *CHLAMYDIA*

The most common sexually transmitted disease in North America, chlamydia is caused by the organism *Chlamydia trachomatis*. Identification of this parasite requires cultivation in the laboratory. After incubation, *Chlamydia*-infected cells can be detected by fluorescein isothiocyanate-conjugated monoclonal antibodies or by iodine stain. Detection in cell cultures of *C. psittaci* and *C. pneumoniae* requires specific technical manipulations and reagents.

Culture is the detection method of choice, but rapid noncultural (antigen detection) procedures are also available.

Purpose
• To confirm infections caused by *C. trachomatis*

Patient preparation
• Explain the purpose of the test to the patient.
• Describe the procedure for collecting a specimen for culture.
• If the specimen will be collected from the patient's genital tract, instruct

the patient not to urinate for 1 hour before the specimen is taken.
• Tell a female patient not to douche for 24 hours before the test.

Equipment
Gloves, sterile cotton swabs, wire bacteriologic loop or thin urogenital alginate swabs (for male), vaginal speculum, sucrose phosphate (2SP) transport medium

Procedure and posttest care
• Obtain a specimen of the epithelial cells from the infected site. In adults, these sites may include the eye, urethra (rather than from the purulent exudate that may be present), endocervix, and rectum.
• Obtain a urethral specimen by inserting a cotton-tipped applicator ¾″ to 2″ (2 to 5 cm) into the urethra.
• To collect a specimen from the endocervix, use a microbiologic transport swab or cytobrush.
• Extract the specimen into 2SP transport medium.
• Specimens collected from the throat, eye, or nasopharynx and aspirates from infants should be extracted into 2SP transport medium. The specimens are sent to the laboratory at 39.2° F (4° C).
• If the anticipated time between specimen collection and inoculation into cell culture is more than 24 hours, freeze the 2SP transport medium and send it to the laboratory with dry ice.

Note: In patients suspected of being sexually abused, be sure to process specimens by culture rather than by antigen detection methods.
• Advise the patient to avoid all sexual contact until after test results are available.
• If the culture confirms infection, provide counseling for the patient regarding treatment of sexual partners.

Precautions
• Place the male patient in the supine position to prevent falling if vasovagal syncope occurs when the cotton swab or wire loop is introduced into the urethra. Observe for profound hypotension, bradycardia, pallor, and sweating.
• Wear gloves when performing the procedures and handling the specimens.
• Collect a urethral specimen at least 1 hour after the patient has voided to prevent loss of urethral secretions.
• After collecting the specimens, carefully dispose of gloves, swabs, and speculum to prevent staff exposure.

Normal findings
Normally, no *C. trachomatis* appears in the culture.

Abnormal findings
A positive culture confirms *C. trachomatis* infection.

Interfering factors
• Using an antimicrobial drug within a few days before specimen collection (possible inability to recover *C. trachomatis*)
• In males, voiding within 1 hour of specimen collection; in females, douching within 24 hours of specimen collection (fewer organisms available for culture)
• Failure to use proper collection technique
• Contamination of the specimen due to fecal material in a rectal culture

CHAPTER 9

Biopsy

RESPIRATORY SYSTEM   460

460   Lung biopsy   461   Pleural biopsy

GASTROINTESTINAL SYSTEM   463

463   Small-bowel biopsy   465   Percutaneous liver biopsy

REPRODUCTIVE SYSTEM   467

467   Breast biopsy   471   Cervical biopsy
469   Prostate gland biopsy

SKELETAL SYSTEM   472

472   Bone biopsy   478   Synovial membrane biopsy
474   Bone marrow aspiration and
      biopsy

OTHER ORGAN-SPECIFIC BIOPSIES   479

479   Thyroid biopsy   484   Skin biopsy
481   Lymph node biopsy   485   Percutaneous renal biopsy
482   Sentinel lymph node biopsy

RESPIRATORY SYSTEM

LUNG BIOPSY

In biopsy of the lung, a specimen of pulmonary tissue is excised by closed or open technique for histologic examination. Closed technique, performed under local anesthesia, includes both needle and transbronchial biopsies; open technique, performed under general anesthesia in the operating room, includes both limited and standard thoracotomies. Needle biopsy is appropriate when the lesion is readily accessible, originates in the lung parenchyma and is confined to it, or is affixed to the chest wall; it provides a much smaller specimen than the open technique. Transbronchial biopsy, the removal of multiple tissue specimens through a fiber-optic bronchoscope, may be used in patients with diffuse infiltrative pulmonary disease or tumors or when severe debilitation contraindicates open biopsy. Open biopsy is appropriate for the study of a well-circumscribed lesion that may require resection.

Generally, a biopsy of the lung is recommended after chest X-rays, computed tomography scan, and bronchoscopy have failed to identify the cause of diffuse parenchymal pulmonary disease or a pulmonary lesion. Complications of lung biopsy include bleeding, infection, and pneumothorax.

Purpose
● To confirm a diagnosis of diffuse parenchymal pulmonary disease and pulmonary lesions

Patient preparation
● Explain to the patient that this test is used to confirm or rule out a diagnostic finding in the lung.
● Describe the procedure to the patient, and answer any questions.
● Tell the patient that a chest X-ray and blood studies (prothrombin time, activated partial thromboplastin time, and platelet count) will be performed before the biopsy.
● Tell him who will perform the biopsy and where.
● Instruct the patient to fast after midnight before the procedure. (Sometimes the patient is permitted to have clear liquids the morning of the test.)
● Make sure the patient or an appropriate family member has signed an informed consent form.
● Check the patient's history for hypersensitivity to the local anesthetic.
● Administer a mild sedative 30 minutes before the biopsy to help the patient relax. You may also administer codeine to suppress the cough reflex. Tell him that he'll receive a local anesthetic but may experience a sharp, transient pain when the biopsy needle touches the lung.

Procedure and posttest care
● After the biopsy site is selected, lead markers are placed on the patient's skin.
● Position the patient on the fluoroscopy table so that the needle is perpendicular to the lesion by the shortest distance. Depending on the location of the lesion, the patient may be on his back, side, or stomach.
● Prepare the skin over the biopsy site and drape the appropriate area.
● With a 25G needle, the local anesthetic is injected just above the rib below the selected site to prevent damage to the intercostal nerves and vessels.

- Using a 22G needle, the examiner anesthetizes the intercostal muscles and parietal pleura.
- A short 20G needle to be used as the guide is inserted into the chest wall at the previously marked location. This needle doesn't puncture the pleura.
- The aspiration needle is passed through the guide, punctures the pleura, and is guided fluoroscopically to the lesion.
- The specimen is divided immediately: The tissue for histology is placed in a properly labeled bottle containing 10% neutral buffered formaldehyde solution; the tissue for microbiology is placed in a sterile container.
- Exert pressure on the biopsy site to stop the bleeding, and apply a small bandage.

   CLINICAL ALERT Check vital signs every 15 minutes for 1 hour, every hour for 4 hours, and then every 4 hours. Watch for bleeding, dyspnea, elevated pulse rate, diminished breath sounds on the biopsy side and, eventually, cyanosis. Complications include pneumothorax and bleeding. Make sure the chest X-ray is repeated as soon as the biopsy has been completed.
- Inform the patient that he may resume his normal diet.

Precautions
- Needle biopsy is contraindicated in patients with a lesion that's separated from the chest wall or that's accompanied by emphysematous bullae, cysts, or gross emphysema and in patients with coagulopathy, hypoxia, pulmonary hypertension, or cardiac disease with cor pulmonale.
- During biopsy, observe for signs of respiratory distress — shortness of breath, elevated pulse rate, and cyanosis (late sign). If such signs develop, report them immediately.

- Because coughing and movement during biopsy can cause tearing of the lung by the biopsy needle, keep the patient calm and still.

Normal findings
Normal pulmonary tissue shows uniform texture of the alveolar ducts, alveolar walls, bronchioles, and small vessels.

Abnormal findings
Histologic examination of a pulmonary tissue specimen can reveal squamous cell or oat cell carcinoma and adenocarcinoma and supplements the results of microbiologic cultures, deep-cough sputum specimens, chest X-rays, and bronchoscopy and the patient's physical history in confirming cancer or parenchymal pulmonary disease.

Interfering factors
- Failure to obtain a representative tissue specimen
- Failure to store the specimen in the appropriate containers

PLEURAL BIOPSY

Pleural biopsy is the removal of pleural tissue by needle biopsy or open biopsy for histologic examination. Needle pleural biopsy is performed under local anesthesia. It generally follows or is done in conjunction with thoracentesis (aspiration of pleural fluid), which is performed when the cause of the effusion is unknown, but it can be performed separately.

   Open pleural biopsy, performed in the absence of pleural effusion, permits direct visualization of the pleura and the underlying lung. It's performed in the operating room.

Purpose
- To differentiate between nonmalignant and malignant disease
- To diagnose viral, fungal, or parasitic disease and collagen vascular disease of the pleura

Patient preparation
- Describe the procedure to the patient and answer his questions.
- Explain that this test permits microscopic examination of pleural tissue.
- Tell him who will perform the biopsy and where.
- Explain that blood studies will precede the biopsy and chest X-rays will be taken before and after the biopsy.
- Make sure the patient or an appropriate family member has signed an informed consent form.
- Check the patient's history for hypersensitivity to the local anesthetic.
- Tell him that he'll receive an anesthetic and should experience little pain.
- Just before the procedure, record vital signs.

Procedure and posttest care
- Seat the patient on the side of the bed, with his feet resting on a stool and his arms on the overbed table or supported by his upper body. Tell him to hold this position and remain still during the procedure.
- Prepare the skin and drape the area.
- The local anesthetic is then administered.
- In a *Vim-Silverman needle biopsy,* a needle is inserted through the appropriate intercostal space into the biopsy site, with the outer tip distal to the pleura and the central portion pushed in deeper and held in place. In *Cope's needle biopsy,* a trocar is introduced through the appropriate intercostal space into the biopsy site. To obtain the specimen, a hooked stylet is inserted through the trocar.

- Put the specimen immediately into a 10% neutral buffered formaldehyde solution in a labeled specimen bottle, and send it to the laboratory immediately.
- Clean the skin around the biopsy site, and apply an adhesive bandage.
- Make sure the chest X-ray is repeated immediately after the biopsy.
- Check vital signs every 15 minutes for 1 hour and then every hour for 4 hours or until stable.

▶ **CLINICAL ALERT** Watch for signs of respiratory distress (dyspnea), shoulder pain, and complications such as pneumothorax (immediate), pneumonia (delayed), and hemorrhage.

Precautions
- Pleural biopsy is contraindicated in patients with severe bleeding disorders.

Normal findings
The normal pleura consists primarily of mesothelial cells that are flattened in a uniform layer. Layers of areolar connective tissue that contain blood vessels, nerves, and lymphatics lie below.

Abnormal findings
Histologic examination of the tissue specimen can reveal malignant disease, tuberculosis, and viral, fungal, parasitic, or collagen vascular disease. Primary neoplasms of the pleura are generally fibrous and epithelial.

Interfering factors
- Failure to use the proper fixative or to obtain an adequate specimen
- Patient's inability to remain still, keep from coughing, or follow instructions, such as "Hold your breath," during the procedure

GASTROINTESTINAL SYSTEM

SMALL-BOWEL BIOPSY

Small-bowel biopsy is used to evaluate diseases of the intestinal mucosa, which may cause malabsorption or diarrhea. It produces larger specimens than those produced by endoscopic biopsy and allows removal of tissue from areas beyond an endoscope's reach. (See *Endoscopic biopsy of the GI tract,* page 464.)

Several similar types of capsules are available for tissue collection. In each, a mercury-weighted bag is attached to one end of the capsule; a thin polyethylene tube about 5' (1.5 m) long is attached to the other end. When the bag, capsule, and tube are in place in the small bowel, suction on the tube draws the mucosa into the capsule and closes it, cutting off the piece of tissue within. Although this is an invasive procedure, it causes little pain and rarely causes complications.

Small-bowel biopsy verifies diagnosis of some diseases, such as Whipple's disease, and may help confirm others, such as tropical sprue.

Purpose
- To help diagnose diseases of the intestinal mucosa

Patient preparation
- Explain to the patient that this test is used to identify intestinal disorders.
- Describe the procedure to the patient, and answer any questions.
- Instruct him to restrict food and fluids for at least 8 hours before the test.

- Tell him who will perform the biopsy and where.
- Make sure the patient or a responsible family member has signed an informed consent form.
- Ensure that coagulation tests have been performed and that the results are recorded on the patient's chart.
- Withhold aspirin and anticoagulants, as ordered. If these drugs must be continued, note this on the laboratory slip.

Procedure and posttest care
- Check the tubing and the mercury bag for leaks.
- Lightly lubricate the tube and capsule with a water-soluble lubricant, and moisten the mercury bag with water.
- Spray the back of the patient's throat with a local anesthetic to decrease gagging.
- Ask the patient to sit upright.
- The capsule is placed in his pharynx, and he's asked to flex his neck and swallow as the tube is advanced.
- If a local anesthetic is used to control the gag reflex, the patient mustn't receive any fluids to help him swallow the capsule.
- Place the patient on his right side; the tube is then advanced another 20″ (50 cm). The tube's position is checked by fluoroscopy or by instilling air through the tube and listening with a stethoscope for air to enter the stomach.
- Next, the tube is advanced 2″ to 4″ (5 to 10 cm) at a time to pass the capsule through the pylorus. (Talk to the patient about food to stimulate the pylorus and help the capsule pass.)
- When fluoroscopy confirms that the capsule has passed the pylorus, keep the patient on his right side to allow the capsule to move into the second and third portions of the small bowel.

ENDOSCOPIC BIOPSY OF THE GI TRACT

Endoscopy allows direct visualization of the GI tract and any site that requires biopsy of tissue specimens for histologic analysis. This relatively painless procedure helps detect, support diagnosis of, or monitor GI tract disorders. Its complications, notably hemorrhage, perforation, and aspiration, are rare.

Patient preparation

Careful patient preparation is vital for this procedure. Describe the procedure to the patient and reassure him that he'll be able to breathe with the endoscope in place. Tell him to fast for at least 8 hours before the procedure. For lower GI biopsy, clean the bowel. Make sure the patient or a responsible family member has signed an informed consent form.

Just before the procedure, administer the prescribed sedative to the patient. He should be relaxed but not asleep because his cooperation is necessary to promote smooth passage of the endoscope. Spray the back of his throat with a local anesthetic to suppress his gag reflex. Have suction equipment and bipolar cauterizing electrodes available to prevent aspiration and excessive bleeding.

Obtaining the sample

After the endoscope is passed into the upper or lower GI tract and a lesion, node, or other abnormal area is visualized, a biopsy forceps is pushed through a channel in the endoscope until this, too, can be seen. The forceps are then opened, positioned at the biopsy site, and closed on the tissue. The closed forceps and tissue specimen are removed from the endoscope, and the tissue is taken from the forceps. Then the forceps may be used to cauterize any remaining abnormal tissue or stop bleeding.

The specimen is placed mucosal side up on fine mesh gauze or filter paper and then placed in a labeled biopsy bottle containing fixative. When all specimens have been collected, the endoscope is removed. Specimens are sent to the laboratory immediately.

Endoscopic biopsy of the GI tract can be used to diagnose cancer, lymphoma, amyloidosis, candidiasis, and gastric ulcers; to support diagnosis of Crohn's disease, chronic ulcerative colitis, gastritis, esophagitis, and melanosis coli in laxative abuse; and to monitor progression of Barrett's esophagus, multiple gastric polyps, colon cancer and polyps, and chronic ulcerative colitis.

• Tell the patient that he may hold the tube loosely to one side of his mouth if it makes him more comfortable.
• Capsule position is checked again by fluoroscopy. When the capsule is at or beyond the ligament of Treitz, the biopsy sample can be taken. (The doctor will determine the biopsy site.)

• Place the patient in a supine position so that the capsule's position can be verified fluoroscopically.
• The specimen is gently removed with forceps, placed mucosal side up on a piece of mesh, and then placed in a biopsy bottle with required fixative.
• Resume the patient's diet after confirming return of the gag reflex.

• Although complications are rare, watch for signs of hemorrhage, bacteremia with transient fever and pain, and bowel perforation. Tell the patient to report abdominal pain or bleeding.

Precautions
• Send the specimen to the laboratory immediately.
• Keep suction equipment nearby to prevent aspiration if the patient vomits.
• Don't allow the patient to bite the tubing.
• Handle the tissue carefully and place it correctly on the slide.
• Biopsy is contraindicated in uncooperative patients, those taking aspirin or anticoagulants, and those with uncontrolled coagulation disorders.

Normal findings
A normal small-bowel biopsy specimen consists of fingerlike villi, crypts, columnar epithelial cells, and round cells.

Abnormal findings
Small-bowel tissue that reveals histologic changes in cell structure may indicate Whipple's disease, abetalipoproteinemia, lymphoma, lymphangiectasia, eosinophilic enteritis, and such parasitic infections as giardiasis and coccidiosis. Abnormal specimens may also suggest celiac sprue, tropical sprue, infectious gastroenteritis, intraluminal bacterial overgrowth, folate and vitamin B_{12} deficiency, radiation enteritis, and malnutrition, but such disorders require further studies.

Interfering factors
• Failure to observe pretest restrictions (possible poor specimen or vomiting and aspiration)
• Mechanical failure of the biopsy capsule or hole in the tubing (possible difficulty in removing tissue specimen)

• Patient's inability to remain still or keep from coughing during the procedure
• Incorrect handling or positioning of the specimen or failure to place it in a fixative
• Delay in transporting the specimen to the laboratory

PERCUTANEOUS LIVER BIOPSY

Percutaneous biopsy of the liver is the needle aspiration of a core of tissue for histologic analysis. This procedure is performed under local or general anesthesia. Findings may help to identify hepatic disorders after ultrasonography, computed tomography, and radionuclide studies have failed to detect them. Because many patients with hepatic disorders have clotting defects, testing for hemostasis should precede liver biopsy.

Purpose
• To diagnose hepatic parenchymal disease, cancer, and granulomatous infections

Patient preparation
• Explain to the patient that this test is used to diagnose liver disorders.
• Describe the procedure to the patient, and answer any questions.
• Instruct the patient to restrict food and fluids for 4 to 8 hours before the test.
• Tell him who will perform the biopsy and where.
• Make sure the patient or an appropriate family member has signed an informed consent form.

• Check the patient's history for hypersensitivity to the local anesthetic.
• Make sure coagulation studies have been performed and that the results are recorded on the patient's chart.
• Just before the biopsy, tell the patient to void; then, record vital signs.
• Inform him that he'll receive a local anesthetic but may experience pain similar to that of a punch in his right shoulder as the biopsy needle passes the phrenic nerve.

Procedure and posttest care
• For aspiration biopsy using the Menghini needle, place the patient in a supine position, with his right hand under his head. Instruct him to maintain this position and remain as still as possible during the procedure.
• The liver is palpated, the biopsy site is selected and marked, and the anesthetic is then injected.
• The needle flange is set to control the depth of penetration, and 2 ml of sterile normal saline solution are drawn into the syringe.
• The syringe is attached to the biopsy needle, and the needle is introduced into the subcutaneous tissue through the right eighth or ninth intercostal space at the midaxillary line and advanced up to the pleura.
• Next, 1 ml of normal saline solution is injected to clear the needle and the plunger; then the plunger is drawn back to the 4-ml mark to create negative pressure.
• At this point in the procedure, ask the patient to take a deep breath, exhale, and hold his breath at the end of expiration to prevent movement of the chest wall.
• As the patient holds his breath, the biopsy needle is quickly inserted into the liver and withdrawn in 1 second.
• For patients who are unable to hold their breath, the biopsy needle is

quickly inserted and withdrawn at the end of expiration.
• After the needle is withdrawn, tell the patient to resume normal respirations.
• The tissue specimen is then placed in a properly labeled specimen cup containing 10% formaldehyde solution.
• Again, 1 ml of normal saline solution is injected to clear the needle of the tissue specimen.
• Apply pressure to the biopsy site to stop bleeding.
• Position the patient on his right side for 2 to 4 hours, with a small pillow or sandbag under the costal margin to provide extra pressure. Advise bed rest for at least 5 hours. Restrict activity for the rest of the day.
• Check the patient's vital signs every 15 minutes for 1 hour and then every 30 minutes for 4 hours. Throughout, observe carefully for signs of shock.

▶ **CLINICAL ALERT** Immediately report bleeding or signs of bile peritonitis, such as tenderness and rigidity around the biopsy site. Be alert for symptoms of pneumothorax, such as rising respiratory rate, depressed breath sounds, dyspnea, persistent shoulder pain, and pleuritic chest pain. Report such complications promptly.
• If the patient experiences pain, which may persist for several hours after the test, administer an analgesic.
• Inform the patient that he may resume his normal diet.

Precautions
• Percutaneous liver biopsy is contraindicated in a patient with a platelet count below 100,000/μl; prothrombin time longer than 15 seconds; empyema of the lungs, pleurae, peritoneum, biliary tract, or liver; vascular tumor; hepatic angiomas; hydatid cyst; or tense ascites. If extrahepatic obstruction is suspected, ultrasonography or subcuta-

neous transhepatic cholangiography should rule out this condition before the biopsy is considered.
- Send the specimen to the laboratory immediately.

Normal findings
The normal liver consists of sheets of hepatocytes supported by a reticulin framework.

Abnormal findings
Examination of the hepatic tissue may reveal diffuse hepatic disease, such as cirrhosis or hepatitis, or granulomatous infections, such as tuberculosis. Primary malignant tumors include hepatocellular carcinoma, cholangiocellular carcinoma, and angiosarcoma, but hepatic metastasis is more common.

Nonmalignant findings with a known focal lesion require further studies, such as laparotomy or laparoscopy with biopsy.

Interfering factors
- Failure to obtain a representative specimen
- Failure to place the specimen in the proper preservative
- Failure to send the specimen to the laboratory immediately

REPRODUCTIVE SYSTEM

BREAST BIOPSY

Breast biopsy is performed to confirm or rule out breast cancer after clinical examination, mammography, or thermography has identified a mass. Fine-needle aspiration is usually done on a mass that has been identified by ultrasonography as being fluid-filled. Solid masses are assessed by one of four methods: ultrasound-guided core biopsy, stereotactic breast biopsy, needle or wire localization biopsy, or excisional biopsy. An incisional biopsy is seldom performed. Stereotactic breast biopsy immobilizes the breast and allows the computer to calculate the exact location of the mass, based on X-rays from two angles. Needle or wire localization biopsy is used to localize a nonpalpable lesion for excisional biopsy.

All four techniques require only local anesthesia, although an excisional biopsy may be done under general anesthesia. If sufficient tissue is obtained and the mass is found to be a malignant tumor, specimens are sent for estrogen and progesterone receptor assays to assist in determining future therapy and the prognosis.

Because breast cancer remains the most prevalent cancer in women, genetic researchers are continually working to identify women at risk. (See *BRCA testing*, page 468.)

Purpose
- To differentiate between benign and malignant breast tumors

Patient preparation
- Describe the procedure to the patient, and explain that this test permits microscopic examination of a breast tissue specimen. Offer her emotional support, and assure her that breast masses don't always indicate cancer.
- If the patient is to receive a local anesthetic, tell her that she needn't restrict food, fluids, or medication before the biopsy.
- If she is to receive a general anesthetic, advise her to fast from midnight before the test until after the biopsy.

BRCA TESTING

Recently, genetic researchers located two genes, BRCA1 and BRCA2, that have been linked to certain forms of breast cancer. BRCA testing can detect the presence of BRCA gene mutations, which may increase an individual's susceptibility to some breast cancers.

The test, performed on a blood sample, is available for women with a family history of breast cancer. Controversy continues over whether or not BRCA testing should be made available to the general public.

• Tell her who will perform the biopsy and where.
• Make sure the patient or an appropriate family member has signed an informed consent form.
• Check the patient's history for hypersensitivity to anesthetics.

Procedure and posttest care

Ultrasound-guided core biopsy
• Instruct the patient to undress to the waist and put on a gown. Have her lie on her back on the ultrasound table. Position her additionally as needed, such as with her arms over her head, depending on the location of the mass to be biopsied.
• Ultrasonography of the breast is performed, the mass is localized, and its position is marked on the skin.
• The area is cleaned, and local anesthetic is injected.
• The biopsy needle is then inserted at the previously marked spot and a tissue specimen obtained.

• After the needle is removed, apply pressure for 10 minutes and then apply a dressing and an ice bag.

Stereotactic breast biopsy
• Instruct the patient to undress to the waist, put on a gown, and lie face-down on the special breast biopsy table. Position her breast through the round opening in the table. Mammography equipment located under the table is used for the procedure.
• The breast is compressed by a paddle, as with a regular mammogram, and remains compressed throughout the procedure. Films are then taken from two angles and visualized on the computer.
• The computer calculates the exact position of the mass and the insertion site for the needle.
• Next, the skin is cleaned and a local anesthetic injected.
• The biopsy probe is inserted, and X-ray images are taken to confirm proper placement.
• A tissue specimen is obtained using a punch biopsy needle or a Mammotome probe.
• After the probe is removed, apply pressure for 10 minutes, dress the site, and apply ice.

Needle or wire localization biopsy
• The suspicious area is identified, using craniocaudal and mediolateral X-ray views of the breast.
• The area is anesthetized and a double-lumen needle inserted.
• X-rays are obtained to ensure proper needle placement, and areas may be marked with blue dye or a radiopaque contrast medium.
• The outer needle is then removed, leaving in place a small hooked wire. The wire is taped to the patient's skin to identify the excisional biopsy site.

Excisional biopsy
• After the patient receives an anesthetic, her skin is prepared and draped.

• A curvilinear incision is made over the palpable mass or the area identified by the localization wire.

• The mass as well as a margin of normal tissue around it are removed, and the skin is sutured.

• A dressing is applied, and the patient is observed for at least 1 hour before discharge.

All procedures

• Tissue specimens are placed in 10% formaldehyde solution and sent for frozen-section and receptor assays.

• Check vital signs, and provide medication for pain. If the patient has received a general anesthetic, check vital signs every 30 minutes for the first 4 hours, every hour for the next 4 hours, and then every 4 hours.

• Watch for and report bleeding, tenderness, and redness at the biopsy site.

• Provide emotional support to the patient who is awaiting diagnosis.

Precautions

• Excisional breast biopsy is contraindicated in patients with conditions that preclude surgery.

• Send the specimen to the laboratory immediately.

Normal findings

Normally, breast tissue consists of cellular and noncellular connective tissue, fat lobules, and various lactiferous ducts. It's pink, more fatty than fibrous, and shows no abnormal development of cells or tissue elements.

Abnormal findings

Abnormal breast tissue may exhibit a wide range of malignant or benign pathology. Breast tumors are common in women and account for 32% of female cancers; such tumors are rare in men (0.2% of male cancers). Benign tumors include fibrocystic disease, adenofibroma, intraductal papilloma, mammary fat necrosis, and plasma cell mastitis (mammary duct ectasia). Malignant tumors include adenocarcinoma, cystosarcoma, intraductal carcinoma, infiltrating carcinoma, inflammatory carcinoma, medullary or circumcribed carcinoma, colloid carcinoma, lobular carcinoma, sarcoma, and Paget's disease.

Interfering factors

• Patient's inability to lie flat on her stomach or back

• Pain due to continuous compression of the breast during stereotactic biopsy

• Failure to obtain an adequate tissue specimen

• Failure to place the specimen in the proper solution and to send it to the laboratory immediately

PROSTATE GLAND BIOPSY

Prostate gland biopsy is the needle excision of a prostate tissue specimen for histologic examination. Indications include potentially malignant prostatic hypertrophy and prostatic nodules. Most prostate gland biopsies are performed using transrectal ultrasound guidance. Occasionally, a transurethral approach may be used if the transrectal approach is contraindicated.

Purpose

• To confirm prostate cancer

• To determine the cause of prostatic hyperplasia

Patient preparation

• Describe the procedure to the patient, answer his questions, and tell him that the test provides a tissue specimen for microscopic study.

• Tell him who will perform the biopsy and where.

• Make sure the patient or an appropriate family member has signed an informed consent form.

• Check the patient's history for hypersensitivity to the anesthetic or other drugs.

• For a transrectal approach, administer enemas until the return is clear and administer an antibacterial agent to minimize the risk of infection. This approach may be performed on outpatients without an anesthetic.

• Just before the biopsy, check vital signs and administer a sedative.

• Administer a prophylactic antibiotic, as ordered.

• Instruct the patient to remain still during the procedure and to follow instructions.

Procedure and posttest care

Transrectal approach

• Place the patient in the left lateral position.

• A digital rectal examination is performed before an ultrasound probe is inserted. A curved needle guide is attached to the finger palpating the rectum. The biopsy needle is pushed along the guide into the prostate that was localized by ultrasonography.

• As the needle enters the prostate, the patient may experience pain. Biopsies are obtained from the base, midgland, and apex on both sides of the prostate.

• If an abnormality in the rectum is identified, that area is localized by ultrasonography and a specimen is collected from there as well.

• The specimen is immediately placed in a labeled specimen bottle containing 10% formaldehyde solution.

Transurethral approach

• An endoscopic instrument is passed through the urethra, permitting direct viewing of the prostate and passage of a cutting loop.

• The loop is rotated to obtain tissue and then withdrawn.

• The specimen is placed immediately in a labeled specimen bottle containing 10% formaldehyde solution.

Both approaches

• Check vital signs immediately after the procedure, every 2 hours for 4 hours, and then every 4 hours.

• Observe the patient for signs and symptoms of hematoma and infection, such as redness, swelling, and pain. Watch for urine retention, urinary frequency, and hematuria.

Precautions

• Complications may include transient, painless hematuria and bleeding into the prostatic urethra and bladder.

Normal findings

Normally, the prostate gland consists of a thin, fibrous capsule surrounding the stroma, which is made up of elastic and connective tissues and smooth-muscle fibers. The epithelial glands found in these tissues and muscle fibers drain into the chief excreting ducts.

Abnormal findings

Histologic examination can confirm cancer. Further tests — bone scans, bone marrow biopsy, tests for prostate-specific antigen, and serum acid phosphatase and prostatic acid phosphatase determinations — identify the extent of the cancer. Acid phosphatase levels usually rise in metastatic prostatic carcinoma; they tend to be low in carcinoma that's confined to the prostatic capsule. In the latter case, radical surgery and irradiation, although controversial, can provide a high cure rate. If discovery of cancer is delayed, treatment necessitates estrogen therapy because tumor growth depends on testosterone secretion.

Histologic examination can also be used to detect benign prostatic hyperplasia, prostatitis, tuberculosis, lymphomas, and rectal or bladder cancer.

Interfering factors
• Patient's inability to follow instructions or to lie still
• Inadequate bowel preparation
• Failure to obtain an adequate tissue specimen
• Failure to place the specimen in formaldehyde

CERVICAL BIOPSY

Cervical biopsy is the excision by sharp forceps of a tissue specimen from the cervix for histologic examination. Two types of cervical biopsy are performed to evaluate abnormal lesions of the cervix or abnormalities revealed on a Papanicolaou (Pap) test. One is a cervical biopsy that's performed during colposcopy. The other is a cone biopsy often performed during a loop electrosurgical excision procedure. The biopsy site is selected by direct visualization of the cervix with a colposcope, and the biopsy is performed when the cervix is least vascular, usually 1 week after menses.

Purpose
• To evaluate suspicious cervical lesions
• To diagnose cervical cancer

Patient preparation
• Describe the procedure to the patient, and explain that it provides a cervical tissue specimen for microscopic study.
• Tell her who will perform the biopsy and where.
• Advise the outpatient to have someone accompany her home after the biopsy.
• Make sure the patient or a responsible family member has signed an informed consent form.
• Just before the biopsy, ask the patient to void.

Procedure and posttest care
• Place the patient in the lithotomy position, and tell her to relax as the unlubricated speculum is inserted.
• For direct visualization, the colposcope is inserted through the speculum, the biopsy site is located, and the cervix is cleaned with a swab soaked in 3% acetic acid solution. The biopsy forceps are then inserted through the speculum or the colposcope, and tissue is removed from any lesion or from selected sites, starting from the posterior lip to avoid obscuring other sites with blood. Each specimen is immediately put in 10% formaldehyde solution in a labeled bottle. To control bleeding after biopsy, the cervix is swabbed with 5% silver nitrate solution (cautery or sutures may be used instead). If bleeding persists, the examiner may insert a tampon.
• If a cone biopsy is to be performed, a local anesthetic may be injected into the cervix.
• Record the patient's and doctor's names and the biopsy sites on the laboratory slip.
• Instruct the patient to avoid strenuous exercise for 24 hours after the biopsy. Encourage the outpatient to rest briefly before leaving the office.

Tell her to avoid heavy lifting for a few days.

● If a tampon or vaginal packing was inserted after the biopsy, tell the patient to leave it in place for 8 to 24 hours. Inform her that some bleeding may occur, but tell her to report heavy bleeding (heavier than menses). Warn the patient to avoid using tampons, which can irritate the cervix and provoke bleeding.

● Tell the patient to avoid douching and intercourse for 2 weeks, or as directed.

● Inform the patient that a foul-smelling, gray-green vaginal discharge is normal for several days after the biopsy and may persist for 3 weeks.

Precautions

● Send the specimens to the laboratory immediately.

Normal findings

Normal cervical tissue is composed of columnar and squamous epithelial cells, loose connective tissue, and smooth-muscle fibers with no dysplasia or abnormal cell growth.

Abnormal findings

Histologic examination of a cervical tissue specimen is used to identify abnormal cells and to differentiate the tissue as intraepithelial neoplasia or invasive cancer. If the cause of an abnormal Pap test isn't demonstrated by cervical biopsy or if the specimen shows advanced dysplasia or carcinoma in situ, a cone biopsy is performed under general anesthesia to obtain a larger tissue specimen and to allow a more accurate evaluation of dysplasia.

Interfering factors

● Menses

● Patient's inability to assume the lithotomy position

● Failure to obtain representative specimens or to place them in the preservative immediately

SKELETAL SYSTEM

BONE BIOPSY

Bone biopsy is the removal of a piece or a core of bone for histologic examination. It's performed either by using a special drill needle under local anesthesia or by surgical excision under general anesthesia.

Bone biopsy is indicated in patients with bone pain and tenderness after bone scan, computed tomography scan, X-ray, or arteriography reveals a mass or deformity. Excision provides a larger specimen than drill biopsy and permits immediate surgical treatment if quick histologic analysis of the specimen reveals cancer.

Possible complications include bone fracture, damage to surrounding tissue, infection (osteomyelitis) and, possibly, contamination of normal tissue with tumor cells.

Purpose

● To distinguish between benign and malignant bone tumors

Patient preparation

● Describe the procedure to the patient, and answer any questions.

● Explain that this test permits microscopic examination of a bone specimen.

● If the patient is to have a drill biopsy, he needn't restrict food or fluids; if he's to have open biopsy, he must fast overnight before the test.

• Tell him who will perform the biopsy and where.

• Tell the patient that he'll receive a local anesthetic but will still experience discomfort and pressure when the biopsy needle enters the bone.

• Explain that a special drill forces the needle into the bone; if possible, show him a photograph of the bone drill. Stress the importance of his cooperation during the biopsy.

• Make sure the patient or a responsible family member has signed an informed consent form.

• Check the patient's history for hypersensitivity to the local anesthetic.

Procedure and posttest care

Drill biopsy

• The patient is properly positioned, and the biopsy site is shaved and meticulously prepared.

• After the local anesthetic is injected, a small incision (usually about 3 mm) is made and the biopsy needle is pushed with a pointed trocar into the bone; then it's rotated about 180 degrees.

• When the bone core is obtained, the trocar is withdrawn, and the specimen is placed in a properly labeled bottle containing 10% formaldehyde solution. Then pressure is applied to the site with a sterile gauze pad.

• When bleeding stops, apply a topical antiseptic (povidone-iodine ointment) and an adhesive bandage or other sterile covering to close the wound and prevent infection.

Excisional biopsy

• The patient is anesthetized, and the biopsy site is shaved, cleaned with surgical soap, and disinfected with an iodine wash and alcohol.

• An incision is made, and a piece of bone is removed and sent to the histology laboratory immediately for analysis. Further surgery can then be performed, depending on findings.

Both procedures

• Check vital signs and the dressing at the biopsy site. Determine how much drainage is expected and report excessive drainage.

• If the patient experiences pain, administer an analgesic.

• For several days after the biopsy, watch for and report indications of bone infection: fever, headache, pain on movement, and redness or abscess near the biopsy site.

• Advise the patient that he may resume his usual diet.

Precautions

• Bone biopsy should be performed cautiously in patients with coagulopathy.

Normal findings

Normal bone tissue consists of fibers of collagen, osteocytes, and osteoblasts. It may be compact or cancellous. Compact bone has dense, concentric layers of mineral deposits, or lamellae. Cancellous bone has widely spaced lamellae, with osteocytes and red and yellow marrow between them.

Abnormal findings

Histologic examination of a bone specimen can reveal benign or malignant tumors. Benign tumors, generally well circumscribed and nonmetastasizing, include osteoid osteoma, osteoblastoma, osteochondroma, unicameral bone cyst, benign giant-cell tumor, and fibroma. Malignant tumors, which spread irregularly and rapidly, most commonly include both multiple myeloma and osteosarcoma; the most lethal is Ewing's sarcoma. Most malignant tumors spread to the bone through the blood and lymphatic system from the breasts, lungs, prostate, thyroid, or kidneys.

Interfering factors
• Failure to obtain a representative bone specimen
• Failure to use the proper fixative
• Failure to send the specimen to the laboratory immediately

BONE MARROW ASPIRATION AND BIOPSY

The histologic and hematologic examination of bone marrow provides reliable diagnostic information about blood disorders. Marrow may be removed by aspiration or needle biopsy under local anesthesia. In aspiration biopsy, a fluid specimen in which pustulae of marrow are suspended is removed from the bone marrow. In needle biopsy, a core of marrow cells (not fluid) is removed. These methods are often used concurrently to obtain the best possible marrow specimens. Red marrow, which constitutes about 50% of an adult's marrow, actively produces stem cells that ultimately evolve into red blood cells, white blood cells, and platelets. Yellow marrow contains fat cells and connective tissue and is inactive, but it can become active in response to the body's needs.

Bleeding and infection may result from bone marrow biopsy at any site, but the most serious complications occur at the sternum. Such complications are rare but include puncture of the heart and major vessels, causing severe hemorrhage, and puncture of the mediastinum, causing mediastinitis or pneumomediastinum.

Purpose
• To diagnose thrombocytopenia, leukemias, and granulomas as well as aplastic, hypoplastic, and pernicious anemias
• To diagnose primary and metastatic tumors
• To determine the cause of infection
• To aid staging of disease, such as Hodgkin's disease
• To evaluate the effectiveness of chemotherapy and monitor myelosuppression

Patient preparation
• Explain to the patient that the test permits microscopic examination of a bone marrow specimen.
• Describe the procedure to the patient, and answer any questions.
• Inform the patient that he needn't restrict food or fluids before the test.
• Tell him who will perform the biopsy and where.
• Inform him that more than one bone marrow specimen may be required and that a blood sample will be collected before biopsy for laboratory testing.
• Make sure the patient or a responsible family member has signed an informed consent form.
• Check the patient's history for hypersensitivity to the local anesthetic.
• Tell the patient which bone — the sternum, anterior or posterior iliac crest, vertebral spinous process, rib, or tibia — will be the biopsy site.
• Inform him that he'll receive a local anesthetic but will feel pressure on insertion of the biopsy needle and a brief, pulling pain on removal of the marrow. Administer a mild sedative 1 hour before the test.

Procedure and posttest care
• After positioning the patient, instruct him to remain as still as possible.

• Offer emotional support during the biopsy by talking quietly to the patient, describing what's being done and answering any questions.

Aspiration biopsy

• After the skin over the biopsy site is prepared and the area is draped, the local anesthetic is injected. With a twisting motion, the marrow aspiration needle is inserted through the skin, the subcutaneous tissue, and the cortex of the bone.

• The stylet is removed from the needle, and a 10- to 20-ml syringe is attached. The examiner aspirates 0.2 to 0.5 ml of marrow and then withdraws the needle.

• Apply pressure to the site for 5 minutes, while the marrow slides are being prepared. (If the patient has thrombocytopenia, apply pressure to the site for 10 to 15 minutes.)

• The biopsy site is cleaned again, and a sterile adhesive bandage is applied.

• If an adequate marrow specimen is not obtained on the first attempt, the needle may be repositioned within the marrow cavity or removed and reinserted in another site within the anesthetized area. If the second attempt fails, a needle biopsy may be needed.

Needle biopsy

• After preparing the biopsy site and draping the area, the examiner marks the skin at the site with an indelible pencil or marking pen.

• A local anesthetic is then injected intradermally, subcutaneously, and at the surface of the bone.

• The biopsy needle is inserted into the periosteum, and the needle guard is set, as indicated. The needle is advanced with a steady boring motion until the outer needle passes through the cortex of the bone.

• The inner needle with trephine tip is inserted into the outer needle. By alternately rotating the inner needle clock-wise and counterclockwise, the examiner directs the needle into the marrow cavity and then removes a tissue plug.

• The needle assembly is withdrawn, and the marrow is expelled into a labeled bottle containing Zenker's acetic acid solution.

• After the biopsy site is cleaned, a sterile adhesive bandage or a pressure dressing is applied.

Both procedures

• Check the biopsy site for bleeding and inflammation.

• Observe the patient for signs of hemorrhage and infection, such as rapid pulse rate, low blood pressure, and fever.

Precautions

• Bone marrow biopsy is contraindicated in patients with severe bleeding disorders.

• Send the tissue specimen or slides to the laboratory immediately.

Normal findings

Yellow marrow contains fat cells and connective tissue; red marrow contains hematopoietic cells, fat cells, and connective tissue. An adult has a large hematopoietic capacity. An infant's marrow is mainly red, reflecting a small hematopoietic capacity.

In addition, special stains that are used to detect hematologic disorders produce these normal findings: The iron stain, which is used to measure hemosiderin (storage iron), has a +2 level; the Sudan black B (SBB) fat stain, which shows granulocytes, is negative; and the periodic acid–Schiff (PAS) stain, which is used to detect glycogen reactions, is negative.

Abnormal findings

Histologic examination of a bone marrow specimen can be used to detect myelofibrosis, granulomas, lymphoma,

BONE MARROW: NORMAL VALUES AND IMPLICATIONS OF ABNORMAL FINDINGS

CELL TYPES	NORMAL MEAN VALUES			CLINICAL IMPLICATIONS
	Adults	**Children**	**Infants**	
Normoblasts, total	25.6%	23.1%	8.0%	*Elevated values:* polycythemia vera
Pronormoblasts	0.2% to 1.3%	0.5%	0.1%	*Depressed values:* vitamin B_{12} or folic acid deficiency; hypoplastic or aplastic anemia
Basophilic	0.5% to 2.4%	1.7%	0.34%	
Polychromatic	17.9% to 29.2%	18.2%	6.9%	
Orthochromatic	0.4% to 4.6%	2.7%	0.54%	
Neutrophils, total	56.5%	57.1%	32.4%	*Elevated values:* acute myeloblastic or chronic myeloid leukemia
Myeloblasts	0.2% to 1.5%	1.2%	0.62%	*Depressed values:* lymphoblastic, lymphatic, or monocytic leukemia; aplastic anemia
Promyelocytes	2.1% to 4.1%	1.4%	0.76%	
Myelocytes	8.2% to 15.7%	18.3%	2.5%	
Metamyelocytes	9.6% to 24.6%	23.3%	11.3%	
Bands	9.5% to 15.3%	0	14.1%	
Segmented	6.0% to 12.0%	12.9%	3.6%	
Eosinophils	3.1%	3.6%	2.6%	*Elevated values:* bone marrow carcinoma, lymphadenoma, myeloid leukemia, eosinophilic leukemia, pernicious anemia (in relapse)

BONE MARROW: NORMAL VALUES AND IMPLICATIONS OF ABNORMAL FINDINGS *(continued)*

CELL TYPES	NORMAL MEAN VALUES			CLINICAL IMPLICATIONS
	Adults	Children	Infants	
Plasma cells	1.3%	0.4%	0.02%	*Elevated values:* myeloma, collagen disease, infection, antigen sensitivity, cancer
Basophils	0.01%	0.06%	0.07%	*Elevated values:* no relation between basophil count and symptoms *Depressed values:* no relation between basophil count and symptoms
Lymphocytes	16.2%	16.0%	49.0%	*Elevated values:* B- and T-cell chronic lymphocytic leukemia, other lymphatic leukemias, lymphoma, mononucleosis, aplastic anemia, macroglobulinemia
Megakaryo-cytes	0.1%	0.1%	0.05%	*Elevated values:* old age, chronic myeloid leukemia, polycythemia vera, megakaryocytic myelosis, infection, autoimmune thrombocytopenic purpura, thrombocytopenia *Depressed values:* pernicious anemia
Myeloid-erythroid ratio	2.3	2.9	4.4	*Elevated values:* myeloid leukemia, infection, leukemoid reactions, depressed hematopoiesis *Depressed values:* agranulocytosis, hematopoiesis after hemorrhage or hemolysis, iron deficiency anemia, polycythemia vera

and cancer. Hematologic analysis, including the differential count and myeloid-erythroid ratio, can implicate a wide range of disorders. (See *Bone marrow: Normal values and implications of abnormal findings*.)

In an iron stain, decreased hemosiderin levels may indicate a true iron deficiency. Increased levels may accompany other types of anemias and blood disorders. A positive SBB stain can differentiate acute granulocytic leukemia from acute lymphocytic leukemia (SBB-negative) or may indicate granulation in myeloblasts. A positive PAS stain may indicate acute or chronic lymphocytic leukemia, amyloidosis, thalassemia, lymphomas, infectious mononucleosis, iron deficiency anemia, or sideroblastic anemia.

Interfering factors
- Failure to obtain a representative specimen
- Failure to use a fixative for histologic analysis
- Failure to send the specimen to the laboratory immediately

SYNOVIAL MEMBRANE BIOPSY

Biopsy of the synovial membrane is needle excision of a tissue specimen for histologic examination of the thin epithelium lining the diarthrodial joint capsules. In a large joint, such as the knee, preliminary arthroscopy can aid selection of the biopsy site. Synovial membrane biopsy is performed when analysis of synovial fluid — a viscous, lubricating fluid contained within the synovial membrane — proves nondiagnostic or when the fluid is absent.

Purpose
- To diagnose gout, pseudogout, bacterial infections and lesions, and granulomatous infections
- To aid diagnosis of systemic lupus erythematosus (SLE), rheumatoid arthritis, or Reiter's disease and to monitor joint pathology

Patient preparation
- Explain to the patient that this test provides a tissue specimen from the membrane that lines the affected joint.
- Describe the procedure to the patient, and ask if he has any questions.
- Advise him that he needn't restrict food or fluids.
- Tell him who will perform the procedure and where.
- Inform the patient that complications include infection and bleeding into the joint, but they are rare.
- Make sure the patient or an appropriate family member has signed an informed consent form.
- Check the patient's history for hypersensitivity to the local anesthetic.
- Inform the patient which site — knee (most common), elbow, wrist, ankle, or shoulder — has been chosen for this biopsy (usually, the most symptomatic joint is selected).
- Administer a sedative to help him relax.

Procedure and posttest care
- Place the patient in the proper position, clean the biopsy site, and drape the area.
- The local anesthetic is injected into the joint space; then, the trocar is forcefully thrust into the joint space.
- The biopsy needle is inserted through the trocar. The hooked notch side of the biopsy needle is positioned against the synovium, and suction is applied with a 50-ml luer-lock syringe.
- While the trocar is held stationary, the biopsy needle is twisted to cut off a tissue segment.
- The biopsy needle is withdrawn, and the specimen is placed in a properly labeled sterile container or a specimen bottle containing absolute ethyl alcohol, as indicated.
- By changing the angle of the biopsy needle, several specimens can be obtained without reinserting the trocar.

• The trocar is then removed, the biopsy site is cleaned, and a pressure bandage is applied.

• Watch for signs of bleeding into the joint (swelling and tenderness) every hour for 4 hours and then every 4 hours for 12 hours.

• Administer medication if the patient experiences pain.

• Tell the patient to rest the joint for 1 day before resuming normal activity.

Precautions

• Send a specimen in a container with absolute ethyl alcohol to the histology laboratory immediately or send one in a sterile container to the microbiology laboratory.

Normal findings

The synovial membrane contains cells that are identical to those found in other connective tissue. The membrane surface is relatively smooth, except for villi, folds, and fat pads that project into the joint cavity. The membrane tissue produces synovial fluid and contains a capillary network, lymphatic vessels, and a few nerve fibers. A pathologic condition of the synovial membrane also affects the cellular composition of the synovial fluid.

Abnormal findings

Histologic examination of synovial tissue can diagnose coccidioidomycosis, gout, pseudogout, hemochromatosis, tuberculosis, sarcoidosis, amyloidosis, pigmented villonodular synovitis, synovial tumors, and synovial cancer (rare). Such examination can also aid diagnosis of rheumatoid arthritis, SLE, and Reiter's disease.

Interfering factors

• Failure to obtain several biopsy specimens

• Failure to obtain the specimens away from the infiltration site of the anesthetic

• Failure to store the specimens in the appropriate solution or to send them to the laboratory immediately

• Patient's inability to remain still

• Hypocellular marrow

OTHER ORGAN-SPECIFIC BIOPSIES

THYROID BIOPSY

Thyroid biopsy is the excision of a thyroid tissue specimen for histologic examination. This procedure is indicated in patients with thyroid enlargement or nodules, breathing and swallowing difficulties, vocal cord paralysis, weight loss, hemoptysis, and a sensation of fullness in the neck. It's commonly performed when noninvasive tests, such as thyroid ultrasonography and scans, are abnormal or inconclusive. Coagulation studies should always precede thyroid biopsy.

Thyroid tissue may be obtained with a hollow needle under local anesthesia or during open (surgical) biopsy under general anesthesia. Open biopsy provides more information than needle biopsy; it also permits direct examination and immediate excision of suspicious tissue.

Purpose

• To differentiate between benign and malignant thyroid disease

• To help diagnose Hashimoto's thyroiditis, subacute granulomatous thyroiditis, hyperthyroidism, and nontoxic nodular goiter

Patient preparation

- Describe the procedure to the patient, and answer any questions.
- Explain that this test permits microscopic examination of a thyroid tissue specimen.
- Inform the patient that he needn't restrict food or fluids (unless he receives a general anesthetic).
- Tell him who will perform the biopsy and where.
- Make sure the patient or an appropriate family member has signed an informed consent form.
- Check the patient's history for hypersensitivity to anesthetics or analgesics.
- Check the results of the patient's coagulation studies and make sure they're on his chart.
- Advise him that he may have a sore throat the day after the test.
- Administer a sedative to the patient 15 minutes before biopsy.

Procedure and posttest care

- For needle biopsy, place the patient in the supine position, with a pillow under his shoulder blades. (This position pushes the trachea and thyroid forward and allows the neck veins to fall backward.)
- Prepare the skin over the biopsy site.
- As the examiner prepares to inject the local anesthetic, warn the patient not to swallow.
- After the anesthetic is injected, the carotid artery is palpated and the biopsy needle is inserted parallel to the thyroid cartilage to prevent damage to the deep structures and the larynx.
- When the specimen is obtained, the needle is removed and the specimen is immediately placed in formaldehyde.
- Apply pressure to the biopsy site to stop bleeding. If bleeding continues for more than a few minutes, press on the site for up to an additional 15 minutes. Apply an adhesive bandage. (Bleeding

may persist in a patient with prolonged prothrombin time [PT] or prolonged activated partial thromboplastin time [APTT] or in a patient with a large, vascular thyroid with distended veins.)

- To make the patient more comfortable, place him in the semi-Fowler position; tell him to avoid straining the biopsy site by putting both hands behind his neck when he sits up.
- Watch for tenderness or redness, and report signs of bleeding at the biopsy site. Check the back of the neck and the patient's pillow for bleeding every hour for 8 hours. Observe for difficult breathing due to edema or hematoma, with resultant tracheal collapse.
- Keep the biopsy site clean and dry.

Precautions

- Thyroid biopsy should be used cautiously in patients with coagulation defects, as indicated by prolonged PT or APTT.
- The specimen must be placed immediately in formaldehyde solution because cell breakdown in the tissue specimen begins immediately after excision.

Normal findings

Histologic examination of normal tissue shows fibrous networks dividing the gland into pseudolobules that are made up of follicles and capillaries. Cuboidal epithelium lines the follicle walls and contains the protein thyroglobulin, which stores thyroxine and triiodothyronine.

Abnormal findings

Malignant tumors appear as well-encapsulated, solitary nodules of uniform but abnormal structure. Papillary carcinoma is the most common thyroid cancer. Follicular carcinoma, a less common form, strongly resembles normal cells.

Benign tumors, such as nontoxic nodular goiter, demonstrate hypertrophy, hyperplasia, and hypervascularity. Distinct histologic patterns characterize subacute granulomatous thyroiditis, Hashimoto's thyroiditis, and hyperthyroidism.

Because thyroid tumors are frequently multicentric and small, a negative histologic report doesn't rule out cancer.

Interfering factors
- Failure to obtain a representative tissue specimen
- Failure to immediately place the specimen in formaldehyde solution

LYMPH NODE BIOPSY

Lymph node biopsy is the surgical excision of an active lymph node or the needle aspiration of a nodal specimen for histologic examination. Both techniques usually use a local anesthetic and sample the superficial nodes in the cervical, supraclavicular, axillary, or inguinal region. Excision is preferred because it yields a larger specimen.

Although lymph nodes swell during infection, biopsy is indicated when nodal enlargement is prolonged and accompanied by backache, leg edema, breathing and swallowing difficulties and, later, weight loss, weakness, severe itching, fever, night sweats, cough, hemoptysis, and hoarseness. Generalized or localized lymph node enlargement is typical of such diseases as chronic lymphatic leukemia, Hodgkin's disease, infectious mononucleosis, and rheumatoid arthritis.

Complete blood count, liver function studies, liver and spleen scans, and X-rays should precede this test.

Purpose
- To determine the cause of lymph node enlargement
- To distinguish between benign and malignant lymph node processes
- To stage certain cancers or metastatic carcinoma

Patient preparation
- Explain to the patient that this test allows microscopic study of lymph node tissue.
- Describe the procedure to the patient, and answer any questions.
- For excisional biopsy, instruct the patient to restrict food from midnight and to drink only clear liquids on the morning of the test (if general anesthesia is needed for deeper nodes, he must also restrict fluids).
- For needle biopsy, inform him that he needn't restrict food or fluids. Tell him who will perform the biopsy and where.
- Make sure the patient or a responsible family member has signed an informed consent form.
- Check the patient's history for hypersensitivity to the anesthetic.
- If the patient will receive a local anesthetic, explain that he may experience discomfort during the injection.
- Just before the biopsy, record baseline vital signs.

Procedure and posttest care
Excisional biopsy
- After the skin over the biopsy site is prepared and draped, the anesthetic is administered.
- The examiner makes an incision, removes an entire node, and places it in a properly labeled bottle containing normal saline solution.
- The wound is sutured and dressed.
Needle biopsy
- After preparing the biopsy site and administering a local anesthetic, the

examiner grasps the node between his thumb and forefinger, inserts the needle directly into the node, and obtains a small core specimen.

• The needle is removed, and the specimen is placed in a properly labeled bottle containing normal saline solution.

• Pressure is exerted at the biopsy site to control bleeding, and an adhesive bandage is applied.

Both procedures

• Check vital signs, and watch for bleeding, tenderness, and redness.

• Inform the patient that he may resume his usual diet.

Precautions

• Storing the tissue specimen in normal saline solution instead of 10% formaldehyde solution allows part of the specimen to be used for cytologic impression smears, which are studied along with the biopsy specimen.

Normal findings

The normal lymph node is encapsulated by collagenous connective tissue and divided into smaller lobes by tissue strands called trabeculae. It has an outer cortex, composed of lymphoid cells and nodules or follicles containing lymphocytes, and an inner medulla, composed of reticular phagocytic cells that collect and drain fluid.

Abnormal findings

Histologic examination of the tissue specimen distinguishes between malignant and nonmalignant causes of lymph node enlargement. Lymphatic cancer accounts for up to 5% of all cancers and is slightly more prevalent in males than in females. Hodgkin's disease, a lymphoma affecting the entire lymph system, is the leading cancer affecting adolescents and young

adults. Lymph node cancer may also result from metastasizing carcinoma.

When histologic results aren't clear or nodular material isn't involved, mediastinoscopy or laparotomy can provide another nodal specimen. Occasionally, lymphangiography can furnish additional diagnostic information.

Interfering factors

• Failure to obtain a representative tissue specimen

• Improper specimen storage

• Inability to differentiate nodal pathology

SENTINEL LYMPH NODE BIOPSY

Sentinel lymph node biopsy is considered experimental for breast cancer patients but has become part of the standard of care for melanoma patients. A sentinel lymph node is defined as the first node in the lymphatic basin into which a primary tumor site drains. Hypothetically, the histology of the sentinel node will reflect the histology of the rest of the nodes in that basin. Hence, if that sentinel node is identified and found to be negative for tumor invasion, it's hypothesized that the rest of the nodes are also negative for tumor. In breast cancer, if the hypothesis is proven true, axillary lymph node dissections and their resulting morbidity could be avoided.

Sentinel lymph node biopsy is performed using one of two techniques; in most cases, the techniques are combined to increase the likelihood of identifying the sentinel node. One technique is lymphoscintigraphy, performed in nuclear medicine using injected technetium-99 (^{99}Tc), a radioactive isotope. The second technique uses the injection of blue dye.

Purpose
• To identify the sentinel lymph node and evaluate it for the presence or absence of tumor cells indicating nodal metastasis

Patient preparation
• Explain to the patient that this test evaluates a particular lymph node to determine if cancer has spread into the lymph system. Tell her that it's usually done in conjunction with lumpectomy or mastectomy.
• Tell the patient that a radioactive substance will be injected under the skin. Assure her that she won't be radioactive and that the amount of radiation exposure will be less than that of a routine chest X-ray.

Procedure and posttest care
• The patient is positioned on the table in the nuclear medicine suite.
• A standard dose of ^{99}Tc is injected circumferentially around the margins of a palpable mass, using a 25G needle. For a nonpalpable mass, injections are guided with ultrasound or mammographic techniques. If the tumor has already been excised, the injections are made around the tumor bed.
• Images of the axilla are taken with a gamma camera. The location of the sentinel node is marked on the skin in indelible ink and noted on a data sheet.
• The patient is then transported to the operating room and placed under appropriate anesthesia.
• Blue dye is injected circumferentially in the tissue immediately surrounding the biopsy site, using a 25G needle.
• Within 10 to 15 minutes of the dye injection, a small incision is made in

the axilla over the suspected location of the sentinel lymph node. The surgeon follows the trail of stained lymphatics to the sentinel lymph node. The node is identified by the blue dye and by using an intraoperative gamma probe that measures radioactivity; the node having the highest radioactivity is deemed the sentinel node and removed.
• The axilla is then checked for remaining radioactivity; if none is noted, the surgical procedure concludes.
• Because of the radioactivity, the sentinel lymph node is maintained in formaldehyde for 24 to 48 hours before it can be processed.
• Other than routine postoperative care, no special posttest care is required for this procedure.

Precautions
• Because ^{99}Tc is a radioactive substance, all radiation precautions must be implemented. Staff members need to be monitored for radiation exposure. Radiation levels need to be determined in both the nuclear medicine suite and the operating room postsurgically.
• Rare cases of allergy to the ^{99}Tc or blue dye have been noted; patients should be observed for signs of allergic reaction (skin changes and respiratory difficulties).

Normal findings
Normal findings are the same as for a normal lymph node biopsy.

Abnormal findings
Sentinel lymph node biopsy is performed only in breast cancer and melanoma, so abnormal findings mean the identification of melanoma or breast cancer cells. Their presence indicates lymph node metastasis and guides the prognosis and treatment.

Interfering factors
- Allergy to radioactive substance
- Inability to raise arm to allow access to axilla
- Inability to obtain adequate specimen
- Improper specimen storage

SKIN BIOPSY

Skin biopsy is the removal of a small piece of tissue under local anesthesia from a lesion suspected of being malignant or from other dermatoses. One of three techniques may be used: shave biopsy, punch biopsy, or excisional biopsy. Shave biopsy uses a scalpel to slice a superficial specimen from the site. Punch biopsy removes an oval core from the center of a lesion down to the dermis or subcutaneous tissue. Excisional biopsy removes the entire lesion with a small border of normal skin.

Lesions suspected of being malignant usually have changed color, size, or appearance or fail to heal properly after injury. Fully developed lesions should be selected for biopsy whenever possible because they provide more diagnostic information than lesions that are resolving or in early developing stages.

Purpose
- To provide differential diagnosis among basal cell carcinoma, squamous cell carcinoma, malignant melanoma, and benign growths
- To diagnose chronic bacterial or fungal skin infections

Patient preparation
- Explain to the patient that the biopsy provides a specimen for microscopic study.
- Describe the procedure to the patient, and answer any questions.
- Inform him that he needn't restrict food or fluids.
- Tell him who will perform the procedure and where.
- Have the patient or an appropriate family member sign an informed consent form.
- Check the patient's history for hypersensitivity to the local anesthetic.

Procedure and posttest care
- Position the patient comfortably, and clean the biopsy site before the local anesthetic is administered.

Shave biopsy
- The protruding growth is cut off at the skin line with a #15 scalpel and the tissue is placed immediately in a properly labeled specimen bottle containing 10% formaldehyde solution.
- Apply pressure to the area to stop the bleeding.

Punch biopsy
- The skin surrounding the lesion is pulled taut, and the punch is firmly introduced into the lesion and rotated to obtain a tissue specimen. The plug is lifted with forceps or a needle and severed as deeply into the fat layer as possible.
- The specimen is placed in a properly labeled specimen bottle containing 10% formaldehyde solution or in a sterile container, if indicated.
- Closing the wound depends on the size of the punch: A 3-mm punch requires only an adhesive bandage, a 4-mm punch requires one suture, and a 6-mm punch requires two sutures.

Excisional biopsy
- A #15 scalpel is used to excise the entire lesion; the elliptical incision is made as wide and as deep as necessary and includes a margin of apparently normal skin.

• The tissue specimen is removed and placed immediately in a properly labeled specimen bottle containing 10% formaldehyde solution.
• Apply pressure to the site to stop the bleeding.
• The wound is closed using 4-0 suture. If the incision is large, skin graft may be required.
All procedures
• Check the biopsy site for bleeding.
• If the patient experiences pain, administer an analgesic.
• Advise the patient with sutures to keep the area as clean and dry as possible. Facial sutures are removed in 3 to 5 days; trunk sutures, in 7 to 14 days. Tell the patient with adhesive strips to leave them in place for 14 to 21 days.

Precautions
• Send the specimen to the laboratory immediately.

Normal findings
Normal skin consists of squamous epithelium (epidermis) and fibrous connective tissue (dermis).

Abnormal findings
Histologic examination of the tissue specimen may reveal a benign or malignant lesion. Benign growths include cysts, seborrheic keratoses, warts, pigmented nevi (moles), keloids, dermatofibromas, and multiple neurofibromas.

Malignant tumors include basal cell carcinoma, squamous cell carcinoma, and malignant melanoma. Basal cell carcinoma occurs on hair-bearing skin; the most common location is the face, including the nose and its folds. Squamous cell carcinoma most often appears on the lips, mouth, and genitalia. Malignant melanoma, the deadliest skin cancer, can spread through the body by way of the lymphatic system and blood.

Cultures can be used to detect chronic bacterial and fungal infections in which flora are relatively sparse.

Interfering factors
• Improper selection of the biopsy site
• Failure to use the appropriate fixative or a sterile container
• Failure to send the specimen to the laboratory immediately

PERCUTANEOUS RENAL BIOPSY

Percutaneous renal biopsy is the needle excision of a core of kidney tissue for histologic examination. This biopsy may help assess histologic changes caused by acute or chronic glomerulonephritis, pyelonephritis, renal vein thrombosis, amyloid infiltration, and systemic lupus erythematosus. In the case of a mass, results can differentiate a primary renal cancer from a metastatic lesion.

Complications of percutaneous biopsy include bleeding, hematoma, arteriovenous fistula, and infection. This procedure is safer than open biopsy, which is the preferred method for sampling a solid lesion, but noninvasive procedures, especially renal ultrasonography and computed tomography, have replaced percutaneous renal biopsy in many hospitals. (See *Urinary tract brush biopsy*, page 486.)

Purpose
• To obtain information about glomerular and tubular function or to evaluate a solid renal mass
• To aid diagnosis of renal parenchymal disease

Urinary tract brush biopsy

Retrograde brush biopsy of the urinary tract may be used to obtain a renal tissue specimen when X-rays show a lesion in the renal pelvis or calyx. It can also be used to obtain specimens from other areas of the urinary tract. Retrograde brush biopsy is contraindicated in patients with acute urinary tract infection or an obstruction at or below the biopsy site.

Patient preparation
To prepare the patient for brush biopsy, describe the procedure and tell him that he may experience some discomfort. Inform him who will perform the biopsy and when. Reassure the patient that the procedure will take only 30 to 60 minutes.

Make sure the patient or a responsible family member has signed an informed consent form. Because this procedure requires use of a contrast medium and a general, local, or spinal anesthetic, check the patient's history for hypersensitivity to anesthetics, contrast media, or iodine-containing foods such as shellfish. Just before the biopsy procedure, administer a sedative to the patient.

Obtaining the biopsy
After the patient has received a sedative and an anesthetic, place him in the lithotomy position. Using a cystoscope, a guide wire is passed up the ureter and a urethral catheter is passed over the guide wire. Contrast medium is instilled through the catheter, which is positioned next to the lesion under fluoroscopic guidance. The contrast medium is washed out with normal saline solution to prevent cell distortions from the dye. A nylon or steel brush is passed up the catheter and the lesion is brushed. This procedure is repeated at least six times, using a new brush each time.

As each brush is removed from the catheter, a smear is made for Papanicolaou staining and the brush tip is cut off and placed in formaldehyde for 1 hour. The biopsy material is then removed from the brush tip for histologic examination. When the last brush is withdrawn, the catheter is irrigated with normal saline solution to remove additional cells. These cells are also sent for histologic examination.

Results differentiate between malignant and benign lesions, which may appear the same on X-rays.

Posttest care
Because brush biopsy may cause complications, such as perforation, hemorrhage, sepsis, and contrast medium extravasation, carefully monitor the patient's vital signs. Be sure to record the time, color, and amount of voiding, being alert for hematuria and abdominal or flank pain. Report any abnormal findings immediately, and administer analgesics and antibiotics.

• To monitor the progression of renal disease and assess the effectiveness of therapy
• To determine the histology of a solid mass

Patient preparation
• Explain to the patient that this test is used to diagnose kidney disorders.
• Describe the procedure to the patient, and answer any questions.
• Instruct the patient to restrict food and fluids for 8 hours before the test.

• Tell him who will perform the biopsy and where.

• Ensure that blood samples and urine specimens are collected and tested before the biopsy and that results of other tests to determine the biopsy site, such as excretory urography, ultrasonography, and an erect film of the abdomen, are available.

• Check the patient's history for hemorrhagic tendencies and hypersensitivity to the local anesthetic.

• Administer a mild sedative 30 minutes to 1 hour before the biopsy to help the patient relax.

• Inform the patient that he'll receive a local anesthetic but may experience a pinching pain when the needle is inserted through the back into the kidney.

• Check vital signs, and tell the patient to void just before the test.

Procedure and posttest care

• Place the patient in a prone position on a firm surface with a sandbag beneath his abdomen.

• Tell him to take a deep breath while his kidney is being palpated.

• A 7″ 20G needle is used to inject the local anesthetic into the skin at the biopsy site. Instruct the patient to hold his breath and remain still as the needle is inserted through the back muscles, the deep lumbar fascia, the perinephric fat, and the kidney capsule. After the needle is inserted, tell the patient to take several deep breaths. If the needle swings smoothly during deep breathing, it has penetrated the kidney capsule. After the penetration depth is marked on the needle shaft, instruct the patient to hold his breath and remain as still as possible while the needle is withdrawn.

• After a small incision is made in the anesthetized skin, instruct the patient to hold his breath and remain still while the Vim-Silverman needle or a

Tru-cut needle with stylet is inserted to the measured depth. An 18G spring-loaded biopsy gun may also be used.

• Tell the patient to breathe deeply. Then tell him to remain still while the tissue specimen is obtained.

• The tissue is examined immediately under a hand lens to ensure that the specimen contains tissue from both cortex and medulla. Then it's placed on a saline-soaked gauze pad and placed in a properly labeled container.

• If an adequate tissue specimen hasn't been obtained, the procedure is repeated immediately.

• After an adequate specimen is secured, apply pressure to the biopsy site for 3 to 5 minutes to stop superficial bleeding. Then, apply a pressure dressing.

• Instruct the patient to lie flat on his back without moving for at least 12 hours to prevent bleeding. Check vital signs every 15 minutes for 4 hours, then every 30 minutes for 4 hours, then every hour for 4 hours and, finally, every 4 hours. Report any changes.

• Examine all urine for blood; small amounts may be present after the biopsy but should disappear within 8 hours. Hematocrit may be monitored after the procedure to screen for internal bleeding.

• Encourage fluid ingestion to minimize colic and obstruction from blood clotting within the renal pelvis.

• Inform the patient that he may resume his normal diet.

Precautions

• Percutaneous renal biopsy is contraindicated in a patient with a severe bleeding disorder, markedly reduced plasma or blood volume, severe hypertension, hydronephrosis, perinephric abscess, advanced renal failure with uremia, or only one kidney.

- Instruct the patient to hold his breath and remain still whenever the needle or prongs are advanced into or retracted from the kidney.
- Send the specimen to the laboratory immediately.

Normal findings

Normally, a section of kidney tissue shows Bowman's capsule — the area between two layers of flat epithelial cells — the glomerular tuft, and the capillary lumen. The tubule sections differ, depending on the area of tubule involved. The proximal tubule is one layer of epithelial cells with microvilli that form a brush border. The descending loop of Henle has flat squamous epithelial cells. The ascending, distal convoluted, and collecting tubules are lined with squamous epithelial cells.

Abnormal findings

Histologic examination of renal tissue can reveal cancer or renal disease. Malignant tumors include Wilms' tumor, which is usually present in early childhood, and renal cell carcinoma, which is most prevalent in people over age 40. Diseases indicated by characteristic histologic changes include disseminated lupus erythematosus, amyloid infiltration, acute or chronic glomerulonephritis, renal vein thrombosis, and pyelonephritis.

Interfering factors

- Failure to obtain an adequate tissue specimen
- Failure to store the specimen properly
- Failure to send the specimen to the laboratory immediately

CHAPTER 10

Endoscopy

RESPIRATORY SYSTEM 490

490 Direct laryngoscopy
491 Bronchoscopy

494 Mediastinoscopy
495 Thoracoscopy

GASTROINTESTINAL SYSTEM 496

496 Esophagogastroduodenoscopy
499 Colonoscopy

501 Proctosigmoidoscopy
504 Endoscopic ultrasound

REPRODUCTIVE SYSTEM 505

505 Colposcopy

506 Gynecologic laparoscopy

SKELETAL SYSTEM 508

508 Arthroscopy

RESPIRATORY SYSTEM

DIRECT LARYNGOSCOPY

This test allows visualization of the larynx by the use of a fiber-optic endoscope or laryngoscope passed through the mouth and pharynx to the larynx. It's indicated for children, patients with strong gag reflexes due to anatomic abnormalities, and those who have had no response to short-term therapy for symptoms of pharyngeal or laryngeal disease, such as stridor and hemoptysis. Secretions or tissue may be removed during this procedure for further study. The test is usually contraindicated in patients with epiglottitis but may be performed on them in an operating room with resuscitative equipment available.

Purpose
• To detect lesions or strictures and to remove benign lesions or foreign bodies from the larynx
• To aid diagnosis of laryngeal cancer
• To examine the larynx when indirect laryngoscopy is inadequate

Patient preparation
• Explain to the patient that this test is used to detect laryngeal abnormalities.
• Instruct the patient to fast for 6 to 8 hours before the test.
• Tell him who will perform the procedure and where it will be performed.
• Inform the patient that he'll receive a sedative to help him relax, medication to reduce secretions and, during the procedure, a general or local anesthet-

ic. Reassure him that this procedure won't obstruct his airway.
• Make sure the patient or a responsible family member has signed an informed consent form.
• Check the patient's history for hypersensitivity to the anesthetic.
• Obtain baseline vital signs.
• Administer the sedative and other medication (usually 30 minutes to 1 hour before the test).
• Before the patient receives the sedative, instruct him to remove dentures, contact lenses, and jewelry and ask him to void.

Equipment
Laryngoscope, sedative, atropine, local anesthetic (spray or jelly) or general anesthetic, sterile container for microbiology specimen, sterile gloves, Coplin jar with 95% ethyl alcohol for cytology smears, container with 10% formaldehyde solution for histology specimen, forceps for biopsy, emesis basin, suction and resuscitation equipment

Procedure and posttest care
• Place the patient in the supine position.
• Encourage him to breathe through his nose and to relax with his arms at his sides.
• A general anesthetic is administered, or the patient's mouth and throat are sprayed with a local anesthetic.
• A laryngoscope is introduced through the patient's mouth, the larynx is examined for abnormalities, and a specimen or secretions may be removed for further study; minor surgery, such as removal of polyps or nodules, may be performed at this time.
• Place the specimens in their respective containers.
• Place the conscious patient in semi-Fowler's position; place the uncon-

scious patient on his side with his head slightly elevated to prevent aspiration.

• Check vital signs every 15 minutes until the patient is stable and then every 30 minutes for 4 hours, every hour for the next 4 hours, and then every 4 hours for 24 hours. Immediately report to the doctor any adverse reaction to the anesthetic or sedative.

• Apply an ice collar to minimize laryngeal edema.

• Provide an emesis basin, and instruct the patient to spit out saliva rather than swallow it. Observe sputum for blood, and report excessive bleeding immediately.

• Instruct the patient to refrain from clearing his throat and coughing to prevent hemorrhaging at the biopsy site.

• Advise the patient to avoid smoking until vital signs are stable and there is no evidence of complications.

• Immediately report subcutaneous crepitus around the patient's face and neck, which may indicate tracheal perforation.

• Listen to the patient's neck with a stethoscope for signs of stridor and airway obstruction.

CLINICAL ALERT Observe the patient with epiglottitis for signs of airway obstruction, and immediately report signs of respiratory difficulty. Keep emergency resuscitation equipment available; keep a tracheotomy tray nearby for 24 hours.

• Restrict food and fluids to avoid aspiration until the gag reflex returns (usually within 2 hours). Then the patient may resume his usual diet, beginning with sips of water.

• Reassure the patient that voice loss, hoarseness, and sore throat are temporary. Provide throat lozenges or a soothing liquid gargle when his gag reflex returns.

Precautions
• Send the specimens to the laboratory immediately.

Normal findings
A normal larynx shows no evidence of inflammation, lesions, strictures, or foreign bodies.

Abnormal findings
Indirect laryngoscopy may reveal inflammation, lesions, or polyps. The combined results of direct laryngoscopy, biopsy, and radiography may indicate laryngeal carcinoma. Direct laryngoscopy also may show benign lesions, strictures, congenital abnormalities, and foreign bodies.

Interfering factors
• Failure to place the specimens in appropriate containers or to send them to the laboratory immediately
• Patient's inability to cooperate with the procedure

BRONCHOSCOPY

This test allows direct visualization of the larynx, trachea, and bronchi through a flexible fiber-optic bronchoscope or a rigid metal bronchoscope. Although a flexible fiber-optic bronchoscope allows a wider view and is used more often, the rigid metal bronchoscope is required to remove foreign objects, excise endobronchial lesions, and control massive hemoptysis. A brush, biopsy forceps, or catheter may be passed through the bronchoscope to obtain specimens for cytologic examination.

Purpose

- To visually examine a tumor, an obstruction, secretions, bleeding, or a foreign body in the tracheobronchial tree
- To help diagnose bronchogenic carcinoma, tuberculosis, interstitial pulmonary disease, and fungal or parasitic pulmonary infection by obtaining a specimen for bacteriologic and cytologic examination
- To remove foreign bodies, malignant or benign tumors, mucus plugs, and excessive secretions from the tracheobronchial tree

Patient preparation

- Explain to the patient that this test is used to examine the lower airways.
- Describe the procedure, and instruct the patient to fast for 6 to 12 hours before the test.
- Tell him who will perform the test and where and that the procedure takes 45 to 60 minutes.
- Tell the patient that a chest X-ray and blood studies will be performed before the bronchoscopy and afterward, if appropriate.
- Advise him that he may receive a sedative I.V. to help him relax.
- If the procedure isn't being performed under general anesthesia, inform the patient that a local anesthetic will be sprayed into his nose and mouth to suppress the gag reflex. Warn him that the spray has an unpleasant taste and that he may experience discomfort during the procedure.
- Reassure him that his airway won't be blocked during the procedure and that oxygen will be administered through the bronchoscope.
- Make sure the patient or a responsible family member has signed a consent form.
- Check the patient's history for hypersensitivity to the anesthetic.

- Obtain baseline vital signs.
- Administer the preoperative sedative.
- If the patient is wearing dentures, have him remove them before he receives the sedative.

Equipment

Flexible fiber-optic bronchoscope, sedative, local anesthetic (spray, jelly, or liquid), sterile gloves, sterile container for microbiology specimen, container with 10% formaldehyde solution for histology specimen, Coplin jar with 95% ethyl alcohol for cytology smears, six glass slides (frosted, if possible, or with frosted tips), emesis basin, hand-held resuscitation bag with face mask, oral and endotracheal airways, continuous suction equipment, laryngoscope, oxygen delivery equipment, ventilating bronchoscope for a patient requiring controlled mechanical ventilation

Procedure and posttest care

- Place the patient in the supine position, or have him sit upright in a chair.
- Tell him to remain relaxed with his arms at his sides and to breathe through his nose.
- Provide supplemental oxygen by nasal cannula, if necessary.
- After the local anesthetic is sprayed into the patient's throat and takes effect, a bronchoscope is introduced; it's used to inspect the anatomic structure of the trachea and bronchi, observe the color of the mucosal lining, and note masses or inflamed areas.
- Biopsy forceps may be used to remove a tissue specimen from a suspect area, a bronchial brush may be used to obtain cells from the surface of a lesion, and a suction apparatus may be used to remove foreign bodies or mucus plugs.
- After collection, place the specimens in their respective, properly labeled

containers and send them to the laboratory at once.

• Check vital signs every 15 minutes until the patient is stable and then every 30 minutes for 4 hours, every hour for the next 4 hours, and then every 4 hours for 24 hours. Immediately notify the doctor of any adverse reactions to the anesthetic or sedative.

• Place the conscious patient in semi-Fowler's position; place the unconscious patient on his side with his head slightly elevated to prevent aspiration.

• Provide an emesis basin, and instruct the patient to spit out saliva rather than swallow it. Observe sputum for blood, and report excessive bleeding immediately.

• Tell the patient who has had a biopsy to refrain from clearing his throat and coughing, which may dislodge the clot at the biopsy site and cause hemorrhaging.

• Immediately report subcutaneous crepitus around the patient's face and neck because this may indicate tracheal or bronchial perforation.

CLINICAL ALERT Watch, listen for, and immediately report symptoms of respiratory difficulty resulting from laryngeal edema or laryngospasm, such as laryngeal stridor and dyspnea. Observe for signs of hypoxemia, pneumothorax, bronchospasm, and bleeding.

• Restrict food and fluids to avoid aspiration until the gag reflex returns (usually in 1 to 2 hours). Then the patient may resume his usual diet, beginning with sips of clear liquid or ice chips.

• Reassure the patient that hoarseness, loss of voice, and sore throat are temporary. Provide lozenges or a soothing liquid gargle to ease discomfort when his gag reflex returns.

Precautions

• A patient with respiratory failure who can't breathe adequately by himself should be placed on a ventilator before bronchoscopy.

• Send the specimens to the laboratory immediately.

Normal findings

The trachea normally consists of smooth muscle containing C-shaped rings of cartilage at regular intervals, and it's lined with ciliated mucosa. The bronchi appear structurally similar to the trachea; the right bronchus is slightly larger and more vertical than the left. Smaller segmental bronchi branch off the main bronchi.

Abnormal findings

Bronchial wall abnormalities include inflammation, swelling, and tumors. Endotracheal abnormalities include stenosis, compression, and abnormal bifurcation due to diverticulum.

Abnormal substances in the trachea or bronchi include blood, secretions, and foreign bodies. They'll be removed and sent for culture and cytologic examination.

Results of tissue and cell studies may indicate interstitial pulmonary disease, bronchogenic carcinoma, tuberculosis, or other pulmonary infections, such as *Pneumocystis carinii* pneumonia and aspergillosis. Correlation of radiographic, bronchoscopic, and cytologic findings with clinical signs and symptoms is essential.

Interfering factors

• Failure to observe pretest restrictions
• Failure to place specimens in the appropriate containers or to send them to the laboratory immediately
• Patient's inability to cooperate if the procedure is done under local anesthesia

MEDIASTINOSCOPY

Using an exploring speculum with built-in fiber light and side slit, mediastinoscopy allows direct viewing of mediastinal structures. It also permits palpation and biopsy of paratracheal and carinal lymph nodes. This surgical procedure is indicated when other tests, such as sputum cytology, lung scans, radiography, and bronchoscopic biopsy, fail to confirm the diagnosis.

Scarring of the area from previous mediastinoscopy contraindicates this procedure.

Purpose
● To detect bronchogenic carcinoma, lymphoma (including Hodgkin's disease), and sarcoidosis
● To determine stages of lung cancer

Patient preparation
● Explain to the patient that this test is used to evaluate the lymph nodes and other structures in the chest. Review the patient's history for previous mediastinoscopy because repeat examination is contraindicated.
● Describe the procedure and answer any questions.
● Instruct the patient to fast after midnight before the test.
● Tell him who will perform the procedure and where, that he'll be given general anesthesia, and that the procedure takes about 1 hour.
● Tell him that he may have temporary chest pain, tenderness at the incision site, or a sore throat (from intubation).
● Reassure him that complications are rare with this procedure.
● Make sure the patient or a responsible family member has signed a consent form.

● Check the patient's history for hypersensitivity to the anesthetic.
● Give a sedative the night before the test and again before the procedure.

Procedure and posttest care
● After the endotracheal tube is in place, a small transverse suprasternal incision is made and the surgeon palpates the lymph nodes.
● The mediastinoscope is inserted, and tissue specimens are collected and sent to the laboratory for frozen section examination.
● If analysis confirms malignancy of a resectable tumor, thoracotomy and pneumonectomy may follow immediately.
● Monitor postoperative vital signs for 24 hours, and check dressings for bleeding and fluid drainage.
● Observe for the following complications: fever (a sign of mediastinitis); crepitus (a sign of subcutaneous emphysema); dyspnea, cyanosis, and diminished breath sounds on the affected side (signs of pneumothorax); tachycardia and hypotension (signs of hemorrhage).
● Administer the prescribed analgesic, as needed.

Normal findings
Lymph nodes appear normal with no evidence of disease.

Abnormal findings
A lymph node biopsy may indicate carcinoma and allow for staging lung cancer and evaluating the extent of metastasis. A biopsy may also identify sarcoidosis and infections such as histoplasmosis.

Interfering factor
● Previous mediastinoscopy (makes dissection of nodes difficult or impossible)

THORACOSCOPY

In this test, an endoscope is inserted directly into the chest wall to view the pleural space, thoracic walls, mediastinum, and pericardium. It's used for both diagnostic and therapeutic purposes and can sometimes replace traditional thoracotomy. Thoracoscopy reduces morbidity (by reducing the use of open chest surgery) and postoperative pain, decreases surgical and anesthesia time, and allows faster recovery.

Purpose
• To diagnose pleural disease
• To obtain biopsy specimens
• To treat pleural conditions, such as cysts, blebs, and effusions
• To perform wedge resections or laser procedures

Patient preparation
• Explain to the patient that this procedure permits visual examination of the chest wall to view the pleural space, thoracic wall, mediastinum, and pericardium.
• Describe the procedure. Caution the patient that an open thoracotomy may still be needed for diagnosis or treatment and that general anesthesia may be required.
• Instruct the patient not to eat or drink for 8 to 12 hours before the procedure.
• Make sure that the appropriate preoperative tests (such as pulmonary function and coagulation tests, electrocardiography, and chest X-ray) have been performed and that a consent form has been signed.
• Tell the patient that he'll have a chest tube and drainage system in place after surgery. Reassure him that analgesics will be available and that complications are rare.

Equipment
Monitors, videocassette recorder, camera, light source, insufflator, cautery, suction and irrigation equipment, trocars, endostaplers, endosutures, Cope's needle, Abram's fine needle, Wang needle

Procedure and posttest care
• The patient is anesthetized, and a double-lumen endobronchial tube is inserted.
• The lung on the operative side is collapsed, and a small intercostal incision is made, through which a trocar is inserted.
• A lens is then inserted to view the area and assess thoracoscopy access.
• Two or three more small incisions are made, and trocars are placed for insertion of suction and dissection instruments.
• The camera lens and instruments are moved from site to site as needed.
• After thoracoscopy, the lung is reexpanded, a chest tube is placed through one incision site, and a water-sealed drainage system is attached. The other incisions are closed with adhesive strips and dressed.
• Monitor postoperative vital signs every 15 minutes for 1 hour, every 30 minutes for 2 hours, every hour for 2 hours, and then every 4 hours.
• Assess respiratory status and the patency of the chest drainage system.
• Give analgesics as needed for pain.

Precautions
• Send specimens to the laboratory immediately.

CLINICAL ALERT Don't clamp chest tubes unless specifically ordered to do so.
• Complications, although rare, include hemorrhage, nerve injury, perforation of the diaphragm, air emboli, and tension pneumothorax.

Normal findings

A normal pleural cavity contains a small amount of lubricating fluid that facilitates movement of the lung and chest wall. The parietal and visceral layers are lesion-free and able to separate from each other.

Abnormal findings

Lesions, such as tumors, ulcers, and bleeding sites, adjacent to or involving the pleura or mediastinum can be seen and biopsies can be taken. Diagnosis may include carcinoma, empyema, pleural effusion, tuberculosis, or an inflammatory process. Areas of blebs can be removed by wedge resection to reduce the risk of repeat episodes of spontaneous pneumothorax.

Interfering factors

● Extensive or inaccessible pathology, coagulopathies or lesions near major blood vessels, previous thoracic surgery, and inadequate oxygenation with one lung (possible contraindications)
● Excessive bleeding during the procedure (may require open thoracotomy)

GASTROINTESTINAL SYSTEM

ESOPHAGOGASTRO-DUODENOSCOPY

Esophagogastroduodenoscopy (EGD) permits visual examination of the lining of the esophagus, stomach, and upper duodenum using a flexible fiberoptic or video endoscope. It's indicated for patients with GI bleeding, hematemesis, melena, substernal or epigastric pain, gastroesophageal reflux disease (GERD), dysphagia, anemia, strictures, or peptic ulcer disease; those requiring foreign body retrieval; and postoperative patients with recurrent or new symptoms.

EGD eliminates the need for extensive exploratory surgery and can be used to detect small or surface lesions missed by radiography. Because the scope provides a channel for biopsy forceps or a cytology brush, it permits laboratory evaluation of abnormalities detected by radiography. Similarly, it allows removal of foreign bodies by suction (for small, soft objects) or by electrocautery snare or forceps (for large, hard objects).

Purpose

● To diagnose inflammatory disease, malignant and benign tumors, ulcers, Mallory-Weiss syndrome, structural abnormalities, and stages of GERD
● To evaluate the stomach and duodenum postoperatively
● To obtain emergency diagnosis of duodenal ulcer or esophageal injury, such as that caused by ingestion of chemicals
● To treat varices with laser therapy or thermal coagulation
● To treat strictures or polyps

Patient preparation

● Explain to the patient that this procedure permits visual examination of the lining of the esophagus, stomach, and upper duodenum.
● Check the patient's medical history for allergies, medications, and information pertinent to the current complaint.
● Instruct him to fast for 6 to 8 hours before the test.
● Tell him that a flexible instrument with a camera on the end will be passed through his mouth; explain who

will perform this procedure and where and that it takes about 30 minutes.

• If an emergency EGD is to be performed, tell the patient that stomach contents may be aspirated through a nasogastric tube.

• Inform the patient that a bitter-tasting local anesthetic will be sprayed into his mouth and throat or that he'll be given a pill to suck on to calm the gag reflex, and that his tongue and throat may feel swollen, making swallowing seem difficult. Advise him to let the saliva drain from the side of his mouth; a suction machine may be used to remove saliva, if necessary.

• Explain that a mouth guard will be inserted to protect his teeth and the endoscope; assure him that this won't obstruct his breathing.

• Inform him that an I.V. line will be started and a sedative will be administered before the endoscope is inserted to help him relax. If the procedure is being done on an outpatient basis, advise the patient to arrange for someone to drive him home. Warn him that conscious sedation may affect his reflexes and reaction time, even though he may feel fine.

• Tell the patient that he may experience pressure in the stomach as the endoscope is moved about and a feeling of fullness when air or carbon dioxide is insufflated (insufflation distends and flattens the stomach wall to aid visualization).

• Make sure the patient or a responsible family member has signed an informed consent form.

• Just before the procedure, instruct the patient to remove dentures, eyeglasses, and constricting undergarments.

Equipment

Monitors, flexible fiber-optic video endoscope, cautery, suction and irrigation equipment

Procedure and posttest care

• Obtain baseline vital signs, and leave the blood pressure cuff in place for monitoring throughout the procedure. Observe the patient's skin color, temperature, and dryness; abdominal distention; level of consciousness; and pain tolerance.

• Ask the patient to hold his breath while his mouth and throat are sprayed with a local anesthetic, if requested by the doctor.

• Remind the patient to let saliva drain from the side of his mouth. Provide an emesis basin to spit out saliva and tissues to wipe saliva from his mouth, or use oropharyngeal suction as needed.

• The patient is placed in a left lateral position, his head is bent forward, and he's asked to open his mouth.

• The examiner guides the tip of the endoscope to the back of the throat and downward. As the endoscope passes through the posterior pharynx and the cricopharyngeal sphincter, the patient's neck is slowly extended.

• When the endoscope is well into the esophagus (about 12″ [30 cm]), the patient's head is positioned with his chin toward the table so that saliva can drain out of his mouth.

• After examination of the esophagus and the cardiac sphincter, the endoscope is advanced to allow examination of the stomach and duodenum. During the examination, air or water may be introduced through the endoscope and suction may be applied to remove insufflated air and secretions.

• A measuring tube may be passed through the endoscope to determine the size of a lesion.

• Biopsy forceps or a cytology brush may be passed through the scope to obtain specimens for hisologic or cytologic study. A laser, a cauterizing device, or a sclerosing agent may be used to treat areas of bleeding or polyps.

• The endoscope is slowly withdrawn, and suspicious-looking areas of the gastric and esophageal lining are reexamined.

• Place tissue specimens immediately in a specimen bottle containing 10% formaldehyde solution; cell specimens are smeared on glass slides and placed in a Coplin jar containing 95% ethyl alcohol. Tissue specimens may also be obtained to test for *Helicobacter pylori*.

CLINICAL ALERT Observe the patient for possible perforation. Perforation in the cervical area of the esophagus produces pain on swallowing and with neck movement; thoracic perforation causes substernal or epigastric pain that increases with breathing or movement of the trunk; diaphragmatic perforation produces shoulder pain and dyspnea; gastric perforation causes abdominal or back pain, cyanosis, fever, and pleural effusion.

• Monitor vital signs, and document according to the facility's policy.

• Test the gag reflex by touching the back of the throat with a tongue blade. Withhold food and fluids until the gag reflex returns (usually in 1 hour), and then allow fluids and a light meal.

• Tell the patient that he may burp some insufflated air and have a sore throat for 1 to 2 days. Throat lozenges and warm saline gargles may ease his discomfort.

• If the patient experiences soreness at the I.V. site, apply warm soaks.

• Instruct him to notify the doctor immediately if he experiences persistent difficulty in swallowing, pain, fever, black stools, or bloody vomitus.

Precautions
• If tissue or cell specimens are obtained during the procedure, label and send them to the appropriate laboratory immediately.

• This procedure is generally safe but can cause perforation of the esophagus, stomach, or duodenum, especially if the patient is restless or uncooperative.

• EGD is usually contraindicated in patients with Zenker's diverticulum, a large aortic aneurysm, or recent ulcer perforation.

• EGD shouldn't be performed within 2 days after an upper GI series.

CLINICAL ALERT Observe closely for adverse effects of the sedative: respiratory depression, apnea, hypotension, excessive diaphoresis, bradycardia, and laryngospasm. Have available emergency resuscitation equipment and a narcotic antagonist such as naloxone. Be prepared to intervene as necessary.

Normal findings
The smooth mucosa of the esophagus is normally yellow-pink and marked by a fine vascular network. A pulsation on the anterior wall of the esophagus between 8″ and 10″ (20 and 25 cm) from the incisor teeth represents the aortic arch. The orange-red mucosa of the stomach begins at the "Z" line, an irregular transition line slightly above the esophagogastric junction.

Unlike the esophagus, the stomach has rugal folds, and its blood vessels aren't visible beneath the gastric mucosa. The reddish mucosa of the duodenal bulb is marked by a few shallow longitudinal folds. The mucosa of the distal duodenum has prominent circular folds, is lined with villi, and appears velvety.

Abnormal findings
EGD, coupled with the results of histologic and cytologic tests, may indicate

acute or chronic ulcers, benign or malignant tumors, and inflammatory disease, including esophagitis, gastritis, and duodenitis. This test may demonstrate varices, Mallory-Weiss syndrome, esophageal and pyloric stenoses, and esophageal hiatal hernia. Although EGD can evaluate gross abnormalities of esophageal motility, as occur in achalasia, manometric studies are more accurate.

Interfering factors
• Esophogeal stricture that hinders endoscope
• Severe cervical arthritis that prevents mobility of the head
• Failure to adhere to pretest restrictions or to send specimens to the laboratory immediately
• Patient's inability to cooperate, preventing optimal visualization

COLONOSCOPY

This test uses a flexible fiber-optic video endoscope to permit visual examination of the lining of the large intestine. It's indicated for patients with a history of constipation or diarrhea, persistent rectal bleeding, and lower abdominal pain when the results of proctosigmoidoscopy and a barium enema test are negative or inconclusive.

Purpose
• To detect or evaluate inflammatory and ulcerative bowel disease
• To locate the origin of lower GI bleeding
• To aid diagnosis of colonic strictures and benign or malignant lesions
• To evaluate the colon postoperatively for recurrence of polyps and malignant lesions

Patient preparation
• Tell the patient that this test permits examination of the lining of the large intestine.
• Instruct him to maintain a clear liquid diet the evening before the test and to fast the morning of the procedure, according to the doctor's orders.
• Describe the procedure, and tell the patient who will perform it and where. Inform the patient that the test usually takes 30 to 60 minutes.
• Explain that the large intestine must be thoroughly cleaned to be clearly visible. Instruct the patient to perform the prescribed bowel preparation (for example, consuming Co-lyte, Fleet Phospho-Soda, or magnesium citrate) usually the night before the procedure.
• Inform the patient that an I.V. line will be started before the procedure and that a sedative will be administered just before the procedure. Advise him to arrange for someone to drive him home because conscious sedation may affect his reflexes and reaction time, even if he feels fine.
• Assure him that the colonoscope is well lubricated to ease its insertion, that it initially feels cool, and that he may feel an urge to defecate when it's inserted and advanced.
• Explain that air may be introduced through the colonoscope to distend the intestinal wall and to facilitate viewing the lining and advancing the instrument. Tell him that flatus normally escapes around the instrument because of air insufflation and that he should not attempt to control it.
• Tell him that suction may be used to remove blood or liquid stools that obscure vision but that this won't cause discomfort.
• Check the patient's medical history for allergies, medications, and information pertinent to the current complaint.

• Make sure the patient or a responsible family member has signed an informed consent form.

Procedure and posttest care

• Place the patient on his left side with his knees flexed, and drape him.

• Obtain baseline vital signs and leave the blood pressure cuff in place for monitoring during the procedure. Observe the patient's skin color, temperature, and dryness; abdominal distention; level of consciousness; and pain tolerance throughout the procedure.

• Instruct the patient to breathe deeply and slowly through his mouth as the doctor palpates the mucosa of the anus and rectum and inserts the colonoscope.

• The doctor inserts the lubricated colonoscope through the patient's anus and rectum into the sigmoid colon.

• Assist the doctor as necessary in passing the colonoscope through the transverse colon, through the hepatic flexure, and into the ascending colon and cecum.

• Abdominal palpation or fluoroscopy may be used to help guide the colonoscope through the large intestine.

• Suction may be used to remove blood and secretions that obscure vision.

• Biopsy forceps or a cytology brush may be passed through the colonoscope to obtain specimens for histologic or cytologic examination; an electrocautery snare may be used to remove polyps. A laser, Bicap, or Argon Plasma Coagulator may be used to treat areas of bleeding and polyps.

• If the examiner removes a tissue specimen, immediately place it in a specimen bottle containing 10% formaldehyde; immediately place cytology smears in a Coplin jar containing 95% ethyl alcohol. Send specimens to the laboratory immediately.

• Observe the patient closely for signs of bowel perforation. Report such signs immediately.

• Check vital signs, and document them according to facility policy.

• After the patient has recovered from sedation, he may resume his usual diet unless the doctor orders otherwise.

• Provide privacy while the patient rests after the test; tell him that he may pass large amounts of flatus after insufflation.

• If a polyp has been removed, inform the patient that his stool may contain some blood.

Precautions

• Although it's usually a safe procedure, colonoscopy can cause perforation of the large intestine, excessive bleeding, and retroperitoneal emphysema.

• This procedure is contraindicated in patients who have ischemic bowel disease, acute diverticulitis, peritonitis, fulminant granulomatous colitis, or fulminant ulcerative colitis.

CLINICAL ALERT Watch closely for adverse effects of the sedative. Have available emergency resuscitation equipment and a narcotic antagonist, such as naloxone, for I.V. use, if necessary.

• If a polyp is removed but not retrieved during the examination, give enemas and strain stools to retrieve it, if the doctor requests it.

Normal findings

Normally, the mucosa of the large intestine beyond the sigmoid colon appears light pink-orange and is marked by semilunar folds and deep tubular pits. Blood vessels are visible beneath the intestinal mucosa, which glistens from mucus secretions.

Abnormal findings

Visual examination of the large intestine, coupled with histologic and cytologic test results, may indicate polyps, inflammation, ulceration, strictures, presence of a foreign body, granulomatous or ulcerative colitis, Crohn's disease, and malignant or benign lesions. Diverticular disease or the site of lower GI bleeding can be detected through visual examination alone.

Interfering factors

• Fulminant colitis, peritonitis, acute severe diverticulitis, existing perforation, coagulopathy, and serious cardiac problems, such as unstable cardiomyopathy or recent myocardial infarction

• Fixation of the sigmoid colon due to inflammatory bowel disease, surgery, or radiation therapy (may hinder passage of the colonoscope)

• Blood from acute colonic hemorrhage (hinders visualization)

• Insufficient bowel preparation or barium retained in the intestine from previous diagnostic studies (makes accurate visual examination impossible)

• Failure to place histologic or cytologic specimens in the appropriate preservative or to send the specimens to the laboratory immediately

• Patient's inability to cooperate or to physically tolerate the procedure

PROCTOSIGMOIDOSCOPY

This procedure uses a proctoscope, sigmoidoscope, or colonoscope and digital examination to evaluate the lining of the distal sigmoid colon, rectum, and anal canal. It's indicated in patients with recent changes in bowel habits, lower abdominal and perineal pain,

prolapse on defecation, pruritus, and passage of mucus, blood, or pus in the stool. Specimens may be obtained from suspicious areas of the mucosa by biopsy, lavage or cytology brush, or culture swab.

Possible complications of this procedure include rectal bleeding and, rarely, bowel perforation.

Purpose

• To aid diagnosis of inflammatory, infectious, and ulcerative bowel disease

• To diagnose malignant and benign neoplasms

• To detect hemorrhoids, hypertrophic anal papilla, polyps, fissures, fistulas, and abscesses in the rectum and anal canal

Patient preparation

• Explain to the patient that this procedure allows visual examination of the lining of the distal sigmoid colon, rectum, and anal canal.

• Tell him that the test requires passage of two special instruments through the anus, who will perform the procedure and where, and that it takes 15 to 30 minutes.

• Check the patient's history for allergies, medications, and information pertinent to the current complaint. Find out if he has had a barium test within the past week because barium in the colon hinders accurate examination.

• Because dietary and bowel preparations for this procedure vary according to the doctor's preference, follow the orders carefully. If a special bowel preparation is ordered, explain to the patient that this clears the intestine to ensure a better view.

• Instruct the patient to maintain a clear liquid diet the evening before the test and to fast the morning of the procedure, according to the doctor's preference.

• Describe the position the patient will be asked to assume, and assure him that he'll be adequately draped.

• Tell him that he may be secured to a tilting table that rotates into horizontal and vertical positions.

• Tell the patient that the examiner's finger and the instrument are well lubricated to ease insertion, that the instrument initially feels cool, and that he may experience the urge to defecate when the instrument is inserted and advanced. Instruct the patient to breathe deeply and slowly through his mouth to relax the abdominal muscles; this reduces the urge to defecate and eases discomfort.

• Inform him that the instrument may stretch the intestinal wall and cause transient muscle spasms or colicky lower abdominal pain.

• Explain to the patient that air may be introduced through the endoscope into the intestine to distend its walls. Tell him that this causes flatus to escape around the endoscope, and he should not attempt to control it.

• Inform him that a suction machine may remove blood, mucus, or liquid stool that obscures vision but that it won't cause discomfort.

• Inform the patient that an I.V. line will be started if an I.V. sedative is to be used. If the procedure is being done on an outpatient basis and the patient is receiving conscious sedation, advise him to arrange for someone to drive him home. Conscious sedation may affect his reflexes and reaction time, even though he may feel fine.

• Make sure the patient or a responsible family member has signed a consent form.

• If the patient has rectal inflammation, provide a local anesthetic about 15 to 20 minutes before the procedure to minimize discomfort.

Procedure and posttest care

• Obtain baseline vital signs, and leave the blood pressure cuff in place if the patient is to receive I.V. conscious sedation. Monitor the patient throughout the procedure and observe his skin color, temperature, and dryness; abdominal distention; level of consciousness; and pain tolerance.

• Place the patient in a knee-chest or left lateral position with knees flexed, and drape him.

• If a left lateral position is used, a sandbag may be placed under the patient's left hip so that the buttocks project over the edge of the table. The right buttock is gently raised, and the anus and perianal region are examined.

• Instruct the patient to breathe deeply and slowly through his mouth as the examiner palpates the anal canal, rectum, and rectal mucosa for induration and tenderness; the examiner then withdraws his finger and checks for the presence of blood, mucus, or stool.

• The sigmoidoscope is lubricated, and the patient is told that the instrument is about to be inserted. The right buttock is raised, and the sigmoidoscope is inserted into the anus. As the scope is passed with steady pressure through the anal sphincters, instruct the patient to bear down as though defecating to aid its passage. The sigmoidoscope is advanced through the anal canal into the rectum.

• At the rectosigmoid junction, a small amount of air may be insufflated to open the bowel lumen. The scope is then gently advanced to its full length into the distal sigmoid colon.

• As the sigmoidoscope is slowly withdrawn, air is carefully insufflated, and the intestinal mucosa is thoroughly examined.

• If stool obscures vision, the eyepiece on the scope is removed, a cotton swab is inserted through the scope, and the bowel lumen is swabbed.

• To obtain specimens from suspicious areas of the intestinal mucosa, a biopsy forceps, cytology brush, or culture swab is passed through the sigmoidoscope.

• A laser, Bicap, or Argon Plasma Coagulator may be used to treat areas of bleeding or polyps.

• Polyps may be removed for histologic examination by inserting an electrocautery snare through the sigmoidoscope.

• Specimens are immediately placed in a specimen bottle containing 10% formaldehyde; cytology slides are placed in a Coplin jar containing 95% ethyl alcohol; culture swabs are placed in a culture tube.

• Depending on the facility and the doctor's preference, after the sigmoidoscope is withdrawn, the proctoscope is lubricated and the patient is told that it's about to be inserted. Assure him that he'll experience less discomfort during passage of the proctoscope.

• The right buttock is raised, and the proctoscope is inserted through the anus and gently advanced to its full length.

• The obturator is removed, and the light source is inserted through the proctoscope handle.

• As the instrument is slowly withdrawn, the rectal and anal mucosa are carefully examined. Specimens may be obtained from suspicious areas of the intestinal mucosa.

• If a biopsy of the anal canal is required, a local anesthetic may be administered first.

• After the examination is completed, the proctoscope is withdrawn.

• If the patient has been examined in a knee-chest position, instruct him to rest in a supine position for several minutes before standing to prevent postural hypotension.

• Observe the patient closely for signs of bowel perforation and for vasovagal attack due to emotional stress. Report such signs immediately.

• If air was introduced into the intestine, tell the patient that he may pass large amounts of flatus. Provide privacy while he rests after the test.

• If a biopsy or polypectomy was performed, inform the patient that blood may appear in his stool.

Precautions

• If a tissue specimen or culture swab has been obtained, label it and send it to the appropriate laboratory immediately.

Normal findings

The mucosa of the sigmoid colon appears light pink-orange and is marked by semilunar folds and deep tubular pits. The rectal mucosa is redder due to its rich vascular network, deepens to a purple hue at the pectinate line (the anatomic division between the rectum and anus), and has three distinct valves. The lower two-thirds of the anus (anoderm) is lined with smooth gray-tan skin and joins with the hair-fringed perianal skin.

Abnormal findings

Visual examination and palpation demonstrate abnormalities of the anal canal and rectum, including internal and external hemorrhoids, hypertrophic anal papilla, anal fissures, anal fistulas, and anorectal abscesses. The examination may also reveal inflammatory bowel diseases, polyps, cancer, and other tumors. Biopsy, culture, and other laboratory tests are often necessary to detect various disorders.

Interfering factors

- Barium in the intestine from previous diagnostic studies (hinders visualization)
- Large amounts of stool in the intestine (hinders visual examination and advancement of the endoscope)
- Failure to place histologic or cytologic specimens in the appropriate preservative or to send the specimens to the laboratory immediately

ENDOSCOPIC ULTRASOUND

Endoscopic ultrasound (EUS) combines ultrasonography and endoscopy to visualize the GI wall and adjacent structures. The incorporation of the ultrasound probe at the distal end of the ultrasonic endoscope allows ultrasound imaging with high resolution.

Purpose

- To evaluate or stage lesions of the esophagus, stomach, duodenum, pancreas, ampulla, biliary ducts, and rectum
- To evaluate submucosal tumors and large folds
- To localize endocrine tumors

Patient preparation

- Explain to the patient that this procedure permits visual examination of tumors and large folds in the GI tract.
- Check the patient's medical history for allergies, medications, and information pertinent to the current complaint.
- Instruct the patient to fast for 6 to 8 hours before the test.

- Describe the procedure to the patient. Tell him who will perform it and where and that the test generally takes 30 to 90 minutes.
- For an esophagogastroduodenoscopy (EGD) EUS, explain that a flexible instrument will be passed through the mouth and into the esophagus, as in an EGD.
- If a sigmoid EUS is to be performed, tell the patient that the scope is well lubricated to ease its insertion through the anus, that it initially feels cool, and that he may feel an urge to defecate when it's inserted and advanced.
- For the sigmoid EUS, the patient may have to take a laxative the evening before, if ordered.
- Inform the patient that he may receive an I.V. sedative to help him relax before the endoscope is inserted. If the procedure is being done on an outpatient basis, advise the patient to arrange for someone to drive him home because conscious sedation may affect his reaction time and reflexes, even though he may feel fine.
- Make sure the patient or a responsible family member has signed the consent form.

Procedure and posttest care

- Obtain baseline vital signs and leave the blood pressure cuff in place for monitoring throughout the procedure, according to facility policy. Throughout the procedure, observe the patient's skin color, temperature, and dryness; abdominal distention; level of consciousness; and pain tolerance.
- Follow the procedures for EGD or sigmoidoscopy, depending on which type of EUS is to be performed.

Precautions

• This procedure is generally safe but can cause perforation of the esophagus, stomach, or duodenum, as in EGD, or of the intestine, as in sigmoidoscopy or colonoscopy.

Normal findings

EUS usually reveals normal anatomy with no evidence of tumor.

Abnormal findings

Refer to the abnormal findings for EGD, colonoscopy, endoscopy, and sigmoidoscopy.

Interfering factors

• Esophageal stricture (hinders passage of the endoscope)
• All interfering factors listed under EGD — endoscopy, colonoscopy, and sigmoidoscopy

REPRODUCTIVE SYSTEM

COLPOSCOPY

In this test, the cervix and vagina are visually examined by an instrument containing a magnifying lens and a light (colposcope). Colposcopy is primarily used to evaluate abnormal cytology or grossly suspicious lesions and to examine the cervix and vagina after a positive Papanicolaou (Pap) test.

During the examination, a biopsy may be performed and photographs taken of suspicious lesions with the colposcope and its attachments. Risks of biopsy include bleeding (especially during pregnancy) and infection.

Purpose

• To help confirm cervical intraepithelial neoplasia (CIN) or invasive carcinoma after a positive Pap test
• To evaluate vaginal or cervical lesions
• To monitor conservatively treated CIN
• To monitor patients whose mothers received diethylstilbestrol during pregnancy

Patient preparation

• Explain to the patient that this test magnifies the image of the vagina and cervix, providing more information than a routine vaginal examination.
• Inform the patient that she needn't restrict food or fluids.
• Tell her who will perform the examination and where, that it's safe and painless, and that it takes 10 to 15 minutes.
• Tell the patient that a biopsy may be performed during colposcopy and that this may cause minimal but easily controlled bleeding. If a biopsy is performed, tell the patient to expect cramping comparable to menstrual cramps.
• Make sure the patient or a responsible family member has signed an informed consent form.

Equipment

Colposcopy: gloves, colposcope, vaginal speculum, 3% to 5% acetic acid solution, swabs

Biopsy: gloves, biopsy forceps, endocervical curette, forceps for uterine dressing, tenaculum, ring forceps, Monsel's (ferric subsulfate) solution, biopsy bottle and preservative, sterile cotton balls, Pap test equipment (glass slide, wooden spatula, swabs, and fixative)

Procedure and posttest care

● The examiner puts on gloves. With the patient in the lithotomy position, the examiner inserts the speculum and, if indicated, performs a Pap test. Help the patient relax during insertion by telling her to breathe through her mouth and concentrate on relaxing her abdominal muscles.

● The cervix is gently swabbed with a dry or saline-soaked swab and then with acetic acid solution to remove mucus.

● After the cervix and vagina are examined, biopsy is performed on areas that appear abnormal.

● Bleeding is stopped by applying pressure or hemostatic solutions.

● After a biopsy, instruct the patient to abstain from intercourse and to avoid inserting anything in her vagina (except a tampon) until healing of the biopsy site is confirmed.

Normal findings

Normally, cervical vessels show a network and hairpin capillary pattern, with about 100 microns between them. Squamous epithelium is smooth and pink; columnar epithelium appears grapelike. Different tissue types are sharply demarcated. The transformation zone, the area between the squamous and columnar epithelium, should be visualized.

Abnormal findings

Abnormal colposcopy findings include white epithelium (leukoplakia) or punctate and mosaic patterns, which may indicate underlying CIN; keratinization in the transformation zone, which may indicate CIN or invasive carcinoma; and atypical vessels, which may indicate invasive carcinoma.

Other abnormalities visible on colposcopic examination include inflammatory changes (usually from infection), atrophic changes (usually from aging or, less often, the use of oral contraceptives), erosion (probably from increased pathogenicity of vaginal flora due to changes in vaginal pH), and papilloma and condyloma (possibly from viruses).

Histologic study of the biopsy specimen confirms colposcopic findings. If the results of the examination and biopsy are inconsistent with the results of the Pap test and biopsy of the squamocolumnar junction, conization of the cervix for biopsy may be indicated.

Interfering factors

● Failure to clean the cervix of menstrual blood or foreign materials, such as creams and medications (possible obstruction to visualization)

● Patient's inability to lie in the lithotomy position

GYNECOLOGIC LAPAROSCOPY

This test permits visualization of the peritoneal cavity by the insertion of a small fiber-optic telescope (laparoscope) through the anterior abdominal wall. This surgical technique may be used diagnostically to detect abnormalities, such as cysts, adhesions, fibroids, and infection. It can also be used therapeutically to perform procedures such as lysis of adhesions; ovarian biopsy; tubal sterilization; removal of ectopic pregnancies, fibroids, hydrosalpinx, and foreign bodies; and fulguration of endometriotic implants.

Although laparoscopy has largely replaced laparotomy, the latter is usually preferred when extensive surgery is indicated. Potential risks of laparoscopy include a punctured visceral organ, causing bleeding or spilling of intestinal contents into the peritoneum.

Purpose
- To identify the cause of pelvic pain
- To help detect endometriosis, ectopic pregnancy, and pelvic inflammatory disease (PID)
- To evaluate pelvic masses or the fallopian tubes of infertile patients
- To stage carcinoma

Patient preparation
- Explain the procedure to the patient, and tell her that the test is used to detect abnormalities of the uterus, fallopian tubes, and ovaries.
- Instruct her to fast for at least 8 hours before surgery.
- Tell her who will perform the procedure and that it takes 15 to 30 minutes.
- Tell the patient whether she'll receive a local or general anesthetic and whether the procedure will require an outpatient visit or overnight hospitalization.
- Warn her that she may experience pain at the puncture site and in the shoulder.
- Make sure the patient or a responsible family member has signed an informed consent form.
- Check the patient's history for hypersensitivity to the anesthetic.
- Make sure all laboratory work is completed and results are reported before the test.

Equipment
Indwelling urinary or straight catheter; sterile tray with scalpel, hemostats, needle holder, suture, and suture scissors; Verees needle; gas insufflator; laparoscope; fiber-optic light source and cable; laparoscope sheath and tro-

car; electrosurgical generator; tenaculum and intrauterine manipulator; probes, scissors, or forceps; adhesive bandages

Procedure and posttest care
- The patient is anesthetized and placed in the lithotomy position.
- The examiner catheterizes the bladder and then performs a bimanual examination of the pelvic area to detect abnormalities that may contraindicate the test and to ensure that the bladder is empty.
- The tenaculum is placed on the cervix and a uterine manipulator is inserted; an incision is made at the inferior rim of the umbilicus.
- The Verees needle is inserted into the peritoneal cavity, and 2 to 3 L of carbon dioxide or nitrous oxide is insufflated to distend the abdominal wall and provide an organ-free space for trocar insertion; the needle is removed and a trocar and sheath are inserted into the peritoneal cavity; another trocar may be inserted at the pubic hairline to allow other instruments.
- After removal of the trocar, the laparoscope is inserted through the sheath to examine the pelvis and abdomen.
- To evaluate tubal patency, the examiner infuses a dye through the cervix and observes the tubes for spillage.
- After the examination, minor surgical procedures, such as ovarian biopsy, may be performed.
- Monitor vital signs and urine output. Report sudden changes immediately; they may indicate complications.
- Monitor the patient for adverse or allergic reactions. After administration of a general anesthetic, monitor electrolyte balance, hemoglobin level, and hematocrit. Help the patient ambulate after recovery.
- Tell the patient that she may resume her usual diet.

• Instruct her to restrict activity for 2 to 7 days, as necessary. However, she'll need to walk postoperatively to help expel gas.

• Reassure the patient that some abdominal and shoulder pain is normal and should disappear within 24 to 36 hours. For mild pain, provide a mild pain reliever such as acetaminophen. For moderate to severe pain, provide an analgesic such as Percocet.

Precautions

• Laparoscopy is contraindicated in patients with advanced abdominal wall cancer, advanced pulmonary or cardiovascular disease, intestinal obstruction, palpable abdominal mass, large abdominal hernia, chronic tuberculosis, or a history of peritonitis.

Normal findings

The uterus and fallopian tubes are of normal size and shape, free of adhesions, and mobile. The ovaries are of normal size and shape; cysts and endometriosis are absent. Dye injected through the cervix flows freely from the fimbria.

Abnormal findings

An ovarian cyst appears as a bubble on the surface of the ovary. The cyst may be clear if filled with follicular fluid or serous or mucous material, or it may be red, blue, or brown if filled with blood. Adhesions may appear as thick and fibrous tissue or as almost transparent strands of tissue.

Endometriosis resembles small, blue powder burns on the peritoneum or the serosa of any pelvic or abdominal structure. Fibroids appear as lumps on the uterus; hydrosalpinx as an enlarged fallopian tube; and ectopic pregnancy as an enlarged or ruptured fallopian tube. In PID, infection or abscess is evident.

Interfering factors

• Adhesions or marked obesity (possible obstruction to visualization)

• Tissue or fluid becoming attached to the lens (possible obstruction to visualization)

• Soft tissues or the inside of a hollow viscus (impossible to palpate)

SKELETAL SYSTEM

ARTHROSCOPY

Arthroscopy is the visual examination of the interior of a joint (most often the knee) with a specially designed fiberoptic endoscope that's inserted through a cannula in the joint cavity. It usually follows and confirms a diagnosis made through physical examination, radiography, and arthrography.

Arthroscopy may be performed under local anesthesia, but it's usually performed under a spinal or general anesthesia, particularly when surgery is anticipated. A camera may be attached to the arthroscope to photograph areas for later study. (See *Arthroscopy of the knee.*)

Complications associated with arthroscopy are rare and may include infection, hemarthrosis, swelling, thrombophlebitis, and joint injury.

Purpose

• To detect and diagnose meniscal, patellar, condylar, extrasynovial, and synovial diseases

• To monitor disease progression

• To perform joint surgery

• To monitor effectiveness of therapy

Arthroscopy of the Knee

With the patient's knee flexed about 40 degrees, the arthroscope is introduced into the joint. The examiner flexes, extends, and rotates the knee to view the joint space. Counterclockwise from the top right, these illustrations show a normal patellofemoral joint with smooth joint surfaces; the articular surface of the patella, showing chondromalacia; and a tear in the anterior cruciate ligament.

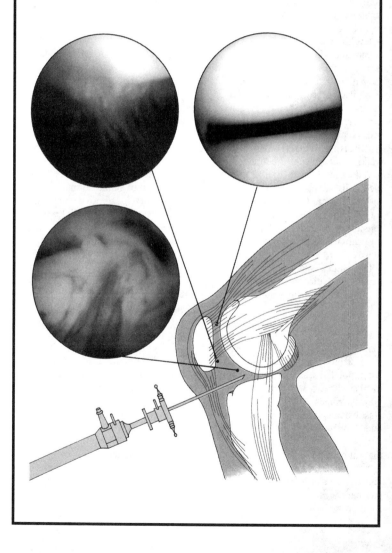

Patient preparation

- Explain to the patient that this test is used to examine the interior of the joint, to evaluate joint disease, or to monitor his response to therapy.
- Describe the procedure to the patient, and answer any questions.
- If surgery or another treatment is anticipated, explain that this may be accomplished during arthroscopy.
- Instruct the patient to fast after midnight before the procedure.
- Tell him who will perform this procedure and where.
- If local anesthesia is to be used, tell the patient that he may experience transient discomfort from the injection of the local anesthetic and the pressure of the tourniquet on his leg.
- If the patient is expected to need crutches after surgery, teach crutch-walking *before* the procedure.
- Make sure the patient or a responsible family member has signed an informed consent form.
- Check the patient's history for hypersensitivity to the anesthetic.
- Obtain baseline and peripheral pulses.
- The surgical site is prepared, and the patient is positioned and draped, according to the facility's protocols.
- Insert an I.V. line.

Equipment

Skin antiseptic (povidone-iodine solution), arthroscope and accessory equipment, pointed scalpel, sterile gloves, local anesthetic, sterile needle, 12- and 60-ml syringes, waterproof stockinette, elastic bandages, pneumatic tourniquet, epinephrine (1:100,000 in 1% lidocaine solution), 500-ml sterile normal saline solution, continuous drainage system, sponges, 2″ × 2″ sterile gauze pads, sterile drapes, small adhesive bandages

Procedure and posttest care

Although arthroscopic techniques vary, depending on the surgeon and the type of arthroscope used, the following procedure is typical for knee arthroscopy.

- After the patient is placed in the supine position on the operating table, a pneumatic tourniquet is placed around his leg but not tightened.
- The patient's leg is scrubbed according to standard surgical procedure, and a waterproof stockinette is applied.
- The patient's leg is elevated and wrapped from toes to lower thigh with an elastic bandage to drain as much blood from the leg as possible.
- The tourniquet is inflated and the elastic bandage removed; the tourniquet may be used at 300 mm Hg and may remain in place during the procedure, depending on the surgeon's preference and the patient's comfort. (For techniques that don't require a tourniquet, 50 ml of sterile normal saline solution with lidocaine and epinephrine is instilled into the patient's knee immediately before insertion of the arthroscope to distend the knee and reduce bleeding.)
- The foot of the table is lowered so that the patient's knee is bent at about 45 degrees, the stockinette is opened, and the local anesthetic is administered.
- A pointed scalpel is used to make a 3- to 5-mm incision in either the anteromedial or anterolateral aspect of the knee, above the tibial plateau.
- If the procedure is being performed under a local anesthetic, warn the patient that he'll feel a thumping sensation as the cannula with sharp trocar is inserted into the capsule at a point medial to the patellar tendon.
- The trocar is removed and replaced with a blunt obturator, which penetrates the synovia, causing transient pain.

- The arthroscope is then inserted through the cannula.
- A viewing medium — a solution of normal saline solution and epinephrine — is introduced into the joint through the arthroscope and drained into a container on the floor.
- The arthroscope is inserted in and out of various joint spaces or is held steady as the knee is bent, extended, and turned to aid visualization. The entire joint can be viewed from one puncture site, but an obstruction may require additional punctures. In most cases, examination of the tibial plateaus, the back recesses of the joint, the menisci, the posterior two-thirds of the femoral condyles, the cruciate structures, and the undersurface of the patella takes about 10 minutes.
- After visual examination, a synovial biopsy or surgery may be performed or treatment applied, as indicated.
- When the examination is completed, the arthroscope is removed, the joint is irrigated by way of the cannula, the cannula is removed, and gentle manual pressure is applied to the knee to remove the normal saline solution.
- An adhesive strip and compression dressing are applied over the incision site.
- Watch for fever, swelling, increased pain, and localized inflammation at the incision site. If the patient reports discomfort, provide a mild pain reliever, such as acetaminophen.
- Tell the patient that he may walk as soon as he's fully awake but should avoid excessive use of the joint for a few days. Tell him that he may resume his usual diet.

Precautions
- Arthroscopy is contraindicated in a patient with fibrous ankylosis with flexion of less than 50 degrees.

- A patient with local skin or wound infections has a risk of subsequent joint involvement. Sepsis in any part of the body will increase the risk of joint infection during this procedure.
- Postoperatively, instruct the patient to watch for symptoms of thrombophlebitis, such as calf tenderness, pain, or heat, and to immediately report these symptoms to the doctor.

■ CLINICAL ALERT Warn the patient not to massage the affected area.

- Teach the patient the signs and symptoms of compartment syndrome, and demonstrate the neurovascular checks to be done for 24 hours. Tell him to report signs or symptoms to the doctor.

Normal findings
The knee is a typical diarthrodial joint surrounded by muscles, ligaments, cartilage, and tendons and lined with synovial membrane. In children, the menisci are smooth and opaque, with their thick outer edges attached to the joint capsule and their inner edges lying snugly against the condylar surfaces, unattached. Articular cartilage appears smooth and white; ligaments and tendons appear cable-like and silvery. The synovium is smooth and marked by a fine vascular network. Degenerative changes begin during adolescence.

Abnormal findings
Arthroscopic examination can reveal meniscal disease, such as a torn medial or lateral meniscus or other meniscal injuries; chondromalacia or fracture; condylar disease, such as osteochondritis dissecans and loose bodies; and extrasynovial disease, such as torn anterior cruciate or tibial collateral ligaments and ganglionic cyst.

Depending on test findings, appropriate treatment or surgery can follow arthroscopy. If arthroscopic surgery can't be performed, arthrotomy is the procedure of choice.

Interfering factors
• Failure to use the arthroscope properly
• Fibrous ankylosis with flexion of less than 50 degrees (inability to flex the knee to 40 degrees)

CHAPTER 11

Ultrasonography

CARDIOVASCULAR SYSTEM 514

514 Echocardiography
517 Transesophageal echocardiography

519 Doppler ultrasonography
523 Ultrasonography of the abdominal aorta

GASTROINTESTINAL SYSTEM 524

524 Ultrasonography of the gallbladder and biliary system
526 Ultrasonography of the liver

528 Ultrasonography of the spleen
530 Ultrasonography of the pancreas

MISCELLANEOUS TESTS 531

531 Thyroid ultrasonography
532 Pelvic ultrasonography
533 Renal ultrasonography

535 Transcranial Doppler studies
536 Vaginal ultrasonography

CARDIOVASCULAR SYSTEM

ECHOCARDIOGRAPHY

Echocardiography is a noninvasive test that shows the size, shape, and motion of cardiac structures. It's useful for evaluating patients with chest pain, enlarged cardiac silhouettes on X-ray films, electrocardiographic changes unrelated to coronary artery disease, and abnormal heart sounds on auscultation.

In this test, a transducer directs ultra-high-frequency sound waves toward cardiac structures, which reflect these waves. The echoes are converted to images that are displayed on a monitor and recorded on a strip chart or videotape. Results are correlated with clinical history, physical examination, and findings from additional tests.

The techniques most commonly used in echocardiography are M-mode (motion-mode), for recording the motion and dimensions of intracardiac structures, and two-dimensional (cross-sectional), for recording lateral motion and providing the correct spatial relationship between cardiac structures. (See *M-mode echocardiograms.*)

Purpose
• To diagnose and evaluate valvular abnormalities
• To measure the size of the heart's chambers
• To evaluate chambers and valves in congenital heart disorders
• To aid diagnosis of hypertrophic and related cardiomyopathies
• To detect atrial tumors

• To evaluate cardiac function or wall motion after myocardial infarction
• To detect pericardial effusion

Patient preparation
• Explain to the patient that this test is used to evaluate the size, shape, and motion of various cardiac structures.
• Inform him that he needn't restrict food or fluids before the test.
• Tell him who will perform the test and where, that it usually takes 15 to 30 minutes, and that it's safe, painless, and noninvasive.
• Explain that the room may be darkened slightly to aid visualization on the monitor screen, and that other procedures (electrocardiography and phonocardiography) may be performed simultaneously to time events in the cardiac cycle.
• Describe the procedure and instruct the patient to remain still during the test because movement may distort results.
• Inform the patient that he may be asked to inhale a gas with a slightly sweet odor (amyl nitrite) while changes in heart function are recorded; describe the possible adverse effects of amyl nitrite (dizziness, flushing, and tachycardia), but assure the patient that such symptoms quickly subside.

Procedure and posttest care
• The patient is placed in a supine position.
• Conductive gel is applied to the third or fourth intercostal space to the left of the sternum, and the transducer is placed directly over it.
• The transducer is systematically angled to direct ultrasonic waves at specific parts of the patient's heart.
• Significant findings are recorded on a strip chart recorder (M-mode echocardiography) or on a videotape recorder (two-dimensional echocardiography).

M-MODE ECHOCARDIOGRAMS

In the normal motion-mode echocardiogram of the mitral valve shown below (top), valve movement appears as a characteristic lopsided M-shaped tracing. The anterior and posterior mitral valve leaflets separate (D) in early diastole, quickly reach maximum separation (E), then close during rapid ventricular filling (E-F).

Leaflet separation varies during mid-diastole, and the valve opens widely again (A) following atrial contraction. The valve starts to close with atrial relaxation (A-B) and is completely closed during the start of ventricular systole (C). The steepness of the E-F slope indirectly shows the speed of ventricular filling, which is normally rapid.

Normal echocardiogram
Chest wall

Right ventricle

Anterior mitral valve leaflet

Posterior mitral valve leaflet

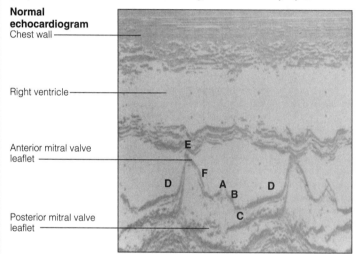

Abnormal echocardiogram
Mitral stenosis is evident in the abnormal echocardiogram shown at right. The E-F slope (dashed line) is very shallow, indicating slowed left ventricular filling.

• For a different view of the heart, the transducer is placed beneath the xiphoid process or directly above the sternum.

• For a left lateral view, the patient may be positioned on his left side.

• To record heart function under various conditions, the patient is asked to inhale and exhale slowly, to hold his breath, or to inhale amyl nitrite.

• Remove the conductive gel from the patient's skin.

Normal findings

An echocardiogram can reveal both the motion pattern and structure of the four cardiac valves. Anterior and posterior mitral valve leaflets normally separate in early diastole, with the anterior leaflet moving toward the chest wall and the posterior leaflet moving away from it. The leaflets attain maximum excursion rapidly, then move toward each other during ventricular diastole; after atrial contraction, they come together and remain so during ventricular systole. On an M-mode echocardiogram, the leaflets appear as two fine lines within the echo-free, blood-filled left ventricular cavity.

The aortic valve cusps lie between the parallel walls of the aortic root, which move anteriorly during systole and posteriorly during diastole. During ventricular systole, these cusps separate and appear as a boxlike configuration on an M-mode echocardiogram. They remain open throughout systole and normally demonstrate a characteristic fine fluttering motion. During diastole, the cusps come together and appear as a single or double line within the aortic root on an M-mode echocardiogram.

The motion of the tricuspid valve resembles that of the mitral valve. The motion of the pulmonic valve — particularly the posterior cusp — is different: During diastole, this cusp gradual-

ly moves posteriorly; during atrial systole, it's displaced posteriorly; during ventricular systole, it quickly moves posteriorly; and during right ventricular ejection, the cusp moves anteriorly, attaining its most anterior position during diastole.

The left ventricular cavity normally appears as an echo-free space between the interventricular septum and the posterior left ventricular wall. Echoes produced by the chordae tendineae and the mitral leaflet appear within this cavity. The right ventricular cavity normally appears as an echo-free space between the anterior chest wall and the interventricular septum.

Abnormal findings

Valvular abnormalities readily appear on the echocardiogram. In mitral stenosis, the valve narrows abnormally due to the leaflets' thickening and disordered motion. Instead of moving in opposite directions during diastole, both mitral valve leaflets move anteriorly. In mitral valve prolapse, one or both leaflets balloon into the left atrium during systole.

Aortic valve abnormalities — especially aortic insufficiency — can also affect the mitral valve because the anterior mitral leaflet is just below the aortic cusps. When blood regurgitates through the aortic valve during diastole, it strikes this leaflet, causing the flutter seen in M-mode. Although the aortic valve may appear normal, this characteristic fluttering confirms aortic insufficiency. In stenosis, due to conditions such as rheumatic fever or bacterial endocarditis, the aortic valve thickens and thus generates more echoes. However, in rheumatic fever, the valve may thicken slightly and allow normal motion during systole, or it may thicken severely and curtail motion. In bacterial endocarditis, valve motion is disrupted, and shaggy or fuzzy echoes usually appear on or near the valve.

Other chamber or valve abnormalities may indicate a congenital heart disorder, such as aortic stenosis, which may require further tests. A large chamber size may indicate cardiomyopathy, valvular disorders, or heart failure; a small chamber, restrictive pericarditis.

Idiopathic hypertrophic subaortic stenosis can also be identified by the echocardiogram, with systolic anterior motion of the mitral valve and asymmetric septal hypertrophy.

Left atrial tumors are usually on a pedicle and can thus shift in and out of the mitral opening. During diastole, the tumor appears as a mass of echoes against the anterior mitral valve leaflet; during ventricular systole, these echoes shift back into the body of the atrium.

In coronary artery disease, ischemia or infarction may cause absent or paradoxical motion in ventricular walls that normally move together and thicken during systole. These affected areas may also fail to thicken or may become thinner, particularly if scar tissue is present.

The echocardiogram is especially sensitive in detecting pericardial effusion. Normally, the epicardium and pericardium are continuous membranes, and thus produce a single or near-single echo. When fluid accumulates between these membranes, it causes an abnormal echo-free space to appear. In large effusions, pressure exerted by excess fluid can restrict pericardial motion.

Interfering factors

• Incorrect transducer placement and excessive movement
• Thick chest or chest wall abnormalities (possible poor imaging)
• Chronic obstructive pulmonary disease (possible poor imaging)

• Arrhythmias (may invalidate test results)
• Hyperinflation of lungs with mechanical ventilation, especially positive end-expiratory pressure > 10 cm H_2O (may invalidate test results)

TRANSESOPHAGEAL ECHOCARDIOGRAPHY

Transesophageal echocardiography combines ultrasound with endoscopy to give a better view of the heart's structures. In this procedure, a small transducer is attached to the end of a gastroscope and inserted into the esophagus, allowing images to be taken from the posterior aspect of the heart. This causes less tissue penetration and interference from chest wall structures and produces high-quality images of the thoracic aorta, except for the superior ascending aorta, which is shadowed by the trachea.

This test is appropriate for both inpatients and outpatients, for patients under general anesthesia, and for critically ill, intubated patients.

Purpose

To visualize and evaluate:
• thoracic and aortic disorders, such as dissection and aneurysm
• valvular disease, especially in the mitral valve and in prosthetic devices
• endocarditis
• congenital heart disease
• intracardiac thrombi
• cardiac tumors
• valvular repairs.

Patient preparation

• Explain to the patient that this test allows visual examination of heart function and structures.

• Tell him who will perform the test, when it's scheduled, and that he'll need to fast for 6 hours beforehand.

• Review the patient's medical history for possible contraindications to the test, such as esophageal obstruction or varices, GI bleeding, previous mediastinal radiation therapy, or severe cervical arthritis.

• Ask the patient about any allergies and note them on the chart.

• Before the test, have the patient remove any dentures or oral prostheses, and note any loose teeth.

• Explain that his throat will be sprayed with a topical anesthetic and that he may gag when the tube is inserted.

• Tell him that an I.V. line will be inserted to administer sedation before the procedure and that he may feel some discomfort from the needle puncture and the pressure of the tourniquet. Reassure him that he'll be made as comfortable as possible during the procedure and that his blood pressure and heart rate will be monitored continuously.

• Make sure the patient or a responsible family member signs a consent form, if required.

Equipment

Cardiac monitor, sedative, topical anesthetic, bite block, gastroscope, ultrasonography equipment, suction equipment, resuscitation equipment

Procedure and posttest care

• Connect the patient to a cardiac monitor, the automated blood pressure cuff, and pulse oximetry probe so that all parameters can be assessed during the procedure.

• Help him lie down on his left side, and administer the prescribed sedative.

• The back of the patient's throat is sprayed with a topical anesthetic.

• A bite block is placed in his mouth, and he's instructed to close his lips around it.

• A gastroscope is introduced and advanced 12″ to 14″ (30 to 35 cm) to the level of the right atrium. To visualize the left ventricle, the scope is advanced 16″ to 18″ (40 to 45 cm).

• Ultrasound images are recorded and then reviewed after the procedure.

• Monitor the patient's vital signs and oxygen levels for any changes.

• Keep the patient supine until the sedative wears off.

• Encourage the patient to cough after the procedure, either while lying on his side or sitting upright.

• Don't give food or water until the patient's gag response returns.

• If the procedure is done on an outpatient basis, make sure someone is available to drive the patient home.

• Treat sore throat symptomatically.

Precautions

• Keep resuscitation equipment readily available.

• Have suction equipment nearby to avoid aspiration if vomiting occurs.

• Vasovagal responses may occur with gagging, so observe the cardiac monitor closely.

• Use pulse oximetry to detect hypoxia.

• If bleeding occurs, stop the procedure immediately.

• Laryngospasm, arrhythmias, or bleeding increase the risk of complications. If any of these occurs, postpone the test.

Normal findings

Transesophageal echocardiography should reveal no cardiac problems.

Abnormal findings

This test can reveal thoracic and aortic disorders, endocarditis, congenital heart disease, intracardiac thrombi, or tumors, and it can evaluate valvular disease or repairs. Findings may include aortic dissection or aneurysm, mitral valve disease, or congenital defects such as patent ductus arteriosus.

Interfering factors
• Uncooperative patient
• Transesophageal approach (restricted visualization of the left atrial appendage and ascending or descending aorta)
• Hyperinflation of lungs due to such causes as chronic obstructive pulmonary disease or mechanical ventilation (possible poor imaging)

DOPPLER ULTRASONOGRAPHY

Doppler ultrasonography is a noninvasive test used to evaluate blood flow in the major veins and arteries of the arms and legs and in the extracranial cerebrovascular system. An alternative to arteriography and venography, it's safer, less costly, and faster than invasive tests.

In Doppler ultrasonography, a handheld transducer directs high-frequency sound waves to the artery or vein being tested. The sound waves strike moving red blood cells and are reflected back to the transducer, allowing direct listening and graphic recording of blood flow. (See *How to detect thrombi with a Doppler probe,* page 520.)

Measurement of systolic pressure during this test is used to detect the presence, location, and extent of peripheral arterial occlusive disease. Changes in sound wave frequency during respiration are observed to detect venous occlusive disease. Compression maneuvers detect occlusion of the veins and occlusion or stenosis of

carotid arteries. Compression maneuvers are also highly sensitive to deep vein thrombosis in the thigh.

Pulse volume recorder testing may be performed with Doppler ultrasonography to record changes in blood volume or flow in an extremity or organ.

Purpose
• To aid diagnosis of chronic venous insufficiency and superficial and deep vein thromboses (popliteal, femoral, iliac)
• To aid diagnosis of peripheral artery disease and arterial occlusion
• To monitor patients who have had arterial reconstruction and bypass grafts
• To detect abnormalities of carotid artery blood flow associated with conditions such as aortic stenosis
• To evaluate possible arterial trauma

Patient preparation
• Explain to the patient that this test is used to evaluate blood flow in the arms and legs or neck.
• Tell the patient who will perform the test and that it takes about 20 minutes.
• Reassure the patient that the test doesn't involve risk or discomfort.
• Tell him that he'll be asked to move his arms to different positions and to perform breathing exercises as measurements are taken. If the lower extremities are being evaluated, his calves may be squeezed during the test. A small ultrasonic probe resembling a microphone is placed at various sites along veins or arteries, and blood pressure is checked at several sites.
• Check with the vascular laboratory about special equipment or instructions.

Procedure and posttest care
• Water-soluble conductive gel is applied to the tip of the transducer.

How to Detect Thrombi with a Doppler Probe

The Doppler probe is typically used to detect venous thrombi by first positioning the transducer and then occluding the blood vessel by compression (as illustrated with the normal leg at right). Water-soluble conductive gel is applied to the tip of the transducer to provide coupling between the skin and the transducer.

When pressure is released, allowing blood flow to resume, the transducer picks up the sudden augmentation of the flow sound and permits graphic recording of blood flow. If a thrombus is present, a compression maneuver fails to produce the augmented flow sound because the blood flow (as shown at right in the femoral vein) is significantly impaired.

Peripheral arterial evaluation
● The usual test sites in each leg are the common femoral, superficial femoral, popliteal, posterior tibial, and dorsalis pedis arteries; in each arm the test sites are usually the subclavian, brachial, radial, ulnar and, occasionally, the palmar arch and digital arteries.

● The patient is instructed to remove all clothing above or below the waist, depending on the test site, and he's placed in a supine position on the examining table or bed, with his arms at his sides.

- Brachial blood pressure is measured, and the transducer is placed at various points along the test arteries.
- The signals are monitored and the waveforms recorded for later analysis.
- Segmental limb blood pressure is obtained to localize arterial occlusive disease.
- During lower extremity tests, a blood pressure cuff is wrapped around the calf, pressure readings are obtained, and waveforms are recorded from the dorsalis pedis and posterior tibial arteries. Then the cuff is wrapped around the thigh, and waveforms are recorded at the popliteal artery.
- In upper extremity tests, examination is performed on one arm, with the patient first supine and then sitting; it's then repeated on the other arm. A blood pressure cuff is wrapped around the forearm, pressure readings are taken, and waveforms are recorded over both the radial and ulnar arteries. Then, the cuff is wrapped around the upper arm, pressure readings are taken, and waveforms are recorded with the transducer over the brachial artery. Blood pressure readings and waveform recordings are repeated with the arm in extreme hyperextension and hyperabduction to check for possible compression factors that may interfere with arterial blood flow.

Peripheral venous evaluation
- Usual test sites include the popliteal, superficial femoral, and common femoral veins in the leg and the posterior tibial vein at the ankle; the brachial, axillary, and subclavian veins in the arm; jugular veins; and, occasionally, the inferior and superior vena cava.
- The patient is instructed to remove all clothing above or below the waist, depending on the test site.
- He's placed in the supine position and instructed to breathe normally.
- The transducer is placed over the appropriate vein, waveforms and compressibility are recorded, and respiratory modulations noted.
- Proximal limb compression maneuvers are performed and augmentation noted after release of compression, to evaluate venous valve competency.
- Changes in respiration are monitored.
- During lower extremity tests, the patient is asked to perform Valsalva's maneuver, and venous blood flow is recorded.
- The procedure is repeated for the other arm or leg.

Extracranial cerebrovascular evaluation
- Usual test sites include the supraorbital, common carotid, external carotid, internal carotid, and vertebral arteries.
- The patient is placed in supine position on the examining table or bed, with a pillow beneath his head for support.
- Brachial blood pressure is then recorded using the Doppler probe.
- The transducer is positioned over the test artery, and blood flow velocity is monitored and recorded.
- The influence of compression maneuvers on blood flow velocity is measured, and the procedure is repeated on the opposite side.

All procedures
- Remove the conductive gel from the patient's skin.

Precautions
- Don't place the Doppler probe over an open or draining lesion.

Normal findings
Arterial waveforms of the arms and legs are triphasic, with a prominent systolic component and one or more diastolic sounds. The ankle-arm pressure index (API) — the ratio between ankle systolic pressure and brachial systolic pressure — is normally equal to or greater than 1. (The API is also

known as arterial ischemia index, the ankle-brachial index, or the pedal-brachial index.) Proximal thigh pressure is normally 20 to 30 mm Hg higher than arm pressure, but pressure measurements at adjacent sites are similar. In the arms, pressure readings should remain unchanged despite postural changes.

Venous blood flow velocity is normally phasic with respiration, and is of a lower pitch than arterial flow. Distal compression or release of proximal limb compression increases blood flow velocity. In the legs, abdominal compression eliminates respiratory variations, but release increases blood flow; Valsalva's maneuver also interrupts venous flow velocity.

In cerebrovascular testing, a strong velocity signal is present. In the common carotid artery, blood flow velocity increases during diastole due to low peripheral vascular resistance of the brain. The direction of periorbital arterial flow is normally anterograde out of the orbit.

Abnormal findings

Arterial stenosis or occlusion diminishes the blood flow velocity signal, with no diastolic sound and a less prominent systolic component distal to the lesion. At the lesion, the signal is high-pitched and, occasionally, turbulent. If complete occlusion is present and collateral circulation has not taken over, the velocity signal may be absent.

A pressure gradient exceeding 20 to 30 mm Hg at adjacent sites of measurement in the leg may indicate occlusive disease. Specifically, low proximal thigh pressure signifies common femoral or aorto-iliac occlusive disease. An abnormal gradient between the proximal thigh and the above- or below-knee cuffs indicates superficial femoral or popliteal artery occlusive

disease; an abnormal gradient between the below-knee and ankle cuffs indicates tibiofibular disease. Abnormal gradients of arm and forearm pressure readings may indicate brachial artery occlusion.

An abnormal API is directly proportional to the degree of circulatory impairment.

If venous blood flow velocity is unchanged by respirations, doesn't increase in response to compression or Valsalva's maneuver, or is absent, venous thrombosis is indicated. In chronic venous insufficiency and varicose veins, the flow velocity signal may be reversed. Confirmation of results may require venography.

Inability to identify Doppler signals during cerebrovascular examination implies total arterial occlusion. Reversed periorbital arterial flow indicates significant arterial occlusive disease of the extracranial internal carotid artery. In addition, the audible signal may take on the acoustic characteristics of a normal peripheral artery. Stenosis of the internal carotid artery causes turbulent signals. Collateral circulation can be assessed by compression maneuvers outside the neck.

Oculoplethysmography, carotid phonoangiography, or carotid imaging can further evaluate cerebrovascular disease. Retrograde blood velocity in the vertebral artery can indicate subclavian steal syndrome. A weak velocity signal on comparison of contralateral vertebral arteries can indicate diffuse vertebral artery disease.

Interfering factors

● Uncooperative patient
● Failure to correctly place the transducer
● Abnormally large, muscular neck (poor imaging)

ULTRASONOGRAPHY OF THE ABDOMINAL AORTA

In ultrasonography of the abdominal aorta, a transducer directs high-frequency sound waves into the abdomen over a wide area from the xiphoid process to the umbilical region. The echoing sound waves are displayed on a monitor to indicate internal organs, the vertebral column, and the size and course of the abdominal aorta and other major vessels.

Purpose

• To detect and measure a suspected abdominal aortic aneurysm (findings may be supported and refined by angiography or computed tomography angiography)

• To detect and measure expansion of a known abdominal aortic aneurysm and thereby assess risk of rupture

Patient preparation

• Explain to the patient that this test allows examination of the abdominal aorta.

• Instruct the patient to fast for 12 hours before the test to minimize bowel gas and motility.

• Tell him who will perform the test and where, that the lights may be lowered, that he'll feel only slight pressure, and that the test takes 30 to 45 minutes.

• Describe the procedure and reassure the patient with a known aneurysm that the sound waves won't cause rupture.

• Instruct him to remain still during scanning and to hold his breath when requested.

• Give simethicone to reduce bowel gas.

Procedure and posttest care

• The patient is placed in a supine position, and conductive gel or mineral oil is applied to his abdomen.

• Longitudinal scans are made at ⅛" to ⅜" (0.5- to 1-cm) intervals left and right of the midline until the entire abdominal aorta is outlined; transverse scans are made at ⅜" to ¾" (1- to 2-cm) intervals from the xiphoid to the bifurcation at the common iliac arteries.

• The patient may be placed in right and left lateral positions.

• Appropriate views are photographed or videotaped.

• Remove the conductive gel from the patient's skin.

• Instruct the patient to resume his usual diet and medications.

◼ **CLINICAL ALERT** Aneurysms may expand and dissect rapidly, so check the patient's vital signs frequently. Remember that sudden onset of constant abdominal or back pain accompanies rapid expansion of the aneurysm; sudden, excruciating pain with weakness, sweating, tachycardia, and hypotension signals rupture.

Normal findings

In adults, the normal abdominal aorta tapers from about 2.5 to 1.5 cm in diameter along its length from the diaphragm to the bifurcation. It descends through the retroperitoneal space, anterior to the vertebral column and slightly left of the midline. Four of its major branches are usually well visualized: the celiac trunk, the renal arteries, the superior mesenteric artery, and the common iliac arteries.

Abnormal findings

Luminal diameter of the abdominal aorta greater than 1½" (4 cm) suggests aneurysm; greater than 2¾" (7 cm) suggests aneurysm with high risk of rupture.

Interfering factors

The following factors may hinder imaging:

- Bowel gas and motility, excessive body movement, surgical wounds, and severe dyspnea
- Residual barium from GI contrast studies within past 24 hours
- Air introduced during endoscopy within past 12 to 24 hours
- Mesenteric fat in obese patients

GASTROINTESTINAL SYSTEM

ULTRASONOGRAPHY OF THE GALLBLADDER AND BILIARY SYSTEM

In ultrasonography of the gallbladder and biliary system, a focused beam of high-frequency sound waves passes into the right upper quadrant of the abdomen, creating echoes that vary with changes in tissue density. These echoes are converted to images on a screen, indicating the size, shape, and position of the gallbladder and biliary system.

Purpose

- To confirm diagnosis of cholelithiasis (technetium-labeled iminodiacetic acid [^{99m}Tc HIDA] nuclear medicine scan may be performed if ultrasound is inconclusive)
- To diagnose acute cholecystitis
- To distinguish between obstructive and nonobstructive jaundice

Patient preparation

- Explain to the patient that this procedure allows examination of the gallbladder and the biliary system.
- Instruct him to eat a fat-free meal in the evening and then to fast for 8 to 12 hours before the procedure, if possible; this promotes accumulation of bile in the gallbladder and enhances ultrasonic visualization.
- Tell him who will perform the procedure and where and that the test takes 15 to 30 minutes.
- Tell the patient that the room may be darkened slightly to aid visualization on the screen.
- Describe the procedure; assure him that he'll feel only mild pressure as the transducer passes over his skin.
- Instruct him to remain as still as possible during the procedure and to hold his breath when requested to ensure that the gallbladder is in the same position for each scan.

Procedure and posttest care

- The patient is placed in a supine position.
- A water-soluble conductive gel is applied to the face of the transducer.
- Transverse and longitudinal oblique scans of the gallbladder are taken.
- During each scan, the patient is asked to inhale deeply and to hold his breath. (If the gallbladder is positioned deeply under the right costal margin, a scan may be taken through the intercostal spaces while the patient holds his breath.)
- The patient is then placed in a left lateral decubitus position and is scanned beneath the right costal margin. (This position and scanning angle may displace and allow detection of stones lodged in the gallbladder neck and the cystic duct region.)
- Scanning with the patient erect helps demonstrate mobility or fixity of sus-

picious echogenic areas. Views may be photographed for later study.

- Remove the conductive gel from the patient's skin.
- Inform the patient that he may resume his usual diet.

Precautions

- Keep the patient in a fasting state to prevent the excretion of bile in the gallbladder.

Normal findings

The normal gallbladder is sonolucent; it appears circular on transverse scans and pear-shaped on longitudinal scans. Although the size of the gallbladder varies, its outer walls normally appear sharp and smooth. Intrahepatic radicles seldom appear because the flow of sonolucent bile is very fine. The cystic duct may also be indistinct — the result of folds known as Heister's valves that line the cystic duct lumen. When visualized, the cystic duct has a serpentine appearance. The common bile duct, in contrast, has a linear appearance but is sometimes obscured by overlying bowel gas.

Abnormal findings

Gallstones within the gallbladder lumen or the biliary system typically appear as mobile, echogenic areas, usually associated with an acoustic shadow. The size of gallstones generally parallels the size of their shadows; gallstones 5 mm or larger usually produce shadows. However, if the gallbladder is distended with bile, gallstones as small as 1 mm can be detected because of the acoustic contrast between liquid bile and solid gallstones. Detecting stones in the biliary ducts, which contain little bile, may be difficult. When the gallbladder is shrunken or fully impacted with gallstones, inadequate bile may likewise make gallstone detection dif-

ficult, and the gallbladder itself might not be detectable. In this case, an acoustic shadow in the gallbladder fossa indicates cholelithiasis; the presence of such a shadow in the cystic and common bile ducts can also indicate cholelithiasis.

Polyps and carcinoma within the gallbladder lumen are distinguished from gallstones by their fixity. Polyps usually appear as sharply defined, echogenic areas; carcinoma appears as a poorly defined mass, often associated with a thickened gallbladder wall.

Biliary sludge within the gallbladder lumen appears as a fine layer of echoes that slowly gravitates to the dependent portion of the gallbladder as the patient changes position. Although biliary sludge may arise without accompanying pathology, it may also result from obstruction and can predispose to gallstone formation.

Acute cholecystitis is indicated by an enlarged gallbladder with thickened, double-rimmed walls, usually with gallstones within the lumen. There may also be precholecystic fluid. In chronic cholecystitis, the walls of the gallbladder appear thickened; the organ itself, however, is generally contracted. In obstructive jaundice, ultrasonography readily demonstrates a dilated biliary system and, usually, a dilated gallbladder. Dilated intrahepatic radicles appear tortuous and irregular; a dilated gallbladder usually loses its characteristic pear shape, becoming spherical.

Biliary obstruction may result from intrinsic factors, such as a gallstone or small carcinoma within the biliary system. (Ultrasonography cannot distinguish between these two echogenic masses.) Or, it may result from extrinsic factors, such as a mass in the hepatic portal that compresses the cystic duct and interferes with bile drainage from the intrahepatic radicles, or from pathology in the head of the pancreas that obstructs the common bile duct. Such pathology includes carcinoma and pancreatitis, although ultrasonography cannot distinguish between the two. When ultrasonography fails to clearly define the site of biliary obstruction, percutaneous transhepatic cholangiography or endoscopic retrograde cholangiopancreatography should be performed.

Interfering factors
• Failure to observe pretest dietary restrictions
• Overlying bowel gas or retained barium from a previous test (possible poor imaging)
• Deficiency of body fluids in a dehydrated patient, obscuring boundaries between organs and tissue structures (possible poor imaging)

ULTRASONOGRAPHY OF THE LIVER

Ultrasonography of the liver produces images by channeling high-frequency sound waves into the right upper quadrant of the abdomen. Resultant echoes are converted to cross-sectional images on a monitor; different shades of gray depict various tissue densities. Ultrasonography can show intrahepatic structures and organ size, shape, and position.

This procedure is indicated in patients with jaundice of unknown etiology, with unexplained hepatomegaly and abnormal biochemical test results, with suspected metastatic tumors and elevated serum alkaline phosphatase levels, and with recent abdominal trauma.

When used with liver-spleen scanning, ultrasonography can define cold spots (focal defects that fail to pick up the radionuclide) as tumors, abscesses, or cysts; it also provides better views of the periportal and perihepatic spaces than liver-spleen scanning. If ultrasonography fails to provide definitive diagnosis, computed tomography, gallium scanning, or liver biopsy may yield more information.

Purpose
• To distinguish between obstructive and nonobstructive jaundice
• To screen for hepatocellular disease
• To detect hepatic metastases and hematoma
• To define cold spots as tumors, abscesses, or cysts

Patient preparation
• Explain to the patient that this procedure allows examination of the liver.
• Instruct him to fast for 8 to 12 hours before the test to reduce bowel gas, which hinders transmission of ultrasound.
• Describe the procedure; tell him who will perform the test and where and that the test takes 15 to 30 minutes.
• Assure him that this test isn't harmful or painful, although he may feel mild pressure as the transducer is pressed against his skin.
• Instruct him to remain as still as possible during the procedure and to hold his breath when requested.

Procedure and posttest care
• The patient is placed in a supine position.
• A water-soluble conductive gel is applied to the face of the transducer.
• Transverse scans between the costal margins demonstrate the left lobe of the liver and part of the right lobe; sector scans through the intercostal spaces

are used to view the remainder of the right lobe.

• Scans are taken longitudinally from the right border of the liver to the left.

• For better demonstration of the right lateral dome, oblique cephalad-angled scans may be taken beneath the right costal margin.

• Scans are then taken parallel to the hepatic portal, at a 45-degree angle toward the superior right lateral dome, to examine the peripheral anatomy, portal venous system, common bile duct, and biliary tree. Clear images are photographed for later study.

• During each scan, ask the patient to hold his breath briefly in deep inspiration to displace the liver caudally from the costal margin and the ribs, to aid visualization.

• Remove the conductive gel from the patient's skin.

• Inform the patient that he may resume his usual diet.

Normal findings

The liver normally demonstrates a homogeneous, low-level echo pattern, interrupted only by the different echo patterns of its portal and hepatic veins, the aorta, and the inferior vena cava. Hepatic veins appear completely sonolucent; portal veins have margins that are highly echogenic.

Abnormal findings

In obstructive jaundice, ultrasonography shows dilated intrahepatic biliary radicles and extrahepatic ducts. Conversely, in nonobstructive jaundice, ultrasonography shows a biliary tree of normal diameter.

Ultrasonographic characteristics of hepatocellular disease are generally nonspecific, and disorders in early stages can escape detection; liver-spleen scanning is a more sensitive diagnostic tool. In cirrhosis, ultrasonography may demonstrate variable liver size; dilated, tortuous portal branches associated with portal hypertension; and an irregular echo pattern with increased echo amplitude, causing overall increased attenuation. Demonstration of splenomegaly by spleen ultrasonography or liver-spleen scanning aids diagnosis. In fatty infiltration of the liver, ultrasonography may show hepatomegaly and a regular echo pattern that, although greater in echo amplitude than that of normal parenchyma, doesn't alter attenuation.

Ultrasonographic characteristics of metastases in the liver vary widely; metastases may appear either hypoechoic or echogenic, poorly defined or well defined. For example, metastatic lymphomas and sarcomas are generally hypoechoic; mucin-secreting adenocarcinoma of the colon is highly echogenic. Liver biopsy is necessary to confirm tumor type. Serial ultrasonography may be used to monitor the effectiveness of therapy.

Primary hepatic tumors also present a varied appearance and may mimic metastases, requiring angiography and liver biopsy for definitive diagnosis. Hepatomas are the most common malignant tumors in adults; hepatoblastomas are most common in children. Benign tumors are far less common than malignant ones.

Abscesses usually appear as sonolucent masses with ill-defined, slightly thickened borders and accentuated posterior wall transmission; scattered internal echoes, caused by necrotic debris, may also be present. Because they produce similar echo patterns, intrahepatic abscesses are occasionally mistaken for hematomas, necrotic metastases, or hemorrhagic cysts. Gas-containing intrahepatic abscesses, which may be echogenic, are sometimes confused with solid intrahepatic lesions.

Subphrenic abscesses occur between the diaphragm and the liver; subhepatic abscesses appear inferior to the liver and anterior to the upper pole of the right kidney. Ascitic fluid resembles a subhepatic abscess, but lacks internal echoes and has a more regular border.

Cysts usually appear as spherical, sonolucent areas with well-defined borders and accentuated posterior wall transmission. When a cyst cannot be distinguished from an abscess or necrotic metastases, gallium scanning, computed tomography, and angiography should be performed.

Hematomas — either intrahepatic or subcapsular — usually result from trauma. Intrahepatic hematomas appear as poorly defined, relatively sonolucent masses and may have scattered internal echoes due to clotting; serial ultrasonography can differentiate between a hematoma and a cyst or tumor as the hematoma becomes smaller. Subcapsular hematoma may appear as a focal, sonolucent mass on the periphery of the liver or as a diffuse, sonolucent area surrounding part of the liver.

Interfering factors

• Overlying ribs and gas or residual barium in the stomach or colon (possible misleading results)
• Deficiency of body fluids in a dehydrated patient, obscuring boundaries between organs and tissue structures (possible misleading results)

ULTRASONOGRAPHY OF THE SPLEEN

In ultrasonography of the spleen, a focused beam of high-frequency sound waves passes into the left upper quad-

rant of the abdomen, creating echoes that vary with changes in tissue density. These are displayed on a monitor as real-time images that indicate the size, shape, and position of the spleen and surrounding viscera.

Ultrasonography is indicated in patients with an upper left quadrant mass of unknown origin; with known splenomegaly, to evaluate changes in splenic size; with left upper quadrant pain and local tenderness; and with recent abdominal trauma.

Purpose

• To demonstrate splenomegaly
• To monitor progression of primary and secondary splenic disease and to evaluate effectiveness of therapy
• To evaluate the spleen after abdominal trauma
• To help detect splenic cysts and subphrenic abscess

Patient preparation

• Explain to the patient that this procedure allows examination of the spleen.
• Tell him who will perform this test and where, that the room may be darkened slightly to aid visualization on the monitor, and that this procedure takes approximately 15 to 30 minutes.
• Instruct him to fast for 8 to 12 hours before the procedure, if possible; this reduces the amount of gas in the bowel, improving the transmission of sound waves.
• Describe the procedure and assure him that he'll feel only mild pressure.
• Instruct him to remain as still as possible during the procedure and to hold his breath when requested, to aid visualization.

Procedure and posttest care

• Because the procedure for ultrasonography varies, depending on the size of the spleen and the patient's physique, the patient is usually repositioned several times; the transducer scanning angle or path is also changed.

• Generally, the patient is first placed in a supine position, with his chest uncovered.

• A water-soluble conductive gel is applied to the face of the transducer, and transverse scans of the spleen are taken at ⅜″ to ¾″ (1- to 2-cm) intervals.

• The patient is then placed in a right lateral decubitus position, and transverse scans are taken through the intercostal spaces using a sectoring motion.

• A pillow may be placed under the patient's right side to help separate the intercostal spaces, making it easier to position the transducer face between them.

• Longitudinal scans are taken from the axilla toward the iliac crest.

• To prevent rib artifacts and to obtain the best view of the splenic parenchyma, oblique scans are taken by passing the transducer face along the intercostal spaces.

• During each scan, the patient may be asked to hold his breath briefly at various stages of inspiration.

• Good views are photographed for later study.

• Remove the conductive gel from the patient's skin.

• Inform the patient that he may resume his usual diet.

Normal findings

The splenic parenchyma normally demonstrates a homogeneous, low-level echo pattern; its individual vascular channels aren't usually apparent. The superior and lateral splenic borders are clearly defined, each having a convex margin. The undersurface and medial borders, in contrast, show indentations from surrounding organs (stomach, left kidney, and pancreas).

The hilar region, where the vascular pedicle enters the spleen, commonly produces an area of highly reflective echoes. The medial surface is generally concave, which helps differentiate between left upper quadrant masses and an enlarged spleen. Even when splenomegaly is present, the spleen generally remains concave medially unless a space-occupying lesion distorts this contour.

Abnormal findings

Ultrasonography can show splenomegaly, but it usually doesn't indicate the cause; a computed tomography (CT) scan can provide more specific information. Splenomegaly is generally accompanied by increased echogenicity. Enlarged vascular channels are commonly visible, especially in the hilar region. If space-occupying lesions distort the splenic contour, liver-spleen scanning should be performed to confirm splenomegaly.

Abdominal trauma may result in splenic rupture or subcapsular hematoma. In splenic rupture, ultrasonography demonstrates splenomegaly and an irregular, sonolucent area (the presence of free intraperitoneal fluid); however, these findings must be confirmed by arteriography. In subcapsular hematoma, ultrasonography shows splenomegaly, as well as a double contour, altered splenic position, and a relatively sonolucent area on the periphery of the spleen. The double contour results from blood accumulation between the splenic parenchyma and the intact splenic capsule. As the spleen enlarges, a transverse section shows its anterior margin extending more anteriorly than the aorta. Ultrasonography may be difficult and painful after abdominal trauma because the transducer may have to pass across fractured ribs and contusions; CT scanning, which differentiates blood and fluid in the peritoneal space, should be used instead.

In subphrenic abscess, ultrasonography shows a sonolucent area beneath the diaphragm. Clinical findings may differentiate between abscess and blood or fluid accumulation.

Used with liver-spleen scanning, ultrasonography differentiates cold spots as cystic or solid lesions. It shows cysts as spherical, sonolucent areas with well-defined, regular margins with acoustic enhancement behind them. When ultrasonography fails to identify a cyst as splenic or extrasplenic — especially if the cyst is located in the upper pole of the left kidney and the adrenal gland, or in the tail of the pancreas — a CT scan and arteriography are used. Ultrasonography can readily clarify cystic cold spots, but using a CT scan with a contrast medium is superior for evaluating primary and metastatic tumors. Ultrasonography usually fails to identify tumors associated with lymphoma and chronic leukemias because these resemble tumors of the splenic parenchyma.

Interfering factors

• Overlying ribs, aerated left lung, gas or residual barium in the colon or the stomach (possible poor imaging)
• Deficiency of body fluids in a dehydrated patient, obscuring boundaries between organs and tissue structures (possible poor imaging)
• Physique affecting the spleen's shape or adjacent masses displacing the spleen (possible poor imaging, may be mistaken for splenomegaly)
• Patient with splenic trauma (possible difficulty in tolerating the procedure)

ULTRASONOGRAPHY OF THE PANCREAS

In ultrasonography of the pancreas, cross-sectional images of the pancreas are produced by channeling high-frequency sound waves into the epigastric region and converting the resultant echoes to real-time images, which are displayed on a monitor. The pattern varies with tissue density and indicates the size, shape, and position of the pancreas and surrounding viscera.

Purpose

• To help detect anatomic abnormalities and aid diagnosis of pancreatitis, pseudocysts, and pancreatic carcinoma
• To guide insertion of biopsy needles

Patient preparation

• Explain to the patient that this procedure permits examination of the pancreas.
• Instruct him to fast for 8 to 12 hours before the procedure to reduce bowel gas.
• Tell him who will perform the procedure and where, that the room is darkened slightly to aid visualization, and that this test takes 30 minutes.
• If the patient is a smoker, ask him to abstain before the test; this eliminates the risk of swallowing air while inhaling, which interferes with test results.
• Describe the procedure and assure him that it isn't harmful or painful, but that he may experience mild pressure.
• Tell him he'll be asked to inhale deeply during scanning, and instruct him to remain still during the procedure.

Procedure and posttest care

- The patient is placed in a supine position.
- A water-soluble conductive gel or mineral oil is applied to the abdomen and, with the patient at full inspiration, transverse scans are taken at 1-cm intervals, starting from the xiphoid and moving caudally; longitudinal scans are taken to view the head, body, and tail of the pancreas in sequence; scanning the right anterior oblique view allows imaging of the head and body of the pancreas; oblique sagittal scans are used to view the portal vein; and scanning from the sagittal view images the vena cava.
- Good views are photographed for later study.
- Remove the conductive gel from the patient's skin.
- Inform the patient that he may resume his usual diet.

Normal findings

The pancreas normally demonstrates a coarse, uniform echo pattern and usually appears more echogenic than the adjacent liver.

Abnormal findings

Alterations in the size, contour, and parenchymal texture of the pancreas characterize pancreatic disease. An enlarged pancreas with decreased echogenicity and distinct borders suggests pancreatitis; a well-defined mass with an essentially echo-free interior indicates pseudocyst; an ill-defined mass with scattered internal echoes or a mass in the head of the pancreas (obstructing the common bile duct) and a large noncontracting gallbladder suggest pancreatic carcinoma.

Subsequent computed tomography scan and biopsy of the pancreas may be necessary to confirm a diagnosis.

Interfering factors

- Gas or residual barium in the stomach and intestine (possible poor imaging)
- Deficiency of body fluids in a dehydrated patient, obscuring boundaries between organs and tissue structures (possible poor imaging)
- Obesity (possible poor imaging)
- Fatty infiltration of pancreas (possible poor imaging)

MISCELLANEOUS TESTS

THYROID ULTRASONOGRAPHY

In thyroid ultrasonography, high-frequency sound waves emitted from a transducer are directed at the thyroid gland and reflected back to produce structural images on a monitor.

When a mass is located by palpation or by thyroid imaging, thyroid ultrasonography can differentiate between a cyst and a tumor larger than 3/8″ (1 cm) with a high degree of accuracy. This test is also used to evaluate thyroid nodules during pregnancy because it doesn't require use of radioactive iodine.

Purpose

- To evaluate thyroid structure
- To differentiate between a cyst and a solid tumor
- To monitor the size of the thyroid gland during suppressive therapy

Patient preparation
- Describe the procedure to the patient, and explain that this test defines the size and shape of the thyroid gland.
- Inform him that he needn't restrict food or fluids before the test.
- Tell him who will perform the procedure and where, that it takes approximately 30 minutes, that it's painless and safe, and that test results are usually available within 24 hours.

Procedure and posttest care
- The patient is placed in a supine position, with a pillow under his shoulder blades to hyperextend his neck.
- His neck is coated with water-soluble conductive gel, and scanning proceeds.
- The image on the monitor is photographed for subsequent examination.
- Accurate visualization of the anterior portion of the thyroid requires use of a short-focused transducer.
- Thoroughly clean the patient's neck to remove the conductive gel.

Normal findings
Normally, thyroid ultrasonography exhibits a uniform echo pattern throughout the gland.

Abnormal findings
Cysts appear as smooth-bordered, echo-free areas with enhanced sound transmission; adenomas and carcinomas appear either solid and well demarcated with identical echo patterns or, less frequently, solid with cystic areas. Carcinoma infiltrating the gland may not be well demarcated.

Identification of a tumor is generally followed up by fine needle aspiration or an excisional biopsy to determine malignancy.

Interfering factors
- None significant

PELVIC ULTRASONOGRAPHY

In pelvic ultrasonography, high-frequency sound waves are reflected to a transducer to provide images of the interior pelvic area on a monitor. Techniques of sound imaging include A-mode (amplitude modulation, recorded as spikes), B-mode (brightness modulation), gray scale (a representation of organ texture in shades of gray), and real-time imaging (instantaneous images of the tissues in motion, similar to fluoroscopic examination). Selected views may be photographed for later examination and a permanent record of the test.

Purpose
- To evaluate symptoms that suggest pelvic disease and to confirm tentative diagnosis
- To detect foreign bodies and distinguish between cystic and solid masses (tumors)
- To measure organ size
- To evaluate fetal viability, position, gestational age, and growth rate
- To detect multiple pregnancy
- To confirm fetal abnormalities and maternal abnormalities
- To guide amniocentesis by determining placental location and fetal position

Patient preparation
- Describe the test to the patient, and tell her the reason it's being performed.
- Assure her that this procedure is safe, noninvasive, and painless.
- Because this test requires a full bladder as a landmark to define pelvic organs, instruct the patient to drink liquids and not to void before the test.

• Tell her who will perform the procedure and where and that it can vary in length from a few minutes to several hours.

• Explain that a water enema may be necessary to produce a better outline of the large intestine.

• Explain that sometimes a transvaginal sonogram may be performed to enhance visualization of pelvic structures.

• Reassure the patient that the test won't harm the fetus, and provide emotional support throughout.

Procedure and posttest care

• With the patient in a supine position, the pelvic area is coated with mineral oil or water-soluble conductive gel to increase sound wave conduction.

• The transducer is guided over the area, images are observed on the monitor, and good images are photographed.

• Remove the conductive gel from the patient's skin.

• Allow the patient to immediately empty her bladder after the test.

Normal findings

The uterus is normal in size and shape. The ovaries' size, shape, and sonographic density are normal. No other masses are visible. If the patient is pregnant, the gestational sac and fetus are of normal size in relation to gestational age.

Abnormal findings

Both cystic and solid masses have homogeneous densities, but solid masses (such as fibroids) appear more dense. Inappropriate fetal size may indicate miscalculated conception or delivery date, fetal anomalies, or a dead fetus. Abnormal echo patterns may indicate foreign bodies (such as an intrauterine device), multiple pregnancy, maternal abnormalities (such as placenta previa

or abruptio placentae), fetal abnormalities (such as molar pregnancy or abnormalities of the arms and legs, spine, heart, head, kidneys, and abdomen), fetal malpresentation (such as breech or shoulder presentation), and cephalopelvic disproportion.

Interfering factors

• Failure to fill the bladder, obesity, or fetal head deep in the pelvis (possible poor imaging)

RENAL ULTRASONOGRAPHY

In renal ultrasonography, high-frequency sound waves are transmitted from a transducer to the kidneys and perirenal structures. The resulting echoes are displayed on a monitor as anatomic images.

Renal ultrasonography can be used to detect abnormalities or clarify those detected by other tests. It's especially useful in cases in which excretory urography is ruled out. Unlike excretory urography, this test isn't dependent on renal function and therefore may be useful in patients with renal failure. Ultrasonography of the ureter, bladder, and gonads also may be used to evaluate urologic disorders.

Purpose

• To determine the size, shape, and position of the kidneys, their internal structures, and perirenal tissues

• To evaluate and localize urinary obstruction and abnormal fluid accumulation

• To assess and diagnose complications after kidney transplantation

Patient preparation

• Explain to the patient that this test is used to detect kidney abnormalities.
• Inform him that he needn't restrict food or fluids before the test.
• Tell him who will perform the test and where, that it takes about 30 minutes, and that it's safe and painless.

Procedure and posttest care

• The patient is placed in prone position, the area to be scanned is exposed, and conductive gel is applied to the area.
• The longitudinal axis of the kidneys is located by using measurements from excretory urography or by performing transverse scans through the upper and lower renal poles.
• These points are marked on the skin and connected with straight lines. Sectional images ⅜″ to ¾″ (1 to 2 cm) apart can then be obtained.
• During the test, the patient may be asked to breathe deeply to assess the kidneys' movement during respiration.
• Remove the conductive gel from the patient's skin.

Normal findings

The kidneys are located between the superior iliac crests and the diaphragm. The renal capsule should be outlined sharply; the cortex should produce more echoes than the medulla. In the center of each kidney, the renal collecting systems appear as irregular areas of higher density than surrounding tissue. The renal veins and, depending on the scanner, some internal structures can be visualized. If the bladder is also being evaluated, its size, shape, position, and urine content can be determined.

Abnormal findings

Cysts are usually fluid-filled, circular structures that don't reflect sound waves. Tumors produce multiple echoes and appear as irregular shapes. Abscesses found within or around the kidneys usually echo sound waves poorly; their boundaries are slightly more irregular than those of cysts. A perirenal abscess may displace the kidney anteriorly.

Generally, acute pyelonephritis and glomerulonephritis aren't detectable unless the renal parenchyma is significantly scarred and atrophied. In such patients, the renal capsule appears irregular and the kidney may appear smaller than normal; also, an increased number of echoes may arise from the parenchyma due to fibrosis.

In patients with hydronephrosis, renal ultrasonography may show a large, echo-free, central mass that compresses the renal cortex. Calyceal echoes are usually circularly diffused and the pelvis significantly enlarged. This test can also be used to detect congenital anomalies, such as horseshoe, ectopic, or duplicated kidneys. Ultrasonography clearly detects renal hypertrophy.

Following renal transplantation, compensatory hypertrophy of the transplanted kidney is normal but an acute increase in size indicates rejection.

This test allows identification of abnormal accumulations of fluid within or around the kidneys that sometimes arise from an obstruction. It also allows evaluation of perirenal structures and can identify abnormalities of the adrenal glands, such as tumors, cysts, and adrenal dysfunction. However, a normal adrenal gland is difficult to define ultrasonically because of its small size.

Renal ultrasonography can be used to detect changes in the shape of the bladder that result from masses and can assess urine volume. Increased urine volume or residual urine postvoiding may indicate bladder outlet obstruction.

Interfering factors
• Retained barium from a previous test (possible poor imaging)
• Obese patient (possible poor imaging)

TRANSCRANIAL DOPPLER STUDIES

Transcranial Doppler studies provide information about the presence, quality, and changing nature of circulation to an area of the brain by measuring the velocity of blood flow through cerebral arteries. Narrowed blood vessels produce high velocities, indicating possible stenosis or vasospasm. High velocities may also indicate an arteriovenous malformation.

Purpose
• To measure the velocity of blood flow through certain cerebral vessels
• To detect and monitor the progression of cerebral vasospasm
• To determine whether collateral blood flow exists before surgical ligation or radiologic occlusion of diseased vessels
• To help determine brain death

Patient preparation
• Explain the purpose of the study to the patient (or to his family).
• Tell him that the test will be done while he lies on a bed or stretcher or sits in a reclining chair (or it can be performed at the bedside if he's too ill to be moved to the laboratory).
• Describe the procedure and tell the patient that it usually takes less than 1 hour, depending on the number of vessels to be examined and any interfering factors (in a complete study, the middle cerebral arteries, anterior cerebral arteries, posterior cerebral arteries, ophthalmic arteries, carotid siphon, vertebral arteries, and basilar artery are studied).
• Tell the patient that fasting isn't required before the test.

Equipment
Transcranial Doppler unit, probe, conductive gel

Procedure and posttest care
• The patient reclines in a chair or on a stretcher or bed.
• A small amount of conductive gel is applied to the transcranial window (an area where bone is thin enough to allow the Doppler signal to enter and be detected); the most common approaches are temporal, transorbital, and through the foramen magnum.
• The technician directs the signal toward the artery being studied and records the velocities detected; waveforms may be printed for later analysis.
• The Doppler signal can be transmitted to varying depths.
• When the study is completed, wipe away the conductive gel.

Precautions
• Be sure to remove turban head dressings or thick dressings over the test site.

Normal findings
The type of waveforms and velocities obtained indicate whether or not pathology exists.

Abnormal findings
Although this test often isn't definitive, high velocities are typically abnormal and suggest that blood flow is too turbulent or the vessel is too narrow.

After the transcranial Doppler study and before surgery, the patient may undergo cerebral angiography to further define cerebral blood flow patterns and locate the exact vascular abnormality.

Interfering factor
• Failure to remove dressings over the test site (possible poor imaging)

VAGINAL ULTRASONOGRAPHY

In vaginal ultrasonography, a probe inserted into the vagina reflects high-frequency sound waves to a transducer, forming an image of the pelvic structures. This study allows better evaluation of pelvic anatomy and earlier diagnosis of pregnancy. It also circumvents the poor visualization encountered with obese patients.

Purpose
• To establish pregnancy with fetal heart motion as early as the 5th to 6th week of gestation
• To determine ectopic pregnancy
• To evaluate abnormal pregnancy
• To diagnose fetal abnormalities and placental location
• To visualize retained products of conception
• To evaluate adnexal pathology, such as tubo-ovarian abscess, hydrosalpinx, and ovarian masses
• To evaluate the uterine lining (in cases of dysfunctional uterine bleeding and postmenopausal bleeding)
• To monitor follicular growth during infertility treatment

Patient preparation
• Describe the procedure to the patient, and explain the reason for the test.

• Assure her that the procedure is safe.

Procedure and posttest care
• The patient is placed in the lithotomy position. If the sonographer is a male, a female assistant should be present during the examination.
• Water-soluble conductive gel is placed on the transducer tip to allow better sound transmission, and a protective sheath is placed over the transducer.
• Place more lubricant on the sheathed transducer tip to allow for its gentle insertion into the vagina by the patient or the sonographer. Allowing the patient to introduce the probe may decrease her anxiety.
• To observe the pelvic structures, rotate the probe 90 degrees to one side and then the other.

Normal findings
If the patient is not pregnant, the uterus and ovaries are normal in size and shape. If the patient is pregnant, the gestational sac and fetus are of normal size for the gestational dates.

Abnormal findings
Vaginal ultrasonography may reveal an empty uterus, if the patient was pregnant. Free peritoneal fluid may be visible in the pelvic cavity, indicating possible peritonitis. Ectopic pregnancies may also be visible in the pelvic cavity.

Interfering factors
• Mistaking the bowel for the ovaries
• Small tubal mass (possible difficulty in detecting ectopic pregnancies)
• Patient positioning (decreased visibility of structures)

CHAPTER 12

Radiography

NEUROLOGIC SYSTEM   539

539   Skull radiography   542   Myelography
540   Cerebral angiography

EYE   545

545   Orbital radiography   546   Fluorescein angiography

RESPIRATORY SYSTEM   548

548   Chest radiography   554   Chest tomography
551   Paranasal sinus radiography   555   Bronchography
553   Fluoroscopy   557   Pulmonary angiography

CARDIOVASCULAR SYSTEM   558

558   Cardiac radiography   560   Lower limb venography

GASTROINTESTINAL SYSTEM   562

562   Barium swallow   576   Postoperative cholangiography
564   Upper GI and small-bowel series 577   Endoscopic retrograde
567   Barium enema   cholangiopancreatography
570   Hypotonic duodenography   580   Celiac and mesenteric
572   Oral cholecystography   arteriography
574   Percutaneous transhepatic
      cholangiography

GENITOURINARY SYSTEM   583

583   Kidney-ureter-bladder   592   Antegrade pyelography
      radiography   594   Excretory urography
584   Nephrotomography   596   Renal angiography
587   Retrograde urethrography   598   Renal venography
588   Retrograde cystography   601   Voiding cystourethrography
590   Retrograde ureteropyelography 602   Whitaker test

REPRODUCTIVE SYSTEM 604

604 Mammography
606 Hysterosalpingography

SKELETAL SYSTEM 607

607 Vertebral radiography
608 Bone densitometry
609 Arthrography

MISCELLANEOUS TESTS 611

611 Lymphangiography

NEUROLOGIC SYSTEM

SKULL RADIOGRAPHY

Although skull radiography is of limited value in assessing patients with head injuries, skull X-rays are extremely valuable for studying abnormalities of the base of the skull and the cranial vault, congenital and perinatal anomalies, and systemic diseases that produce bone defects of the skull. For more accurate assessment of head injuries as well as of skull and head abnormalities, nonenhanced computed tomography studies of the head are done.

Skull radiography evaluates the three groups of bones that comprise the skull: the calvaria (vault), the mandible (jaw bone), and the facial bones. The calvaria and the facial bones are closely connected by immovable joints with irregular serrated edges called sutures. The bones of the skull form an anatomic structure so complex that a complete skull examination requires several radiologic views of each area.

Purpose

• To detect fractures in patients with head trauma
• To aid diagnosis of pituitary tumors
• To detect congenital anomalies

Patient preparation

• Explain to the patient that his head will be immobilized and that several X-rays of his skull will be taken from various angles.
• Tell him that this test helps determine the presence of fractures, tumors, or other anomalies.

• Explain that a radiologic technician will perform the test. Describe where it will take place (usually the radiology department).
• Explain that he needn't restrict food or fluid before the test.
• Tell him to remove glasses, dentures, jewelry, or any metal objects that would be in the X-ray field.

Procedure and posttest care

• Have the patient recline on the X-ray table or sit in a chair.
• Tell him to remain still during the procedure.
• Use foam pads, sandbags, or a headband to immobilize the patient's head and increase comfort.
• Five views of the skull are routinely taken: left and right lateral, anteroposterior Townes, posteroanterior Caldwell, and axial (or base).
• Films are developed and checked for quality before the patient leaves the area.

Normal findings

A radiologist interprets the X-rays, evaluating the size, shape, thickness, and position of the cranial bones as well as the vascular markings, sinuses, and sutures. All should be normal for the patient's age.

Abnormal findings

Skull radiography is often used to diagnose fractures of the vault or base, although basilar fractures may not show on the film if the bone is dense. This test may confirm congenital anomalies and may show erosion, enlargement, or decalcification of the sella turcica that result from increased intracranial pressure (ICP). A marked rise in ICP may cause the brain to expand and press against the inner bony table of the skull, yielding visible marks or impressions.

In conditions such as osteomyelitis (with possible calcification of the skull itself) and chronic subdural hematomas, X-rays may show abnormal areas of calcification. The X-rays can detect neoplasms within brain substance that contains calcium (such as oligodendrogliomas or meningiomas) or the midline shifting of a calcified pineal gland caused by a space-occupying lesion.

Radiography may also detect other changes in bone structure, for example, those that arise from metabolic disorders such as acromegaly or Paget's disease.

Interfering factors
● Improper positioning of the patient and excessive head movement (possible poor imaging)
● Failure to remove radiopaque objects from the X-ray field (possible poor imaging)

CEREBRAL ANGIOGRAPHY

Cerebral angiography involves injecting a contrast medium to allow radiographic examination of the cerebral vasculature. Possible injection sites include the femoral, carotid, and brachial arteries. Because it allows visualization of four vessels (the carotid and the vertebral arteries), the femoral artery is used most often.

Usually, this test is performed on patients with suspected abnormality of the cerebral vasculature; abnormalities may be suggested by intracranial computed tomography or lumbar puncture.

Purpose
● To detect cerebrovascular abnormalities such as aneurysm or arteriovenous malformation, thrombosis, narrowing, or occlusion
● To study vascular displacement caused by tumor, hematoma, edema, herniation, vasospasm, increased intracranial pressure (ICP), or hydrocephalus
● To locate clips applied to blood vessels during surgery and to evaluate the postoperative status of affected vessels

Patient preparation
● Explain to the patient that this test shows blood circulation in the brain.
● Describe the test, including who will administer it, where it'll take place, and its duration (usually 2 to 4 hours, depending on the tests ordered).
● Tell the patient to fast for 8 to 10 hours before the test.
● Explain that he'll wear a gown and that he must remove all jewelry, dentures, hairpins, and other radiopaque objects before the test.
● If appropriate, administer a sedative and an anticholinergic drug 30 to 45 minutes before the test.
● Make sure the patient voids before leaving his room. Keep in mind that the patient may benefit from an indwelling urinary catheter.
● Tell him that he'll be positioned on an X-ray table, with his head immobilized, and that he should remain still when told.
● Explain that a local anesthetic will be administered at the angiocatheter insertion site (some patients — especially children — receive a general anesthetic).
● Describe possible adverse effects associated with the contrast medium, such as a transient burning sensation as the medium is injected; a warm, flushed feeling; transient headache; a salty or metallic taste in his mouth; or

nausea and vomiting after the dye is injected.

• Make sure a consent form has been signed, if required.

CLINICAL ALERT Check the patient's history for hypersensitivity to iodine, iodine-containing substances (such as shellfish), or other contrast media. Note any hypersensitivities on his chart and report them as appropriate.

Equipment
Contrast medium, automatic contrast injector, arterial needles (18G or 19G, 2½″ needle for adults; 20G, 1½″ needle for children), femoral arterial catheters for femoral injection

Procedure and posttest care
• Have the patient recline on an X-ray table, and instruct him to lie still with his arms at his sides.

• Shave the injection site (femoral, carotid, or brachial artery) and clean it with alcohol and povidone-iodine.

• A local anesthetic is injected. Then the artery is punctured with the appropriate needle and catheterized.

• *In the femoral artery approach,* a catheter is threaded to the aortic arch.

• *In the carotid artery approach,* the patient's neck is hyperextended, a rolled towel or sandbag is placed under his shoulders, and his head is immobilized with a restraint or tape.

• *In the brachial artery approach* (least common), a blood pressure cuff is placed distal to the puncture site and inflated before injection to prevent the contrast medium from flowing into the forearm and hand.

• After X-rays or fluoroscopy verifies placement of the needle or catheter, the contrast medium is injected. Observe the patient for a reaction, such as hives, flushing, or laryngeal stridor.

• An initial series of lateral and anteroposterior X-rays is taken, developed, and reviewed. Depending on the results, more contrast medium may be injected and another series taken.

• During the test, maintain arterial catheter patency by continuous or periodic flushing. Monitor vital and neurologic signs.

• When a satisfactory series of X-rays is obtained, the needle (or catheter) is withdrawn. Apply firm pressure to the puncture site for 15 minutes.

• After the test, observe the patient for bleeding, check distal pulses, and apply a pressure bandage.

• Typically, the patient will be on bed rest for 12 to 24 hours. Administer prescribed pain medications and monitor his vital signs and neurologic status for 24 hours (hourly for the first 4 hours, and then every 4 hours).

• Observe the puncture site for signs of extravasation (redness, swelling) and apply an ice bag to ease the patient's discomfort and minimize swelling. If bleeding occurs, apply firm pressure to the puncture site and inform the doctor.

• If the femoral approach was used, keep the affected leg straight for 12 hours or longer and routinely check pulses distal to the site (dorsalis pedis, popliteal). Monitor the leg for temperature, color, and sensation. Thrombosis or hematoma can occlude blood flow; extravasation can also impede the flow of blood by exerting pressure on the artery.

• If the carotid artery was used, monitor the patient for dysphagia or respiratory distress possibly resulting from hematoma or extravasation.

• Monitor for disorientation and weakness or numbness in the extremities (signs of thrombosis or hematoma) and for arterial spasms, which may produce symptoms of transient ischemic attacks.

• If the brachial approach was used, immobilize the affected arm for

6 hours or longer and routinely check the radial pulse.

• Place a sign near the patient's bed warning personnel not to take blood pressure readings from the affected arm.

• Observe the arm and hand for any changes in color, temperature, or sensation. If they become pale, cool, or numb, report these changes at once.

• After the test, tell the patient he may resume his usual diet. Encourage him to drink fluids to help him pass the contrast dye.

Precautions

• Cerebral angiography is contraindicated in patients with hepatic, renal, or thyroid disease.

• This test is also contraindicated in patients with hypersensitivity to iodine or contrast media.

• If the patient has been receiving aspirin or other anticoagulants daily, take extra care when compressing the puncture site.

CLINICAL ALERT Monitor the catheter puncture site frequently and closely for hemorrhage or hematoma formation. If either occurs, notify the doctor immediately.

Normal findings

During the arterial phase of perfusion, the contrast medium fills and opacifies superficial and deep arteries and arterioles; it opacifies superficial and deep veins during the venous phase. The finding of apparently normal (symmetrical) cerebral vasculature must be correlated with the patient's history and clinical status.

Abnormal findings

Changes in the caliber of vessel lumina suggest vascular disease, possibly due to spasms, plaques, fistulas, arteriovenous malformation, or arteriosclerosis.

Diminished blood flow to vessels may be related to increased ICP.

Vessel displacement may reflect the presence and size of a tumor, areas of edema, or obstruction of the cerebrospinal fluid pathway. Cerebral angiography may also show circulation within a tumor, often giving precise information on the tumor's position and nature. Meningeal blood supply originating in the external carotid artery may indicate an extracerebral tumor but usually designates a meningioma. Such a tumor may arise outside the brain substance, but it may still be within the cerebral hemisphere.

Interfering factors

• Head movement during the test (possible poor imaging)

• Failure to remove metal objects from the X-ray field (possible poor imaging)

MYELOGRAPHY

Myelography uses fluoroscopy and radiography to evaluate the spinal subarachnoid space after injection of a contrast medium. Because the contrast medium is heavier than cerebrospinal fluid (CSF), it flows through the subarachnoid space to the dependent area when the patient, lying prone on a fluoroscopic table, is tilted up or down. The fluoroscope allows the doctor to see the flow of the contrast medium and the outline of the subarachnoid space. X-rays are taken to provide a permanent record. If not contraindicated, magnetic resonance imaging (MRI) of the spine provides more detailed imaging of the subarachnoid space.

Purpose

- To identify lesions, such as tumors and herniated intervertebral disks, that partially or totally block the flow of CSF in the subarachnoid space
- To help detect arachnoiditis, spinal nerve root injury, or tumors in the posterior fossa of the skull

Patient preparation

- Explain to the patient that this test reveals obstructions in the spinal cord.
- Tell him that his food and fluid intake will be restricted for 8 hours before the test. If the test is scheduled for the afternoon, and facility policy permits, the patient may have clear liquids before the test.
- Describe the test, including who will administer it, where it will take place, and its duration (1 hour or more).
- Describe likely adverse effects, such as a transient burning sensation as the contrast medium is injected; a warm, flushed feeling; transient headache; a salty taste; or nausea and vomiting after the dye is injected. Explain that he may feel some pain caused by his positioning, needle insertion and, in some cases, removal of the contrast medium.
- Make sure the patient or a responsible family member has signed the appropriate consent form.

 CLINICAL ALERT Check the patient's history for hypersensitivity to iodine and iodine-containing substances (for example, shellfish), radiographic contrast media, and associated medications. Notify the radiologist if the patient has a history of epilepsy or phenothiazine use. If metrizamide is to be used as a contrast medium, discontinue phenothiazine 48 hours before the test.

- Tell the patient to remove jewelry, metal, or other radiopaque material before the test.

- Perform pretest procedures and administer prescribed medications. For example, a cleansing enema may be prescribed, and a sedative and anticholinergic (such as atropine sulfate) may be prescribed to reduce swallowing during the procedure.

Equipment

Alcohol, 1% lidocaine solution, lumbar puncture tray, contrast medium (iophendylate or metrizamide sodium), two 10-ml syringes, spinal needle (18G for iophendylate or 11G for metrizamide), povidone-iodine solution, sterile gloves, small adhesive bandage

Procedure and posttest care

- Computed tomography of the head may be obtained before the procedure to check for increased intracranial pressure.
- Position the patient on his side at the edge of the table, with his chin on his chest and knees drawn up to his abdomen. (If the patient has lumbar deformity or infection at the puncture site, cisternal puncture may be done.)
- After the lumbar puncture is performed, the fluoroscope is used to verify proper positioning of the needle in the subarachnoid space. Some CSF may be removed for routine laboratory analysis.
- Turn the patient to the prone position and secure him with straps across his upper back, under his arms, and across his ankles. Hyperextend his chin to prevent contrast medium from flowing into the cranium; place a towel or sponge under his chin for comfort.
- If the patient complains of a headache or trouble swallowing or reports that he's not breathing deeply enough, provide reassurance and explain that he'll be able to rest periodically during the procedure.

• The contrast medium is injected and the table tilted so that the dye flows through the subarachnoid space. (In rare circumstances, air is used as a negative contrast medium; however, this is typically reserved for patients with suspected congenital abnormalities, such as syringomyelia.)

• The flow of the contrast medium is observed by fluoroscope and X-rays are taken. If an obstruction in the subarachnoid space blocks the upward flow of the contrast medium, a cisternal puncture may be performed.

• The contrast medium is withdrawn, if necessary, after satisfactory X-rays are obtained, and the needle is removed. Clean the puncture site with povidone-iodine solution, and apply a small adhesive bandage.

• Based on the contrast medium used during the test, position the patient as follows: If metrizamide was used, tell him to stay in bed for the next 12 to 16 hours. Keep the head of his bed elevated for the first 6 to 8 hours. If an oil-based contrast medium was used, tell him to remain flat in bed for 6 to 24 hours.

• Monitor vital signs and neurologic status at least every 30 minutes for the first 4 hours, then every 4 hours for 24 hours.

• Encourage the patient to drink extra fluids. He should void within 8 hours after returning to his room.

• If there are no complications or adverse reactions, tell the patient that he may resume his usual diet and activities the day after the test.

• Monitor for radicular pain, fever, back pain, or signs of meningeal irritation, such as headache, irritability, or stiff neck. If these signs or symptoms occur, keep the room quiet and dark and administer an analgesic or antipyretic as needed.

Precautions

• Generally, myelography is contraindicated for patients with increased intracranial pressure, hypersensitivity to iodine or contrast media, or infection at the puncture site.

• Improper positioning after the test may affect recovery.

Normal findings

Normally, the contrast medium flows freely through the subarachnoid space, showing no obstruction or structural abnormalities.

Abnormal findings

Myelography can identify and localize lesions within or surrounding the spinal cord or subarachnoid space. Examples of common extradural lesions include herniated intervertebral disks and metastatic tumors. Neurofibromas and meningiomas are common lesions within the subarachnoid space, and ependymomas and astrocytomas are common within the spinal cord.

If the test confirms a spinal tumor, the patient may be taken directly to the operating room. Immediate surgery also may be necessary if the contrast medium causes a total block of the subarachnoid space.

Myelography may help locate or confirm a ruptured disk, spinal stenosis, or abscess and, occasionally, confirm the need for surgery. This test may also detect syringomyelia (a congenital abnormality marked by fluid-filled cavities within the spinal cord and widening of the cord itself), arachnoiditis, spinal nerve root injury, and tumors in the posterior fossa of the skull. Test results must be correlated with the patient's history and clinical status.

Interfering factors
- Incorrect needle placement
- Uncooperative patient

EYE

ORBITAL RADIOGRAPHY

Orbital radiography evaluates the orbit, the bony cavity that houses the eye and the lacrimal glands, as well as blood vessels, nerves, muscles, and fat. Because portions of the orbit are composed of thin bone that fractures easily, X-rays are commonly taken following facial trauma. They are also useful in diagnosing ocular and orbital pathologies. Special radiographic techniques can reveal foreign bodies in the orbit or eye that are invisible to an ophthalmoscope. In some cases, radiography is used in conjunction with computed tomography (CT) scans and ultrasonography to better define an abnormality.

Purpose
- To aid in diagnosis of orbital fractures and pathologies
- To help locate intraorbital or intraocular foreign bodies

Patient preparation
- Explain that this test involves taking several X-rays to assess the condition of the bones around the eye.
- Describe the test, including who will perform it, where it will be performed, and the expected duration (about 15 minutes).
- Reassure the patient that the procedure is usually painless unless he has suffered facial trauma, in which case positioning may cause some discomfort. Explain that he'll be asked to turn his head from side to side and to flex or extend his neck.
- Instruct him to remove all metal objects, jewelry, and other radiopaque materials from the X-ray field.

Procedure and posttest care
- Have the patient recline on the X-ray table or sit in a chair.
- Instruct him to remain still while the X-rays are taken.
- Usually, a series of orbital X-rays includes a lateral view, posteroanterior view, submentovertical (base) view, stereo Waters' views (views from both sides), Towne's (half-axial) projection, and optic canal projections. If enlargement of the superior orbital fissure is suspected, apical views are obtained.
- The films are developed and inspected before the patient leaves the radiography department.

Normal findings
Each orbit is composed of a roof, a floor, and medial and lateral walls. The bones of the roof and floor are very thin (the floor can be less than 1-mm thick). The medial walls, which parallel each other, are slightly thicker, except for the portion formed by the ethmoid bone. The lateral walls are the thickest part of the orbit and are strongest at the orbital rim.

The superior orbital fissure, at the back of the orbit between the lateral wall and the roof, is actually a gap between the greater and lesser wings of the sphenoid bone. The optic canal, which carries the optic nerve and ophthalmic artery, is an opening in the lesser wing of the sphenoid bone located at the apex of the orbit.

Abnormal findings
Orbital fractures associated with facial trauma are most common in the thin

structures of the floor and ethmoid bone. Abnormalities are detected by comparing the size and shape of orbital structures on the affected side with those on the opposite side.

Generally, orbit enlargement indicates the presence of a lesion that has caused proptosis due to increased intraorbital pressure. Any growing tumor can produce these changes. Superior orbital fissure enlargement can result from orbital meningioma, from intracranial conditions such as pituitary tumors or, more characteristically, from vascular anomalies. Optic canal enlargement may result from extraocular extension of a retinoblastoma or, in children, from an optic nerve glioma. In adults, only prolonged pathology can increase orbital size; however, in children, even a rapidly growing lesion can cause orbital enlargement because orbital bones are not fully developed. A decrease in the size of the orbit may follow childhood enucleation of the eye or conditions such as congenital microphthalmia.

Destruction of the orbital walls may indicate a malignant neoplasm or an infection. A benign tumor or cyst produces a clear-cut local indentation of the orbital wall. Lesions of adjacent structures may also produce radiographic changes due to enlargement and erosion of the orbit.

Increased bone density may be seen in conditions such as osteoblastic metastasis, sphenoid ridge meningioma, or Paget's disease. To confirm orbital pathology, however, radiographic findings must be supplemented with results from other appropriate tests and procedures.

Interfering factors
• None significant

FLUORESCEIN ANGIOGRAPHY

In fluorescein angiography, a special camera takes rapid-sequence photographs of the fundus following I.V. injection of sodium fluorescein (a contrast medium), thereby recording the appearance of blood vessels within the eye. This technique provides enhanced visibility of the microvascular structures of the retina and choroid, which permits evaluation of the entire retinal vascular bed, including retinal circulation.

Purpose
• To document retinal circulation when evaluating intraocular abnormalities, such as retinopathy, tumors, and circulatory or inflammatory disorders

Patient preparation
• Explain that this procedure takes about 30 minutes and evaluates the small blood vessels in the eyes.
• Make sure the patient or an appropriate family member has signed a consent form.
• Check the patient's history for glaucoma and hypersensitivity reactions, especially to contrast media and dilating eyedrops. If necessary, tell a patient with glaucoma not to use miotic eyedrops on the day of the test.
• Explain that eyedrops will be instilled to dilate his pupils and that a dye will be injected into his arm. Tell him that his eyes will be photographed with a special camera before and after the injection. Stress that these are photographs, not X-rays.
• Warn him that his skin and urine may appear yellow for 24 to 48 hours after the procedure.

Equipment

Fundus camera and film, mydriatic eyedrops, alcohol swabs, tourniquet, 21G scalp-vein needle, 5- to 10-ml syringe, 2 ml of 25% sodium fluorescein or 5 ml of 10% sodium fluorescein, small sterile dressing, emesis basin, emergency resuscitation kit

Procedure and posttest care

• Administer mydriatic eyedrops. Usually, two instillations are necessary to achieve maximum mydriasis within 15 to 40 minutes.

• Following mydriasis, seat the patient comfortably in the examining chair, facing the camera.

• Have him loosen or remove any restrictive clothing around his neck.

• Tell the patient to place his chin in the chin rest and his forehead against the bar. Tell him to open his eyes wide and stare straight ahead, while keeping his teeth together and maintaining normal breathing and blinking.

• The antecubital vein is prepared and punctured; however, dye isn't injected yet. At this time, a few photographs may be taken. Make sure the patient keeps his arm extended; if necessary, use an arm board.

• Warn the patient that the dye will be injected rapidly. Remind him to maintain his position and to continue to stare straight ahead. Then, inject the dye.

• The patient may experience nausea and a feeling of warmth. Provide reassurance and observe for hypersensitivity reactions, such as vomiting, dry mouth, metallic taste, suddenly increased salivation, sneezing, lightheadedness, fainting, or hives. In rare instances, anaphylactic shock may occur.

• As the dye is injected, 25 to 30 photographs are taken in rapid sequence.

Each photograph is taken 1 second after the other.

• The needle and syringe are removed carefully; pressure and a dressing are applied to the injection site.

• If late-phase photographs are needed, tell the patient to sit and relax for 20 minutes, then reposition him for 5 to 10 photographs. If necessary, photographs may be taken up to 1 hour after the injection.

• Remind the patient that his skin and urine will be slightly discolored for 24 to 48 hours after the test.

• Explain that his near vision will be blurred for up to 12 hours and that he should avoid direct sunlight and refrain from driving during this time.

Precautions

• Don't leave the patient unattended. He may experience mild adverse reactions, such as nausea, vomiting, sneezing, paresthesia of the tongue, and dizziness.

CLINICAL ALERT Have emergency resuscitation equipment at hand. Serious adverse effects (laryngeal edema, bronchospasm, and respiratory arrest) are possible. If a reaction occurs, note it on the patient's allergy history.

• The needle must be placed in the vein correctly; extravasation of dye around the injection site is painful.

Normal findings

After rapid injection into the antecubital vein, sodium fluorescein reaches the retina in 12 to 15 seconds (filling phase). As the choroidal vessels and choriocapillaries fill, the background of the retina fluoresces, taking on an evenly mottled appearance known as the choroidal flush. Then the dye fills the arteries (arterial phase). The arteriovenous phase lasts from the complete filling of the arteries and capillaries to the earliest evidence of dye in the veins. The time the arteries begin to empty to the time the veins fill and empty is known as the venous phase. Finally, the recirculation phase occurs 30 to 60 minutes after the injection, when the fluorescein — if at all present — is barely detectable in the retinal vessels. Normally, there is no leakage from the retinal vessels.

Abnormal findings

The varying and complex findings after fluorescein angiography require interpretation by a highly skilled ophthalmologist with extensive experience in the diagnosis of retinal disorders.

Abnormalities detected in the early filling phase may include microaneurysms, arteriovenous shunts, and neovascularization. The test may identify arterial occlusion by showing delayed or absent flow of the dye through the arteries, stenosis, and prolonged venous drainage. Venous occlusion may be associated with dilation of the vessels and fluorescein leakage. Chronic obstruction may produce recanalization and collateral circulation.

In hypertensive retinopathy, abnormalities may include areas of increased vascular tortuosity, microaneurysms around zones of capillary nonperfusion, and generalized suffusion of the dye in the retina. Aneurysms and capillary hemangiomas may leak fluorescein and are often surrounded by hard yellow exudate. Tumors exhibit variable fluorescein patterns, depending on histologic type. Retinal edema or inflammation and fibrous tissue may show variable degrees of fluorescence. Papilledema produces vascular leakage in the disk area.

Interfering factors

● Inadequate view of the fundus due to insufficient pupillary dilation (possible poor imaging)

● Cataract, media opacity, or inability to keep eyes open and to maintain fixation (possible poor imaging)

RESPIRATORY SYSTEM

CHEST RADIOGRAPHY

In chest radiography, X-rays or electromagnetic waves penetrate the chest and cause an image to form on specially sensitized film. Normal pulmonary tissue is radiolucent, whereas abnormalities — such as infiltrates, foreign bodies, fluids, and tumors — appear as densities on the film. A chest X-ray is most useful when compared with prior films to detect changes. (See *Selected clinical implications of chest X-ray films.*)

Purpose

● To detect pulmonary disorders, such as pneumonia, atelectasis, pneumothorax, pulmonary bullae, and tumors
● To detect mediastinal abnormalities, such as tumors, and cardiac disease, such as heart failure
● To determine the location and size of a lesion
● To help assess pulmonary status

Patient preparation

● Explain that this test assesses respiratory status.
● Tell the patient he needn't restrict food or fluid before the test.
● Describe the test, including who will perform it, where it will take place, and its expected duration.
● Provide a gown without snaps, and instruct the patient to remove jewelry

SELECTED CLINICAL IMPLICATIONS OF CHEST X-RAY FILMS

NORMAL ANATOMIC LOCATION AND APPEARANCE	POSSIBLE ABNORMALITY	IMPLICATIONS
Trachea		
Visible midline in the anterior mediastinal cavity; translucent tubelike appearance	• Deviation from midline	• Tension pneumothorax, atelectasis, pleural effusion, consolidation, mediastinal nodes or, in children, enlarged thymus
	• Narrowing with hourglass appearance and deviation to one side	• Substernal thyroid
Heart		
Visible in the anterior left mediastinal cavity; solid appearance due to blood contents; edges may be clear in contrast with surrounding air density of the lung	• Large central pulmonary arteries, right ventricular enlargement	• Cor pulmonale
	• Cardiomegaly, increased pulmonary vascular markings, interstitial edema	• Heart failure
Aortic knob		
Visible as water density; formed by the arch of the aorta	• Solid densities, possibly indicating calcifications	• Atherosclerosis
	• Tortuous shape	• Atherosclerosis
Mediastinum (mediastinal shadow)		
Visible as the space between the lungs; shadowy appearance that widens at the hilum of the lungs	• Deviation to nondiseased side; deviation to diseased side by traction	• Pleural effusion or tumor, fibrosis or collapsed lung
	• Gross widening	• Neoplasms of esophagus, bronchi, lungs, thyroid tissue; aortic aneurysm; mediastinitis; cor pulmonale
Ribs		
Visible as thoracic cavity encasement	• Break or misalignment	• Fractured sternum or ribs
	• Widening of intercostal spaces	• Emphysema
Spine		
Visible midline in the posterior chest; straight bony structure	• Spinal curvature	• Scoliosis, kyphosis
	• Break or misalignment	• Fractures

(continued)

SELECTED CLINICAL IMPLICATIONS OF CHEST X-RAY FILMS *(continued)*

NORMAL ANATOMIC LOCATION AND APPEARANCE	POSSIBLE ABNORMALITY	IMPLICATIONS
Clavicles		
Visible in upper thorax; intact and equidistant in properly centered X-ray films	• Break or misalignment	• Fractures
Hila (lung roots)		
Visible above the heart, where pulmonary vessels, bronchi, and lymph nodes join the lungs; appear as small, white, bilateral densities	• Shift to one side, accentuated shadows	• Atelectasis, pneumothorax, emphysema, pulmonary abscess, tumor, enlarged lymph nodes
Mainstem bronchus		
Visible; part of the hila with translucent tubelike appearance	• Spherical or oval density	• Bronchogenic cyst
Bronchi		
Usually not visible	• Visible	• Bronchial pneumonia
Lung fields		
Usually not visible throughout, except for the blood vessels	• Visible • Irregular	• Atelectasis • Resolving pneumonia, infiltrates, silicosis, fibrosis, metastatic neoplasm
Hemidiaphragm		
Rounded, visible; right side ⅜″ to ¾″	• Elevation of diaphragm (difference in elevation can be measured on inspiration and expiration to detect movement) • Flattening of diaphragm • Elevation of left side only	• Active tuberculosis, pneumonia, pleurisy, acute bronchitis, active disease of the abdominal viscera, bilateral phrenic nerve involvement, atelectasis • Asthma, emphysema • Possible unilateral phrenic nerve paresis • Perforated ulcer (rare), gas distention of stomach or splenic flexure of colon, free air in abdomen

and other metal objects that may be in the X-ray field.

• Explain that he'll be asked to take a deep breath and to hold it momentarily while the film is being taken to provide a clearer view of pulmonary structures.

Procedure and posttest care

• If a stationary X-ray machine is used, the patient stands or sits in front of the machine, so films can be taken of the posteroanterior and left lateral views.

• If a portable X-ray machine is used at the patient's bedside, the patient is moved to the top of the bed, if his tolerance permits. The head of the bed is elevated for maximum upright positioning.

• Move cardiac monitoring lead wires, I.V. tubing from central lines, pulmonary artery catheter lines, and safety pins as far from the X-ray field as possible.

Precautions

• Chest radiography is usually contraindicated during the first trimester of pregnancy; however, when radiography is absolutely necessary, a lead apron placed over the patient's abdomen can shield the fetus.

• If the patient is intubated, check that no tubes have been dislodged during positioning.

• To avoid exposure to radiation, leave the room or the immediate area while the films are being taken. If you must stay in the area, wear a lead-lined apron or protective clothing.

Findings

For an overview of normal and abnormal chest radiography findings, see the accompanying chart. For an accurate diagnosis, radiography findings must be correlated with the results of additional radiologic and pulmonary tests as well as physical assessment findings. For example, pulmonary hyperin-

flation with low diaphragm and generalized increased radiolucency may suggest emphysema but may also occur in a healthy person.

Interfering factors

• Portable chest X-rays (possibly lower quality image than stationary X-rays)

• Portable chest X-rays taken in the anteroposterior position (may show larger cardiac shadowing than other X-rays due to shorter distance between beam and anterior structures)

• Patient in supine position (hides fluid levels that are visible in decubitus views)

• Patient's inability to take a full inspiration

• Underexposure or overexposure of films

PARANASAL SINUS RADIOGRAPHY

The paranasal sinuses — air-filled cavities lined with mucous membrane — lie within the maxillary, ethmoid, sphenoid, and frontal bones. Sinus abnormalities resulting from inflammation, trauma, cysts, mucoceles, granulomatosis, and other conditions may include distorted bony sinus walls, altered mucous membranes, and fluid or masses within the cavities. In paranasal sinus radiography, X-rays or electromagnetic waves penetrate the paranasal sinuses and react on specially sensitized film, forming a film image that differentiates sinus structures.

When surrounding facial structures that are superimposed on the paranasal sinuses interfere with visualization of relevant areas, computed tomography scanning may be performed to provide further information.

Abnormal Findings in Paranasal Sinus Radiography

DISORDER	ABNORMAL FINDINGS
Paranasal sinus trauma or fracture	• Edema or hemorrhage in mucous membrane lining or sinus cavity • Clouded sinus air cells • Air-fluid level • Radiolucent, linear bone defects • Irregular, overriding bone edges • Depression or displacement of bone fragments • Foreign bodies
Acute sinusitis	• Swollen, inflamed mucous membrane • Inflammatory exudate • Hazy to opaque sinus air cells • Air-fluid level
Chronic sinusitis	• Thickened mucous membrane • Hazy to opaque sinus air cells • Air-fluid level • Thickening or sclerosis of bony wall of affected sinus
Wegener's granulomatosis	• Clouded to opaque sinus air cells • Destruction of bony sinus wall
Malignant neoplasm	• Rounded or lobulated soft-tissue mass, projecting into sinus • Destruction of bony sinus wall
Benign bone tumor	• Distortion of bony sinus wall in specific patterns
Cyst, polyp, or benign tumor	• Rounded or lobulated soft-tissue mass, projecting into sinus
Mucocele	• Clouded sinus air cells • Destruction of bony sinus wall resulting in various degrees of radiolucency

Purpose
• To detect unilateral or bilateral abnormalities, possibly indicating trauma or disease
• To confirm diagnosis of neoplastic or inflammatory paranasal sinus disease
• To determine the location and size of a malignant neoplasm

Patient preparation
• Explain that this test helps evaluate abnormalities of the paranasal sinuses.

• Describe the test, including who will perform it, where it will take place, and its expected duration (usually 10 to 15 minutes).
• Tell the patient that his head may be immobilized in a foam vise during the test to help him maintain the correct position but that the vise doesn't hurt.
• Explain that he'll be asked to sit upright and avoid moving while the X-rays are being taken to prevent blurring of the image and to allow visualization of air-fluid levels, if present.

Emphasize the importance of his cooperation.

• Instruct him to remove dentures, all jewelry, and metal objects in the X-ray field.

Procedure and posttest care

• Have the patient sit upright (his head may be placed in a foam vise) between the X-ray tube and a film cassette.

• During the test, the X-ray tube is positioned at specific angles, and the patient's head is placed in various standard positions, while his paranasal sinuses are filmed from different angles. If necessary, assist with positioning the patient.

Precautions

• Paranasal sinus radiography is usually contraindicated during pregnancy; however, when it's absolutely necessary, a lead-lined apron placed over the patient's abdomen can shield the fetus.

• To avoid exposure to radiation, leave the room or the immediate area during the test; if you must stay in the area, wear a lead-lined apron.

Normal findings

Normal paranasal sinuses are radiolucent and filled with air, which appears black on films.

Abnormal findings

See *Abnormal findings in paranasal sinus radiography.*

Interfering factors

• Presence of dentures, jewelry, or other metal objects in X-ray field, or presence of numerous metallic foreign bodies around paranasal sinuses (possible poor imaging)

• Patient movement (possible poor imaging)

• Patient unable to sit upright (may require supine position, reducing diagnostic value of test)

• Superimposition of the surrounding facial structures on the film (obscures paranasal sinuses)

FLUOROSCOPY

In fluoroscopy, a continuous stream of X-rays passes through the patient, casting shadows of the heart, lungs, and diaphragm on a fluorescent screen. Because fluoroscopy reveals less detail than standard chest radiography, it's indicated only when diagnosis requires visualization of physiologic or pathologic motion of thoracic contents — for example, to rule out paralysis in patients with diaphragmatic elevation.

Purpose

• To assess lung expansion and contraction during quiet breathing, deep breathing, and coughing

• To assess movement and paralysis of the diaphragm (sniff test)

• To detect bronchial obstructions and pulmonary disease

Patient preparation

• Explain to the patient that this test assesses respiratory structures and their motion.

• Describe the test, including who will perform it, where it will take place, and its expected duration (usually 5 minutes).

• Tell the patient that he'll be asked to follow specific instructions — for example, to breathe deeply and cough — while X-ray images depict his breathing.

• Instruct him to remove all jewelry within the X-ray field.

Procedure and posttest care

• If necessary, assist with positioning the patient.

● Move cardiac monitoring cables, I.V. tubing from subclavian lines, pulmonary artery catheter lines, and safety pins as far from the X-ray field as possible.
● During the test, the patient's cardiopulmonary motion is observed on a screen. Special equipment may be used to intensify the images, or a videotape recording of the fluoroscopy may be made for later study.

Precautions
● Fluoroscopy is contraindicated during pregnancy.
● If the patient is intubated, check that no tubes have been dislodged during positioning.
● To avoid exposure to radiation, leave the room or the immediate area during the test; if you must stay in the area, wear a lead-lined apron.

Normal findings
Normal diaphragmatic movement is synchronous and symmetrical. Normal diaphragmatic excursion ranges from $\frac{3}{4}''$ to $1\frac{5}{8}''$ (2 to 4 cm).

Abnormal findings
Diminished diaphragmatic movement may indicate pulmonary disease. Increased lung translucency may indicate loss of elasticity or bronchial obstruction. In elderly patients, the lowest part of the trachea may be displaced to the right by an elongated aorta.

Diminished or paradoxical diaphragmatic movement may indicate paralysis of the diaphragm; however, fluoroscopy may not detect such paralysis in patients who compensate for diminished diaphragm function by forcefully contracting their abdominal muscles to aid expiration.

Interfering factor
● Failure to remove all metal objects within the X-ray field (possible poor imaging)

CHEST TOMOGRAPHY

Also called laminagraphy, planigraphy, stratigraphy, or body section roentgenography, chest tomography provides clearly focused radiographic images of selected body sections otherwise obscured by shadows of overlying or underlying structures. In this procedure, the X-ray tube and film move around the patient in opposite directions (a motion called the linear tube sweep), producing exposures in which a selected body plane appears sharply defined and the areas above and below it are blurred. Because tomography emits high radiation levels, it's used only for evaluation of chest lesions.

Purpose
● To demonstrate pulmonary densities (for cavitation, calcification, and presence of fat), tumors (especially those obstructing the bronchial lumen), or lesions (especially those located deep within the mediastinum, such as at lymph nodes at the hilum)

Patient preparation
● Explain to the patient that this test helps evaluate lesions inside the chest.
● Describe the test, including who will perform it, where it will take place, and its duration (30 to 60 minutes).
● Tell him that he needn't restrict food or fluids before the test.
● Warn the patient that the equipment is noisy because of rapidly moving metal-on-metal parts and that the X-ray tube swings overhead.

• Advise him to breathe normally during the test but to remain immobile; tell him that foam wedges will be used to help him maintain a comfortable, motionless position.

• Suggest that he close his eyes to prevent involuntary movement.

• Instruct him to remove all jewelry within the X-ray field.

Procedure and posttest care

• The patient is placed in a supine position or in different degrees of lateral rotation on the X-ray table. The X-ray tube then swings over the patient, taking numerous films from different angles.

• For lung tomography, the X-ray tube is usually moved in a linear direction but may be moved in a hypocycloid, circular, elliptic, trispiral, or figure-eight pattern. Multidirectional films aid diagnosis of mediastinal lesions or tumors.

Precautions

• Tomography is contraindicated during pregnancy.

• To avoid exposure to radiation, leave the room or the immediate area during the test; if you must stay in the area, wear a lead-lined apron.

Normal findings

A normal chest tomogram shows structures equivalent to those seen on a normal chest X-ray film.

Abnormal findings

Central calcification in a nodule suggests a benign lesion; an irregularly bordered tumor suggests malignancy; a sharply defined tumor suggests granuloma or nonmalignancy. Evaluation of the hilum can help differentiate blood vessels from nodes, detect tumor extension into the hilar lung area, and identify bronchial dilation, stenosis, and endobronchial lesions. Tomogra-

phy can also identify extension of a mediastinal lesion to the ribs or spine.

Interfering factors

• Failure to remove all metal objects within the X-ray field (possible poor imaging)

• Uncooperative patient

BRONCHOGRAPHY

Bronchography is X-ray examination of the tracheobronchial tree after instillation of a radiopaque iodine contrast agent through a catheter into the lumens of the trachea and bronchi. The contrast agent coats the bronchial tree, permitting visualization of any anatomic deviations. Bronchography of a localized lung area may be accomplished by instilling contrast dye through a fiber-optic bronchoscope placed in the area to be filmed.

Since the development of computed tomography scanning, bronchography is used less frequently. It may be performed using a local anesthetic instilled through the catheter or bronchoscope, although a general anesthetic may be necessary for children or during a concurrent bronchoscopy.

Purpose

• To help detect bronchiectasis, bronchial obstruction, pulmonary tumors, cysts, and cavities and, indirectly, to pinpoint the cause of hemoptysis

• To provide permanent films of pathologic findings

Patient preparation

• Explain to the patient that this test helps evaluate abnormalities of the bronchial structures.

• Instruct the patient to fast for 12 hours before the test.

- Tell him to perform good oral hygiene the night before and the morning of the test.
- Explain who will perform the test, where it will take place, and its expected duration.
- Make sure the patient or a responsible family member has signed a consent form.
- Check the patient's history for hypersensitivity to anesthetics, iodine, or contrast media.
- If the patient has a productive cough, administer a prescribed expectorant and perform postural drainage 1 to 3 days before the test.
- If the procedure is to be performed under a local anesthetic, tell the patient he'll receive a sedative to help him relax and to suppress the gag reflex. Prepare him for the unpleasant taste of the anesthetic spray. Warn him that he may experience some difficulty breathing during the procedure, but reassure him that his airway won't be blocked and that he'll receive enough oxygen. Tell him the catheter or bronchoscope will pass more easily if he relaxes.
- If bronchography is to be performed under a general anesthetic, inform the patient that he'll receive a sedative before the test to help him relax.
- Just before the test, instruct the patient to remove his dentures and to void.

Equipment
Tilting table, sedative, anesthetic, catheter or bronchoscope, radiopaque oils or water-soluble contrast agent, emergency resuscitation equipment

Procedure and posttest care
- After a local anesthetic is sprayed into the patient's mouth and throat, a bronchoscope or catheter is passed into the trachea, and the anesthetic and contrast medium are instilled.

- The patient is placed in various positions during the test to promote movement of the contrast medium into different areas of the bronchial tree. After X-rays are taken, the contrast medium is removed through postural drainage and by having the patient cough it up.

▶ CLINICAL ALERT Watch for signs of laryngeal spasms (dyspnea) or edema (hoarseness, dyspnea, laryngeal stridor) secondary to traumatic intubation.

▶ CLINICAL ALERT Immediately report signs of allergic reaction to the contrast medium or anesthetic, such as itching, dyspnea, tachycardia, palpitations, excitation, hypotension, hypertension, or euphoria.

- Withhold food, fluids, and oral medications until the gag reflex returns (usually in 2 hours). Fluid intake before the gag reflex returns may cause aspiration.
- Encourage gentle coughing and postural drainage to facilitate clearing of the contrast medium. A postdrainage film is usually done in 24 to 48 hours.
- Watch for signs of chemical or secondary bacterial pneumonia — fever, dyspnea, crackles, or rhonchi — the result of incomplete expectoration of the contrast medium.
- If the patient has a sore throat, reassure him that it's only temporary, and provide throat lozenges or a liquid gargle when his gag reflex returns.
- Advise the outpatient not to resume his usual activities until the next day.

Precautions
- Bronchography is contraindicated during pregnancy, in persons with hypersensitivity to iodine or contrast media, and usually in persons with respiratory insufficiency.
- Observe the patient with asthma for laryngeal spasm secondary to the instillation of the contrast medium.

• Observe the patient with chronic obstructive pulmonary disease for airway occlusion secondary to the instillation of the contrast medium.

Normal findings

The right mainstem bronchus is shorter, wider, and more vertical than the left bronchus. Successive branches of the bronchi become smaller in diameter and are free of obstruction or lesions.

Abnormal findings

Bronchography may demonstrate bronchiectasis or bronchial obstruction due to tumors, cysts, cavities, or foreign objects. Findings must be correlated with physical examination, patient history, and perhaps other pulmonary studies.

Interfering factors

• Presence of secretions, inability to suppress coughing, or improper patient positioning (possible poor imaging due to inadequate filling of bronchial tree)

PULMONARY ANGIOGRAPHY

Also called pulmonary arteriography, pulmonary angiography is the radiographic examination of the pulmonary circulation following injection of a radiopaque iodine contrast agent into the pulmonary artery or one of its branches.

Possible complications include arterial occlusion, myocardial perforation or rupture, ventricular arrhythmias from myocardial irritation, and acute renal failure from hypersensitivity to the contrast agent.

Purpose

• To detect pulmonary embolism in a patient who is symptomatic but whose lung scan is indeterminate or normal, especially before anticoagulant therapy or in patients in whom anticoagulant therapy is contraindicated

• To evaluate pulmonary circulation preoperatively in the patient with congenital heart disease

Patient preparation

• Describe the procedure to the patient. Explain that this test permits evaluation of the blood vessels to help identify the cause of his symptoms.

• Instruct him to fast for 8 hours before the test or as prescribed. Tell him who will perform the test and where and that it will take approximately 1 hour.

• Tell the patient a small incision will be made in the right arm where blood samples are usually drawn, or in the right groin, and that a local anesthetic will be used to numb the area. Inform him that a small catheter will then be inserted into the blood vessel and passed into the right side of the heart and then to the pulmonary artery.

• Tell him the contrast agent will then be injected into this artery. Warn him that he may experience an urge to cough, a flushed feeling, nausea, or a salty or metallic taste for approximately 5 minutes after the injection.

• Inform him that his heart rate will be monitored continuously during the procedure.

• Make sure the patient or a responsible family member has signed a consent form. Check the patient's history for hypersensitivity to anesthetics, iodine, seafood, or radiographic contrast agents.

Equipment

50 ml of 60% meglumine diatrizoate or of 45% diatrizoate; 60 ml of thimeros-

al; 60 ml of 70% alcohol; 500 ml of physiologic saline solution; epinephrine for emergency administration; 30 ml of 2% procaine; 3-ml, 6-ml, and 20-ml syringes; two 2½″ 18G needles; polyethylene catheter; extension tubing (Venotube) with stopcock; two sterile graduated cups; knife blade and handle; mechanical contrast agent injector; radiographic equipment

Procedure and posttest care

• After the patient is placed in a supine position, the local anesthetic is injected and the cardiac monitor is attached to the patient.

• An incision is made, and a catheter is introduced into the antecubital or femoral vein. As the catheter passes through the right atrium, the right ventricle, and the pulmonary artery, pressures are measured and blood samples are drawn from various regions of the pulmonary circulatory system.

• The contrast agent is injected and circulates through the pulmonary artery and lung capillaries while X-rays are taken.

• Apply a pressure dressing over the catheter insertion site, and note any bleeding.

• Maintain bed rest for about 6 hours.

• Observe for signs of myocardial perforation or rupture by monitoring vital signs.

• Be alert for signs of acute renal failure, such as sudden onset of oliguria, nausea, and vomiting.

• Check the catheter insertion site for inflammation or hematoma formation and report symptoms of a delayed hypersensitivity response to the contrast agent or to the local anesthetic (dyspnea, itching, tachycardia, palpitations, hypotension or hypertension, excitation, or euphoria).

• Advise the patient about any restriction of activity. Tell him that he may re-

sume his usual diet after the test, and encourage him to drink lots of fluids.

Precautions

◤ **CLINICAL ALERT** Pulmonary angiography is contraindicated during pregnancy and in patients who are hypersensitive to iodine, seafood, or radiographic contrast agents.

• Monitor for ventricular arrhythmias due to myocardial irritation from passage of the catheter through the heart chambers.

• Observe for signs of hypersensitivity to the contrast agent, such as dyspnea, nausea, vomiting, sweating, increased heart rate, and numbness of extremities.

• Keep emergency equipment available in case of a hypersensitivity reaction to the contrast agent.

Normal findings

Normally, the contrast agent flows symmetrically and without interruption through the pulmonary circulatory system.

Abnormal findings

Interruption of blood flow may result from emboli and from other types of pulmonary vascular abnormalities.

Interfering factors

• None significant

CARDIOVASCULAR SYSTEM

CARDIAC RADIOGRAPHY

Among the most frequently used tests for evaluating cardiac disease and its effects on the pulmonary vasculature, cardiac radiography provides images of the thorax, mediastinum, heart, and lungs. In a routine evaluation, postero-anterior and left lateral views are taken. The posteroanterior view is preferable to the anteroposterior view because it places the heart slightly closer to the plane of the film, providing a sharper, less distorted image. Cardiac radiography may be performed on a bedridden patient using portable equipment, but such equipment can provide only anteroposterior views.

Purpose

• To help detect cardiac disease and abnormalities that change the size, shape, or appearance of the heart and lungs

• To ensure correct positioning of pulmonary artery and cardiac catheters and of pacemaker wires

Patient preparation

• Explain to the patient that this test reveals the size and shape of the heart. Tell him who will perform the test and where. Reassure him that the test uses little radiation and is harmless.

• Instruct the patient to remove jewelry, other metal objects, and clothing above his waist and to put on a gown that has ties instead of metal snaps.

Procedure and posttest care

Posteroanterior view

• The patient stands erect about 6′ (2 m) from the X-ray machine with his back to the machine and his chin resting on top of the film cassette holder.

• The holder is adjusted to slightly hyperextend the patient's neck. The patient places his hands on his hips, with his shoulders touching the holder, and centers his chest against it.

• The patient is asked to take a deep breath and hold it during the X-ray film exposure.

Left lateral view

• The patient is positioned with his arms extended over his head and his left torso flush against the cassette and centered.

• The patient is asked to take a deep breath and hold it during the X-ray film exposure.

Anteroposterior view of a bedridden patient

• The head of the bed is elevated as much as possible.

• The patient is assisted to an upright position to reduce visceral pressure on the diaphragm and other thoracic structures.

• The film cassette is centered under the patient's back. Although the distance between the patient and the X-ray machine may vary a little, the path between the two should be clear.

• The patient is instructed to take a deep breath and hold it during the X-ray film exposure.

Precautions

• Cardiac radiography is usually contraindicated during the first trimester of pregnancy. If it's performed during pregnancy, a lead shield or apron should cover the patient's abdomen and pelvic area during the X-ray exposure.

• When testing an ambulatory patient, make sure the radiographic order stipulates a posteroanterior view and not an anteroposterior view. Include on the order any pertinent findings from previous cardiac radiographs as well as the indication for this test.

• When testing a bedridden patient, make sure anyone else in the room is protected from X-rays by a lead shield, a room divider, or sufficient distance.

• Films obtained while the patient is in the supine position may reveal findings that appear to be abnormal.

Normal findings

Normally, in the posteroanterior view, the thoracic cage appears at least twice as wide as the heart. However, in the anteroposterior view, relative heart size and position may look different, and the cardiac silhouette and vascular markings may increase.

If cardiac radiography is performed to evaluate the position of cardiac catheters and pacemakers, the films should confirm accurate placement.

Abnormal findings

Cardiac X-ray films must be evaluated in light of the patient's history, physical examination, electrocardiography results, and results of previous radiographic tests for cardiac abnormalities.

An abnormal cardiac silhouette usually reflects left or right ventricular or left atrial enlargement, or even a multichamber enlargement. In left ventricular enlargement, the posteroanterior view shows the border of the left side of the heart to be rounded and convex, with lateral extension of the lower left border; the lateral view shows posterior bulging of the left ventricle. In right ventricular enlargement, the posteroanterior view shows secondary prominence of the pulmonary artery segment at the border of the left side of the heart; the lateral view shows anterior bulging in the region of the right ventricular outflow tract.

In left atrial enlargement, the posteroanterior view shows double density of the enlarged left atrium, straightening of the border of the left side of the heart, elevation of the left mainstem bronchus and, rarely, lateral extension of the border of the right side of the heart superior to the right ventricle; the lateral view shows a posterior bulge at the level of the left atrium.

In the posteroanterior view, dilation of pulmonary venous shadows in the superior lateral aspect of the hilus and vascular shadows horizontally and inferiorly along the margin of the right side of the heart may be the first signs of pulmonary vascular congestion. Chronic pulmonary venous hypertension produces an antler pattern, caused by dilated superior pulmonary veins and normal or constricted inferior pulmonary veins. Acute alveolar edema may produce a butterfly appearance, with increased densities in central lung fields; interstitial pulmonary edema, a cloudy or cotton-puff appearance.

Interfering factors

• Patient's failure to maintain inspiration or to remain motionless
• Patient's chest off-center on the film cassette (may hinder viewing of costophrenic angle on X-ray)
• Thoracic deformity, such as scoliosis (possible misleading results)
• Underexposure or overexposure of films

LOWER LIMB VENOGRAPHY

Lower limb venography, or ascending contrast phlebography, is the radiographic examination of a vein. Commonly used to assess the condition of the deep leg veins after injection of a contrast medium, it's the definitive test for deep vein thrombosis (DVT). Venography shouldn't be used for routine screening because it exposes the patient to relatively high doses of radiation and can cause complications, such as phlebitis, local tissue damage and, occasionally, DVT itself. Color Doppler ultrasonography is now the first test used to diagnose DVT. (See *Acu-Tect: New way to diagnose DVT.*)

Venography is also expensive and is not easily repeated. A combination of three noninvasive tests — Doppler ultrasonography, impedance plethysmography, and ^{125}I fibrinogen scan — is an acceptable though less accurate alternative to venography. Radionuclide tests, such as the ^{125}I fibrinogen scan, are used to screen for DVT or to attempt to detect the disorder in a patient who is too ill for venography or is hypersensitive to the contrast medium.

Purpose
• To confirm a diagnosis of DVT
• To distinguish clot formation from venous obstruction (a large tumor of the pelvis impinging on the venous system, for example)
• To evaluate congenital venous abnormalities
• To assess deep vein valvular competence (especially helpful in identifying underlying causes of leg edema)
• To locate a suitable vein for arterial bypass grafting

Patient preparation
• Explain to the patient that this test helps detect abnormal conditions in the veins of the legs.
• Instruct him to restrict food and to drink only clear liquids for 4 hours before the test.
• Describe the test, including who will perform it, where it will take place, and its expected duration (30 to 45 minutes).
• Warn the patient that he may feel a burning sensation in his leg on injection of the contrast medium and some discomfort during the procedure.
• Make sure the patient or a responsible family member has signed a consent form.

ACUTECT: NEW WAY TO DIAGNOSE DVT

The Food and Drug Administration's advisory committee has recommended approval for Acu-Tect, a new method of diagnosing deep vein thrombosis (DVT). In this procedure, an injected peptide travels through the bloodstream as doctors use an imaging technique to monitor its path. The peptide seeks out and attaches to any fresh clot, thus distinguishing between old and new clots.

In recommending approval, the advisory committee also called for more studies to confirm the test's accuracy and reliability.

• Check the patient's history for hypersensitivity to iodine or iodine-containing foods or to contrast media. Mark any sensitivities on the chart.
• Reassure the patient that contrast media complications are rare, but tell him to report nausea, severe burning or itching, constriction in the throat or chest, or dyspnea immediately. Restrict anticoagulant therapy, as appropriate.
• Just before the test, instruct the patient to void, to remove all clothing below the waist, and to put on a gown.
• Administer a prescribed sedative to an anxious or uncooperative patient.

Procedure and posttest care
• The patient is positioned on a tilting radiographic table so that the leg being tested doesn't bear any weight. He's instructed to relax this leg and keep it still; a tourniquet may be tied around the ankle to expedite venous filling.

- A superficial vein in the dorsum of the patient's foot is injected with normal saline solution.
- When needle placement is correct, the contrast medium is slowly injected.
- If a suitable superficial vein can't be found (due to edema), a surgical cutdown of the vein may be performed.
- Using a fluoroscope, the distribution of the contrast medium is monitored, and spot films are taken from the anteroposterior and oblique projections and over the thigh and femoroiliac regions. Then, overhead films are taken of the calf, knee, thigh, and femoral area.
- After filming, the patient is repositioned horizontally, the leg is quickly elevated, and normal saline solution infused to flush the contrast medium from the veins.
- The fluoroscope is checked to confirm complete emptying. Then the needle is removed.
- Apply an adhesive bandage to the injection site.
- Monitor vital signs until stable; check the pulse rate on the dorsalis pedis, popliteal, and femoral arteries.
- Administer prescribed analgesics to counteract the irritating effects of the contrast medium.
- Watch for an allergic reaction to the contrast medium, hematoma, redness, bleeding, or infection (especially if a cutdown of the vein was performed) at the puncture site, and replace the dressing when necessary.
- If the venogram indicates DVT, initiate prescribed therapy (heparin infusion, bed rest, leg elevation or support, or blood chemistry tests).
- Tell the patient he may resume his usual diet and medications.

Precautions

 CLINICAL ALERT Most allergic reactions to the contrast medium

occur within 30 minutes of injection. Carefully observe for signs of anaphylaxis (flushing, urticaria, laryngeal stridor).

Normal findings

A normal venogram shows steady opacification of the superficial and deep vasculature with no filling defects.

Abnormal findings

A venogram that shows consistent filling defects on repeat views, abrupt termination of a column of contrast material, unfilled major deep veins, or diversion of flow (through collaterals, for example) is diagnostic of DVT.

Interfering factors

- Patient placing weight on the leg being tested (possible filling of leg veins with contract medium)
- Movement of the leg being tested
- Excessive tourniquet constriction
- Insufficient injection of contrast medium
- Delay between injection and radiography

GASTROINTESTINAL SYSTEM

BARIUM SWALLOW

Barium swallow (esophagography) is the cineradiographic, radiographic, or fluoroscopic examination of the pharynx and the fluoroscopic examination of the esophagus after ingestion of thick and thin mixtures of barium sulfate. This test, most commonly performed as part of the upper GI series, is indicated in patients with histories of dysphagia and regurgitation. Further testing is usually required for definitive diagnosis.

Cholangiography and the barium enema test, if necessary, should precede the barium swallow because ingested barium may obscure anatomic detail on the X-rays.

Purpose

• To diagnose hiatus hernia, diverticula, and varices
• To detect strictures, ulcers, tumors, polyps, and motility disorders
• To verify gastroesophageal reflux disease

Patient preparation

• Explain to the patient that this test evaluates the function of the pharynx and esophagus.
• Instruct him to fast after midnight the night before the test. (If the patient is an infant, delay feeding to ensure complete digestion of barium).
• Describe the test, including who will perform it, where it will take place, and its expected duration (approximately 30 minutes).
• Describe the milk shake consistency and chalky taste of the barium preparation he is required to ingest. Although it's flavored, he may find it unpleasant to swallow. Tell the patient he'll first receive a thick mixture, then a thin one, and that he must drink 12 to 14 oz (355 to 415 ml) during the examination.
• For a double-contrast study (barium and air), the patient may be asked to eat effervescent granules ("fizzies"). Tell the patient to avoid burping.
• Inform him that he'll be placed in various positions on a tilting X-ray table and that X-rays will be taken.

• Withhold antacids if gastric reflux is suspected.
• Just before the procedure, instruct the patient to put on a gown without snap closures and to remove jewelry, dentures, hair clips, or other radiopaque objects from the X-ray field.

Procedure and posttest care

• The patient is placed in an upright position behind the fluoroscopic screen and his heart, lungs, and abdomen are examined.
• He is then instructed to take one swallow of the thick barium mixture, and the pharyngeal action is recorded using cineradiography. (This action occurs too rapidly for adequate fluoroscopic evaluation.)
• The patient is then told to take several swallows of the thin barium mixture. The passage of the barium is examined fluoroscopically and spot films of the esophageal region are taken from lateral angles and from right and left posteroanterior angles. Esophageal strictures and obstruction of the esophageal lumen by the lower esophageal ring are best detected when the patient is upright. To accentuate small strictures or demonstrate dysphagia, the patient may be requested to swallow a special "barium marshmallow" (soft white bread that has been soaked in barium), or a barium pill.
• The patient is then secured to the X-ray table and is rotated to the Trendelenburg position to evaluate esophageal peristalsis or demonstrate hiatus hernia and gastric reflux.
• He's instructed to take several swallows of barium while the esophagus is examined fluoroscopically, and spot films of significant findings are taken when indicated. After the table is rotated to a horizontal position, the patient is told to take several swallows of bari-

um so that the esophagogastric junction and peristalsis may be evaluated. The passage of the barium is fluoroscopically observed, and spot films of significant findings are taken with the patient in supine and prone positions.

• During fluoroscopic examination of the esophagus, the cardia and fundus of the patient's stomach are also carefully studied because neoplasms in these areas may invade the esophagus and cause obstruction.

• Check that additional spot films and repeat fluoroscopic evaluation haven't been ordered before allowing the patient to resume his usual diet.

• Administer a cathartic, if prescribed.

• Inform the patient that stools will be chalky and light colored for 24 to 72 hours. Record description of all stools passed by the patient in the hospital.

• Barium retained in the intestine may harden, causing obstruction or fecal impaction. Notify the doctor if the patient fails to expel barium in 2 or 3 days.

Precautions

• Barium swallow is usually contraindicated in a patient with intestinal obstruction.

Normal findings

After the barium sulfate is swallowed, the bolus pours over the base of the tongue into the pharynx. A peristaltic wave propels the bolus through the entire length of the esophagus in about 2 seconds. When the peristaltic wave reaches the base of the esophagus, the cardiac sphincter opens, allowing the bolus to enter the stomach. After passage of the bolus, the cardiac sphincter closes. Normally, the bolus evenly fills and distends the lumen of the pharynx and esophagus, and the mucosa appears smooth and regular.

Abnormal findings

Barium swallow may reveal hiatus hernia, diverticula, and varices. Aspiration into the lungs will also be revealed. Although strictures, tumors, polyps, ulcers, and motility disorders (pharyngeal muscular disorders, esophageal spasms, and achalasia) may be detected, definitive diagnosis commonly requires endoscopic biopsy or, for motility disorders, manometric studies.

Interfering factor

• Aspiration of barium into lungs due to poor swallowing reflex

UPPER GI AND SMALL-BOWEL SERIES

The upper GI and small-bowel series is the fluoroscopic examination of the esophagus, stomach, and small intestine after the patient ingests barium sulfate, a contrast agent. As the barium passes through the digestive tract, fluoroscopy outlines peristalsis and the mucosal contours of the respective organs, and spot films record significant findings. This test is indicated in patients who have upper GI symptoms (difficulty in swallowing, regurgitation, burning or gnawing epigastric pain), signs of small-bowel disease (diarrhea, weight loss), signs of small-bowel obstruction (SBO), and signs of GI bleeding (hematemesis, melena).

Although this test can detect various mucosal abnormalities, subsequent biopsy is often necessary to rule out malignancy or distinguish specific inflammatory diseases. Oral cholecystography, barium enema, and routine X-rays should always precede this test because retained barium clouds anatomic detail on X-ray films.

Purpose

- To detect hiatus hernia, diverticula, and varices
- To aid diagnosis of strictures, ulcers, tumors, regional enteritis, and malabsorption syndrome
- To help detect motility disorders

Patient preparation

- Explain to the patient that this procedure uses ingested barium and X-ray films to examine the esophagus, stomach, and small intestine.
- Tell him to consume a low-residue diet for 2 or 3 days before the test and then to fast and avoid smoking after midnight the night before the test.
- Describe the test, including who will perform it, where it will take place, and its expected duration (up to 6 hours).
- Encourage the patient to bring reading material.
- Inform the patient that he'll be placed on an X-ray table that rotates into vertical, semivertical, and horizontal positions.
- Explain that he'll be adequately secured and that he'll be assisted to supine, prone, and side-lying positions.
- Describe the milk shake consistency and chalky taste of the barium mixture. Although it's flavored, he may find its taste unpleasant, but tell him he must drink 16 to 20 oz (475 to 590 ml) for a complete examination.
- Inform him that his abdomen may be compressed to ensure proper coating of the stomach or intestinal walls with barium, or to separate overlapping bowel loops.
- As prescribed, withhold most oral medications after midnight and anticholinergics and narcotics for 24 hours because these drugs affect small intestinal motility. Antacids are also

sometimes withheld for several hours if gastric reflux is suspected.
- Just before the procedure, instruct the patient to put on a gown without snap closures and to remove jewelry, dentures, hair clips, or other objects that might obscure anatomic detail on the X-ray films.

Procedure and posttest care

- After the patient is secured in a supine position on the X-ray table, the table is tilted until the patient is erect, and the heart, lungs, and abdomen are examined fluoroscopically.
- The patient is instructed to take several swallows of the barium suspension, and its passage through the esophagus is observed. (Occasionally, the patient is given a thick barium suspension, especially when esophageal pathology is strongly suspected.)
- During fluoroscopic examination, spot films of the esophagus are taken from lateral angles and from right and left posteroanterior angles.
- When barium enters the stomach, the patient's abdomen is palpated or compressed to ensure adequate coating of the gastric mucosa with barium.
- To perform a double-contrast examination, the patient is instructed to eat effervescent granules ("fizzies"). Instruct the patient *not* to burp because the double-contrast test requires air in the stomach. As the patient eats the granules, a small amount of air is also introduced into the stomach; this permits detailed examination of the gastric rugae, and spot films of significant findings are taken. The patient is then instructed to ingest the remaining barium suspension, and the filling of the stomach and emptying into the duodenum are observed fluoroscopically.
- Two series of spot films of the stomach and duodenum are taken from posteroanterior, anteroposterior, lateral,

and oblique angles, with the patient erect and then supine.

• The passage of barium into the remainder of the small intestine is then observed fluoroscopically, and spot films are taken at 30- to 60-minute intervals until the barium reaches the region of the ileocecal valve. If abnormalities in the small intestine are detected, the area is palpated and compressed to help clarify the defect, and a spot film is taken. The examination ends when the barium enters the cecum.

• Make sure additional X-rays haven't been ordered before allowing the patient food, fluids, and oral medications (if applicable).

• Administer a cathartic or enema to the patient. Tell him his stool will be light colored for 24 to 72 hours. Record and describe any stool passed by the patient in the hospital. Retention of barium in the intestine may cause obstruction or fecal impaction. Also, it may affect scheduling of other GI tests.

Precautions

• The upper GI and small-bowel series may be contraindicated in patients with obstruction or perforation of the digestive tract. Barium may intensify the obstruction or seep into the abdominal cavity. Sometimes a small-bowel series is performed to find a "transition zone." If a perforation is suspected, gastrografin rather than barium may be used.

Normal findings

After the barium suspension is swallowed, it pours over the base of the tongue into the pharynx and is propelled by a peristaltic wave through the entire length of the esophagus in about 2 seconds. The bolus evenly fills and distends the lumen of the pharynx and esophagus, and the mucosa appears smooth and regular. When the peristaltic wave reaches the base of the esophagus, the cardiac sphincter opens, allowing the bolus to enter the stomach. After passage of the bolus, the cardiac sphincter closes.

As barium enters the stomach, it outlines the characteristic longitudinal folds called rugae, which are best observed using the double-contrast technique. When the stomach is completely filled with barium, its outer contour appears smooth and regular without evidence of flattened, rigid areas suggestive of intrinsic or extrinsic lesions.

After barium enters the stomach, it quickly empties into the duodenal bulb through relaxation of the pyloric sphincter. Although the mucosa of the duodenal bulb is relatively smooth, circular folds become apparent as barium enters the duodenal loop. These folds deepen and become more numerous in the jejunum. The barium temporarily lodges between these folds, producing a speckled pattern on the X-ray film. As barium enters the ileum, the circular folds become less prominent and, except for their broadness, resemble those in the duodenum. The film also shows that the diameter of the small intestine tapers gradually from the duodenum to the ileum.

Abnormal findings

X-ray studies of the esophagus may reveal strictures, tumors, hiatus hernia, diverticula, varices, and ulcers (particularly in the distal esophagus). Benign strictures usually dilate the esophagus, whereas malignant ones cause erosive changes in the mucosa. Tumors produce filling defects in the column of barium, but only malignant ones change the mucosal contour. Nevertheless, biopsy is necessary for definitive diagnosis of both esophageal strictures and tumors.

Motility disorders, such as esophageal spasm, are usually difficult to detect because spasms are erratic and transient; manometry, which measures the length and pressure of peristaltic contractions and evaluates the function of the cardiac sphincter, is generally performed to detect such disorders. However, achalasia (cardiospasm) is strongly suggested when the distal esophagus has a beaking appearance. Gastric reflux appears as a backflow of barium from the stomach into the esophagus.

X-ray studies of the stomach may reveal tumors and ulcers. Malignant tumors, usually adenocarcinomas, appear as filling defects on the X-ray film and usually disrupt peristalsis. Benign tumors, such as adenomatous polyps and leiomyomas, appear as outpouchings of the gastric mucosa and generally don't affect peristalsis. Ulcers occur most commonly in the stomach and duodenum (particularly in the duodenal bulb), and these two areas are thus examined together. Benign ulcers usually demonstrate evidence of partial or complete healing and are characterized by radiating folds extending to the edge of the ulcer crater. Malignant ulcers, usually associated with a suspicious mass, generally have radiating folds that extend beyond the ulcer crater to the edge of the mass. However, biopsy is necessary for definitive diagnosis of both tumors and ulcers.

Occasionally, this test detects signs that suggest pancreatitis or pancreatic carcinoma. Such signs include edematous changes in the mucosa of the antrum or duodenal loop or dilation of the duodenal loop. These findings mandate further studies for pancreatic disease, such as endoscopic retrograde cholangiopancreatography, abdominal ultrasonography, or computed tomography scanning.

X-ray studies of the small intestine may reveal regional enteritis, malabsorption syndrome, and tumors. Although regional enteritis may not be detected in its early stages, small ulcerations and edematous changes develop in the mucosa as the disease progresses. Edematous changes, segmentation of the barium column, and flocculation characterize malabsorption syndrome. Filling defects occur with Hodgkin's disease and lymphosarcoma.

Interfering factors

● Failure to observe pretest restrictions (may invalidate results)

● Excess air in the small bowel (possible poor imaging)

● Failure to remove radiopaque objects in X-ray field (possible poor imaging)

BARIUM ENEMA

Also called lower GI examination, barium enema is the radiographic examination of the large intestine after rectal instillation of barium sulfate (single-contrast technique) or barium sulfate and air (double-contrast technique). It's indicated in patients with histories of altered bowel habits, lower abdominal pain, or the passage of blood, mucus, or pus in the stool. It may also be indicated after colostomy or ileostomy; in these patients, barium (or barium and air) is instilled through the stoma. Complications include perforation of the colon, water intoxication, barium granulomas and, rarely, intraperitoneal and extraperitoneal extravasation of barium and barium embolism.

The single-contrast technique provides a profile view of the large intestine; the double-contrast technique provides profile and frontal views. The latter technique best detects small intraluminal tumors (especially polyps), the early mucosal changes of inflammatory disease, and the subtle intestinal bleeding caused by ulcerated polyps or the shallow ulcerations of inflammatory disease.

Although barium enema clearly outlines most of the large intestine, proctosigmoidoscopy provides the best view of the rectosigmoid region. Barium enema should precede the barium swallow and upper GI and small-bowel series because barium ingested in the latter procedure may take several days to pass through the GI tract and thus may interfere with subsequent X-ray studies.

Purpose
• To aid diagnosis of colorectal cancer and inflammatory disease
• To detect polyps, diverticula, and structural changes in the large intestine

Patient preparation
• Explain to the patient that this test permits examination of the large intestine through X-ray films taken after a barium enema.
• Describe the test, including who will perform it, where it will take place, and its expected duration (30 to 45 minutes).
• Because residual fecal material in the colon obscures normal anatomy on X-rays, instruct the patient to carefully follow the prescribed bowel preparation, which may include diet, laxatives, or cleansing enemas. However, in certain conditions, such as ulcerative colitis and active GI bleeding, their use may be prohibited.
• Stress that accurate test results depend on the patient's cooperation with prescribed dietary restrictions and bowel preparation. A common bowel preparation technique includes restrict-

ed intake of dairy products and maintenance of a liquid diet for 24 hours before the test. The patient is encouraged to drink five 8-oz glasses of water or clear liquids 12 to 24 hours before the test.
• Advise the patient to administer prescribed enemas until return is clear.
• Tell him not to eat breakfast before the procedure; if the test is scheduled for late afternoon (or delayed), he may have clear liquids.
• Tell the patient that he'll be placed on a tilting X-ray table and adequately draped. During the test, he'll be secured to the table and assisted to various positions.
• Tell the patient that he may experience cramping pains or the urge to defecate as the barium or air is introduced into the intestine. Instruct him to breathe deeply and slowly through his mouth to ease this discomfort.
• Tell him to keep his anal sphincter tightly contracted against the rectal tube; this holds the tube in position and helps prevent leakage of barium. Stress the importance of retaining the barium enema; if the intestinal walls aren't adequately coated with barium, test results may be inaccurate.
• Assure the patient that the barium enema is fairly easy to retain because of its cool temperature.

Procedure and posttest care
• After the patient is in a supine position on a tilting X-ray table, scout films of the abdomen are taken.
• The patient is assisted to Sims' position and a well-lubricated rectal tube is inserted through the anus. If the patient has anal sphincter atony or severe mental or physical debilitation, a rectal tube with a retaining balloon may be inserted.
• The barium is administered slowly, and the filling process is monitored

fluoroscopically. To aid filling, the table may be tilted or the patient assisted to supine, prone, and lateral decubitus positions.

• As the flow of barium is observed, spot films are taken of significant findings. When the intestine is filled with barium, overhead films of the abdomen are taken. The rectal tube is withdrawn, and the patient is escorted to the toilet or provided with a bedpan and is instructed to expel as much barium as possible.

• After evacuation, an additional overhead film is taken to record the mucosal pattern of the intestine and to evaluate the efficiency of colonic emptying.

• A double-contrast barium enema may directly follow this examination or may be performed separately. If it's performed immediately, a thin film of barium remains in the patient's intestine, coating the mucosa, and air is carefully injected to distend the bowel lumen.

• When the double-contrast technique is performed separately, a colloidal barium suspension is instilled, filling the patient's intestine to either the splenic flexure or the middle of the transverse colon. The suspension is then aspirated, and air is forcefully injected into the intestine. If the intestine is filled to the lower descending colon, air is forcefully injected without prior aspiration of the suspension.

• The patient is then assisted to erect, prone, supine, and lateral decubitus positions in sequence. Barium filling is monitored fluoroscopically, and spot films are taken of significant findings. After the required films are taken, the patient is escorted to the toilet or provided with a bedpan.

• Make sure further studies haven't been ordered before allowing the patient food and fluids. Encourage extra fluid intake because bowel preparation and the test itself can cause dehydration.

• Encourage rest because this test and the bowel preparation that precedes it exhaust most patients.

• Because retention of barium after this test can cause intestinal obstruction or fecal impaction, administer a mild cathartic or a cleansing enema. Tell the patient his stool will be light colored for 24 to 72 hours. Record and describe any stool passed by the patient in the hospital.

Precautions

• Barium enema is contraindicated in patients with tachycardia, fulminant ulcerative colitis associated with systemic toxicity and megacolon, toxic megacolon, or suspected perforation.

• This test should be performed cautiously in patients with obstruction, acute inflammatory conditions (such as ulcerative colitis and diverticulitis), acute vascular insufficiency of the bowel, acute fulminant bloody diarrhea, and suspected pneumatosis cystoides intestinalis.

Normal findings

In the single-contrast enema, the intestine is uniformly filled with barium, and colonic haustral markings are clearly apparent. The intestinal walls collapse as the barium is expelled, and the mucosa has a regular, feathery appearance on the postevacuation film. In the double-contrast enema, the intestine is uniformly distended with air and has a thin layer of barium providing excellent detail of the mucosal pattern. As the patient is assisted to various positions, the barium collects on the dependent walls of the intestine by the force of gravity.

Abnormal findings

Although most colonic cancers occur in the rectosigmoid region and are best detected by proctosigmoidoscopy, X-ray films may reveal adenocarcinoma and, rarely, sarcomas occurring higher in the intestine. Carcinoma usually appears as a localized filling defect, with a sharp transition between the normal and the necrotic mucosa. If it's circumferential, it will have an "apple core" appearance. These characteristics help distinguish carcinoma from the more diffuse lesions of inflammatory disease, but endoscopic biopsy may be necessary to confirm the diagnosis.

X-ray studies demonstrate and define the extent of inflammatory disease, such as diverticulitis, ulcerative colitis, and granulomatous colitis. Ulcerative colitis usually originates in the anal region and ascends through the intestine; granulomatous colitis usually originates in the cecum and terminal ileum, and then descends through the intestine. However, biopsy may be necessary to confirm diagnosis.

Barium X-ray films may also reveal saccular adenomatous polyps, broad-based villous polyps, structural changes in the intestine (such as intussusception, telescoping of the bowel, sigmoid volvulus [360-degree turn or greater], and sigmoid torsion [up to 180-degree turn]), gastroenteritis, irritable colon, vascular injury due to arterial occlusion, and selected cases of acute appendicitis.

Interfering factors

• Inadequate bowel preparation (possible poor imaging)
• Barium retained from previous studies (possible poor imaging)
• Patient's inability to retain barium enema

HYPOTONIC DUODENOGRAPHY

Hypotonic duodenography is the fluoroscopic examination of the duodenum after instillation of barium sulfate and air through an intestinal catheter. This test is indicated in patients with symptoms of duodenal or pancreatic pathology, such as persistent upper abdominal pain.

After the catheter is passed through the patient's nose into the duodenum, I.V. infusion of glucagon or I.M. injection of propantheline bromide (or other anticholinergic) induces duodenal atony. Instillation of barium and air distends the relaxed duodenum, flattening its deep circular folds; spot films then record the precise delineation of the duodenal anatomy. Although these films readily demonstrate small duodenal lesions and tumors of the head of the pancreas that impinge on the duodenal wall, differential diagnosis requires further studies.

Purpose

• To detect small postbulbar duodenal lesions, tumors of the head of the pancreas, and tumors of the ampulla of Vater
• To aid diagnosis of chronic pancreatitis

Patient preparation

• Explain to the patient that this test permits examination of the duodenum and pancreas after the instillation of barium and air.
• Instruct him to fast after midnight the night before the test.
• Describe the test, including who will perform it, where it will take place, and its expected duration (approximately 60 minutes).

• Inform the patient that a tube will be passed through his nose into the duodenum to serve as a channel for the barium and air.

• Tell him that he may experience a cramping pain as air is introduced into the duodenum. Instruct him to breathe deeply and slowly through his mouth if he experiences this pain to help relax the abdominal muscles.

• If glucagon or an anticholinergic is to be administered during the procedure, describe the possible adverse effects of glucagon (nausea, vomiting, hives, and flushing) or of anticholinergics (dry mouth, thirst, tachycardia, urine retention, and blurred vision). If an anticholinergic is administered to an outpatient, advise him to have someone accompany him home.

• Just before the test, tell the patient to remove dentures, glasses, necklaces, hairpins, combs, and constricting undergarments.

• Instruct him to void.

Procedure and posttest care

• While the patient is in a sitting position, a catheter is passed through his nose into the stomach. He is then placed in a supine position on an X-ray table, and the catheter is advanced into the duodenum, under fluoroscopic guidance.

• Glucagon I.V. is administered, which quickly induces duodenal atony for approximately 20 minutes, or an anticholinergic is injected I.M.

• Barium is instilled through the catheter, and spot films are taken of the duodenum.

• Some of the barium is then withdrawn and air is instilled; then additional spot films are taken.

• When the required films have been obtained, the catheter is removed.

• Throughout the procedure, observe the patient for adverse reactions. Be aware that such reactions may follow administration of glucagon or an anticholinergic. If an anticholinergic was given, make sure the patient voids within a few hours after the test. Advise the outpatient to rest in a waiting area until his vision clears (about 2 hours) unless someone can take him home.

• Administer a cathartic, as prescribed.

• Tell the patient he may burp instilled air or pass flatus, and that the barium colors the stool chalky white for 24 to 72 hours.

• Record description of any stool passed by the patient in the hospital.

Precautions

CLINICAL ALERT Anticholinergics are contraindicated in patients with severe cardiac disorders or glaucoma.

CLINICAL ALERT Glucagon is contraindicated in brittle diabetes and relatively contraindicated in type 1 (insulin-dependent) diabetes mellitus.

• Patients with strictures in the upper GI tract, particularly those associated with ulcerations or large masses, shouldn't undergo this procedure.

• Monitor elderly or very ill patients for gastric reflux.

Normal findings

When barium and air distend the atonic duodenum, the mucosa normally appears smooth and even. The regular contour of the head of the pancreas also appears on the duodenal wall.

Abnormal findings

Irregular nodules or masses on the duodenal wall could mean duodenal lesions, tumors of the ampulla of Vater, tumors of the head of the pancreas, or chronic pancreatitis. Differential diagnosis requires further tests, such as endoscopic retrograde cholangiopancreatography, serum and urine amylase determinations, ultrasonography of the pancreas, and computed tomography of the pancreas.

Interfering factors
• None significant

ORAL CHOLECYSTOGRAPHY

Oral cholecystography is the radiographic examination of the gallbladder after administration of a contrast medium. This test is now often replaced by nuclear medicine [99]technetium-labeled scan, ultrasound, and computerized tomography. It's indicated in patients with symptoms of biliary tract disease, such as right upper quadrant epigastric pain, fat intolerance, and jaundice, and is most commonly performed to confirm gallbladder disease.

After the contrast medium is ingested, it's absorbed by the small intestine, filtered by the liver, excreted in the bile, and then concentrated and stored in the gallbladder. Full gallbladder opacification usually occurs 12 to 14 hours after ingestion, and a series of X-ray films then records gallbladder appearance. Additional information is obtained by giving the patient a fat stimulus, causing the gallbladder to contract and empty the contrast-laden bile into the common bile duct and small intestine. Films are then taken to record this emptying and to evaluate patency of the common bile duct.

Oral cholecystography should precede barium studies because retained barium may cloud subsequent X-ray films.

Purpose
• To detect gallstones
• To aid diagnosis of inflammatory disease and tumors of the gallbladder

Patient preparation
• Explain to the patient that this procedure permits examination of the gallbladder through X-ray films taken after ingestion of a contrast medium.
• Instruct the patient to eat a meal containing fat at noon the day before the test and a fat-free meal in the evening. The former stimulates release of bile from the gallbladder, preparing it to receive the contrast-laden bile; the latter inhibits gallbladder contraction, promoting accumulation of bile.
• After the evening meal, instruct the patient to restrict food and fluids, except water.
• Give the patient six tablets (3 g) of iopanoic acid 2 or 3 hours after the evening meal, as necessary. (Other commercial contrast agents are available, such as sodium ipodate, but iopanoic acid is most commonly used.) Have the patient swallow the tablets one at a time at 5-minute intervals, with one or two mouthfuls of water for a total of 8 oz (240 ml) of water. Thereafter, withhold water, cigarettes, and gum.
• Describe the test, including who will perform it, where it will take place, and its expected duration (usually 30 to 45 minutes, but a longer test may be necessary).
• Tell the patient he'll be placed on an X-ray table, and that films will be taken of his gallbladder.
• Check the patient's history for hypersensitivity to iodine, seafood, or contrast media used for other diagnostic tests.
• Inform him that the possible adverse effects of dye ingestion include diarrhea (common) and, rarely, nausea,

vomiting, abdominal cramps, and dysuria. Tell him to report such symptoms immediately if they develop.

● Examine any vomitus or diarrhea for undigested tablets. If any tablets were expelled, notify the X-ray department.

● Administer a cleansing enema the morning of the test, if prescribed. This clears the GI tract of interfering shadows that may obscure the gallbladder.

Procedure and posttest care

● After the patient is in a prone position on the radiographic table, the abdomen is examined fluoroscopically to evaluate gallbladder opacification, and films are taken of significant findings.

● The patient is then examined while in left lateral decubitus and erect positions to detect possible layering or mobility of any filling defects, and additional films are taken.

● The patient may then be given a fat stimulus, such as a high-fat meal or a synthetic fat-containing agent (for example, sincalide).

● Fluoroscopy is used to observe the emptying of the gallbladder in response to the fat stimulus, and spot films are taken at 15- and 30-minute intervals to visualize the common bile duct. If the gallbladder empties slowly or not at all, these films are also taken at 60 minutes.

● If the test results are normal, tell the patient he may resume his usual diet. Nonopacification and repeat cholecystography require continuation of a low-fat diet until definitive diagnosis can be made.

● If gallstones are discovered during opacification, the patient will need an appropriate diet — usually one that restricts fat intake — to help prevent acute attacks.

Precautions

● Oral cholecystography is contraindicated in patients with severe renal or hepatic damage and in those with a hypersensitivity to iodine, seafood, or contrast media.

Normal findings

The gallbladder is normally opacified and appears pear-shaped, with smooth, thin walls. Although its size is variable, its basic structure — neck, infundibulum, body, and fundus — is clearly outlined on film.

Abnormal findings

When the gallbladder is opacified, filling defects (typically appearing within the lumen as negative shadows that show mobility) indicate the presence of gallstones. Fixed defects, on the other hand, may indicate the presence of cholesterol polyps or a benign tumor such as an adenomyoma.

When the gallbladder fails to opacify or when only faint opacification occurs, inflammatory disease such as cholecystitis — with or without gallstone formation — may be present. Gallstones may obstruct the cystic duct and prevent the contrast medium from entering the gallbladder; inflammation may impair the concentrating ability of the gallbladder mucosa and prevent or diminish opacification.

When the gallbladder fails to contract following stimulation by a fatty meal, cholecystitis or common bile duct obstruction may be present. If the X-ray films are inconclusive, oral cholecystography will have to be repeated the following day.

Interfering factors

● Failure to follow dietary restrictions

● Failure to ingest the full dose of contrast medium or partial loss of contrast

medium through emesis or diarrhea (may invalidate test results)
● Inadequate absorption of the contrast medium in the small intestine or barium retained from previous studies (may invalidate test results)
● Decreased excretion of the contrast medium into the bile due to impaired hepatic function and moderate jaundice (possible poor imaging)

PERCUTANEOUS TRANSHEPATIC CHOLANGIOGRAPHY

Percutaneous transhepatic cholangiography is the fluoroscopic examination of the biliary ducts after injection of an iodinated contrast medium directly into a biliary radicle. This test is especially useful for evaluating patients with persistent upper abdominal pain after cholecystectomy and for evaluating patients with severe jaundice.

Although computed tomography scan or ultrasonography is usually performed first when obstructive jaundice is suspected, percutaneous transhepatic cholangiography may provide the most detailed view of the obstruction; however, this invasive procedure carries a potential risk of complications that include bleeding, septicemia, bile peritonitis, extravasation of the contrast medium into the peritoneal cavity, and subcapsular injection.

Purpose
● To determine the cause of upper abdominal pain following cholecystectomy
● To distinguish between obstructive and nonobstructive jaundice

● To determine the location, the extent, and often the cause of mechanical obstruction

Patient preparation
● Explain to the patient that this procedure allows examination of the biliary ducts through X-ray films taken after a contrast medium is injected into the liver.
● Instruct him to fast for 8 hours before the test.
● Describe the test, including who will perform it, where it will take place, and its duration (about 30 minutes).
● Inform the patient that he'll be placed on a tilting X-ray table that rotates into vertical and horizontal positions during the procedure.
● Assure him that he'll be adequately secured to the table and assisted to supine and side-lying positions throughout the procedure.
● Warn him that injection of the local anesthetic may sting the skin and produce transient pain when it punctures the liver capsule.
● Advise him that injection of the contrast medium may produce a sensation of pressure and epigastric fullness and may cause transient upper back pain on his right side.
● If appropriate, advise him that a sedative will be administered just before the procedure begins, and tell him that he must rest for at least 6 hours after the procedure.
● Make sure the patient or a responsible family member has signed a consent form.
● Check the patient's history for hypersensitivity to iodine, seafood, contrast media used in other diagnostic tests, and the local anesthetic. Describe the possible adverse effects of contrast medium administration, such as nausea, vomiting, excessive salivation, flushing, urticaria, sweating and, rarely,

anaphylaxis; tachycardia and fever may accompany intraductal injection.

• Check the patient's history for normal bleeding, clotting, and prothrombin times, and a normal platelet count. If prescribed, administer 1 g of ampicillin I.V. every 4 to 6 hours for 24 hours before the procedure.

• Just before the procedure, administer a sedative, if prescribed.

Procedure and posttest care

• After the patient is placed in a supine position on the X-ray table and is adequately secured, the right upper quadrant of the abdomen is cleaned and draped; the skin, subcutaneous tissue, and liver capsule are infiltrated with a local anesthetic.

• While the patient holds his breath at the end of expiration, the flexible needle is inserted under fluoroscopic guidance through the eighth or ninth intercostal space in the midaxillary line and into the liver.

• The needle is passed deeply into the liver substance and then slowly withdrawn, injecting the contrast medium to locate a biliary radicle. When fluoroscopy reveals placement in a radicle, the needle is held in position and the remaining contrast medium is injected. When the contrast medium enters a biliary radicle, it begins to outline the biliary tree.

• Using a fluoroscope and television monitor, the opacification of the biliary ducts is observed, and spot films of significant findings are taken with the patient in supine and lateral recumbent positions. When the required films have been taken, the needle is removed.

• Apply a sterile dressing to the puncture site.

• Check the patient's vital signs until they're stable.

• Enforce bed rest for at least 6 hours after the test, preferably with the patient lying on his right side, to help prevent hemorrhage.

• Check the injection site for bleeding, swelling, and tenderness. Watch for signs of peritonitis: chills, temperature of 102° to 103° F (38.8° to 39.4°C), and abdominal pain, tenderness, and distention.

• Tell the patient that he may resume his usual diet.

Precautions

• Percutaneous transhepatic cholangiography is contraindicated in patients with cholangitis, massive ascites, uncorrectable coagulopathy, or hypersensitivity to iodine.

Normal findings

The biliary ducts are of normal diameter and appear as regular channels homogeneously filled with contrast medium.

Abnormal findings

Distinguishing between obstructive and nonobstructive jaundice hinges on whether biliary ducts are dilated or of normal size. Obstructive jaundice is associated with dilated ducts; nonobstructive jaundice, with normal-sized ducts. When ducts are dilated, the obstruction site may be defined. Obstruction may result from cholelithiasis, biliary tract carcinoma, or carcinoma of the pancreas or papilla of Vater that impinges on the common bile duct, causing deviation or stricture.

When ducts are of normal size and intrahepatic cholestasis is indicated, liver biopsy may be performed to distinguish among hepatitis, cirrhosis, and granulomatous disease.

Interfering factors
• Marked obesity or gas overlying the biliary ducts (possible poor imaging)

POSTOPERATIVE CHOLANGIOGRAPHY

During cholecystectomy or common bile duct exploration, a T-shaped rubber tube may be inserted into the common bile duct to facilitate drainage. Postoperative cholangiography — radiographic and fluoroscopic examination of the biliary ducts — may be performed 7 to 10 days after surgery.

This procedure requires injection of contrast medium through the T-tube. The contrast medium flows through the biliary ducts and outlines the size and patency of the ducts, revealing any obstruction overlooked during surgery.

Purpose
• To detect calculi, strictures, neoplasms, and fistulae in the biliary ducts

Patient preparation
• Explain to the patient that this procedure permits examination of the biliary ducts through X-ray films taken after the injection of a contrast medium.
• Describe the test, including who will perform it, where it will take place, and its expected duration (approximately 15 minutes).
• Warn the patient that he may feel a bloating sensation (not pain) in the right upper quadrant as the contrast medium is injected.
• Clamp the T-tube the day before the procedure, if necessary. Because bile fills the tube after clamping, this helps prevent air bubbles from entering the ducts.

• Withhold the meal just before the test, and administer a cleansing enema about 1 hour before the procedure.
• Make sure the patient or a responsible family member has signed a consent form.
• Check the patient's history for hypersensitivity to iodine, seafood, or contrast media used in other diagnostic tests. Tell the patient that the adverse effects of intraductal administration may include nausea, vomiting, excessive salivation, flushing, urticaria, sweating and, rarely, anaphylaxis.

Procedure and posttest care
• After the patient is in a supine position on the X-ray table, the injection area of the T-tube is cleaned with sponges soaked with povidone-iodine solution. The T-tube is held in a vertical position, which allows trapped air to surface, and a needle attached to a long transparent catheter is carefully inserted into the end of the T-tube. Care must be taken to avoid injecting air into the biliary tree because air bubbles may affect the clarity of the X-ray films.
• Approximately 5 ml of contrast medium (usually sodium diatrizoate) is injected under fluoroscopic guidance, and a spot film is taken in the anteroposterior position. Additional injections are then administered, and spot films and plain films are taken with the patient in supine and right lateral decubitus positions.
• The T-tube is then clamped, and the patient is assisted to an erect position for additional films; in this position, air bubbles may be distinguished from calculi or other pathology.
• A final film is taken 15 minutes after contrast injection to record the emptying of contrast-laden bile into the duodenum. If emptying is delayed, additional films may be taken.

• If a sterile dressing is applied after removal of the T-tube, observe and record any drainage. Change the dressing, as necessary.

• If the T-tube is left in place, attach it to the drainage system.

Precautions

• Postoperative cholangiography is contraindicated in patients who are hypersensitive to iodine.

Normal findings

Biliary ducts demonstrate homogeneous filling with contrast medium and are normal in diameter. When Oddi's sphincter is functioning properly and the ducts are patent, the contrast flows unimpeded into the duodenum.

Abnormal findings

Negative shadows or filling defects within the biliary ducts associated with dilation may indicate calculi or neoplasms overlooked during surgery. Abnormal channels of contrast medium departing from the biliary ducts indicate fistulae.

Interfering factors

• Marked obesity or gas overlying the biliary ducts (possible poor imaging)

ENDOSCOPIC RETROGRADE CHOLANGIO- PANCREATOGRAPHY

Endoscopic retrograde cholangiopancreatography (ERCP) is the radiographic examination of the pancreatic ducts and hepatobiliary tree after injection of a contrast medium into the duodenal papilla. It's indicated in patients with confirmed or suspected pancreatic disease or obstructive jaundice of unknown etiology. Complications may include cholangitis and pancreatitis.

Purpose

• To evaluate obstructive jaundice

• To diagnose cancer of the duodenal papilla, the pancreas, and the biliary ducts

• To locate calculi and stenosis in the pancreatic ducts and hepatobiliary tree

Patient preparation

• Explain to the patient that this procedure permits examination of the liver, the gallbladder, and the pancreas through X-ray films taken after injection of a contrast medium.

• Instruct him to fast after midnight before the test.

• Describe the test, including who will perform it, where it will take place, and its expected duration (30 to 60 minutes).

• Inform him that a local anesthetic will be sprayed into his mouth to calm the gag reflex. Warn him that the spray has an unpleasant taste and makes the tongue and throat feel swollen, causing difficulty in swallowing.

• Instruct him to let saliva drain from the side of his mouth, and tell him that suction may be used to remove saliva. Tell him a mouth guard will be inserted to protect his teeth and the endoscope; assure him that it won't obstruct his breathing.

• Assure the patient that he'll receive a sedative before insertion of the endoscope to help him relax, but that he'll remain conscious.

• Tell him that he'll also receive an anticholinergic or glucagon I.V. after insertion of the endoscope. Describe the possible adverse effects of anticholinergics (dry mouth, thirst, tachycardia, urine retention, and blurred vision) or of glucagon (nausea, vomiting, urticaria, and flushing).

• Warn him that he may experience transient flushing on injection of the contrast medium. Advise him that he may have a sore throat for 3 or 4 days after the examination.

• Make sure the patient or a responsible family member has signed a consent form.

• Check the patient's history for hypersensitivity to iodine, seafood, or contrast media used for other diagnostic procedures.

• Just before the procedure, obtain baseline vital signs. Instruct the patient to remove all metal or other radiopaque objects and constricting undergarments. Then, tell him to void, to minimize the discomfort of urine retention that may follow the procedure.

Procedure and posttest care

• An I.V. infusion is started with 150 ml of normal saline solution. The local anesthetic is then administered and usually takes effect in about 10 minutes.

• If a spray is used, ask the patient to hold his breath while his mouth and throat are sprayed.

• Place the patient in a left lateral position, and give him an emesis basin; provide tissues. Because the anesthetic causes the patient to lose some control of his secretions and thus increases the risk of aspiration, encourage him to allow saliva to drain from the side of his mouth.

• Insert the mouth guard.

• While the patient remains in the left lateral position, 5 to 20 mg of diazepam is administered I.V.

• When ptosis or dysarthria develops, the patient's head is bent forward, and he's asked to open his mouth.

• The examiner inserts his left index finger in the patient's mouth and guides the tip of the endoscope along his finger to the back of the patient's throat. The scope is then deflected downward with the left index finger and advanced. As the endoscope passes through the posterior pharynx and cricopharyngeal sphincter, the patient's head is slowly extended to assist the advance of the endoscope. The patient's chin must be kept midline. When the endoscope has passed the cricopharyngeal sphincter, the scope is advanced under direct vision. When it's well into the esophagus, the patient's chin is moved toward the table so saliva can drain from the mouth. The endoscope is advanced through the remainder of the esophagus and into the stomach under direct vision.

• When the pylorus is located, a small amount of air is insufflated, and the tip of the endoscope is angled upward and passed into the duodenal bulb.

• After the endoscope is rotated clockwise to enter the descending duodenum, the patient is assisted to a prone position.

• An anticholinergic or glucagon I.V. is administered to induce duodenal atony and to relax the ampullary sphincter.

• A small amount of air is insufflated, and the endoscope is manipulated until the optic lies opposite the duodenal papilla. Then, the cannula filled with contrast medium is passed through the biopsy channel of the endoscope, the duodenal papilla, and into the ampulla of Vater.

• The pancreatic duct is visualized first under fluoroscopic guidance with injection of contrast medium.

• The cannula is repositioned at a more cephalad angle, and the hepatobiliary tree is visualized with injection of contrast medium.

• After each injection, rapid-sequence X-ray films are taken.

• Instruct the patient to remain prone while the films are developed and reviewed. If necessary, additional films may be taken.

• If strictures are detected, a stent may be placed in the common bile duct to relieve the obstruction.

• When the required radiographs have been obtained, the cannula is removed. Before the endoscope is withdrawn, a tissue specimen may be obtained or fluid aspirated for histologic and cytologic examination, respectively.

• Observe closely for signs of cholangitis and pancreatitis. Hyperbilirubinemia, fever, and chills are the immediate signs of cholangitis; hypotension associated with gram-negative septicemia may develop later. Left upper quadrant pain and tenderness, elevated serum amylase levels, and transient hyperbilirubinemia are the usual signs of pancreatitis. Draw blood samples for amylase and bilirubin determinations, if necessary, but remember that these levels usually rise after ERCP.

• Continue to watch for signs of respiratory depression, apnea, hypotension, excessive diaphoresis, bradycardia, and laryngospasm. Check vital signs every 15 minutes for 4 hours, then every hour for 4 hours, and then every 4 hours for 48 hours.

• Withhold food and fluids until the gag reflex returns. Test the gag reflex by touching the back of the throat with a tongue blade. When the gag reflex returns, allow fluids and a light meal.

• Discontinue or maintain the I.V. infusion as appropriate.

• Check for signs of urine retention for the next 8 hours.

• If the patient has a sore throat, provide soothing lozenges and warm saline gargles to ease discomfort.

Precautions

• ERCP is contraindicated in patients with infectious disease, pancreatic pseudocysts, stricture or obstruction of the esophagus or duodenum, and acute pancreatitis, cholangitis, or cardiorespiratory disease.

• Monitor vital signs and airway patency throughout the procedure. Watch for signs of respiratory depression, apnea, hypotension, excessive diaphoresis, bradycardia, and laryngospasm. Be sure to have available emergency resuscitation equipment and a narcotic antagonist, such as naloxone.

Normal findings

The duodenal papilla appears as a small red (or sometimes pale) erosion protruding into the lumen. Its orifice is commonly bordered by a fringe of white mucosa, and a longitudinal fold running perpendicular to the deep circular folds of the duodenum helps mark its location. Although the pancreatic and hepatobiliary ducts usually unite in the ampulla of Vater and empty through the duodenal papilla, separate orifices are sometimes present.

The contrast medium uniformly fills the pancreatic duct, the hepatobiliary tree, and the gallbladder.

Abnormal findings

Obstructive jaundice may result from various abnormalities of the hepatobiliary tree and pancreatic duct. Examination of the hepatobiliary tree may reveal stones, strictures, or irregular deviations that suggest biliary cirrhosis, primary sclerosing cholangitis, or carcinoma of the bile ducts.

Examination of the pancreatic ducts may also show stones, strictures, and irregular deviations that may indicate pancreatic cysts and pseudocysts, pancreatic tumor, carcinoma of the head of the pancreas, chronic pancreatitis, pancreatic fibrosis, carcinoma of the duodenal papilla, and papillary stenosis.

Depending on test findings, a definitive diagnosis may require further studies.

Interfering factor
• Barium in GI tract from previous studies (possible poor imaging)

CELIAC AND MESENTERIC ARTERIOGRAPHY

Celiac and mesenteric arteriography involves the radiographic examination of the abdominal vasculature after intra-arterial injection of contrast medium through a catheter. Most commonly, the catheter is passed through the femoral artery into the aorta and then, using fluoroscopy, is positioned in the celiac, superior mesenteric, or inferior mesenteric artery. Injection of contrast medium into one or more of these arteries provides a map of abdominal vasculature; injection into specific arterial branches, called superselective angiography, permits detailed visualization of a particular area. As the contrast medium flows through the abdominal vasculature, serial radiographs outline abdominal vessels in the arterial, capillary, and venous phases of perfusion.

Celiac and mesenteric arteriography is indicated when endoscopy is unable to locate the source of GI bleeding or when barium studies, ultrasonography, and nuclear medicine or computed tomography scanning prove inconclusive in evaluating neoplasms. It's also used to evaluate cirrhosis and portal hypertension (especially when a portacaval shunt is being considered); to evaluate vascular damage, particularly in the spleen and liver, after abdominal trauma; and to detect vascular abnormalities. Because arteriography can demonstrate the portal vein even when portal venous flow is reversed, it's used more often than splenoportography.

Complications associated with this test include hemorrhage, venous and intracardiac thrombosis, cardiac arrhythmia, and emboli caused by dislodging atherosclerotic plaques.

Purpose
• To locate the source of GI bleeding
• To help distinguish between benign and malignant neoplasms
• To evaluate cirrhosis and portal hypertension
• To evaluate vascular damage after abdominal trauma
• To detect vascular abnormalities

Patient preparation
• Explain to the patient that this test permits examination of the abdominal blood vessels after injection of a contrast medium.
• Instruct him to fast for 8 hours before the test.
• Tell him that he'll receive a local anesthetic and that he may feel a brief, stinging sensation as it's injected. He may also feel pressure when the femoral artery is palpated, but the local anesthetic will minimize the pain when the needle is introduced into the artery.
• Tell him he may feel a transient burning as the contrast medium is injected and that he may experience a transient headache, a salty taste in his mouth, and nausea and vomiting.
• Tell him that the X-ray equipment makes a loud, clacking sound as the films are taken.

- Instruct him to lie still during the test to avoid blurring the films, and inform him that restraints may be used to help him remain still.
- Warn him that he may feel some temporary stiffness after the test from lying still on the hard X-ray table.
- Tell him who will perform the test and where and that it takes 30 minutes to 3 hours, depending on the number of vessels studied.
- Make sure the patient or a responsible family member has signed a consent form, if required.
- Check the patient's history for hypersensitivity to iodine, shellfish, or the contrast medium.
- Make sure blood studies (hemoglobin and hematocrit levels; clotting, prothrombin, and activated partial thromboplastin times; and platelet count) have been completed.
- Make sure that no barium is present from previous studies, such as computed tomography or barium enema. Abdominal scout films may determine this.
- Just before the procedure, instruct the patient to put on a gown and to remove jewelry and other objects that might obscure anatomic detail on X-ray films.
- Tell the patient to void; then record baseline vital signs.
- Administer a sedative, if prescribed.

Procedure and posttest care
- After the patient is placed in a supine position on the X-ray table, an I.V. infusion is started to maintain hydration and to permit emergency administration of medication.
- Scout films of the patient's abdomen are taken, and the peripheral pulses are palpated and marked.
- The puncture site is cleaned with soap and water; the area is shaved,

cleaned with povidone-iodine preparation, and surrounded by sterile drapes.
- The local anesthetic is injected and the femoral artery is located by palpation. The needle is gently inserted until a pulsing blood flow is obtained.
- A guide wire is passed through the needle into the aorta; then the needle is removed, leaving the guide wire in place.
- The angiocath is inserted over the guide wire; the guide wire is withdrawn to inject the contrast medium to check for catheter placement. The guide wire is again inserted into the selected artery for fluoroscopic guidance.
- When the wire is in position, the catheter is advanced over it into the artery. The wire is then removed and placement verified by hand injection of contrast medium.
- The automatic injector is then attached to the catheter. As the contrast medium is injected, a series of films is taken in rapid sequence.
- After injecting into one or more major arteries, superselective catheterization may be performed. Using fluoroscopy, the catheter is repositioned in a specific branch of a major artery, contrast medium is injected, and rapid-sequence films are taken. If necessary, several specific branches may be catheterized.
- If GI bleeding is detected, coils may be placed to occlude the vessel, or vasopressin may be infused.
- If a neoplasm is detected, tumor embolization may be performed.
- After filming, the catheter is withdrawn, and firm pressure is applied to the puncture site for about 15 minutes.
- Observe the puncture site for hematoma formation, and check peripheral pulses.
- Inform the patient that he'll be on bed rest for 4 to 6 hours and that he

must keep the leg with the puncture site straight. Do not raise the bed further than 30 degrees. He'll be able to logroll and may use the unaffected leg to reposition himself to use the bedpan.

• Monitor vital signs until stable, and check peripheral pulses. Note the color and temperature of the leg that was used for the test.

• Check the puncture site for bleeding and hematoma. If bleeding develops, apply pressure to the site. If a hematoma develops, apply warm soaks.

• Confirm whether the patient can resume his usual diet. If the patient isn't receiving I.V. infusions, encourage intake of fluids to speed excretion of the contrast medium.

• Tell the patient that he must be careful when swallowing for 4 to 6 hours after surgery.

Precautions

• Celiac and mesenteric arteriography should be performed cautiously in patients with coagulopathy.

⬛ **CLINICAL ALERT** Most reactions to the contrast medium occur within a half-hour. Watch carefully for cardiovascular shock or arrest, flushing, laryngeal stridor, or urticaria.

Normal findings

X-ray films show the three phases of perfusion — arterial, capillary, and venous. The arteries normally taper regularly, becoming gradually smaller with subsequent divisions. The contrast medium then spreads evenly within the sinusoids. The portal vein appears 10 to 20 seconds after the injection, as the contrast medium empties from the spleen into the splenic vein or from the intestine into the superior mesenteric vein and further into the portal vein.

Abnormal findings

GI hemorrhage appears on the angiogram as the extravasation of contrast medium from the damaged vessels. Upper GI hemorrhage can result from conditions such as Mallory-Weiss syndrome, gastric or peptic ulcer, hemorrhagic gastritis, and eroded hiatal hernia. Esophageal hemorrhage rarely appears on the angiogram because the contrast medium usually fails to fill the esophageal vein. Lower GI hemorrhage can result from conditions such as bleeding diverticula, carcinoma, and angiodysplasia.

Abdominal neoplasms — carcinoid tumors, adenomas, leiomyomas, angiomas, and adenocarcinomas — can disrupt the normal vasculature in several ways. Neoplasms can invade or encase nearby arteries and veins, distorting their regular channel-like appearance and, in late stages, displacing them. Vessels within the neoplasm, known as neovasculature, appear as abnormal vascular areas. Areas of necrosis appear as puddles of contrast medium. Contrast medium may also remain in the neoplasm longer during capillary perfusion, producing a tumor blush or stain on the angiogram. Arteriovenous shunting may also be present, depending on the size and location of the tumor. Because these characteristics aren't uniformly present in all neoplasms, combinations of these characteristics can often distinguish between benign and malignant neoplasms.

In early or mild cirrhosis, portal venous flow to the liver remains relatively unaffected, and the hepatic artery and its branches appear normal. As this disease progresses, portal venous flow diminishes, the hepatic artery and its branches become dilated and tortuous, and collateral veins develop. In advanced cirrhosis, portal venous flow reverses. However, the portal vein still appears on the X-ray film, which may also show thrombi.

Abdominal trauma commonly causes splenic injury; less often, hepatic injury. Splenic rupture often displaces intrasplenic arterial branches, causing contrast medium to leak from splenic arteries into the splenic pulp. When rupture occurs without subcapsular hematoma, the spleen usually maintains its normal size. However, in subcapsular hematoma, the spleen enlarges to displace the splenic artery and vein; the subcapsular hematoma itself appears as a large, avascular mass that stretches intrasplenic arteries and compresses the splenic pulp away from the capsule.

Hepatic injury causes similar vascular distortion, such as displacement of the common hepatic artery and extrahepatic branches. Intrahepatic and subcapsular hematomas displace and stretch intrahepatic arteries. As the hepatic vascular supply is disrupted, an arteriovenous fistula may develop between the hepatic artery and the portal vein.

Various abnormalities affecting the diameter and course of an artery may appear on the angiogram. Atherosclerotic plaques or atheromas — lipid deposits on the intima — narrow the arterial lumen and may even occlude it, resulting in formation of collaterals. Other identifiable vascular abnormalities include aneurysms, thrombi, and emboli.

Interfering factors
• Patient's inability to remain still during the procedure
• Barium, gas, or stool from a previous procedure (possible poor imaging)
• Presence of an atherosclerotic lesion in the vessel to be cannulated (prevents entry and passage of catheter)

GENITOURINARY SYSTEM

KIDNEY-URETER-BLADDER RADIOGRAPHY

Usually the first step in diagnostic testing of the urinary system, kidney-ureter-bladder (KUB) radiography surveys the abdomen to determine the position of the kidneys, ureters, and bladder, and to detect gross abnormalities.

This test doesn't require intact renal function and may aid differential diagnosis of urologic and GI diseases, which often produce similar signs and symptoms. However, KUB radiography has many limitations and nearly always must be followed by more elaborate tests, such as excretory urography or renal computed tomography. KUB radiography should not follow recent instillation of barium.

Purpose
• To evaluate the size, structure, and position of the kidneys
• To screen for abnormalities, such as calcifications, in the region of the kidneys, ureters, and bladder

Patient preparation
• Explain to the patient that this test helps detect urinary system abnormalities.
• Inform him that he needn't restrict food or fluids. Tell him who will perform the test and where and that it takes only a few minutes.

Procedure and posttest care

• The patient is placed in a supine position in correct body alignment on an X-ray table. His arms are extended overhead, and the iliac crests are checked for symmetrical positioning.
• If the patient can't extend his arms or stand, he may lie on his left side with his right arm up.
• A single X-ray is taken.

Precautions

• Male patients should have gonadal shielding to prevent irradiation of the testes. Female patients' ovaries can't be shielded because they're too close to the kidneys, ureters, and bladder.

Normal findings

The shadows of the kidneys appear bilaterally, the right slightly lower than the left. Both kidneys should be approximately the same size, with the superior poles tilted slightly toward the vertebral column, paralleling the shadows (or stripes) produced by the psoas muscles. The ureters are only visible when an abnormality such as calcification is present. Visualization of the bladder depends on the density of its muscular wall and on the amount of urine in it.

Abnormal findings

Bilateral renal enlargement may result from polycystic disease, multiple myeloma, lymphoma, amyloidosis, diabetes, hydronephrosis, or compensatory hypertrophy. Tumor, cyst, or hydronephrosis may cause unilateral enlargement. Abnormally small kidneys may suggest end-stage glomerulonephritis or bilateral atrophic pyelonephritis. An apparent decrease in the size of one kidney suggests possible congenital hypoplasia, atrophic pyelonephritis, or ischemia. Renal displacement may be due to a retroperitoneal tumor, such as an adrenal tumor. Obliteration or bulging of a portion of the psoas muscle stripe may result from tumor, abscess, or hematoma.

Congenital anomalies, such as abnormal location or absence of a kidney, may be detected. Horseshoe kidney may be suggested by renal axes that parallel the vertebral column, especially if the inferior poles of the kidneys cannot be clearly distinguished. A lobulated edge or border may suggest polycystic kidney disease or patchy atrophic pyelonephritis.

Opaque bodies may reflect calculi or vascular calcification due to aneurysm or atheroma; opacification may also suggest cystic tumors, fecaliths, foreign bodies, or abnormal fluid collection. Calcifications may appear anywhere in the urinary system, but positive identification requires further testing. The lone exception is staghorn calculus, which forms a perfect cast of the renal pelvis and calyces.

Interfering factors

• Gas, stool, contrast medium, or foreign bodies in the intestine (possible poor imaging)
• Calcified uterine fibromas or ovarian lesions
• Obesity or ascites (possible poor imaging)

NEPHROTOMOGRAPHY

In nephrotomography, special films are exposed before and after opacification of the renal arterial network and parenchyma with contrast medium. The resulting tomographic slices clearly delineate various linear layers of the kidneys, while blurring structures in front of and behind these selected planes.

Nephrotomography can be performed as a separate procedure or as an adjunct to excretory urography. Nephrotomography is particularly helpful in visualizing space-occupying lesions suggested by excretory urography or retrograde ureteropyelography. Additional films are exposed to define the thickness of the wall of the mass and its interior. Other tests that may resolve nephrotomographic findings include renal angiography and radionuclide renal imaging.

Enhanced computed tomography (CT) of the abdomen and pelvis is increasingly being used instead of nephrotomography.

Purpose
- To differentiate between a simple renal cyst and a solid neoplasm
- To assess renal lacerations as well as posttraumatic nonperfused areas of the kidneys
- To localize adrenal tumors when laboratory tests indicate their presence

Patient preparation
- Explain to the patient that this test provides images of sections or layers of the kidney tissues and blood vessels.
- Instruct him to fast for 8 hours before the test. Tell him who will perform the test and where and that the test takes less than 1 hour.
- Tell him that he'll be positioned on an X-ray table and that he may hear loud, clacking sounds as the films are exposed. Tell him that he may experience transient adverse effects from the injection of the contrast medium — usually a burning or stinging sensation at the injection site, flushing, and a metallic taste.
- Make sure that the patient or a responsible family member has signed a consent form if required.

- Check his history for hypersensitivity to iodine or iodine-containing foods or to contrast media used in other diagnostic tests. If the patient has a history of sensitivity, provide antiallergenic prophylaxis (such as diphenhydramine) or use a non-iodine-containing contrast medium, as necessary. Also check the patient for renal insufficiency; this may contraindicate contrast media study.

Procedure and posttest care
- The test may be performed using either the infusion method or the bolus method. Complications resulting from either technique are minor and infrequent.
- A plain film of the kidneys is exposed to provide general information about their position, size, and shape, and preliminary anteroposterior tomograms are made to determine tomographic levels. Posterior oblique tomograms are made to rule out the presence of radiopaque renal calculi, which would be masked by the contrast medium.

Infusion method
- After test tomograms are reviewed, five vertical slices of renal parenchyma 1 cm apart are selected for filming.
- Contrast medium is then administered through the antecubital vein — the first half in 4 to 5 minutes (rapid phase) and the second half in the following 8 to 10 minutes (slow phase). Serial tomograms are made as soon as the slow phase begins.

Bolus method
- After test tomograms are reviewed, circulation time from arm to tongue is determined by injecting a bolus of a bitter-tasting agent (dehydrocholic acid or sodium dehydrocholate) into the antecubital vein. Arm-to-tongue circulation time is close to arm-to-kidney circulation time.

SIMPLE CYST OR SOLID TUMOR: DIFFERENTIAL DIAGNOSIS IN NEPHROTOMOGRAPHY

FEATURE	CYST	TUMOR
Consistency	Homogeneous	Irregular
Contact with healthy renal tissue	Sharply distinct	Poorly resolved
Density	Radiolucent	Variable radiolucent patches (or same as normal renal parenchyma)
Shape	Spherical	Variable
Wall of lesion	Thin and well defined	Thick and irregular

- With the needle still in place, a loading dose of a conventional urographic contrast medium is injected to perform excretory urography.
- Five minutes after this injection, a loading dose of a contrast medium (such as Renografin-76 or Hypaque-M 75%) is quickly injected to ensure a high concentration of the contrast medium in the kidneys. A multifilm tomographic cassette, exposed at the predetermined arm-to-kidney circulation time, visualizes the main renal vessels and possible vessels within tumors.
- A series of individual tomograms measuring 1 cm are then made in rapid succession through the opacified kidneys.
- If the exposures are poor, this method requires a second infusion of contrast medium because normal kidneys quickly clear the substance.

Both methods
- If a hematoma develops at the injection site, apply warm soaks.
- Monitor vital signs and urine output for 24 hours after the test.

 CLINICAL ALERT Observe for signs of a posttest allergic reaction (flushing, nausea, urticaria, and sneezing). Have epinephrine (1:1,000) and an antihistamine readily available to counter allergic reactions.

Precautions
- Nephrotomography should be performed with extreme caution in patients with hypersensitivity to iodine-based compounds or in those with severe cardiovascular disease or multiple myeloma.

Normal findings
The size, shape, and position of the kidneys appear within normal range, with no space-occupying lesions or other abnormalities.

Abnormal findings
Among the abnormalities detectable through nephrotomography are simple cysts and solid tumors, renal sinus–related lesions, ectopic renal lobes, adrenal tumors, areas of nonperfusion, and renal lacerations following trauma. (See *Simple cyst or solid tumor: Differential diagnosis in nephrotomography.*)

Interfering factor
• Residual barium from a recent enema or other GI studies (possible poor imaging)

RETROGRADE URETHROGRAPHY

Used almost exclusively in men, retrograde urethrography requires instillation or injection of a contrast medium into the urethra and permits visualization of its membranous, bulbar, and penile portions.

Although visualization of the anterior portion of the urethra is excellent with this test alone, the posterior portion is more effectively outlined by retrograde urethrography in tandem with voiding cystourethrography.

Purpose
• To diagnose urethral strictures, outlet obstruction, diverticula, and congenital anomalies
• To assess urethral lacerations or other trauma
• To assist with follow-up examination after surgical repair of the urethra

Patient preparation
• Explain to the patient that this test diagnoses urethral structural problems. Inform him that he needn't restrict food or fluids.
• Describe the test, including who will perform it, where it will take place, and its expected duration (about 30 minutes).
• Inform the patient that he may experience some discomfort when the catheter is inserted and when the contrast medium is instilled through the catheter.

• Tell him that he may hear loud, clacking sounds as the X-ray films are made.
• Make sure the patient or a responsible family member has signed a consent form if required.
• Check the patient's history for hypersensitivity to iodine-containing foods, such as shellfish, or contrast media.
• Just before the procedure, administer any prescribed sedatives and instruct the patient to void before leaving the unit.

Equipment
Penile clamp, 50-ml syringe with tapered universal adapter, indwelling urinary catheter, 1″ (2.5-cm) roller gauze, contrast medium (half-strength preparation)

Procedure and posttest care
For men
• The patient is placed in a recumbent position on the examining table. Anteroposterior exposures of the bladder and urethra are made, and the resulting films studied for radiopaque densities, foreign bodies, or stones.
• The glans and meatus are cleaned with an antiseptic solution. The catheter is filled with the contrast medium before insertion to eliminate air bubbles.
• Although no lubricant should be used, the tip of the catheter may be dipped in sterile water to facilitate insertion.
• The catheter is inserted until the balloon portion is inside the meatus; the balloon is then inflated with 1 to 2 ml of water, which prevents the catheter from slipping during the procedure.
• The patient then assumes the right posterior oblique position, with his right thigh drawn up to a 90-degree angle and the penis placed along its axis. The left thigh is extended.

• The contrast medium is injected through the catheter. After three-fourths of the contrast medium has been injected, the first X-ray film is exposed while the remainder of the contrast medium is being injected. Left lateral oblique views may also be taken.

• Fluoroscopic control may be helpful, especially for evaluating urethral injury.

For women and children

• In women, this test may be used when urethral diverticula are suspected. A double-balloon catheter is used, which occludes the bladder neck from above and the external meatus from below.

• In children, the procedure is the same as for adults except that a smaller catheter is used.

For all patients

• Watch for chills and fever related to extravasation of contrast medium into the general circulation for 12 to 24 hours after retrograde urethrography. Also observe for signs of sepsis and allergic manifestations.

Precautions

• Retrograde urethrography should be performed cautiously in patients with urinary tract infection.

Normal findings

The membranous, bulbar, and penile portions of the urethra — and occasionally the prostatic portion — appear normal in size, shape, and course.

Abnormal findings

Radiographs obtained during retrograde urethrography may show the following abnormalities: urethral diverticula, fistulas, strictures, false passages, calculi, and lacerations; congenital anomalies, such as urethral valves and perineal hypospadias; and

rarely, tumors (in less than 1% of patients).

Interfering factors

• None significant

RETROGRADE CYSTOGRAPHY

Retrograde cystography involves the instillation of contrast medium into the bladder, followed by radiographic examination. This procedure is used to diagnose bladder rupture without urethral involvement because it can determine the location and extent of the rupture. Other indications for retrograde cystography include neurogenic bladder, recurrent urinary tract infections (UTIs, especially in children), suspected vesicoureteral reflux, and vesical fistulas, diverticula, and tumors. This test is also performed when cystoscopic examination is impractical, as in male infants, or when excretory urography has not adequately visualized the bladder. Voiding cystourethrography is often performed concomitantly.

Purpose

• To evaluate the structure and integrity of the bladder

Patient preparation

• Explain to the patient that this test permits radiographic examination of the bladder.

• Inform him that he needn't restrict food or fluids before the test.

• Tell him who will perform the test and where and that the procedure takes about 30 to 60 minutes.

• Inform the patient that he may experience some discomfort when the catheter is inserted and when the contrast medium is instilled through the catheter.

• Tell him that he may hear loud, clacking sounds as the X-ray films are made.

• Make sure the patient or a responsible family member has signed a consent form.

• Check the patient's history for hypersensitivity to contrast media, iodine, or shellfish; mark it on the chart.

Equipment
Drip infusion set or syringes, standard contrast medium, urethral indwelling urinary catheters

Procedure and posttest care
• The patient is placed in a supine position on the X-ray table, and a preliminary kidney-ureter-bladder radiograph is taken.

• The radiograph is developed immediately and scrutinized for renal shadows, calcifications, contours of the bone and psoas muscles, and gas patterns in the lumen of the GI tract.

• The bladder is catheterized, and 200 to 300 ml of sterile contrast medium (50 to 100 ml in an infant) is instilled by gravity or gentle syringe injection. The catheter is then clamped.

• With the patient supine, an anteroposterior film is taken. The patient is then tilted to one side, then the other, and two posterior oblique (and sometimes lateral) views are taken.

• If the patient's condition permits, he's placed in the jackknife position and a posteroanterior film is taken. A space-occupying vesical lesion may require additional exposures. Rarely, to enhance visualization, 100 to 300 ml of air may be insufflated into the bladder by syringe after removal of the contrast medium (double-contrast technique).

• The catheter is then unclamped, the bladder fluid is allowed to drain, and a radiograph is obtained to detect urethral diverticula, reflux into the ureters, fistulous tracts into the vagina, or intraperitoneal or extraperitoneal extravasation of the contrast medium.

• Monitor vital signs every 15 minutes for the first hour, every 30 minutes during the second hour, then every 2 hours for up to 24 hours.

• Record the time of the patient's voidings and the color and volume of the urine. Observe for hematuria that persists after the third voiding.

• Watch for signs of urinary sepsis from UTI (chills, fever, elevated pulse and respiration rates, and hypotension) or similar signs related to extravasation of contrast medium into the general circulation.

Precautions
• Retrograde cystography is contraindicated during exacerbation of an acute UTI or in patients with an obstruction that prevents passage of a urinary catheter.

• This test should not be performed in patients with urethral evulsion or transection, unless catheter passage and flow of contrast medium are monitored fluoroscopically.

Normal findings
Retrograde cystography shows a bladder with normal contours, capacity, integrity, and urethrovesical angle and with no evidence of tumor, diverticula, or rupture. Vesicoureteral reflux should be absent. The bladder should not be displaced or externally compressed; the bladder wall should be smooth, not thick.

Abnormal findings
Retrograde cystography can identify vesical trabeculae or diverticula, space-occupying lesions (tumors), calculi or

gravel, blood clots, high- or low-pressure vesicoureteral reflux, and a hypotonic or hypertonic bladder.

Interfering factors
• Gas, stool, or residual barium from recent diagnostic tests in the bowel (possible poor imaging)

RETROGRADE URETEROPYELOGRAPHY

Retrograde ureteropyelography allows radiographic examination of the renal collecting system after injection of a contrast medium through a ureteral catheter during cystoscopy. The contrast medium is usually iodine-based and, although some of it may be absorbed through the mucous membranes, this test is preferred for patients with hypersensitivity to iodine (in whom I.V. administration of an iodine-based contrast medium, as in excretory urography, is contraindicated). This test is also indicated when visualization of the renal collecting system by excretory urography is inadequate due to inferior films or marked renal insufficiency because retrograde ureteropyelography is not influenced by impaired renal function. (See *Sites and types of obstruction indicated by ureteropyelography*.)

Purpose
• To assess the structure and integrity of the renal collecting system (calyces, renal pelvis, and ureter)

Patient preparation
• Explain to the patient that this test permits visualization of the urinary collecting system.

• If a general anesthetic is to be used, instruct him to fast for 8 hours before the test. Generally, he should be well hydrated to ensure adequate urine flow.
• Tell him who will perform the test and where and that it takes about 1 hour.
• Inform the patient that he'll be positioned on an examinination table, with his legs in stirrups, and that the position may be tiring.
• If he will be awake throughout the procedure, tell him he may feel pressure as the instrument is passed and a pressure sensation in the kidney area when the contrast medium is introduced. Also, he may feel an urgency to void.
• Make sure that the patient or a responsible family member has signed a consent form.
• Just before the procedure, administer any prescribed premedication.

Equipment
Cystoscopy setup, ureteral catheters, 10-ml syringes with ureteral adapters, contrast medium

Procedure and posttest care
• Place the patient in lithotomy position. Care must be taken to avoid pressure points or impairment to circulation while his legs are in the stirrups.
• After the patient is anesthetized, the urologist first performs a cystoscopic examination.
• After visual inspection of the bladder, one or both ureters are catheterized with opaque catheters, depending on the condition or abnormality suspected. Radiographic monitoring allows correct positioning of the catheter tip in the renal pelvis.
• The renal pelvis is emptied by gravity drainage or aspiration. About 4 or 5 ml of contrast medium is then injected slowly through the catheter using the syringe with the special adapter.

• When adequate filling and opacification have occurred, anteroposterior radiographic films are taken and immediately developed. Lateral and oblique films can be taken, as needed, after the injection of more contrast medium.

• After the radiographs of the renal pelvis are examined, a few more milliliters of contrast medium are injected to outline the ureters as the catheter is slowly withdrawn.

• Delayed films (10 to 15 minutes after complete catheter removal) are then taken to check for retention of the contrast medium, indicating urinary stasis.

• If ureteral obstruction is present, the ureteral catheter may be kept in place and, together with an indwelling urinary catheter, connected to a gravity drainage system until posttest urinary flow is corrected or returns to normal.

• Check vital signs every 15 minutes for the first 4 hours, then every hour for the next 4 hours, and then every 4 hours for 24 hours.

• Monitor fluid intake and urine output for 24 hours. Observe each specimen for hematuria. Gross hematuria or hematuria after the third voiding is abnormal and should be reported. If the patient doesn't void for 8 hours after the procedure, or immediately if the patient feels distress and his bladder is distended, urethral catheterization may be necessary.

◤ **CLINICAL ALERT** Be especially attentive to catheter output if ureteral catheters have been left in place, because inadequate output may reflect catheter obstruction, requiring irrigation. Protect ureteral catheters from dislodgment.

• Administer prescribed analgesics, tub baths, and increased fluid intake for dysuria, which commonly occurs after retrograde ureteropyelography.

• Watch for and report severe pain in the area of the kidneys as well as any

SITES AND TYPES OF OBSTRUCTION INDICATED BY URETEROPYELOGRAPHY

Ureteropyelography may detect a stricture, neoplasm, blood clot, or calculus that obstructs urine flow in the calyces, pelvis, or ureter. Small calculi may remain in the calyces and pelvis or pass down the ureter. A staghorn calculus (a cast of the calyceal and pelvic collecting system) may form from a calculus that stays in the kidney.

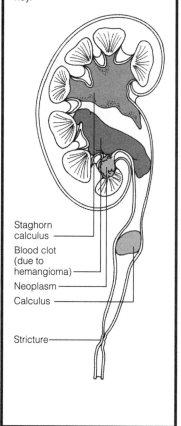

Staghorn calculus

Blood clot (due to hemangioma)

Neoplasm

Calculus

Stricture

signs of sepsis (such as chills, fever, and hypotension).

Precautions
• Retrograde ureteropyelography must be done carefully in patients with urinary stasis caused by ureteral obstruction to prevent further injury to the ureter.

Normal findings
Following a normal cystoscopic examination, ureteral catheterization, and injection of contrast medium through the catheters, opacification of the pelves and calyces should occur immediately. Normal structures should be outlined clearly and should appear symmetrical in bilateral testing. Ureters should fill uniformly and appear normal in size and course. Inspiratory and expiratory exposures, when superimposed, normally create two outlines of the renal pelvis ¾″ (2 cm) apart.

Abnormal findings
Incomplete or delayed drainage reflects an obstruction, most commonly at the ureteropelvic junction. Enlargement of the components of the collecting system or delayed emptying of contrast medium may indicate obstruction due to tumor, blood clot, stricture, or calculi.

Perinephric inflammation or suppuration often causes fixation of the kidney on the same side, resulting in a single sharp radiographic outline of the collecting system when inspiratory and expiratory exposures are superimposed. Upward, downward, or lateral renal displacement can result from renal abscess or tumor or from perinephric abscess. Neoplasms can cause displacement of either pole or of the entire kidney.

Interfering factors
• Previous contrast studies or presence of stool or gas in the bowel (possible poor imaging)

ANTEGRADE PYELOGRAPHY

Antegrade pyelography allows examination of the upper collecting system when ureteral obstruction rules out retrograde ureteropyelography or when cystoscopy is contraindicated. It depends on percutaneous needle puncture for injection of contrast medium into the renal pelvis or calyces.

Renal pressure can be measured during this procedure. Also, urine can be collected for cultures and cytologic studies and for evaluation of renal functional reserve before surgery.

After completion of radiographic studies, a nephrostomy tube can be inserted to provide temporary drainage or access for other therapeutic or diagnostic procedures.

Purpose
• To evaluate obstruction of the upper collecting system by stricture, calculus, clot, or tumor
• To evaluate hydronephrosis revealed during excretory urography or ultrasonography and to enable placement of a percutaneous nephrostomy tube
• To evaluate the function of the upper collecting system after ureteral surgery or urinary diversion
• To assess renal functional reserve before surgery

Patient preparation
• Explain to the patient that this test allows radiographic examination of the kidney.

• Tell him that he may be required to fast for 6 to 8 hours before the test.

• Tell him he may receive antimicrobial drugs before and after the procedure.

• Inform the patient who will perform the test and where and that it will take approximately 1 to 2 hours.

• Explain that a needle will be inserted into the kidney after he's given a sedative and a local anesthetic. Explain that urine may be collected from the kidney for testing and that, if necessary, a tube will be left in the kidney for drainage.

• Tell him that he may feel mild discomfort during injection of the local anesthetic and contrast medium and that he may also feel transient burning and flushing from the contrast medium.

• Warn him that the X-ray machine makes loud, clacking sounds as films are taken.

• Check the patient's history for hypersensitivity reactions to contrast media, iodine, or shellfish. Mark any sensitivities clearly on the chart. Also check the history and recent coagulation studies for indications of bleeding disorders.

• Make sure that the patient or a responsible family member has signed an appropriate consent form.

• Just before the procedure, administer a sedative, if needed.

Equipment
Percutaneous nephrostomy tray, manometer, preparatory tray, gloves and sterile containers for specimens, syringes and needles, contrast medium, local anesthetic, emergency resuscitation equipment

Procedure and posttest care
• The patient is placed prone on the X-ray table. The skin over the kidney is cleaned with antiseptic solution, and a local anesthetic is injected.

• Previous urographic films or ultrasound recordings are studied for anatomic landmarks. (It's important to determine if the kidney to be studied is in normal position. If not, the angle of the needle entry must be adjusted during percutaneous puncture.)

• Under guidance of fluoroscopy or ultrasonography, the percutaneous needle is inserted below the 12th rib at the level of the transverse process of the 2nd lumbar vertebra. Aspiration of urine confirms that the needle has reached the dilated collecting system.

• Flexible tubing is connected to the needle to prevent displacement during the procedure. If intrarenal pressure is to be measured, the manometer is connected to the tubing as soon as it's in place. Urine specimens are then taken if needed.

• An amount of urine equal to the amount of contrast medium to be injected is withdrawn to prevent overdistention of the collecting system.

• The contrast medium is injected under fluoroscopic guidance. Posteroanterior, oblique, and anteroposterior radiographs are taken. Ureteral peristalsis is observed on the fluoroscope screen to evaluate obstruction.

• A percutaneous nephrostomy tube is inserted if drainage is needed because of increased renal pressure, dilation, or intrarenal reflux. If drainage isn't needed, the catheter is withdrawn and a sterile dressing is applied.

• Check vital signs every 15 minutes for the first hour, every 30 minutes for the second hour, and every 2 hours for the next 24 hours.

• Check dressings for bleeding, hematoma, or urine leakage at the puncture site at each check of vital signs. For bleeding, apply pressure. For a hematoma, apply warm soaks. Report urine leakage or the patient's failure to void within 8 hours.

• Monitor fluid intake and urine output for 24 hours. Observe each specimen for hematuria. Report hematuria if it persists after the third voiding.

• Watch for and report signs of sepsis or extravasation of contrast medium (chills, fever, rapid pulse or respirations, and hypotension).

CLINICAL ALERT Also watch for and report signs that adjacent organs have been punctured: pain in the abdomen or flank, or pneumothorax (sudden onset of pleuritic chest pain, dyspnea, tachypnea, decreased breath sounds on the affected side, and tachycardia).

• If a nephrostomy tube is inserted, check to be sure that it's patent and draining well.

• Administer prescribed antibiotics for several days after the procedure and analgesics.

Precautions
• Antegrade pyelography is contraindicated in patients with bleeding disorders.

• Watch for signs of hypersensitivity to the contrast medium.

Normal findings
After injection of contrast medium, the upper collecting system should fill uniformly and appear normal in size and course. Normal structures should be outlined clearly.

Abnormal findings
Enlargements of the upper collecting system and parts of the ureteropelvic junction indicate obstruction. Antegrade pyelography shows the degree of dilation, clearly defines obstructions, and demonstrates intrarenal reflux. In hydronephrosis, the ureteropelvic junction shows marked distention. Results of recent surgery or urinary diversion will be obvious; for example, a ureteral

stent or a dilated stenotic area will be clearly visualized.

Intrarenal pressure greater than 20 cm H_2O indicates obstruction. Cultures or cytologic studies of urine specimens taken during antegrade pyelography can confirm antegrade pyelonephrosis or malignancy.

Interfering factors
• Recent barium procedures, or stool or gas in the bowel (possible poor imaging)

• Obesity (possible difficulty in needle placement)

EXCRETORY UROGRAPHY

The cornerstone of a urologic workup, excretory urography (also called intravenous pyelography) requires I.V. administration of a contrast medium and allows visualization of the renal parenchyma, calyces, and pelvis, as well as the ureters, bladder and, in some cases, the urethra.

In some facilities, a nonenhanced computed tomography scan of the urinary tract is commonly performed instead of this test if urinary tract stones are suspected.

Purpose
• To evaluate the structure and excretory function of the kidneys, ureters, and bladder

• To evaluate suspected renal or urinary tract disease, renal calculi, space-occupying lesions, congenital anomalies, or trauma to the urinary system

• To support a differential diagnosis of renovascular hypertension

Patient preparation

• Explain to the patient that this test helps to evaluate the structure and function of the urinary tract.

• Make sure the patient is well hydrated; then instruct him to fast for 8 hours before the test. Tell him who will perform the test and where.

• Inform the patient that he may experience a transient burning sensation and metallic taste when the contrast medium is injected. Tell him to report any other sensations he may experience.

• Warn him that the X-ray machine may make loud, clacking sounds during the test.

• Make sure that the patient or a responsible family member has signed a consent form.

• Check the patient's history for hypersensitivity to iodine, iodine-containing foods, or contrast media containing iodine. Mark any sensitivities on the chart.

• Administer a laxative, if necessary, the night before the test, to minimize poor resolution of X-ray films due to stool and gas in the GI tract.

Equipment

Contrast medium (sodium diatrizoate or iothalamate, or meglumine diatrizoate or iothalamate); 50-ml syringe (or I.V. container and tubing); 19G to 21G needle, catheter, or butterfly needle; venipuncture equipment (tourniquet, antiseptic, adhesive bandage); emergency resuscitative equipment

Procedure and posttest care

• The patient is placed in a supine position on the X-ray table.

• A kidney-ureter-bladder radiograph is exposed, developed, and studied for gross abnormalities of the urinary system. In the absence of any such abnormality, contrast medium is injected (dosage varies according to age), and

the patient is observed for signs of hypersensitivity (flushing, nausea, vomiting, hives, or dyspnea).

• The first radiograph, visualizing the renal parenchyma, is obtained about 1 minute after the injection, possibly supplemented by tomography if small space-occupying masses, such as cysts or tumors, are suspected.

• Films are then exposed at regular intervals — usually 5, 10, and 15 or 20 minutes after the injection.

• Ureteral compression is performed after the 5-minute film is exposed. This can be accomplished through inflation of two small rubber bladders placed on the abdomen on both sides of the midline, secured by a fastener wrapped around the patient's torso. The inflated bladders occlude the ureters without causing the patient discomfort, and facilitate retention of the contrast medium by the upper urinary tract. (Ureteral compression is contraindicated by ureteral calculi, aortic aneurysm, pregnancy, or recent abdominal trauma or surgical procedure.)

• After the 10-minute film is exposed, ureteral compression is released. As the contrast flows into the lower urinary tract, another film is taken of the lower halves of both ureters and then, finally, one is taken of the bladder.

• At the end of the procedure, the patient voids, and another film is made immediately to visualize residual bladder content or mucosal abnormalities of the bladder or urethra.

• If a hematoma develops at the injection site, ease the patient's discomfort by applying warm soaks.

• Observe for delayed reactions to the contrast medium.

Precautions

• Premedication with corticosteroids may be indicated for patients with severe asthma or a history of sensitivity to the contrast medium.

Normal findings

The kidneys, ureters, and bladder show no gross evidence of soft- or hard-tissue lesions. Prompt visualization of the contrast medium in the kidneys demonstrates bilateral renal parenchyma and pelvicalyceal systems of normal conformity. The ureters and bladder should be outlined, and the postvoiding radiograph should show no mucosal abnormalities and minimal residual urine.

Abnormal findings

Excretory urography can demonstrate many abnormalities of the urinary system, including renal or ureteral calculi; abnormal size, shape, or structure of kidneys, ureters, or bladder; supernumerary or absent kidney; polycystic kidney disease associated with renal hypertrophy; redundant pelvis or ureter; space-occupying lesion; pyelonephritis; renal tuberculosis; hydronephrosis; and renovascular hypertension.

Interfering factors

- End-stage renal disease, stool or gas in the colon (possible poor imaging)
- Insufficient injection of contrast medium, a recent barium enema, GI or gallbladder series (possible poor imaging)

RENAL ANGIOGRAPHY

Renal angiography requires arterial injection of a contrast medium and permits radiographic examination of the renal vasculature and parenchyma. As the contrast pervades the renal vasculature, rapid-sequence radiographs show the vessels during three phases of filling: arterial, nephrographic, and venous.

This procedure virtually always follows standard bolus aortography, which shows individual variations in number, size, and condition of the main renal arteries, aberrant vessels, and the relationship of the renal arteries to the aorta.

Purpose

- To demonstrate the configuration of total renal vasculature before surgical procedures
- To determine the cause of renovascular hypertension, such as from stenosis, thrombotic occlusions, emboli, and aneurysms
- To investigate unilateral or bilateral kidney enlargement, nonfunctioning kidneys in patients with acute renal failure, and intrarenal calcifications of unexplained etiology
- To evaluate chronic renal disease or renal failure
- To investigate renal masses, vascular malformations, pseudotumors, and renal trauma
- To detect complications following renal transplantation, such as a nonfunctioning shunt or rejection of the donor organ

Patient preparation

- Explain to the patient that this test permits visualization of the kidneys, blood vessels, and functional units and aids in diagnosing renal disease or masses.
- Instruct him to fast for 8 hours before the test.
- Tell him who will perform the test and where and that it takes approximately 1 hour.
- Describe the procedure to him, and inform him that he may experience transient discomfort (flushing, burning sensation, and nausea) during injection of the contrast medium.

• Make sure that the patient or a responsible family member has signed a consent form.

• Check the patient's history for hypersensitivity to iodine-based contrast media or iodine-containing foods such as shellfish. Mark sensitivities on the chart. The patient may require prophylactic antiallergenics (diphenhydramine or steroids).

• Administer prescribed medications (usually a sedative and a narcotic analgesic) before the test.

• Instruct the patient to put on a gown and to remove all metallic objects that may interfere with test results.

• Ask him to void before leaving the unit.

Equipment

Pressure-injection device, rapid cassette changer, polyethylene radiopaque vascular catheters, flexible guide wire, contrast material (such as Hypaque, Renografin, Conray, or Isopaque), preparation tray with 70% alcohol or povidone-iodine solution, emergency resuscitative equipment

Procedure and posttest care

• The patient is placed in supine position, and a peripheral I.V. infusion is started. The skin over the arterial puncture site is cleaned with antiseptic solution, and a local anesthetic is injected.

• The femoral artery is punctured and, under fluoroscopic visualization, cannulated. (If a femoral pulse is absent or the artery is convoluted or plaque-ridden, percutaneous transaxillary, transbrachial, or translumbar catheterization may be performed instead.)

• After passing the flexible guide wire through the artery, the cannula is withdrawn, leaving several inches of wire in the lumen.

• A polyethylene catheter is passed over the wire and advanced, under flu-oroscopic guidance, up the femoroiliac vessels to the aorta. The guide wire is removed, and the catheter is flushed with heparin flush solution.

• The contrast medium is injected, and screening aortograms are taken before proceeding.

• On completion of the aortographic study, a renal catheter is exchanged for the vascular catheter.

• To determine the position of the renal arteries and ensure that the tip of the catheter is in the lumen, a test bolus of contrast medium is injected immediately.

• If the patient has no adverse reaction to the contrast medium, 20 to 25 ml of the substance is injected just below the origin of the renal arteries.

• A series of rapid-sequence X-ray films of the filling of the renal vascular tree is exposed.

• If additional selective studies are required, the catheter remains in place while the films are examined. If the films are satisfactory, the catheter is removed.

• Apply a sterile sponge firmly to the puncture site for 15 minutes.

• Before the patient is returned to his room, observe the puncture site for hematoma.

• Keep the patient flat in bed and instruct him to keep the punctured leg straight for at least 6 hours.

• Check vital signs every 15 minutes for 1 hour, then every 30 minutes for 2 hours, and then every hour until they stabilize.

• Monitor popliteal and dorsalis pedis pulses for adequate perfusion at least every hour for 4 hours.

• Watch for bleeding or hematomas at the injection site. Keep the pressure dressing in place, and check for bleeding when you check all vital signs. If bleeding occurs, act promptly and apply direct pressure to the site.

Precautions
• Renal angiography is contraindicated during pregnancy and in patients with bleeding tendencies, allergy to contrast media, and renal failure due to end-stage renal disease.

Normal findings
Renal arteriographs show normal arborization of the vascular tree and normal architecture of the renal parenchyma.

Abnormal findings
Renal tumors usually show hypervascularity; renal cysts typically appear as clearly delineated, radiolucent masses. Renal artery stenosis caused by arteriosclerosis produces a noticeable constriction in the blood vessels, usually within the proximal portion of its length; this is a crucial finding in confirming renovascular hypertension. Renal artery dysplasia, unlike renal artery stenosis, usually affects the middle and distal portions of the vessel. Alternating aneurysms and stenotic regions give this rare disorder a characteristic beads-on-a-string appearance.

In renal infarction, blood vessels may appear to be absent or cut off, with the normal tissue replaced by scar tissue. Another typical finding is the appearance of triangular areas of infarcted tissue near the periphery of the affected kidney. The kidney itself may appear shrunken due to tissue scarring.

Other disorders that may be discovered through renal angiography include renal artery aneurysms (saccular or fusiform) and renal arteriovenous fistula with abnormal widening of and direct passage between the renal artery and renal vein. Destruction, distortion, and fibrosis of renal tissue with areas of reduced and tortuous vascularity may be noted in severe or chronic pyelonephritis, and an increase in capsular

vessels with abnormal intrarenal circulation may indicate renal abscesses or inflammatory masses.

When angiography is used to evaluate renal trauma, it may detect intrarenal hematoma, parenchymal laceration, shattered kidneys, and areas of infarction. Renal angiography may also be useful in distinguishing pseudotumors from tumors or cysts, in evaluating the volume of residual functioning renal tissue in hydronephrosis, and in evaluating donors and recipients before and after renal transplantation.

Interfering factors
• Patient movement
• Recent contrast studies, such as barium enema or an upper GI series (possible poor imaging)
• Presence of stool or gas in the GI tract (possible poor imaging)

RENAL VENOGRAPHY

Renal venography is a relatively simple procedure allowing radiographic examination of the main renal veins and their tributaries. In this test, contrast medium is injected by percutaneous catheter passed through the femoral vein and inferior vena cava into the renal vein. Indications for renal venography include renal vein thrombosis, tumor, and venous anomalies.

Purpose
• To detect renal vein thrombosis
• To evaluate renal vein compression due to extrinsic tumors or retroperitoneal fibrosis
• To distinguish renal parenchymal disease and aneurysms from pressure exerted by an adjacent mass

- To assess renal tumors and detect invasion of the renal vein or inferior vena cava
- To detect venous anomalies and defects
- To differentiate renal agenesis from a small kidney
- To collect renal venous blood samples for evaluation of renovascular hypertension

Patient preparation

- Explain to the patient that this test permits radiographic study of the renal veins.
- If prescribed, instruct him to fast for 4 hours before the test.
- Tell him who will perform the test and where and that it takes about 1 hour.
- Inform him that a catheter will be inserted into a vein in the groin area after he is given a sedative and a local anesthetic.
- Tell him that he may feel mild discomfort during injection of the local anesthetic and contrast medium and that he may feel transient burning and flushing from the contrast medium.
- Warn him that the X-ray equipment may make loud, clacking noises as the films are taken.
- Check his history for hypersensitivity to contrast media, iodine, or iodine-containing foods, such as shellfish. Mark sensitivities on the chart.
- Check his history and any coagulation studies for indications of bleeding disorders.
- If renin assays will be done, check the patient's diet and medications, and consult with the health care team. As necessary, restrict the patient's salt intake and discontinue antihypertensive drugs, diuretics, estrogen, and oral contraceptives.

- Make sure that the patient or a responsible family member has signed a consent form.
- Just before the procedure, administer a sedative if necessary.

Equipment

Renal venography tray with flexible guide wires, polyethylene radiopaque vascular catheters, needle and cannula or 18G needle, three-way stopcock, and flexible tubing; preparatory tray; syringes and needles; contrast medium; local anesthetic; emergency resuscitation equipment

Procedure and posttest care

- The patient is placed in a supine position on the X-ray table, with his abdomen centered over the film. The skin over the right femoral vein near the groin is cleaned with antiseptic solution and draped. (The left femoral vein or jugular veins may be used.)
- A local anesthetic is injected, and the femoral vein is cannulated.
- Under fluoroscopic guidance, a guide wire is threaded a short distance through the cannula, which is then removed. A catheter is passed over the wire into the inferior vena cava.
- When catheterization of the femoral vein is contraindicated, the right antecubital vein is punctured, and the catheter is inserted and advanced through the right atrium of the heart into the inferior vena cava.
- A test bolus of contrast medium is injected to determine that the vena cava is patent. If so, the catheter is advanced into the right renal vein and contrast medium is injected.
- When studies of the right renal vasculature are completed, the catheter is withdrawn into the vena cava, rotated, and guided into the left renal vein.
- If visualization of the renal venous tributaries is indicated, epinephrine can

be injected into the ipsilateral renal artery by catheter before contrast medium is injected into the renal vein. Epinephrine temporarily blocks arterial flow and allows filling of distal intrarenal veins. Obstructing the artery briefly with a balloon catheter produces the same effect.

• After anteroposterior films are made, the patient lies prone for posteroanterior films.

• For renin assays, blood samples are withdrawn under fluoroscopy within 15 minutes after venography. After catheter removal, apply pressure to the site for 15 minutes and put on a dressing.

• Check vital signs and distal pulses every 15 minutes for the first hour, then every 30 minutes for the second hour, and then every 2 hours for 24 hours.

• Observe the puncture site for bleeding or hematoma when checking vital signs; if bleeding occurs, apply pressure. Report bleeding as soon as possible.

• Report signs of vein perforation, embolism, and extravasation of contrast medium. These include chills, fever, rapid pulse and respiration, hypotension, dyspnea, and chest, abdominal, or flank pain. Also report complaints of paresthesia or pain in the catheterized limb — symptoms of nerve irritation or vascular compromise.

• Administer prescribed sedatives and antimicrobials.

• Instruct the patient to resume his normal diet and any discontinued medications.

Precautions

• Renal venography is contraindicated in severe thrombosis of the inferior vena cava.

• The guide wire and catheter should be advanced carefully if severe renal vein thrombosis is suspected.

• Watch for signs of hypersensitivity to the contrast medium.

Normal findings

After injection of the contrast medium, opacification of the renal vein and tributaries should occur immediately.

Normal renin content of venous blood in a supine adult is 1.5 to 1.6 ng/ml/hour.

Abnormal findings

Occlusion of the renal vein near the inferior vena cava or the kidney indicates renal vein thrombosis. If the clot is outlined by contrast medium, it may look like a filling defect. However, a clot can usually be identified because it's within the lumen and less sharply outlined than a filling defect. Collateral venous channels, which opacify with retrograde filling during contrast injection, often surround the occlusion. Complete occlusion prolongs transit of the contrast medium through the renal veins.

A filling defect of the renal vein may indicate obstruction or compression by extrinsic tumor or retroperitoneal fibrosis. A renal tumor that invades the renal vein or inferior vena cava usually produces a filling defect with a sharply defined border.

Venous anomalies are indicated by opacification of abnormally positioned or clustered vessels. Absence of a renal vein differentiates renal agenesis from a small kidney.

Elevated renin content in renal venous blood usually indicates essential renovascular hypertension when assay results correspond for both kidneys. Elevated renin levels in one kidney indicate a unilateral lesion and usually require further evaluation by arteriography.

Interfering factors
• Recent contrast studies or stool or gas in the bowel
• Failure to restrict salt, antihypertensive drugs, diuretics, estrogen, and oral contraceptives

VOIDING CYSTOURETHROGRAPHY

In voiding cystourethrography, a contrast medium is instilled by gentle syringe pressure or gravity into the bladder through a urethral catheter. Fluoroscopic films or overhead radiographs demonstrate bladder filling, and then show excretion of the contrast medium as the patient voids.

Purpose
• To detect abnormalities of the bladder and urethra, such as vesicoureteral reflux, neurogenic bladder, prostatic hyperplasia, or diverticula
• To investigate possible causes of chronic urinary tract infection
• To investigate a suspected congenital anomaly of the lower urinary tract, abnormal bladder emptying, and incontinence
• To assess hypertrophy of the lobes of the prostate, urethral stricture, and the degree of compromise of a stenotic prostatic urethra (in men)

Patient preparation
• Explain to the patient that this test permits assessment of the bladder and the urethra.
• Inform him that he needn't restrict food or fluids before the test.

• Tell him who will perform the test and where and that it takes approximately 30 to 45 minutes.
• Inform the patient that a catheter will be inserted into his bladder and that a contrast medium will be instilled through the catheter.
• Tell him he may experience a feeling of fullness and an urge to void when the contrast medium is instilled. Explain that X-rays will be taken of his bladder and urethra and that he'll be asked to assume various positions.
• Make sure that the patient or a responsible family member has signed a consent form if required.
• Check the patient's history for hypersensitivity to contrast media or iodine-containing foods, such as shellfish; note sensitivities on the chart.
• Just before the procedure, administer a sedative, if prescribed.

Equipment
Accessories for spot-film radiography, indwelling urinary catheter, standard urographic contrast medium (up to 1,000 ml of 15% solution), 50-ml syringe (for infants) or gravity-feed apparatus

Procedure and posttest care
• The patient is placed in a supine position, and an indwelling urinary catheter is inserted into the bladder.
• The contrast medium is instilled through the catheter until the bladder is full.
• The catheter is clamped, and X-ray films are exposed with the patient in supine, oblique, and lateral positions.
• The catheter is removed, and the patient assumes right oblique position (right leg flexed to 90 degrees, left leg extended, penis parallel to right leg) and begins to void.
• Four high-speed exposures of the bladder and urethra, coned down to re-

duce radiation exposure, are usually made on one film during voiding.

• If the right oblique view doesn't delineate both ureters, the patient is asked to stop urinating and to begin again in the left oblique position.

• The most reliable voiding cystourethrograms are obtained with the patient recumbent. Patients who can't void recumbent may do so standing (not sitting).

• Expression cystourethrography may have to be performed, under a general anesthetic, for young children who cannot void on command.

• Observe and record the time, color, and volume of the patient's voidings. Report hematuria if present after the third voiding.

• Encourage the patient to drink large quantities of fluids to reduce burning on urination and to flush out any residual contrast medium.

• Monitor for chills and fever related to extravasation of contrast material or urinary sepsis.

Precautions

• Voiding cystourethrography is contraindicated in patients with an acute or exacerbated urethral or bladder infection, or an acute urethral injury.

• Hypersensitivity to the contrast medium may also contraindicate this test.

• Male patients should wear a lead shield over their testes to prevent irradiation of the gonads; female patients' ovaries can't be shielded without blocking the urinary bladder.

Normal findings

Delineation of the bladder and urethra shows normal structure and function, with no regurgitation of contrast medium into the ureters.

Abnormal findings

Voiding cystourethrography may show urethral stricture, vesical or urethral diverticula, ureterocele, cystocele, prostate enlargement, vesicoureteral reflux, or neurogenic bladder. The severity and location of such abnormalities are then evaluated to determine whether surgical intervention is necessary.

Interfering factors

• Embarrassment (inhibits patient from voiding on command)

• Interrupted or less vigorous voiding, muscle spasm or incomplete sphincter relaxation (due to urethral trauma during catheterization)

• Presence of contrast media from recent tests, stool, or gas in the bowel (possible poor imaging)

WHITAKER TEST

Also called a pressure or flow study, the Whitaker test correlates radiographic findings with measurements of pressure and flow in the kidneys and ureters, and facilitates assessment of the upper urinary tract's efficiency in emptying.

In this procedure, radiographs are taken after urethral catheterization, I.V. administration of a contrast medium, percutaneous cannulation of the kidney, and renal perfusion of the contrast medium. Intrarenal and bladder pressures are then measured.

Purpose

• To detect renal obstruction and to help determine if surgery is needed

• To further evaluate obstruction (following other procedures, such as percutaneous nephrostomy)

Patient preparation

- Explain to the patient that this test helps to evaluate kidney function.
- Instruct him to avoid food and fluids for at least 4 hours before the test.
- Tell him who will perform the test and where and that it will take about 1 hour.
- Describe the procedure to him. Inform him that he'll be given a mild sedative before the test, that he may feel some discomfort during insertion of the urethral catheter and injection of the local anesthetic, and that he may sense transient burning and flushing after injection of the contrast medium.
- Warn him that the X-ray machine makes loud clacking sounds as films are exposed.
- Make sure that the patient or a responsible family member has signed a consent form.
- Check his history and recent coagulation studies for bleeding disorders. Also check for hypersensitivity reactions to iodine, iodine-containing foods such as shellfish, and contrast media. Mark any sensitivities on the chart.
- Just before the procedure, instruct the patient to void, and administer prescribed sedatives.
- Administer prophylactic antimicrobials as prescribed to prevent infection from instrumentation.

Equipment

Perfusion pump with 50-ml luer-lock syringe, transducer and recorder, manometer, three-way and four-way stopcocks, I.V. extension set, manometer lines, one double-male connector to connect urethral catheter and stopcock, sterile water and normal saline solution, contrast medium, local anesthetic, percutaneous puncture tray with 4″ to 6″ 18G Longdwel cannula, gloves, preparatory tray, emergency resuscitation equipment

Procedure and posttest care

- Place the patient in a supine position on the X-ray table. The table must be horizontal and must remain at the same height throughout the test.
- To prepare for measurement of bladder pressure, a urethral catheter is placed in the bladder. The patient's bladder may or may not be emptied, depending on his suspected condition.
- A plain film of the urinary tract is taken to obtain anatomic landmarks.
- The catheter is then connected to a three-way stopcock on a manometer line linked to the transducer and recorder. The line is then filled with sterile water.
- Contrast medium is injected I.V.
- The patient is placed prone and made comfortable with pillows. When urography demonstrates contrast medium in the kidney, the skin is cleaned with antiseptic solution and draped.
- Pressure recording equipment is calibrated. The renal perfusion tubing is filled with sterile water or normal saline solution and held at the level of the kidney.
- Local anesthetic is injected, and an incision is made through the flank for cannulation of the kidney.
- The patient is asked to hold his breath while the needle is inserted into the renal pelvis. Aspiration of urine confirms that the needle is in position.
- The cannula is then connected by a four-way stopcock to the perfusion tubing and the manometer line.
- Perfusion of the contrast medium is begun, serial X-rays are taken, and intrarenal pressure is measured. Bladder pressure is then measured.
- Perfusion continues until bladder pressure is constant. When pressure

holds steady for a few minutes and adequate films have been taken, perfusion is discontinued. Residual fluid is aspirated from the kidney, the cannula is removed, and the wound is dressed.

● Keep the patient in a supine position for 12 hours after the test.

● Check vital signs every 15 minutes for the first hour, every 30 minutes for the next hour, and then every 2 hours for 24 hours.

● Check the puncture site for bleeding, hematoma, or urine leakage each time vital signs are checked. If bleeding occurs, apply pressure. If a hematoma develops, apply warm soaks. Report urine leakage.

● Monitor fluid intake and urine output for 24 hours. Report hematuria that persists after the third voiding.

● Watch for signs of sepsis (chills, fever, tachycardia, tachypnea, or hypotension) or similar signs of extravasation of the contrast medium.

● Inform the patient that colicky pains are transient.

● Administer prescribed analgesics.

● Administer antimicrobials for several days after the test as needed to prevent infection.

Precautions
● Contraindications include bleeding disorders and severe infection.

Normal findings
Visualization of the kidney after gradual perfusion of the contrast medium shows normal outlines of the renal pelvis and calyces. The ureter should fill uniformly and appear normal in size and course.

The normal value for intrarenal pressure is 15 cm H_2O. The normal value for bladder pressure may range from 5 to 10 cm H_2O.

Abnormal findings
Enlargement of the renal pelvis, calyces, or ureteropelvic junction may indicate obstruction. Subtraction of bladder pressure from intrarenal pressure results in a differential that aids diagnosis. A differential of 12 to 15 cm H_2O indicates obstruction. A differential of less than 10 cm H_2O indicates a bladder abnormality, such as hypertonia or neurogenic bladder.

Interfering factors
● Recent barium studies or stool or gas in the bowel (hinders accurate needle placement and visualization of the upper urinary tract)

● Patient movement

REPRODUCTIVE SYSTEM

MAMMOGRAPHY

Mammography is used as a screening test for breast cancer. It helps to detect breast cysts or tumors, especially those not palpable on physical examination. Biopsy of suspicious areas may be required to confirm cancer. Mammography can detect 90% to 95% of breast cancers. New research is being conducted to develop more comfortable alternatives to mammography. (See *Alternatives to mammography.*)

If a mass is present, a mammogram can be done during pregnancy. A shield is used to protect the fetus.

Purpose
● To screen for breast cancer

• To investigate palpable and unpalpable breast masses, breast pain, or nipple discharge

• To help differentiate between benign breast disease and breast cancer

Patient preparation

• Assess the patient's understanding of the test, answer her questions, and correct any misconceptions.

• Tell her who will perform the test and where.

• Inform her that although the test takes only about 15 minutes to perform, she may be asked to wait while the films are checked to make sure they're readable.

• Just before the test, give her a gown to wear that opens in the front, and ask her to remove all jewelry and clothing above the waist.

• Make sure she isn't wearing powders.

Procedure and posttest care

• The patient stands and is asked to rest one of her breasts on a table above an X-ray cassette.

• The compression plate is placed on the breast, and the patient is told to hold her breath. A radiograph is taken of the craniocaudal view. The machine is rotated, the breast is compressed again, and a radiograph of the lateral view is taken.

• The procedure is repeated on the other breast.

• After the films are developed, they're checked to make sure they're readable.

Normal findings

A normal mammogram reveals normal duct, glandular tissue, and fat architecture. No abnormal masses or calcifications should be seen.

ALTERNATIVES TO MAMMOGRAPHY

Researchers are pursuing two new, noninvasive screening techniques that may improve breast cancer detection and reduce the number of surgical biopsies performed.

Clinical trials are set to begin on a noninvasive screening test called computer tomography laser mammography (CTLM). Using laser technology, CTLM creates a three-dimensional image of breast tissue — an image that can be sliced and turned upside down and inside out to inspect suspicious masses more carefully.

A second technique, the Biofield test, has been approved for use in Europe and is undergoing clinical testing in the United States. In this test, electrodes attached on all sides of the breast fire signals through the breast tissue to detect cancerous cells.

Abnormal findings

Well-outlined, regular, and clear spots suggest benign cysts; irregular, poorly outlined, and opaque areas suggest a malignant tumor. Findings that suggest cancer require further tests, such as additional mammographic views or, for confirmation, biopsy.

Interfering factors

• Powders or salves on the breasts (possible false-positive results)

• Failure to remove jewelry and clothing (possible false-positive results or poor imaging)

• Very glandular breasts (common under age 30) and previous breast surgery (possible poor imaging)
• Breast implants (may hinder detection of masses)

HYSTERO-SALPINGOGRAPHY

Hysterosalpingography is a radiologic examination for visualizing the uterine cavity, the fallopian tubes, and the peritubal area. In this procedure, fluoroscopic X-ray films are taken as a contrast medium flows through the uterus and the fallopian tubes.

This test is generally performed as part of an infertility study. Although ultrasonography has virtually replaced hysterosalpingography in the detection of foreign bodies, such as a dislodged intrauterine device, it can't evaluate tubal patency, which is the main purpose of hysterosalpingography. Risks of this test include uterine perforation, intravascular injection of the contrast medium, and exposure to potentially harmful radiation.

Purpose
• To confirm tubal abnormalities, such as adhesions and occlusion
• To confirm uterine abnormalities, such as the presence of foreign bodies, congenital malformations, and traumatic injuries
• To confirm the presence of fistulas or peritubal adhesions
• To help evaluate repeated fetal loss
• To assess the outcome of surgery, especially uterine unification procedures and tubal reanastomosis

Patient preparation
• Explain to the patient that this test confirms uterine and fallopian tube abnormalities.
• Tell her who will perform the test and where and that it takes about 15 minutes.
• Advise the patient that she may experience moderate cramping from the procedure; however, she may receive a mild sedative, such as diazepam.

Equipment
Povidone-iodine solution, sterile needle, contrast medium (oil- or water-based), vaginal speculum, tenaculum, cannula with acorn tip on one end and luer-lock on the other

Procedure and posttest care
• With the patient in lithotomy position, a scout film is taken.
• A speculum is inserted in the vagina, the tenaculum is placed on the cervix, and the cervix is cleaned.
• The cannula is inserted into the cervix and anchored to the tenaculum. After the contrast medium is injected through the cannula, the uterus and the fallopian tubes are viewed fluoroscopically, and radiographs are taken. To take oblique views, the X-ray table may be tilted or the patient asked to change position.
• Watch for signs of infection, such as fever, pain, increased pulse rate, malaise, and muscle ache.
• Assure the patient that cramps and vagal reaction (slow pulse rate, nausea, and dizziness) are transient.

Precautions
• Hysterosalpingography is contraindicated in patients with menses, undiagnosed vaginal bleeding, or pelvic inflammatory disease.

• Watch for an allergic reaction to the contrast medium, such as urticaria, itching, or hypotension.

Normal findings

Normally, radiographs reveal a symmetrical uterine cavity; the contrast medium courses through fallopian tubes of normal caliber, spills freely into the peritoneal cavity, and doesn't leak from the uterus.

Abnormal findings

An asymmetrical uterus suggests intrauterine adhesions or masses, such as fibroids or foreign bodies; impaired contrast flow through the fallopian tubes suggests partial or complete blockage, resulting from intraluminal agglutination, extrinsic compression by adhesions, or perifimbrial adhesions; leakage of the contrast medium through the uterine wall suggests fistulas. Laparoscopy with contrast medium confirms positive or equivocal findings.

Interfering factors

• Tubal spasm or excessive traction (may show as a stricture in normal fallopian tubes)
• Excessive traction (may displace adhesions, making the fallopian tubes appear normal)

SKELETAL SYSTEM

VERTEBRAL RADIOGRAPHY

Vertebral radiography visualizes all or part of the vertebral column. A com-

monly performed test, it's used to evaluate the vertebrae for deformities, fractures, dislocations, tumors, and other abnormalities. Bone films determine bone density, texture, erosion, and changes in bone relationships. X-rays of the cortex of the bone reveal the presence of any widening, narrowing, and signs of irregularity. Joint X-rays can reveal the presence of fluid, spur formation, narrowing, and changes in the joint structure.

Anatomically, the vertebral column is divided in descending order into five segments: cervical, thoracic, lumbar, sacral, and coccygeal. All vertebrae are similar in structure, but vary in size, shape, and articular surface, according to location. The type and extent of vertebral radiography depends on the patient's clinical condition. For example, a patient with lower back pain requires only study of the lumbar and sacral segments.

Purpose

• To detect vertebral fractures, dislocations, subluxations, and deformities
• To detect vertebral degeneration, infection, and congenital disorders
• To detect disorders of the intervertebral disks
• To determine the vertebral effects of arthritic and metabolic disorders

Patient preparation

• Explain to the patient that this test permits examination of the spine.
• Inform him that he needn't restrict food or fluids.
• Tell him the test requires X-ray films, who will perform the test and where, and that the procedure usually takes 15 to 30 minutes.
• Advise him that he'll be placed in various positions for the X-ray films.

• Tell him that although some positions may cause slight discomfort, his cooperation is needed to ensure accurate results.

• Stress that he must keep still and hold his breath during the procedure.

Procedure and posttest care

The procedure varies considerably depending on the vertebral segment being examined.

• Initially, the patient is placed in a supine position on the X-ray table for an anteroposterior view.

• He may be repositioned for lateral or right and left oblique views; specific positioning depends on the vertebral segment or adjacent structure of interest.

• Analgesics or local heat applications may relieve pain.

Precautions

• Vertebral radiography is contraindicated during the first trimester of pregnancy, unless the benefits outweigh the risk of fetal radiation exposure.

• Exercise extreme caution when handling trauma patients with suspected spinal injuries, particularly of the cervical area. Such patients should be filmed while on the stretcher to avoid further injury during transfer to the radiographic table.

Normal findings

Normal vertebrae show no fractures, subluxations, dislocations, curvatures, or other abnormalities. Specific positions and spacing of the vertebrae vary with the patient's age.

In the lateral view, adult vertebrae are aligned to form four alternately concave and convex curves. The cervical and lumbar curves are convex anteriorly; the thoracic and sacral curves are concave anteriorly. Although the structure of the coccyx varies, it usually points forward and downward.

Neonatal vertebrae form only one curve, which is concave anteriorly.

Abnormal findings

The vertebral radiograph readily shows spondylolisthesis, fractures, subluxations, dislocations, wedging, and such deformities as kyphosis, scoliosis, and lordosis.

To confirm other disorders, spinal structures and their spatial relationships on the radiograph must be examined, and the patient's history and clinical status must be considered. These disorders include congenital abnormalities, such as torticollis (wryneck), absence of sacral or lumbar vertebrae, hemivertebrae, and Klippel-Feil syndrome; degenerative processes, such as hypertrophic spurs, osteoarthritis, and narrowed disk spaces; tuberculosis (Pott's disease); benign or malignant intraspinal tumors; ruptured disk and cervical disk syndrome; and systemic disorders, such as rheumatoid arthritis, Charcot's disease, ankylosing spondylitis, osteoporosis, and Paget's disease.

Depending on radiographic results, definitive diagnosis may also require additional tests, such as myelography or computed tomography scanning.

Interfering factors

• Improper positioning of the patient or patient movement (possible poor imaging)

BONE DENSITOMETRY

Bone densitometry assesses bone mass quantitatively. This noninvasive technique, also known as dual energy

X-ray absorptiometry (DEXA), uses an X-ray tube to measure bone mineral density, but exposes the patient to only minimal radiation. The images detected are computer-analyzed to determine bone mineral status. The computer calculates the size and thickness of the bone as well as its volumetric density to determine its potential resistance to mechanical stress. (See *Other diagnostic tools for osteoporosis.*)

Purpose
• To determine bone mineral density
• To identify risk for osteoporosis
• To evaluate clinical response to therapy for reducing the rate of bone loss

Patient preparation
• Reassure the patient that the test is painless and that the exposure to radiation is minimal.
• Tell him that it will take from 10 minutes to 1 hour, depending on the areas to be scanned.
• Tell him who will perform the test and where.

Procedure and posttest care
• Instruct the patient to remove all metal objects from the area to be scanned.
• The patient is positioned on a table under the scanning device, with the radiation source below and the detector above. The detector measures the bone's radiation absorption and produces a digital readout.

Normal findings
Computer-analyzed results of the bone densitometry scan are within normal limits for the patient's age, sex, and height.

OTHER DIAGNOSTIC TOOLS FOR OSTEOPOROSIS

Two new scanning devices help diagnose osteoporosis and other medical conditions that lead to reduced bone density. Soundscan 2000, approved by the Food and Drug Administration (FDA), measures mineral density of the shin bone. The Sahara Clinical Bone Sonometer, which is awaiting FDA approval, uses ultrasound to gauge the mineral density of the heel bone. These measurements, combined with other clinical risk factors, reveal skeletal deterioration and help determine fracture risk in silent disorders that, until recently, remained undiagnosed until a fracture occurred.

Abnormal findings
Values other than normal for the patient's age, sex, race, and height are considered abnormal.

Interfering factors
• Osteoarthritis (possible decrease)
• Fat tissue (poor visualization)

ARTHROGRAPHY

Arthrography allows radiographic examination of a joint after injection of a radiopaque dye, air, or both (double-contrast arthrogram) to outline soft-tissue structures and the contour of the joint. The joint is put through its range of motion while a series of radiographs are taken.

Indications for arthrography include persistent unexplained joint discomfort or pain. Complications may include persistent joint crepitus and allergic reactions to the contrast dye. A magnetic resonance imaging scan of the joint may be used in place of this test.

Purpose
● To identify acute or chronic tears or other abnormalities of the joint capsule or supporting ligaments of the knee, shoulder, ankle, hips, or wrist
● To detect internal joint derangements
● To locate synovial cysts

Patient preparation
● Describe the procedure to the patient, and answer any questions he may have. Explain that this test permits examination of a joint.
● Inform him he needn't restrict food or fluids.
● Tell him who will perform the procedure and where.
● Explain that the fluoroscope allows the doctor to track the contrast medium as it fills the joint space.
● Inform him that standard X-ray films will also be taken after diffusion of the contrast medium.
● Tell him that, although the joint area will be anesthetized, he may experience a tingling sensation or pressure in the joint when the contrast medium is injected.
● Instruct him to remain as still as possible during the procedure, except when following instructions to change position.
● Stress the importance of his cooperation in assuming various positions because films must be taken as quickly as possible to ensure optimum quality.
● Check the patient's history to determine if he's hypersensitive to local anesthetics, iodine, seafood, or the dyes used for other diagnostic tests.

Equipment
Fluoroscope, povidone-iodine solution, local anesthetic, two 2″ 20G needles, two 24G needles, three 3-ml syringes, short lumbar puncture needle (3″ 22G needle for arthrography of the shoulder), water-soluble radiopaque dye (5 to 15 ml), four sterile sponges, elastic knee bandage, sterile towels, sterile specimen container for fluid, culture tube, sterile adhesive bandage, collodion (optional), shave preparation kit

Procedure and posttest care
Knee arthrography
● The knee is cleaned with an antiseptic solution, and the area around the puncture site is anesthetized. (It isn't usually necessary to anesthetize the joint space itself.)
● A 2″ needle is then inserted into the joint space between the patella and femoral condyle, and fluid is aspirated. The aspirated fluid is usually sent to the laboratory for analysis.
● While the needle is still in place, the aspirating syringe is removed and replaced with a syringe containing dye.
● If fluoroscopic examination demonstrates correct placement of the needle, the dye is injected into the joint space.
● After the needle is removed, the site is rubbed with a sterile sponge and the wound may be sealed with collodion.
● The patient is asked to walk a few steps or to move his knee through a range of motion to distribute the dye in the joint space. A film series is quickly taken with the knee held in various positions.
● If the films are clean and demonstrate proper dye placement, the knee is bandaged, possibly with an elastic bandage.
● Tell the patient to keep the bandage in place for several days, and teach him how to rewrap it.

Shoulder arthrography
• The skin is prepared, and a local anesthetic is injected subcutaneously just in front of the acromioclavicular joint.
• Additional anesthetic is injected directly onto the head of the humerus.
• The short lumbar puncture needle is inserted until the point is embedded in the joint cartilage.
• The stylet is removed, a syringe of contrast medium is attached and, using fluoroscopic guidance, about 1 ml of dye is injected into the joint space, as the needle is withdrawn slightly.
• If fluoroscopic examination demonstrates correct needle placement, the remainder of the dye is injected while the needle is slowly withdrawn, and the site is wiped with a sterile sponge.
• A film series is taken quickly to achieve maximum contrast.
Both types
• Tell the patient to rest the joint for at least 12 hours.
• Inform him that he may experience some swelling or discomfort, or may hear crepitant noises in the joint after the test, but that these symptoms usually disappear after 1 or 2 days; tell him to report persistent symptoms.
• Advise him to apply ice to the joint if swelling occurs and to take a mild analgesic for pain.

Precautions
• Arthrography is contraindicated during pregnancy.
• This procedure is also contraindicated in patients with active arthritis, joint infection, or previous sensitivity to radiopaque media.

Normal findings
A normal knee arthrogram shows a characteristic wedge-shaped shadow, pointed toward the interior of the joint, that indicates a normal medial meniscus. A normal shoulder arthrogram shows the bicipital tendon sheath, redundant inferior joint capsule, and subscapular bursa intact.

Abnormal findings
Arthrography accurately detects medial meniscal tears and lacerations in 90% to 95% of cases. Because the entire joint lining is opacified, arthrography can demonstrate extrameniscal lesions, such as osteochondritis dissecans, chondromalacia patellae, osteochondral fractures, cartilaginous abnormalities, synovial abnormalities, tears of the cruciate ligaments, and disruption of the joint capsule and collateral ligaments.

Arthrography can reveal shoulder abnormalities, such as adhesive capsulitis, bicipital tenosynovitis or rupture, and rotator cuff tears. It can also evaluate damage from recurrent dislocations.

Interfering factors
• Dilution of the contrast medium due to incomplete aspiration of joint effusion (possible poor imaging)
• Improper injection technique (possible displacement of contrast medium)

MISCELLANEOUS TESTS

LYMPHANGIOGRAPHY

Lymphangiography (or lymphography) is the radiographic examination of the lymphatic system after the injection of an oil-based contrast medium into a lymphatic vessel in each foot or, less commonly, in each hand. This test is no longer used widely.

Injection into the foot allows visualization of the lymphatics of the leg, inguinal and iliac regions, and the retroperitoneum up to the thoracic duct.

Injection into the hand allows visualization of the axillary and supraclavicular nodes. This procedure may also be used to study the cervical region (retroauricular area), but this is less useful and less common.

X-ray films are taken immediately after injection to demonstrate the filling of the lymphatic system and then again 24 hours later to visualize the lymph nodes. Because the contrast medium remains in the nodes for up to 2 years, subsequent X-ray films can assess progression of disease and monitor effectiveness of treatment.

Purpose
• To detect and stage lymphomas, and to identify metastatic involvement of the lymph nodes (computed tomography is used more frequently for staging)
• To distinguish primary from secondary lymphedema
• To suggest surgical treatment or evaluate the effectiveness of chemotherapy and radiation therapy in controlling malignancy
• To investigate enlarged lymph nodes detected by computed tomography or ultrasonography

Patient preparation
• Explain to the patient that this test permits examination of the lymphatic system through X-ray films taken after the injection of a contrast medium.
• Inform him that he needn't restrict food or fluids before the test.
• Tell him who will perform this procedure and where and that it takes about 3 hours.

• Mention that additional X-ray films are also taken the following day but that these take less than 30 minutes.
• Inform the patient that blue contrast medium will be injected into each foot to outline the lymphatic vessels; that the injection causes transient discomfort; and that the contrast medium discolors urine and stool for 48 hours, and may give his skin and vision a bluish tinge for 48 hours.
• Tell him that a local anesthetic will be injected before a small incision is made in each foot.
• Inform him that the contrast medium is then injected for the next 1½ hours using a catheter inserted into a lymphatic vessel.
• Advise the patient that he must remain as still as possible during injection of the contrast medium, and that he may experience some discomfort in the popliteal or inguinal areas at the beginning of the injection of the contrast medium.
• If this test is performed on an outpatient basis, advise the patient to have a friend or relative accompany him.
• Warn him that the incision site may be sore for several days after lymphangiography.
• Make sure the patient or a responsible family member has signed a consent form.
• Check the patient's history to determine if he is hypersensitive to iodine, seafood, or the contrast media used in other diagnostic tests, such as excretory urography.
• Just before the procedure, instruct the patient to void, and check his vital signs for a baseline. If prescribed, administer a sedative and an oral antihistamine (if hypersensitivity to the contrast medium is suspected).

Procedure and posttest care

- A preliminary X-ray of the chest is taken with the patient in an erect or a supine position.
- The skin over the dorsum of each foot is cleaned with antiseptics.
- Blue contrast dye is injected intradermally into the area between the toes, usually the first and fourth toe webs.
- The contrast medium infiltrates the lymphatic system and within 15 to 30 minutes the lymphatic vessels appear as small blue lines on the upper surface of the instep of each foot.
- A local anesthetic is then injected into the dorsum of each foot, and a transverse incision is made to expose the lymphatic vessel.
- Each vessel is cannulated with a 30G needle attached to polyethylene tubing and a syringe filled with ethiodized oil.
- Once the needles are positioned, the patient is instructed to remain still throughout the injection period to avoid dislodging the needles.
- The syringe is then placed within an infusion pump that injects the contrast medium.
- Fluoroscopy may be used to monitor filling of the lymphatic system.
- The needles are removed, the incisions are sutured, and sterile dressings are applied.
- X-ray films of the legs, pelvis, abdomen, and chest are taken.
- The patient is then taken to his room but must return 24 hours later for additional films.
- Check the patient's vital signs every 4 hours for 48 hours.
- Watch for pulmonary complications, such as shortness of breath, pleuritic pain, hypotension, low-grade fever, and cyanosis, due to embolization of the contrast medium.

- Enforce bed rest for 24 hours, with the patient's feet elevated to help reduce swelling.
- Apply ice packs to the incision sites to help reduce swelling, and administer prescribed analgesics.
- Check the incision sites for infection, and leave the dressings in place for 2 days, making sure the wounds remain dry. Tell the patient the sutures will be removed in 7 to 10 days.
- Prepare the patient for follow-up X-rays, as needed.

Precautions

- Lymphangiography is contraindicated in patients with hypersensitivity to iodine, pulmonary insufficiencies, cardiac diseases, and severe renal or hepatic diseases.

Normal findings

The lymphatic system normally demonstrates homogeneous and complete filling with contrast medium on the initial films. On the 24-hour films, the lymph nodes are fully opacified and well circumscribed; the lymphatic channels are emptied a few hours after injection of the contrast medium.

Abnormal findings

Enlarged, foamy-looking nodes indicate Hodgkin's disease or malignant lymphoma. Filling defects or lack of opacification indicates metastatic involvement of the lymph nodes. The number of nodes affected, unilateral or bilateral involvement, and the extent of extranodal involvement help determine staging of lymphoma. However, definitive staging may require additional diagnostic tests such as computed tomography, ultrasonography, selective biopsy, and laparotomy.

In differential diagnosis of primary and secondary lymphedema, shortened lymphatic vessels and a deficient number of vessels indicate primary lymph-edema. Abruptly terminating lymphatic vessels, caused by retroperitoneal tumors impinging on the vessels, inflammation, filariasis, and trauma resulting from surgery or radiation, indicate secondary lymphedema.

Interfering factor
• Inability to cannulate the lymphatic vessels (precludes use of this test)

CHAPTER 13

Computed Tomography and Magnetic Resonance Imaging

NEUROLOGIC SYSTEM			616
616	Intracranial computed tomography	618	Intracranial magnetic resonance imaging

GASTROINTESTINAL SYSTEM			621
621	Liver and biliary tract computed tomography	623	Pancreatic computed tomography

MUSCULOSKELETAL SYSTEM			625
625	Spinal computed tomography	629	Skeletal magnetic resonance imaging
628	Skeletal computed tomography		

MISCELLANEOUS TESTS			631
631	Orbital computed tomography	634	Cardiac magnetic resonance imaging
632	Thoracic computed tomography	636	Renal computed tomography

NEUROLOGIC SYSTEM

INTRACRANIAL COMPUTED TOMOGRAPHY

Intracranial computed tomography (CT) provides a series of tomograms, translated by a computer and displayed on a monitor, representing cross-sectional images of various layers of the brain. This technique can reconstruct cross-sectional, horizontal, sagittal, and coronal plane images. Hundreds of thousands of readings of radiation levels absorbed by brain tissues may be combined to depict anatomic slices of varying thickness. Intracranial tumors and other brain lesions may be identified as areas of altered density. Intracranial CT scanning has practically eliminated the need for painful and hazardous invasive procedures, such as pneumoencephalography and cerebral angiography.

Purpose
- To diagnose intracranial lesions and abnormalities
- To monitor the effects of surgery, radiation therapy, or chemotherapy on intracranial tumors
- To assess focal neurologic abnormalities and other clinical features that suggest an intracranial mass
- To provide early diagnosis of intracranial hemorrhage in a patient with suspected head injury

Patient preparation
- Explain to the patient that this test permits assessment of the brain.

- Unless contrast enhancement is scheduled, inform him that there are no food or fluid restrictions. If contrast enhancement is scheduled, instruct him to fast for 4 hours before the test.
- Tell him that a series of X-ray films will be taken of his brain. Describe who will perform the test and where it will take place. Explain that the test will cause minimal discomfort and last 15 to 30 minutes.
- Tell him he'll be positioned on a moving CT bed, with his head immobilized and his face uncovered. The head of the table will then be moved into the scanner, which rotates around his head and makes loud clacking sounds.
- If a contrast medium is used, tell him that he may feel flushed and warm and may experience a transient headache, a salty or metallic taste, or nausea and vomiting after the contrast medium is injected.
- Instruct him to wear a gown (outpatients may wear any comfortable clothing) and to remove all metal objects from the CT scan field.
- If the patient is restless or apprehensive, a sedative may be prescribed.
- Check the patient's history for hypersensitivity to shellfish, iodine, or contrast media, and mark your findings on his chart. Report this information as necessary.

Equipment
Contrast medium (meglumine iothalamate or sodium diatrizoate), 60-ml syringe or power injector, 19G to 21G needle, tourniquet

Procedure and posttest care
- Place the patient in a supine position on an X-ray table, with his head immobilized by straps if required, and ask him to lie still.
- The head of the table is moved into the scanner, which rotates around the

patient's head, taking radiographs at 1-degree intervals in a 180-degree arc.
• When this series of radiographs is completed, a contrast medium is administered by I.V. injection. Monitor for hypersensitivity reactions, such as urticaria, respiratory difficulty, or rash. Reactions usually develop within 30 minutes.
• After injection of the contrast medium, another series of scans is taken. Information from the scans is stored on magnetic tapes, fed into a computer, and converted into images on a monitor. Photographs of selected views are taken for further study.
• If a contrast medium was used, watch for residual adverse reactions (headache, nausea, and vomiting), and inform the patient that he may resume his usual diet.

Precautions
• Intracranial CT scanning with contrast enhancement is contraindicated in persons who are hypersensitive to iodine or contrast medium.
• Iodine or contrast medium may be harmful or fatal to a fetus, especially during the first trimester.

Normal findings
The density of tissue determines the amount of radiation that passes through it. Tissue densities appear as white, black, or shades of gray on the computed image obtained by intracranial CT scanning. Bone, the densest tissue, appears white; ventricular and subarachnoid cerebrospinal fluid, the least dense, appears black. Brain matter appears in shades of gray. Structures are evaluated according to their density, size, shape, and position.

Abnormal findings
Areas of altered density (they may be lighter or darker) or displaced vascula-

ture or other structures may indicate intracranial tumor, hematoma, cerebral atrophy, infarction, edema, or congenital anomalies, such as hydrocephalus.

Intracranial tumors vary significantly in appearance and characteristics. Metastatic tumors generally cause extensive edema in early stages and can usually be defined by contrast enhancement. Primary tumors vary in density and in their capacity to cause edema, displace ventricles, and absorb contrast medium in contrast enhancement. Astrocytomas, for example, usually have low densities; meningiomas have higher densities and can generally be defined with contrast enhancement; glioblastomas, usually ill-defined, are also enhanced after injection of a contrast medium.

Because the high density of blood contrasts markedly with low-density brain tissue, it's normally easy to detect both subdural and epidural hematomas and other acute hemorrhages. Contrast enhancement helps locate subdural hematomas, but it isn't needed.

Cerebral atrophy customarily appears as enlarged ventricles with large sulci. Cerebral infarction may appear as low-density areas at the obstruction site or may not be apparent if the infarction is small or doesn't cause edema. With contrast enhancement, the infarcted area may not show in the acute phase but will show clearly after resolution of the lesion. Cerebral edema usually appears as an area of marked generalized decreased density. In children, enlargement of the fourth ventricle generally indicates hydrocephalus.

Normally, the cerebral vessels don't appear on CT images. However, in patients with arteriovenous malformation, cerebral vessels may appear with slightly increased density. Contrast enhancement allows a better view of the abnormal area, but magnetic resonance

PET SCAN OF THE BRAIN

Like computed tomography (CT) scanning and magnetic resonance imaging (MRI), positron emission tomography (PET) scanning provides images of the brain through sophisticated computer reconstruction algorithms. However, PET images detail brain function as well as structure and thus differ significantly from the images provided by these other advanced techniques.

How it works
During positron emission, pairs of gamma rays are emitted; the PET scanner detects them and relays the information to a computer for reconstruction as an image. Positron emitters can be chemically "tagged" to biologically active molecules such as carbon monoxide, neurotransmitters, hormones, and metabolites (especially glucose), enabling study of their uptake and distribution in brain tissue. For example, blood tagged with ^{11}C-carbon monoxide allows study of hemodynamic patterns in brain tissue; tagged neurotransmitters, hormones, and drugs allow mapping of receptor distribution.

Isotope-tagged glucose (which penetrates the blood-brain barrier rapidly) allows dynamic study of brain function because PET scans can pinpoint the sites of glucose metabolism in the brain under various conditions. This may prove to be useful in the diagnosis of psychiatric disorders, transient ischemic attacks, amyotrophic lateral sclerosis, Parkinson's disease, Wilson's disease, multiple sclerosis, seizure disorders, cerebrovascular disease, and Alzheimer's disease. The reason: All of these disorders may alter the location and patterns of cerebral glucose metabolism.

Cost factors
PET scanning is a costly test because the radioisotopes used have very short half-lives and must be produced at an on-site cyclotron and attached quickly to the desired tracer molecules. However, this procedure has already provided significant information about the brain and may someday have widespread clinical applications.

imaging is now the preferred procedure for imaging cerebral vessels.

Another technology for obtaining images of the brain is positron emission tomography. (See *PET scan of the brain*.)

Interfering factors
• Patient's head movement (possible poor imaging)
• Failure to remove metal objects from the scanning field (possible poor imaging)

• Hemorrhage (possible false-negative imaging due to change in hematoma)

INTRACRANIAL MAGNETIC RESONANCE IMAGING

Intracranial magnetic resonance imaging (MRI) produces highly detailed, cross-sectional images of the brain and spine in multiple planes. The primary advantages of MRI is its ability to "see through" bone and to delineate fluid-filled soft tissue. It has proved useful in the diagnosis of cerebral infarction, tumors, abscesses, edema, hemorrhage, nerve fiber demyelination (as in multiple sclerosis), and other disorders that increase the fluid content of affected tissues. It can also show irregularities of the spinal cord with a resolution and detail previously unobtainable. It can also produce images of organs and vessels in motion.

MRI technology makes use of magnetic fields and radio frequency (RF) waves, which are imperceptible by the patient; no harmful effects have been documented. Research continues on the optimal magnetic fields and RF waves for each type of tissue. (See *Current techniques for monitoring cerebral function,* page 620.)

Purpose
• To aid diagnosis of intracranial and spinal lesions and soft-tissue abnormalities

Patient preparation
• Explain to the patient that this test assesses bone and soft tissue. Tell him who will perform the test, where it will be done, and that it takes up to 90 minutes.
• Explain that MRI is painless and involves no exposure to radiation from the scanner.
• Explain to the patient that sedation may be administered if he suffers from claustrophobia or if extensive time is required for scanning.
• Make sure the patient is able to lie flat.
• Tell him that he'll hear the scanner clicking, whirring, and thumping as it moves inside its housing.

• Reassure him that he'll be able to communicate with the technician at all times.
• Instruct the patient to remove all metallic objects, including jewelry, hair pins, and a watch, and ask if he has any surgically implanted joints, pins, clips, valves, pumps, or pacemakers containing metal that could be attracted to the strong MRI magnet. If he does, he may not be able to undergo the test.
• Ensure that the patient or a responsible family member has signed a consent form.

Procedure and posttest care
• The patient is placed in a supine position on a narrow bed, which then slides him to the desired position inside the scanner where RF energy is directed at his head or spine.
• The resulting images are displayed on a monitor and recorded on film or magnetic tape for permanent storage.
• The radiologist may vary RF waves and use the computer to manipulate and enhance the images.
• During the procedure the patient must remain still.
• Tell the patient that he may resume normal activity after the test.
• If the patient was sedated, ensure that a responsible person drives him home.
• If the test took a long time and the patient was lying flat for an extended period, observe him for orthostatic hypotension.
• Provide emotional support to the patient with claustrophobia or anxiety over his diagnosis.

Precautions
• Because MRI works through a powerful magnetic field, it can't be performed on patients with pacemakers, intracranial aneurysm clips, or other ferrous metal implants or on a patient with gunshot wounds to the head.

CURRENT TECHNIQUES FOR MONITORING CEREBRAL FUNCTION

Magnetic resonance imaging (MRI) is used to provide clear images of parts of the brain, such as the brain stem and cerebellum, that are difficult to image by other methods. Ongoing research into MRI applications has produced valuable methods of investigating the brain more completely.

Fast MRI

This highly sensitive process quickly produces a series of images depicting blood flow in the brain and vascular changes that occur as the patient performs tasks. It is currently used to detect vascular lesions and extramedullary spinal disease and to depict areas abnormally susceptible to magnetic resonance, possibly indicating hemorrhage, occult cerebrovascular malformations, hemorrhagic metastasis, or calcification.

Fast MRI distinguishes between oxygen-laden and oxygen-depleted blood. Because active areas of the brain consume more oxygen than inactive areas, this technology may prove useful in identifying areas of the brain that are active during specific activities or emotional states.

Magnetic resonance angiography

This noninvasive technique allows the visualization of blood flowing through the cerebral vessels.

Magnetic resonance spectroscopy

This test creates images over time that show the metabolism of certain chemical markers in a specific area of the brain. Some researchers have dubbed this test a "metabolic biopsy" because it reveals pathologic neurochemistry over time.

Diffusion-perfusion imaging

This MRI technique uses a stronger-than-normal magnetic gradient to reveal areas of focal cerebral ischemia within minutes. Currently used in stroke research, diffusion-perfusion imaging may be used by diagnosticians to distinguish permanent from reversible ischemia.

Neurograms

Neurograms provide a three-dimensional image of nerves. They may be used in the future to find the exact location of nerves that are damaged, crimped, or in disarray.

● Because of the strong magnetic field, metallic or computer-based equipment (for example, oxygen tanks, ventilators, and I.V. pumps) can't enter the MRI area.

Normal findings

MRI can show normal anatomic details of the central nervous system in any plane, without bone interference. Brain and spinal cord structures should appear distinct and sharply defined. Tissue color and shading will vary, depending on the RF energy, magnetic strength, and degree of computer enhancement. MRI can detect white matter abnormalities, especially multiple sclerosis.

Abnormal findings

Because MRI depicts the density (water content) of tissue, it clearly shows structural changes resulting from disorders that increase tissue water content, such as cerebral edema, demyelinating disease, and pontine and cerebellar tumors. Lesions of multiple sclerosis appear as areas of demyelination (curdlike, gray or gray-white areas) around the edges of ventricles. Tumors appear as changes in normal anatomy, which computer enhancement may further delineate.

Interfering factor
• Excessive patient movement (possible poor imaging)

GASTROINTESTINAL SYSTEM

LIVER AND BILIARY TRACT COMPUTED TOMOGRAPHY

In computed tomography (CT) of the biliary tract and liver, multiple X-rays pass through the upper abdomen and are measured while detectors record differences in tissue attenuation. A computer reconstructs this data as a two-dimensional image on a monitor. CT scanning accurately distinguishes the biliary tract and the liver if the ducts are large. Use of I.V. contrast media during CT scanning can accentuate different densities.

Although CT scanning and ultrasonography detect biliary tract and liver disease equally well, the latter technique is performed more often. CT scanning is more expensive than ultrasonography and requires exposure to moderate amounts of radiation. However, it's the test of choice in patients who are obese and in those with livers positioned high under the rib cage because bone and excessive fat hinder ultrasound transmission.

Purpose
• To distinguish between obstructive and nonobstructive jaundice
• To specify focal defects detected by liver-spleen scanning as solid, cystic, inflammatory, and vascular lesions (biopsy may be necessary to rule out malignancy or to distinguish between metastatic and primary tumors)
• To detect suspected hematoma after abdominal trauma

Patient preparation
• Explain to the patient that this test helps detect biliary tract and liver disease.
• Instruct the patient to fast after midnight before the test if receiving an oral contrast medium. If contrast isn't ordered, fasting isn't necessary.
• Tell him who will perform the test and where.
• Inform him that he'll be placed on an adjustable table, which is positioned inside a scanning gantry. Assure him that the test will be painless.
• Tell him he'll be asked to remain still during the test and to hold his breath when instructed. Stress the importance of remaining still during the test, because movement can cause artifacts, thereby prolonging the test and limiting its accuracy.
• If I.V. contrast medium is being used, inform the patient that he may experience transient discomfort from the needle puncture and a localized feeling of warmth on injection. Tell him to immediately report nausea, vomiting, dizziness, headache, and hives.
• Check his history for hypersensitivity to iodine, seafood, or the contrast media used in other diagnostic tests.

• If a contrast medium has been ordered, give him the oral contrast medium supplied by the radiology department.

Procedure and posttest care

• The patient is placed in a supine position on an X-ray table, and the table is positioned within the opening in the scanning gantry.

• A series of transverse X-ray films is taken and recorded on magnetic tape. This information is reconstructed by a computer and appears as images on a television screen.

• These images are studied, and selected ones are photographed. When the first series of films is completed, the images are reviewed.

• Contrast enhancement may be performed. After the contrast medium is injected, a second series of films is taken, and the patient is carefully observed for an allergic reaction.

• Following the procedure, tell the patient that he may resume his usual diet.

Precautions

• CT scanning of the biliary tract and liver is usually contraindicated during pregnancy.

• Use of an I.V. contrast medium is contraindicated in patients with hypersensitivity to iodine or with severe renal or hepatic disease.

Normal findings

Normally, the liver has a uniform density that's slightly greater than that of the pancreas, kidneys, and spleen. Linear and circular areas of slightly lower density, representing hepatic vascular structures, may interrupt this uniform appearance. The portal vein is usually visible; the hepatic artery usually isn't. I.V. contrast medium enhances the isodensity of both vascular structures and the liver parenchyma.

Typically, intrahepatic biliary radicles are not visible, but the common hepatic and bile ducts may be visible as low-density structures. Because bile has the same density as water, use of an I.V. contrast medium improves demarcation of the biliary tract by enhancing surrounding parenchyma and vascular structures.

Like the biliary ducts, the gallbladder is visible as a round or elliptic low-density structure. A contracted gallbladder may be impossible to visualize.

Abnormal findings

Most focal hepatic defects appear less dense than the normal parenchyma, and CT scans can detect small lesions. Use of rapid-sequence scanning with an I.V. contrast medium helps distinguish between the two because the normal parenchyma shows greater enhancement than focal defects.

Primary and metastatic neoplasms may appear as well-circumscribed or poorly defined areas of slightly lower density than the normal parenchyma. However, some lesions have the same density as the liver parenchyma and may be undetectable. Neoplasms that are especially large may distort the liver's contour. Hepatic abscesses appear as relatively low-density, homogeneous areas, usually with well-defined borders. Hepatic cysts appear as sharply defined round or oval structures and have a density lower than abscesses and neoplasms.

The density of a hepatic hematoma varies with its age. A recent clot is as dense as or slightly more dense than the normal parenchyma; a resolving clot is somewhat less dense than the normal parenchyma. Intrahepatic hematomas vary in shape; subcapsular hematomas are usually crescent-shaped and compress the liver away from the capsule.

When distinguishing between obstructive and nonobstructive jaundice, biliary duct dilation indicates the former and an absence of dilation indicates the latter. Dilated intrahepatic bile ducts appear as low-density linear and circular branching structures. Dilation of the common hepatic duct, common bile duct, and gallbladder may also be apparent, depending on the site and severity of obstruction. Use of an I.V. contrast medium helps detect biliary dilation, especially when the ducts are only slightly dilated.

Usually, CT scanning can identify the cause of obstruction — for example, calculi or pancreatic carcinoma. However, if the site of obstruction must be located before surgery, percutaneous transhepatic cholangiography or endoscopic retrograde cholangiopancreatography (less common) may be performed as well.

Interfering factors

• Presence of oral or I.V. contrast media, including barium, in the bile from earlier tests (possible poor imaging)
• Patient movement or incorrect patient positioning
• Extremely obese patient
• Failure to remove metallic objects from the scan area (possible poor imaging)

PANCREATIC COMPUTED TOMOGRAPHY

In computed tomography (CT) of the pancreas, multiple X-rays penetrate the upper abdomen while a detector records the differences in tissue attenuation, which is then displayed as an image on a television screen. A series of cross-sectional views can provide a detailed look at the pancreas. CT scanning accurately distinguishes the pancreas and surrounding organs and vessels if enough fat is present between the structures. Use of an I.V. or oral contrast medium can further accentuate differences in tissue density.

Purpose

• To detect pancreatic carcinoma or pseudocysts
• To detect or evaluate pancreatitis (CT scans may fail to distinguish between carcinoma and pancreatitis)
• To distinguish between pancreatic disorders and disorders of the retroperitoneum

Patient preparation

• Explain to the patient that this test helps detect disorders of the pancreas.
• Instruct him to fast after midnight before the day of the test.
• Describe the test, including who will perform it and where it will take place.
• Tell him that he'll be placed on an adjustable table that is positioned inside a scanning gantry. Assure him that the procedure is painless.
• Explain that he'll have to remain still during the test and periodically hold his breath.
• Inform him that he may be given an I.V. contrast medium, an oral contrast medium, or both to enhance visualization of the pancreas. Describe possible adverse reactions to the medium, such as nausea, flushing, dizziness, and sweating, and tell him to report any of these symptoms.
• Check his history for recent barium studies and for hypersensitivity to iodine, seafood, or contrast media used in prior tests.
• Administer the oral contrast medium.

NORMAL CT SCAN OF THE PANCREAS

This normal pancreatic computed tomography (CT) scan shows the pancreas opacified by contrast medium.

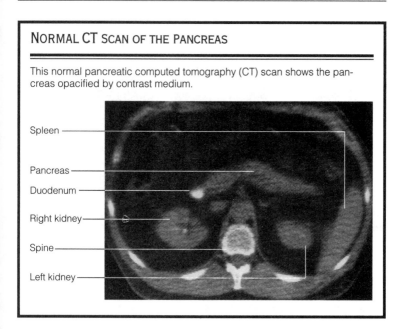

Spleen

Pancreas

Duodenum

Right kidney

Spine

Left kidney

Procedure and posttest care

• Help the patient into the supine position on the X-ray table and position the table within the opening in the scanning gantry.

• A series of transverse X-rays is taken and recorded on magnetic tape. The varying tissue absorption is calculated by a computer, and the information is reconstructed as images on a television screen. These images are studied, and selected ones are photographed.

• After the first series of films is completed, the images are reviewed. Then contrast enhancement may be ordered. After the contrast medium is administered, another series of films is taken, and the patient is observed for an allergic reaction — itching, hypotension, hypertension, diaphoresis, or dyspnea.

• After the procedure, tell the patient he may resume his usual diet.

Precautions

• CT scanning of the pancreas should not be performed during pregnancy or, if a contrast medium is indicated, on patients with a history of hypersensitivity to iodine or severe renal or hepatic disease.

Normal findings

Usually, the pancreatic parenchyma displays a uniform density, especially when an I.V. contrast medium is used. The gland normally thickens from tail to head and has a smooth surface. A contrast medium administered orally opacifies the adjacent stomach and duodenum and helps outline the pancreas, particularly in patients with little peripancreatic fat, such as children and thin adults. (See *Normal CT scan of the pancreas.*)

Abnormal findings

Because the tissue density of pancreatic carcinoma resembles that of the normal parenchyma, changes in pancreatic size and shape help demonstrate carcinoma and pseudocysts. Usually, carcinoma first appears as a localized swelling of the head, body, or tail of the pancreas and may spread to obliterate the fat plane, dilate the main pancreatic duct and common bile duct by obstructing them, and produce low-density focal lesions in the liver from metastasis. Use of an I.V. contrast medium helps detect metastases by opacifying the pancreatic and hepatic parenchyma.

Adenocarcinoma and islet cell tumor are the most common carcinomas of the pancreas. Cystadenomas and cystadenocarcinomas, usually multilocular, occur most frequently in the body and tail of the pancreas and appear as low-density focal lesions marked by internal septa. Contrast medium administered by mouth helps distinguish between bowel loops and tumors in the tail of the pancreas.

Acute pancreatitis, either edematous (interstitial) or necrotizing (hemorrhagic), produces diffuse enlargement of the pancreas. In acute edematous pancreatitis, the density of the parenchyma is uniformly decreased. In acute necrotizing pancreatitis, the density is nonuniform because of the presence of both necrosis and hemorrhage. The areas of tissue necrosis have diminished density. In acute pancreatitis, inflammation often spreads into the peripancreatic fat, causes stranding in the mesenteric fat, and blurs the margin of the gland.

Abscesses, phlegmons, and pseudocysts may occur as complications of acute pancreatitis. Abscesses, either within or outside the pancreas, appear as low-density areas and are most readily detected when they contain gas.

Pseudocysts, which may be unilocular or multilocular, appear as sharply circumscribed, low-density areas that may contain debris. Ascites and pleural effusion may also be apparent in acute pancreatitis.

In chronic pancreatitis, the pancreas may appear normal, enlarged (localized or generalized), or atrophic, depending on the severity of the disease. Calcification of the ducts and dilation of the main pancreatic duct are characteristic. Pseudocysts, obliteration of the fat plane, and secondary complications (such as biliary obstruction) may occur.

Interfering factors

● Barium or other contrast media in the GI tract from earlier tests (possible poor imaging)
● Patient movement or incorrect patient positioning
● Excessive peristalsis
● Extreme obesity
● Failure to remove metallic objects from examination field (possible poor imaging)

MUSCULOSKELETAL SYSTEM

SPINAL COMPUTED TOMOGRAPHY

Much more versatile than conventional radiography, computed tomography (CT) of the spine provides detailed high-resolution images in the cross-sectional, longitudinal, sagittal, and lateral planes. Multiple X-ray beams from a computerized body scanner are directed at the spine from different angles; these pass through the body and strike radiation detectors, producing electrical impulses. A computer then converts these impulses into digital information, which is displayed as a three-dimensional image on a monitor. Storage of the digital information allows electronic recreation and manipulation of the image, creating a permanent record of the images to enable reexamination without repeating the procedure.

Two variations of spinal CT scanning further expand the procedure's diagnostic capabilities. Contrast-enhanced CT scans accentuate spinal vasculature and highlight even subtle differences in tissue density. CT scanning, which involves removing a small amount of cerebrospinal fluid (CSF) and injecting air or contrast material via lumbar puncture, intensifies the contrast between the subarachnoid space and surrounding tissue.

Spinal CT is primarily performed to examine vertebral bodies. If spinal details need to be seen, MRI is the study of choice. If MRI is contraindicated, then enhanced spinal CT may be performed.

Purpose
• To diagnose spinal lesions and abnormalities
• To monitor the effects of spinal surgery or therapy

Patient preparation
• Explain to the patient that this procedure allows visualization of his spine.
• If contrast enhancement isn't ordered, tell him that he needn't restrict food or fluids. If contrast is ordered, instruct him to fast for 4 hours before the test.
• Tell the patient that a series of scans will be taken of his spine. Explain who

will perform the procedure and where and that the test takes 30 to 60 minutes.
• Reassure him that the procedure is painless, but that he may find having to remain still for a prolonged period uncomfortable.
• Explain that he'll be positioned on an X-ray table inside a CT body scanning unit and told to lie still because movement during the procedure may cause distorted images. The computer-controlled scanner will revolve around him taking multiple scans.
• If a contrast medium is used, tell him that he may feel flushed and warm and may experience a transient headache, a salty taste, and nausea or vomiting after injection of the contrast medium. Reassure him that these reactions are normal.
• Instruct the patient to wear a radiologic examining gown and to remove all metal objects and jewelry.
• Check the patient's history for hypersensitivity reactions to iodine, shellfish, or contrast media. If such reactions have occurred, mark them on the patient's chart. The doctor may order prophylactic medications or choose not to use contrast enhancement.
• If the patient appears restless or apprehensive about the procedure, a mild sedative may be prescribed.

Equipment
Recording equipment, contrast medium (meglumine iothalamate or sodium diatrizoate), 60-ml syringe, 19G to 20G needle, tourniquet

Procedure and posttest care
• Place the patient in a supine position on an X-ray table and tell him to lie as still as possible.
• The table slides into the circular opening of the CT scanner and the scanner revolves around the patient,

taking radiographs at preselected intervals.

• After the first set of scans is taken, the patient is removed from the scanner. Contrast medium may be administered.

• Observe the patient for signs and symptoms of a hypersensitivity reaction, including pruritus, rash, and respiratory difficulty, for 30 minutes after the contrast medium has been injected.

• After contrast medium injection, the patient is moved back into the scanner, and another series of scans is taken. The images obtained from the scan are displayed on a monitor during the procedure and stored on magnetic tape.

• After testing with contrast enhancement, observe the patient for residual effects, such as headache, nausea, and vomiting, and inform him that he may resume his usual diet.

Precautions

• Body CT scanning with contrast enhancement is contraindicated in patients who are hypersensitive to iodine, shellfish, or contrast media used in radiographic studies.

• Some patients may experience strong feelings of claustrophobia or anxiety when inside the body CT scanner. For such patients, a mild sedative to help reduce anxiety may be ordered.

• For patients with significant back pain, administer prescribed analgesics before the scan.

Normal findings

In the CT image, spinal tissue appears white, black, or gray, depending on its density. Vertebrae, the densest tissues, are white; CSF is black; soft tissues appear in shades of gray.

Abnormal findings

By highlighting areas of altered density and depicting structural malforma-

tion, CT scanning can reveal all types of spinal lesions and abnormalities. It's particularly useful in detecting and localizing tumors, which appear as masses varying in density. Measuring this density and noting the configuration and location relative to the spinal cord can often identify the type of tumor. For example, a neurinoma (schwannoma) appears as a spherical mass dorsal to the cord. A darker, wider mass lying more laterally or ventrally to the cord may be a meningioma.

CT scans also reveal degenerative processes and structural changes in detail. Herniated nucleus pulposus shows as an obvious herniation of disk material with unilateral or bilateral nerve root compression; if the herniation is midline, spinal cord compression will be evident. Cervical spondylosis shows as cervical cord compression due to bony hypertrophy of the cervical spine; lumbar stenosis as hypertrophy of the lumbar vertebrae, causing cord compression by decreasing space within the spinal column. Facet disorders show as soft-tissue changes, bony overgrowth, and spurring of the vertebrae, which result in nerve root compression. Fluid-filled arachnoidal and other paraspinal cysts show as dark masses displacing the spinal cord. Vascular malformations, evident after contrast enhancement, show as masses or clusters, usually on the dorsal aspect of the spinal cord.

Congenital spinal malformations, such as meningocele, myelocele, and spina bifida, show as abnormally large, dark gaps between the white vertebrae.

Interfering factors

• Excessive patient movement
• Failure to remove metallic objects from the scan area (possible poor imaging)

SKELETAL COMPUTED TOMOGRAPHY

Skeletal computed tomography (CT) provides a series of tomograms, translated by a computer and displayed on a monitor, representing cross-sectional images of various layers (or slices) of bone. This technique can reconstruct cross-sectional, horizontal, sagittal, and coronal plane images.

Taking collimated (parallel) radiographs increases the number of radiation density calculations the computer makes, thereby improving the degree of resolution and thus specificity and accuracy. Hundreds of thousands of readings of radiation levels absorbed by tissues may be combined to depict anatomic slices of varying thickness.

Purpose
● To determine the existence and extent of primary bone tumors, skeletal metastases, and soft-tissue tumors
● To diagnose joint abnormalities difficult to detect by other methods

Patient preparation
● Explain to the patient that this procedure allows visualization of bones and joints. If contrast medium isn't ordered, tell him that he needn't restrict food or fluids. If contrast enhancement is ordered, instruct him to fast for 4 hours before the test.
● Explain who will perform the procedure and where and that the test takes 30 to 60 minutes. Reassure him that the procedure is painless.
● Explain that he'll be positioned on an X-ray table inside a CT scanner and asked to lie still; the computer-controlled scanner will revolve around him taking multiple scans. Stress that he

should lie as still as possible because movement may cause distorted images.
● If a contrast medium is used, tell him that he may feel flushed and warm and may experience a transient headache, a salty or metallic taste, and nausea or vomiting after its injection. Reassure him that these reactions are normal.
● Instruct him to wear a radiologic examining gown and to remove all metal objects and jewelry that may appear in the X-ray field.
● Check his history for hypersensitivity reactions to iodine, shellfish, or contrast media. Mark any such reactions on the chart. The doctor may order prophylactic medications or choose not to use a contrast medium.
● If the patient appears restless or apprehensive about the procedure, a mild sedative may be prescribed.

Equipment
Recording equipment, contrast medium (either meglumine iothalamate or sodium diatrizoate), 60-ml syringe, 19G to 20G needle, tourniquet

Procedure and posttest care
● Place the patient in a supine position on an X-ray table and tell him to lie as still as possible.
● The table is slid into the circular opening of the CT scanner. The scanner revolves around the patient, taking radiographs at preselected intervals.
● After the first set of scans is taken, the patient is removed from the scanner and a contrast medium is administered if necessary.
● Observe the patient for signs and symptoms of a hypersensitivity reaction, including pruritus, rash, and respiratory difficulty, for 30 minutes after the contrast medium has been injected.
● After contrast medium injection, the patient is moved back into the scanner, and another series of scans is taken.

The images obtained from the scan are displayed on a monitor during the procedure and stored on magnetic tape to create a permanent record for subsequent study.

• If contrast media is used, observe for a delayed allergic reaction and treat as necessary. (Diphenhydramine is the drug of choice.)

• Encourage fluids to assist in elimination of the contrast medium.

• Tell the patient that he may resume his usual activity level and diet, if appropriate.

Precautions

• A CT scan with contrast enhancement is contraindicated in patients who are hypersensitive to iodine, shellfish, or contrast media, or in those who have renal insufficiency (if they aren't on dialysis).

• Some patients may experience strong feelings of claustrophobia or anxiety when inside the body CT scanner. For such patients, a mild sedative may be ordered to help reduce anxiety.

• For patients with significant bone or joint pain, administer analgesics so that the patient can lie still comfortably during the scan.

Normal findings

The scan should reveal no pathology in the bones or joints. It produces crisp images of the structure while blurring or eliminating details of surrounding structures.

Abnormal findings

Because of its ability to display cross-sectional anatomy, CT scanning is useful for detecting the shoulder, spine, hip, and pelvis. This cross-sectional view eliminates the confusing shadows of superimposed structures that occur with conventional radiographs. The scan can reveal primary bone tumors

and soft-tissue tumors as well as skeletal metastasis. It can also reveal joint abnormalities difficult to detect by other methods.

Interfering factors

• Claustrophobia (possible interference with patient's ability to lie in scanner for long periods)

• Excessive patient movement

• Failure to remove metallic objects from examination field (possible poor imaging)

SKELETAL MAGNETIC RESONANCE IMAGING

A noninvasive technique, magnetic resonance imaging (MRI) produces clear and sensitive tomographic images of bone and soft tissue. The scan provides superior contrast of body tissues and allows imaging of multiple planes, including direct sagittal and coronal views in regions that can't be easily visualized with X-rays or computed tomography (CT) scans. MRI eliminates any risks associated with exposure to X-ray beams and causes no known harm to cells.

During an MRI scan, the patient is placed on a table that slides into a cylindrical magnet. A radio frequency beam is then introduced into the magnetic field. Resulting energy changes are measured and used to generate images on a monitor.

Purpose

• To evaluate bony and soft-tissue tumors

• To identify changes in bone marrow composition

• To identify spinal disorders

Patient preparation

- Explain to the patient that this test assesses bone and soft tissue. Tell him who will perform the test, where it will be done, and that it takes up to 90 minutes.
- Explain that although MRI is painless and involves no exposure to radiation from the scanner, a contrast medium may be used, depending on the type of tissue being studied.
- Explain to the patient that if he is claustrophobic or if extensive time is required for scanning, a mild sedative may be administered to reduce anxiety.
- Explain to the patient the need to lie flat, and describe the test procedure.
- Explain that he'll hear the scanner clicking, whirring, and thumping as it moves inside its housing.
- Reassure him that he'll be able to communicate with the technician at all times.
- Instruct the patient to remove all metallic objects, including jewelry, hair pins, or watch.
- Ask if he has any surgically implanted joints, pins, clips, valves, pumps, or pacemakers containing metal that could be attracted to the strong MRI magnet. If he does, he may not be able to have the test.

Procedure and posttest care

- At the scanner room door, check the patient one last time for metal objects.
- The patient is placed on a narrow, padded, nonmetallic table that moves into the scanner tunnel. Fans continuously circulate air in the tunnel, and a call bell or intercom is used to maintain verbal contact.
- Remind the patient to remain still throughout the procedure.
- While the patient lies within the strong magnetic field, the area to be studied is stimulated with radio frequency waves.
- If the test is prolonged with the patient lying flat, monitor him for orthostatic hypotension.
- After the test, tell the patient that he may resume normal activity.
- Provide emotional support to the patient with claustrophobia or anxiety over his diagnosis.

Precautions

- MRI can't be performed on patients with pacemakers, intracranial aneurysm clips, or other ferrous metal implants. Ventilators, I.V. infusion pumps, oxygen tanks, and other metallic or computer-based equipment must be kept out of the MRI area.
- If the patient is unstable, make sure an I.V. line without metal components is in place and that all equipment is compatible with MRI imaging. If necessary, monitor oxygen saturation, cardiac rhythm, and respiratory status during the test. An anesthesiologist may be needed to monitor a heavily sedated patient.
- A technician should maintain verbal contact with the conscious patient.

Normal findings

MRI should reveal no pathology in bone, muscles, and joints.

Abnormal findings

MRI is excellent for visualizing diseases of the spinal canal and cord and for identifying primary and metastatic bone tumors. It's beneficial in anatomic delineation of muscles, ligaments, and bones. The images show superior contrast of body tissues and sharply define healthy, benign, and malignant tissues.

Interfering factors

- Excessive patient movement
- Patient unable to fit into scanner

MISCELLANEOUS TESTS

ORBITAL COMPUTED TOMOGRAPHY

Orbital computed tomography (CT) allows visualization of abnormalities not readily seen on standard radiographs, delineating their size, position, and relationship to adjoining structures. A series of tomograms reconstructed by a computer and displayed as anatomic slices on a monitor, the orbital CT scan identifies space-occupying lesions earlier and more accurately than other radiographic techniques and provides three-dimensional images of orbital structures, especially the ocular muscles and the optic nerve.

Purpose

• To evaluate pathologies of the orbit and eye — especially expanding lesions and bone destruction
• To evaluate fractures of the orbit and adjoining structures
• To determine the cause of unilateral exophthalmos
• To aid diagnosis of intracranial lesions that affect vision
• To evaluate a patient with conditions such as suspected circulatory disorders, hemangioma, or subdural hematoma (with contrast enhancement)

Patient preparation

• Describe the procedure to the patient, and explain that this test visualizes the anatomy of the eye and its surrounding structures.
• If contrast enhancement isn't scheduled, inform him that he needn't restrict food or fluids. If contrast enhancement is scheduled, withhold food and fluids from the patient for 4 hours before the test.
• Tell the patient that a series of X-ray films will be taken of his eye and who will perform the test and where.
• Reassure him that the test will cause him no discomfort and will take 15 to 30 minutes to perform.
• Tell the patient that he'll be positioned on an X-ray table and that the head of the table will be moved into the scanner, which will rotate around his head and make loud clacking sounds.
• If a contrast medium will be used for the procedure, tell the patient that he may feel flushed and warm and experience a transient headache, a salty or metallic taste, and nausea or vomiting after the contrast medium is injected. Reassure him that these reactions to contrast media are typical.
• Check his history for hypersensitivity reactions to iodine, shellfish, or contrast media.
• Instruct the patient to remove jewelry, hairpins, or other metal objects in the X-ray field to allow for precise imaging of the orbital structures.

Procedure and posttest care

• The patient is placed in a supine position on the X-ray table, with his head immobilized by straps if required. Ask him to lie still.
• The head of the table is moved into the scanner, which rotates around the patient's head taking radiographs.
• Information obtained is stored on magnetic tapes, and the images are displayed on a monitor. Photographs may be made if a permanent record is desired.
• When this series of radiographs has been taken, contrast enhancement is performed. The contrast medium is in-

jected and a second series of scans is recorded.

• If a contrast medium was used, watch for its residual adverse effects, including headache, nausea, or vomiting. Following the procedure, advise the patient that he may resume his usual diet.

Precautions

• Use of contrast enhancement is contraindicated in those patients with known hypersensitivity reactions to iodine, shellfish, or contrast media used in other tests.

Normal findings

Orbital structures are evaluated for size, shape, and position. Dense orbital bone provides a marked contrast to less dense periocular fat. The optic nerve and the medial and lateral rectus muscles are clearly defined. The rectus muscles appear as thin dense bands on each side, behind the eye. The optic canals should be equal in size.

Abnormal findings

Orbital CT scans can identify intraorbital and extraorbital space-occupying lesions that obscure the normal structures or cause orbital enlargement, indentation of the orbital walls, or bone destruction. This test can also help determine the type of lesion. For example, infiltrative lesions, such as lymphomas and metastatic carcinomas, appear as irregular areas of density. However, encapsulated tumors, such as benign hemangiomas and meningiomas, appear as clearly defined masses of consistent density. CT scans can also visualize intracranial tumors that invade the orbit, thickening of the optic nerve that may occur with gliomas, meningiomas, and secondary tumors

that may cause enlargement of the optic canal.

In evaluating fractures, CT scans allow a complete three-dimensional view of the affected structures. In determining the cause of unilateral exophthalmos, CT scans can show early erosion or expansion of the medial orbital wall that may arise from lesions in the ethmoidal cells. It can also detect space-occupying lesions in the orbit or paranasal sinuses that cause exophthalmos. CT scans can also show thickening of the medial and lateral rectus muscles in proptosis resulting from Graves' disease.

Enhancement with a contrast medium may provide information about the circulation through abnormal ocular tissues.

Interfering factors

• Head movement
• Failure to remove metallic objects from examination field (possible poor imaging)

THORACIC COMPUTED TOMOGRAPHY

Thoracic computed tomography (CT) provides cross-sectional views of the chest by passing an X-ray beam from a computerized scanner through the body at different angles. CT scanning may be done with or without an injected contrast medium, which is primarily used to highlight blood vessels and to allow greater visual discrimination.

This test provides a three-dimensional image and is especially useful in detecting small differences in tissue density. The thoracic CT scan may replace mediastinoscopy in diagnosis of mediastinal masses and Hodgkin's disease; its value in the evaluation of pulmonary pathology is proven.

Purpose

● To locate suspected neoplasms (such as in Hodgkin's disease), especially with mediastinal involvement
● To differentiate coin-sized calcified lesions (indicating tuberculosis) from tumors
● To distinguish tumors adjacent to the aorta from aortic aneurysms
● To detect the invasion of a neck mass in the thorax
● To evaluate primary malignancy that may metastasize to the lungs, especially in patients with primary bone tumors, soft-tissue sarcomas, and melanomas
● To evaluate the mediastinal lymph nodes

Patient preparation

● Explain to the patient that this test provides cross-sectional views of the chest and distinguishes small differences in tissue density.
● If a contrast medium will not be used, inform him that he needn't restrict food or fluids. If the test is to be performed with contrast enhancement, instruct the patient to fast for 4 hours before the test.
● Tell him who will perform the test and where and that the procedure usually takes 90 minutes and won't cause him any discomfort.
● Inform him that he'll be positioned on an X-ray table that moves into the center of a large ring-shaped piece of X-ray equipment and that the equipment may be noisy.
● Inform him that a contrast medium may be injected into a vein in his arm.

If so, he may experience nausea, warmth, flushing of the face, and a salty or metallic taste. Reassure him that these symptoms are normal and that radiation exposure is minimal.
● Tell him not to move during the test, but to breathe normally until told to follow specific breathing instructions. Instruct him to remove all jewelry and metal in the X-ray field.
● Check the patient's history for hypersensitivity to iodine, shellfish, or contrast media.

Procedure and posttest care

● After the patient is placed in a supine position on the X-ray table and the contrast medium has been injected, the machine scans the patient at different angles while the computer calculates small differences in the densities of various tissues, water, fat, bone, and air.
● This information is displayed as a printout of numerical values and as a projection on a monitor. Images may be recorded for further study.
● Watch for signs of delayed hypersensitivity to the contrast medium (itching, hypotension or hypertension, or respiratory distress).
● Following the test, encourage the patient to drink lots of fluids.

Precautions

● Thoracic CT scanning is contraindicated during pregnancy and, if a contrast medium is used, in persons who have a history of hypersensitivity reactions to iodine, shellfish, or contrast media.

Normal findings

Black and white areas on a thoracic CT scan refer, respectively, to air and bone densities. Shades of gray correspond to water, fat, and soft-tissue densities.

Abnormal findings

Abnormal thoracic CT findings include tumors, nodules, cysts, aortic aneurysms, enlarged lymph nodes, pleural effusion, and accumulations of blood, fluid, or fat.

Interfering factors

- Failure to remove all metallic objects from scanning field (possible poor imaging)
- Patient's inability to remain still during the procedure
- Obese patient (may be too heavy for scanning table)

CARDIAC MAGNETIC RESONANCE IMAGING

A great asset in the diagnosis of cardiac disorders, magnetic resonance imaging (MRI) has the ability to "see through" bone and to delineate fluid-filled soft tissue in great detail, as well as produce images of organs and vessels in motion.

In this noninvasive procedure, the patient is placed in a magnetic field, into which a radio frequency (RF) beam is introduced. Resulting energy changes are measured and used by the MRI computer to generate images on a monitor. Cross-sectional images of the anatomy are viewed in multiple planes and recorded for permanent record.

Another technology for evaluating cardiac pathology is positron emission tomography. (See *Cardiac PET scan.*)

Purpose

- To identify anatomic sequelae related to myocardial infarction, such as formation of ventricular aneurysm, ven-

tricular wall thinning, and mural thrombus

- To detect and evaluate cardiomyopathy
- To detect and evaluate pericardial disease
- To identify paracardiac or intracardiac masses
- To detect congenital heart disease, such as atrial or ventricular septal defects, and the degree of malposition of the great vessel
- To identify vascular disease, such as thoracic aneurysm and thoracic dissection
- To assess the structure of the pulmonary vasculature

Patient preparation

- Explain to the patient that this test assesses the heart's function and structure.
- Tell him who will perform the test, where it will be done, and that it takes up to 90 minutes.
- Inform the patient that he'll be positioned on a narrow bed, which slides into a large cylinder that houses the MRI magnets. Tell him that the scanner will make clicking, whirring, and thumping noises as it moves inside its housing.
- Explain to the patient who is claustrophobic or anxious about the test's duration that he'll receive a mild sedative to reduce his anxiety.
- Explain to the patient the need to lie flat.
- Reassure him that he'll be able to communicate with the technician at all times and that the procedure will be stopped if he feels claustrophobic.
- Immediately before the test, have the patient remove all metal objects. Double check to be sure he doesn't have a pacemaker or any surgically implanted joints, pins, clips, valves, or pumps

CARDIAC PET SCAN

Positron emission tomography (PET) scanning combines elements of computed tomography (CT) scanning and conventional radionuclide imaging. This test is used to detect coronary artery disease, to evaluate myocardial metabolism and contractility, and to distinguish viable from infarcted cardiac tissue, especially during early stages of myocardial infarction.

How it works

Like radionuclide imaging, PET scans measure emissions of injected radioisotopes and convert these values to tomographic images. However, PET uses radioisotopes of biologically important elements — oxygen, nitrogen, carbon, and fluorine — which emit particles called positrons. During positron emissions, gamma rays are detected by the PET scanner and reconstructed to form an image. One distinct advantage of PET scans is that positron emitters can be chemically "tagged" to biologically active molecules such as carbon monoxide, neurotransmitters, hormones, and metabolites (particularly glucose), enabling study of their uptake and distribution in tissue.

Patient preparation

When preparing a patient for a PET scan, explain the following key points:
• If the test is ordered to assess myocardial contractility, explain to the patient that the test distinguishes viable tissue from tissue injured by infarction and may also help the doctor assess mitochondrial impairment associated with ischemia or evaluate coronary artery obstruction.
• Explain that he'll be given a radioactive substance, either by injection, inhalation, or I.V., and that a highly specialized camera will detect the radioactive decay of this substance and send this data to a computer, which converts it to a visual image.
• Describe the test, including who will administer it, where it will take place, and its duration (typically 60 to 90 minutes). Take time to describe the equipment.
• Tell him that the test is painless, unless an I.V. infusion is planned, in which case he may experience some discomfort from the needle puncture and the tourniquet. If the radioisotope will be inhaled, explain this painless procedure.
• If a fast is ordered, describe food and fluid restrictions.
• Tell him that he'll undergo an attenuation scan for about 30 minutes. Then he'll receive the appropriate positron emitter and undergo PET scanning.
  Because the radioisotope may be harmful to a fetus, female patients of childbearing age should be screened carefully before undergoing this procedure.

containing metal that could be attracted to the strong MRI magnet. If he does, he may not be able to undergo the test.
• Administer the prescribed sedative.

Procedure and posttest care

• At the scanner room door, check the patient one last time for metal objects.
• The patient is placed supine on a narrow, padded, nonmetallic bed that slides to the desired position inside the

scanner. RF waves are directed at his chest. The resulting images are displayed on a monitor and recorded on film or magnetic tape for permanent storage.

• The radiologist may vary RF waves and use the computer to manipulate and enhance the images.

• Remind the patient to remain still throughout the procedure.

• Assess how he responds to the enclosed environment. Provide reassurance if necessary.

• Monitor the sedated patient's hemodynamic, cardiac, respiratory, and mental status until the effects of the sedative have worn off.

Precautions

• Claustrophobic patients may experience anxiety. Monitor cardiac patients for signs of ischemia (chest pressure, shortness of breath, or changes in hemodynamic status).

• MRI can't be performed on patients with pacemakers or intracranial aneurysm clips.

• If the patient is unstable, make sure an I.V. line with no metal components is in place and that all equipment is compatible with MRI imaging. If necessary, monitor the patient's oxygen saturation, cardiac rhythm, and respiratory status during the test.

• An anesthesiologist may be needed to monitor a heavily sedated patient.

• A nurse or radiology technician should maintain verbal contact with the conscious patient.

Normal findings

MRI should reveal no anatomic or structural dysfunctions in cardiovascular tissue.

Abnormal findings

MRI can detect cardiomyopathy and pericardial disease. It can also detect atrial or ventricular septal defects or other congenital defects. MRI is useful for identifying paracardiac or intracardiac masses. In addition, it can evaluate the extent of pericardial or vascular disease.

Interfering factors

• Patient's inability to remain still during the procedure

• Obese patient (possible poor imaging)

RENAL COMPUTED TOMOGRAPHY

Renal computed tomography (CT) provides a useful image of the kidneys made from a series of tomograms or cross-sectional slices, which are then translated by a computer and displayed on a monitor. The image density reflects the amount of radiation absorbed by renal tissue and permits identification of masses and other lesions. An I.V. contrast medium may be injected to accentuate the renal parenchyma's density and help differentiate renal masses. This highly accurate test is usually performed to investigate diseases found by other diagnostic procedures, such as excretory urography.

Purpose

• To detect and evaluate renal abnormalities, such as tumor, obstruction, calculi, polycystic kidney disease, congenital anomalies, and abnormal fluid accumulation around the kidneys

• To evaluate the retroperitoneum

• To guide needle placement before percutaneous biopsy

• To determine the kidney's size and location in relation to the bladder following a kidney transplant
• To localize renal or perinephric abscesses for drainage

Patient preparation
• Explain to the patient that this test permits examination of the kidneys.
• If contrast enhancement isn't scheduled, inform the patient that he needn't restrict food or fluids. If contrast enhancement is scheduled, instruct him to fast for 4 hours before the test.
• Tell him who will perform the test and where and that the procedure takes about an hour, depending on the purpose of the scan.
• Inform the patient that he'll be positioned on an X-ray table, and that a scanner will take films of his kidneys.
• Warn him that the scanner may make loud, clacking sounds as it rotates around his body.
• Tell him that he may experience transient adverse effects, such as flushing, metallic taste, and headache, after injection of the contrast medium.
• Check the patient's history for hypersensitivity to shellfish, iodine, or contrast media. Mark any sensitivities clearly on the patient's chart.
• Just before the procedure, instruct the patient to put on a gown and to remove any metallic objects that could interfere with the scan.
• Administer prescribed sedatives.

Procedure and posttest care
• The patient is placed in a supine position on the X-ray table and secured with straps.
• The table is moved into the scanner.
• Instruct the patient to lie still.
• The scanner then rotates around the patient, taking multiple images at different angles within each cross-sectional slice.

• When one series of tomograms is complete, contrast enhancement may be performed. Another series of tomograms is then taken.
• After the I.V. contrast medium is administered, monitor for allergic reactions, such as respiratory difficulty, urticaria, or other skin eruption.
• Information from the scan is stored on a disk or on magnetic tape, fed into a computer, and converted into an image for display on a monitor. Radiographs and photographs are taken of selected views.
• After the test, tell the patient who received a contrast medium that he may resume his usual diet.

Precautions
• Watch for signs of hypersensitivity to the contrast medium if contrast enhancement is required.

Normal findings
Normally, the density of the renal parenchyma is slightly higher than that of the liver, but is much less dense than bone, which appears white on a CT scan. The density of the collecting system is generally low (black), unless a contrast medium is used to enhance it to a higher (whiter) density. The position of the kidneys is evaluated according to the surrounding structures; the size and shape of the kidneys are determined by counting cuts between the superior and inferior poles and following the contour of the renal outline.

Abnormal findings
Renal masses appear as areas of different density than normal parenchyma, possibly altering the kidneys' shape or projecting beyond their margins. Renal cysts, for example, appear as smooth, sharply defined masses, with thin walls and a lower density than normal parenchyma. Tumors such as renal cell carci-

noma, however, are usually not as well delineated; they tend to have thick walls and nonuniform density. With contrast enhancement, solid tumors show a higher density than renal cysts but lower density than normal parenchyma. Tumors with hemorrhage, calcification, or necrosis show higher densities. Vascular tumors are more clearly defined with contrast enhancement. Adrenal tumors are confined masses, usually detached from the kidneys and from other retroperitoneal organs.

Renal CT scanning may also identify other abnormalities, including obstructions, calculi, polycystic kidney disease, congenital anomalies, and abnormal accumulations of fluid around the kidneys, such as hematomas, lymphoceles, and abscesses. After nephrectomy, CT scanning can detect abnormal masses, such as recurrent tumors, in a renal fossa that should be empty.

Interfering factors
• Patient's inability to remain still during the procedure
• Presence of contrast media from other recent tests or of foreign bodies such as catheters or surgical clips (possible poor imaging)

CHAPTER 14

Nuclear Medicine Scans

THYROID	640

640 Radioactive iodine uptake test   641 Radionuclide thyroid imaging

RESPIRATORY SYSTEM	643

643 Lung perfusion scan   645 Lung ventilation scan

CARDIOVASCULAR SYSTEM	646

646 Technetium pyrophosphate scanning
647 Thallium imaging

649 Persantine-thallium imaging
650 Cardiac blood pool imaging

MISCELLANEOUS TESTS	651

651 Bone scan
653 Liver-spleen scanning
656 Gallium scanning

658 Red blood cell survival time
660 Radionuclide renal imaging
662 HIDA scan

THYROID

RADIOACTIVE IODINE UPTAKE TEST

The radioactive iodine uptake (RAIU) test evaluates thyroid function by measuring the amount of orally ingested iodine 123 (^{123}I) or iodine 131 (^{131}I) that accumulates in the thyroid gland after 6 and 24 hours. An external single counting probe measures the radioactivity in the thyroid as a percentage of the original dose, thus indicating its ability to trap and retain iodine. The RAIU test accurately diagnoses hyperthyroidism but is less accurate for hypothyroidism. Indications for this test include abnormal results of chemical tests used to evaluate thyroid function.

Purpose
• To evaluate thyroid function
• To help diagnose hyperthyroidism or hypothyroidism
• To help distinguish between primary and secondary thyroid disorders
• To help differentiate Graves' disease from hyperfunctioning toxic adenoma (performed concurrently with radionuclide thyroid imaging and the T_3 resin uptake test)

Patient preparation
• Tell the patient that RAIU testing assesses thyroid function.
• Instruct him to fast beginning at midnight the night before the test.
• Explain that he'll receive radioactive iodine (capsule or liquid) and then be scanned after 6 hours and again after 24 hours.

• Assure him that the test is painless and that the small amount of radioactivity used is harmless.
• Tell him that test results will be available within 24 hours.
• Check the patient's history for iodine exposure, which may interfere with test results. Note any prior radiologic tests using contrast media, nuclear medicine procedures, or current use of iodine preparations or thyroid medications on the film request slip. Iodine hypersensitivity is not considered a contraindication because the amount of iodine used is similar to the amount consumed in a normal diet.

Equipment
Oral dose of ^{123}I or ^{131}I, external single counting probe

Procedure and posttest care
• After ingesting an oral dose of radioactive iodine, the patient's thyroid is scanned at 6 hours and 24 hours by placing the anterior portion of his neck in front of an external single counting probe.
• The amount of radioactivity detected by the probe is compared to the amount of radioactivity contained in the original dose to determine the percent of radioactive iodine retained by the thyroid.
• Instruct the patient to resume a light diet 2 hours after taking the oral dose of radioactive iodine. When the study is complete, the patient may resume a normal diet.

Precautions
• Radioactive iodine uptake testing is contraindicated during pregnancy and lactation because of possible teratogenic effects.

Reference values
At 6 hours, 5% to 20% of the radioactive iodine should accumulate in the

thyroid; at 24 hours, accumulation should be 15% to 40%. The balance of the radioactive iodine is excreted in the urine. Local variations in the normal range of iodine uptake may occur due to regional differences in dietary iodine intake and procedural differences among laboratories.

Abnormal findings
Below-normal iodine uptake may indicate hypothyroidism, subacute thyroiditis, or iodine overload. Above-normal uptake may indicate hyperthyroidism, early Hashimoto's thyroiditis, hypoalbuminemia, lithium ingestion, or iodine-deficient goiter. However, in hyperthyroidism, the rate of turnover may be so rapid that a false normal measurement occurs at 24 hours.

Interfering factors
• Renal failure; diuresis; severe diarrhea; X-ray contrast media studies; ingestion of iodine preparations including iodized salt, cough syrups, and some multivitamins (decrease)
• Thyroid hormones, thyroid hormone antagonists, salicylates, penicillins, antihistamines, anticoagulants, corticosteroids, and phenylbutazone (decrease)
• Phenothiazines or iodine-deficient diet (increase)

RADIONUCLIDE THYROID IMAGING

In radionuclide thyroid imaging, the thyroid is studied by gamma camera after the patient receives a radioisotope (^{123}I, ^{99m}Tc pertechnetate, or ^{131}I). Thyroid imaging typically follows discovery of a palpable mass, an enlarged gland, or an asymmetrical goiter and is performed concurrently with thyroid

uptake tests and measurement of serum triiodothyronine (T_3), thyroid-stimulating hormone (TSH), and serum thyroxine (T_4) levels. Later, thyroid ultrasonography may be performed.

Purpose
• To assess the size, structure, and position of the thyroid gland
• To evaluate thyroid function (in conjunction with specific thyroid uptake studies)

Patient preparation
• Tell the patient that this test helps determine the cause of thyroid dysfunction.
• If ^{123}I or ^{131}I will be used, tell him to fast after midnight the night before the test. Fasting isn't required if an I.V. injection of ^{99m}Tc pertechnetate is used.
• Explain that after he receives the radiopharmaceutical, a gamma camera will be used to produce an image of his thyroid. Tell him that the imaging procedure will take about 30 minutes and assure him that his exposure to radiation is minimal.
• Ask the patient if he has undergone tests that used radiographic contrast media within the past 60 days. Note previous radiographic contrast media exposure on the X-ray request slip.
• Check the patient's diet and medication history. Medications such as thyroid hormones, thyroid hormone antagonists, and iodine preparations (Lugol's solution, some multivitamins, and cough syrups) should be discontinued 2 to 3 weeks before the test. Phenothiazines, corticosteroids, salicylates, anticoagulants, and antihistamines should be discontinued one week before the test. Instruct the patient to stop consuming iodized salt, iodinated salt substitutes, and seafood during this period.
• The patient receives ^{123}I or ^{131}I (oral) or ^{99m}Tc pertechnetate (I.V.). Record the date and the time of administration.

RESULTS OF THYROID IMAGING IN THYROID DISORDERS

CONDITION	FINDINGS	CAUSES
Hypothyroidism	• Glandular damage or absent gland	• Surgical removal of gland • Inflammation • Radiation • Neoplasm (rare)
Hypothyroid goiter	• Enlarged gland • Decreased uptake if glandular destruction is present • Increased uptake possible from congenital error in thyroxine synthesis	• Insufficient iodine intake • Hypersecretion of thyroid-stimulating hormone (TSH) caused by thyroid hormone deficiency
Myxedema (cretinism in children)	• Normal or slightly reduced gland size • Uniform pattern • Decreased uptake	• Defective embryonic development, resulting in congenital absence or underdevelopment of thyroid gland • Maternal iodine deficiency
Hyperthyroidism (Graves' disease)	• Enlarged gland • Uniform pattern • Increased uptake	• Unknown, but may be hereditary • Production of thyroid-stimulating immunoglobulins
Toxic nodular goiter	• Multiple hot spots	• Long-standing simple goiter
Hyperfunctioning adenomas	• Solitary hot spot	• Adenomatous production of T_3 and T_4, suppressing TSH secretion and producing atrophy of other thyroid tissue
Hypofunctioning adenomas	• Solitary cold spot	• Cyst or nonfunctioning nodule
Benign multinodular goiter	• Multiple nodules with variable or no function	• Local inflammation • Degeneration
Thyroid carcinoma	• Usually a solitary cold spot with occasional or no function	• Neoplasm

- Imaging follows oral administration (^{123}I or ^{131}I) by 24 hours, and I.V. injection (^{99m}Tc pertechnetate) by 20 to 30 minutes.
- Just before the test, tell the patient to remove dentures, jewelry, and other materials that may interfere with the imaging process.

Procedure and posttest care
- The patient is placed in a supine position with his neck extended; the thyroid gland is palpated. The gamma camera is positioned above the anterior portion of his neck.
- Images of the patient's thyroid gland are projected on a monitor and are recorded on X-ray film. Three views of the thyroid are obtained: a straight-on anterior view and two bilateral oblique views.
- Following the procedure, tell the patient he may resume medications suspended for the test. Instruct him to resume his normal diet.

Precautions
- Radionuclide thyroid imaging is contraindicated during pregnancy and lactation.

Normal findings
Normally, radionuclide thyroid imaging reveals a thyroid gland that is about 2″ (5 cm) long and 1″ (2.5 cm) wide, with a uniform uptake of the radioisotope and without tumors. The gland is butterfly-shaped, with the isthmus located at the midline. Occasionally, a third lobe called the pyramidal lobe may be present; this is a normal variant.

Abnormal findings
During radionuclide thyroid imaging, hyperfunctioning nodules (areas of excessive iodine uptake) appear as black regions called "hot spots." The presence of hot spots requires a follow-up T_3 (Cytomel) thyroid suppression test to determine if the hyperfunctioning areas are autonomous. Hypofunctioning nodules (areas of little or no iodine uptake) appear as white or light gray regions called "cold spots." If a cold spot appears, subsequent thyroid ultrasonography may be performed to rule out cysts; in addition, fine needle aspiration and biopsy of such nodules may be performed to rule out malignancy. (See *Results of thyroid imaging in thyroid disorders.*)

Interfering factors
- Iodine-deficient diet, phenothiazines (increase)
- Decrease uptake of radioactive iodine due to renal disease; ingestion of iodized salt, iodine preparations, iodinated salt substitutes, or seafood; and use of thyroid hormones, thyroid hormone antagonists, aminosalicylic acid, corticosteroids, multivitamins or cough syrups containing inorganic iodine (decrease)
- Severe diarrhea and vomiting, impairing GI absorption of radioiodine (decrease)

RESPIRATORY SYSTEM

LUNG PERFUSION SCAN

A lung perfusion scan produces an image of pulmonary blood flow after I.V. injection of a radiopharmaceutical, either human serum albumin microspheres or macroaggregated albumin bonded to technetium.

Purpose
• To assess arterial perfusion of the lungs
• To detect pulmonary emboli
• To aid preoperative evaluation of the pulmonary function of a patient with marginal lung reserves
• To help determine ventilation-perfusion ratios (when performed in conjunction with a lung ventilation scan)

Patient preparation
• Tell the patient that this test helps evaluate respiratory function.
• Explain that there are no food or fluid restrictions before the test.
• Describe the test, including who will perform it, where it will take place, and its expected duration (15 to 30 minutes).
• Tell the patient that a radiopharmaceutical will be injected into a vein in his arm and then he'll sit in front of a camera or lie under it. Explain that neither the camera nor the uptake probe emits radiation and that the amount of radioactivity in the radiopharmaceutical is minimal.
• Assure the patient that he'll be comfortable during the test and that he doesn't have to remain perfectly still.
• On the test request slip, note if he has conditions such as chronic obstructive pulmonary disease (COPD), vasculitis, pulmonary edema, tumor, sickle cell disease, or parasitic disease.

Procedure and posttest care
• Half of the radiopharmaceutical is injected I.V. while the patient is in a supine position; the remaining half is injected while the patient is in a prone position.

• After the injection, the gamma camera takes a series of single stationary images in the anterior, posterior, oblique, and both lateral chest views.
• Images, which are projected on an oscilloscope screen, show the distribution of radioactive particles.
• If a hematoma develops at the injection site after the test, apply warm soaks.

Precautions
• A lung scan is contraindicated in patients hypersensitive to the radiopharmaceutical.

Normal findings
Hot spots — areas with normal blood perfusion — show a high uptake of the radioactive substance; a normal lung shows a uniform uptake pattern.

Abnormal findings
Cold spots — areas of low radioactive uptake — indicate poor perfusion, suggesting an embolism; however, a ventilation scan is necessary to confirm diagnosis. Decreased regional blood flow that occurs without vessel obstruction may indicate pneumonitis.

Interfering factors
• Scheduling more than one radionuclide test a day, especially if using different tracing substances (may hinder diffusion of tracer isotope in second test)
• Administering all the radiopharmaceutical while the patient is in sitting position (possible poor imaging due to settling of tracer isotope in lung bases)
• Conditions such as COPD, vasculitis, pulmonary edema, tumor, sickle cell disease, and parasitic disease (possible poor imaging)

LUNG VENTILATION SCAN

The lung ventilation scan is performed after the patient inhales a mixture of air and radioactive gas that delineates areas of the lung ventilated during respiration. The scan records the distribution of the gas during three phases: the buildup of radioactive gas (wash-in phase), the time after rebreathing when radioactivity reaches a steady level (equilibrium phase), and after removal of the radioactive gas from the lungs (wash-out phase).

Purpose

• To help diagnose pulmonary emboli, identify areas of the lung capable of ventilation, help evaluate regional respiratory function, and locate regional hypoventilation (usually caused by smoking or chronic obstructive pulmonary disease)

• To distinguish between parenchymal disease, such as emphysema, sarcoidosis, bronchogenic carcinoma, and tuberculosis, and conditions due to vascular abnormalities such as pulmonary emboli (performed with a lung perfusion scan)

Patient preparation

• Describe the procedure to the patient and explain that this test helps evaluate respiratory function.

• Tell him that he needn't restrict food or fluids.

• Tell him who will perform the test, where it will take place, and that it takes 15 to 30 minutes.

• Ask the patient to remove all jewelry and metal objects from the scanning field.

• Explain that he'll be asked to hold his breath for a short time after inhaling a gas and to remain still while a machine scans his chest.

• Reassure him that a minimal amount of radioactive gas is used.

Procedure and posttest care

• After the patient inhales air mixed with a small amount of radioactive gas through a mask, its distribution in the lungs is monitored on a nuclear scanner.

• The patient's chest is scanned as he exhales.

Precautions

• Watch for leaks in the closed system of radioactive gas, such as through the mask, which can contaminate the surrounding atmosphere.

• In a patient on mechanical ventilation, krypton gas must be used instead of xenon gas.

Normal findings

Normal findings include an equal distribution of gas in both lungs and normal wash-in and wash-out phases.

Abnormal findings

Unequal gas distribution in both lungs indicates poor ventilation or airway obstruction in areas with low radioactivity. When compared with a lung scan (perfusion scan), in vascular obstructions such as pulmonary embolism, the perfusion to the embolized area is decreased, but the ventilation to this area is maintained; in parenchymal disease such as pneumonia, ventilation is abnormal within the areas of consolidation.

Interfering factor

• Failure to remove jewelry and other metal objects from the scanning field (possible poor imaging)

CARDIOVASCULAR SYSTEM

TECHNETIUM PYROPHOSPHATE SCANNING

Technetium pyrophosphate scanning (also called hot spot myocardial imaging or infarct avid imaging) is used to detect a recent myocardial infarction (MI) and to determine its extent. This test uses an I.V. tracer isotope (technetium-99m [^{99m}Tc] pyrophosphate). This isotope accumulates in damaged myocardial tissue (possibly by combining with calcium in the damaged myocardial cells), where it forms a hot spot on a scan made with a scintillation camera. Such hot spots first appear within 12 hours of infarction, are most apparent after 48 to 72 hours, and usually disappear after 1 week. Hot spots that persist longer than 1 week usually suggest ongoing myocardial damage.

Purpose

• To confirm recent MI in patients suffering from obscure cardiac pain or when electrocardiography or serum enzyme studies don't provide sufficient information
• To help define the size and location of an MI
• To aid in determining the prognosis after acute MI

Patient preparation

• Explain to the patient that this test helps assess if the heart muscle is injured.
• Inform the patient that he needn't restrict food or fluids. Tell him who will perform the 30- to 60-minute test and where.
• Inform him that he'll receive a tracer isotope I.V. 2 or 3 hours before the procedure and that multiple images of his heart will be made.
• Reassure him that the injection causes only transient discomfort, that the scan itself is painless, and that the test involves less exposure to radiation than a chest X-ray.
• Instruct him to remain quiet and motionless while he's being scanned.
• Make sure the patient or a responsible family member has signed a consent form.

Procedure and posttest care

• Usually, 20 millicuries of ^{99m}Tc pyrophosphate are injected into the antecubital vein.
• After 2 or 3 hours, the patient is placed in a supine position and electrocardiography electrodes are attached for continuous monitoring during the test.
• Generally, scans are taken with the patient in several positions, including anterior, left anterior oblique, right anterior oblique, and left lateral. Each scan takes 10 minutes.

Normal findings

A normal technetium scan shows no isotope in the myocardium.

Abnormal findings

The isotope is taken up by the sternum and ribs, and their activity is compared with the heart's; 2+, 3+, and 4+ activity (equal to or greater than bone) indicates a positive myocardial scan. The technetium scan can reveal areas of isotope accumulation, or hot spots, in damaged myocardium, particularly 48 to 72 hours after onset of acute MI; however, hot spots are apparent as early as 12 hours after acute MI. In most patients with MI, hot spots disappear after 1 week; in some, they persist for several months if necrosis continues in the area of infarction.

Knowing where the infarct is makes it possible to anticipate complications and to plan patient care. About one-fourth of patients with unstable angina pectoris show hot spots due to subclinical myocardial necrosis, and may require coronary arteriography and bypass grafting.

Interfering factors
• Isotope accumulation (in about 10% of patients, may result from ventricular aneurysm associated with dystrophic calcification, pulmonary neoplasm, recent cardioversion, or valvular heart disease due to severe calcification)

THALLIUM IMAGING

Also called cold spot myocardial imaging or thallium scintigraphy, thallium imaging evaluates myocardial blood flow after I.V. injection of the radioisotope thallium-201. Because thallium, the physiologic analogue of potassium, concentrates in healthy myocardial tissue but not in necrotic or ischemic tissue, areas of the heart with a normal blood supply and intact cells rapidly take it up. Areas with poor blood flow and ischemic cells fail to take up the isotope and appear as cold spots on a scan.

This test is performed in a resting state or after stress. Possible complications of stress testing include arrhythmias, angina pectoris, and myocardial infarction (MI).

Purpose
Resting imaging
• To assess myocardial scarring and perfusion
• To demonstrate the location and extent of acute or chronic MI, including transmural and postoperative infarction
Stress imaging
• To diagnose coronary artery disease (CAD)
• To evaluate the patency of grafts after coronary artery bypass surgery
• To evaluate the effectiveness of antianginal therapy or balloon angioplasty

Patient preparation
• Explain to the patient that these tests help determine if any areas of the heart muscle aren't receiving an adequate supply of blood.
• If the patient will be undergoing stress imaging, instruct him to restrict alcohol, tobacco, and nonprescribed medications for 24 hours before the test and to have nothing by mouth for 3 hours before the test.
• Describe the test, including who will perform it, where it will take place, and its expected duration (45 to 90 minutes). Explain that additional scans may be required.
• Tell him that he'll receive a radioactive tracer I.V. and that multiple images of his heart will be scanned.
• Explain to the patient that it's very important to lie still when images are taken.
• Warn him that he may experience discomfort from skin abrasion during preparation for electrode placement.

Assure him that the test involves minimal radiation exposure.

- Make sure the patient or a responsible family member has signed a consent form.
- Tell the patient undergoing stress imaging to wear walking shoes during the treadmill exercise and to report fatigue, pain, or shortness of breath immediately.

Procedure and posttest care
Resting imaging
- Optimally, within the first few hours of symptoms of MI, the patient receives an injection of thallium I.V. and scanning begins after 3 to 5 minutes.
- If further scanning is required, have the patient rest and restrict food and fluids.

Stress imaging
- The patient, wired with electrodes, walks on a treadmill at a regulated pace that's gradually increased, while the electrocardiogram (ECG), blood pressure, and heart rate are monitored.
- When the patient reaches peak stress, the examiner injects 1.5 to 3 millicuries of thallium into the antecubital vein and then flushes it with 10 to 15 ml of normal saline solution.
- The patient exercises an additional 45 to 60 seconds to permit circulation and uptake of the isotope, and then lies on his back under the scintillation camera.
- If the patient is asymptomatic, the precordial leads are removed. Scanning begins after 3 to 5 minutes with the patient in anterior, 45-degree and 60-degree left anterior oblique, and left lateral positions.
- Additional scans may be taken after the patient rests 3 to 6 hours.

Precautions
- Contraindications include impaired neuromuscular function, pregnancy, locomotor disturbances, acute MI or myocarditis, aortic stenosis, acute infection, unstable metabolic conditions (such as diabetes), digitalis toxicity, and recent pulmonary infarction.
- Stop stress imaging at once if the patient develops chest pain, dyspnea, fatigue, syncope, hypotension, ischemic ECG changes, significant arrhythmias, or critical signs (pale, clammy skin, confusion, or staggering).

Normal findings
Imaging should show normal distribution of the isotope throughout the left ventricle and no defects (cold spots).

Abnormal findings
Persistent defects indicate MI; transient defects (those that disappear after 3 to 6 hours of rest) indicate ischemia from CAD. After coronary artery bypass surgery, improved regional perfusion suggests patency of the graft. Increased perfusion after ingestion of antianginal drugs can show that they relieve ischemia. Improved perfusion after balloon angioplasty suggests increased coronary flow.

Interfering factors
- Cold spots (possible result of sarcoidosis, myocardial fibrosis, cardiac contusion, attenuation due to soft tissue, apical cleft, coronary spasm and artifacts such as implants and electrodes)
- Absence of cold spots in the presence of CAD (possibly due to insignificant obstruction, inadequate stress, delayed imaging, collateral circulation, or single-vessel disease, particularly of the right or left circumflex coronary arteries)

PERSANTINE-THALLIUM IMAGING

Persantine-thallium imaging is an alternative method of assessing coronary vessel function for patients who can't tolerate exercise or stress electrocardiography (ECG). Persantine (dipyridamole) infusion simulates the effects of exercise by increasing blood flow to the collateral circulation and away from the coronary arteries, thereby inducing ischemia. Then thallium infusion allows the examiner to evaluate the cardiac vessels' response. The heart is scanned immediately after the thallium infusion and again 2 to 4 hours later. Diseased vessels can't deliver thallium to the heart, and thallium lingers in diseased areas of the myocardium.

Purpose
• To identify exercise- or stress-induced arrhythmias
• To assess the presence and degree of cardiac ischemia

Patient preparation
• Tell the patient that a painless, 5- to 10-minute baseline ECG will precede the test.
• Explain that he'll need to restrict food and fluids before the test. Tell him to avoid caffeine and other stimulants (which may cause arrhythmias).
• Instruct him to continue to take all his regular medications, with the possible exception of beta blockers, as prescribed.
• Explain that an I.V. line infuses the medications for the study. Tell him who will start the I.V. and when, and that the needle insertion and the tourniquet may cause some discomfort.
• Inform him that he may experience mild nausea, headache, dizziness, or flushing after Persantine administration. Reassure him that these adverse reactions are usually temporary and rarely need treatment.
• Make sure that the patient or a responsible family member has signed a consent form.

Procedure and posttest care
• The patient reclines or sits while a resting ECG is performed. Then Persantine is given either orally or I.V. over 4 minutes. Blood pressure, pulse rate, and cardiac rhythm are monitored continuously.
• After administration of Persantine, the patient is asked to get up and walk. After Persantine takes effect, thallium is injected.
• The patient is placed in a supine position for about 40 minutes while the scan is performed. Then the scan is reviewed. If necessary, a second scan is performed.
• If the patient must return for further scanning, tell him to rest and to restrict food and fluids in the interim.

Precautions
• The patient may experience arrhythmias, angina, ST-segment depression, or bronchospasm. Make sure resuscitation equipment is readily available.
• More common adverse reactions are nausea, headache, flushing, dizziness, and epigastric pain.

Normal findings
Imaging should reveal characteristic distribution of the isotope throughout the left ventricle and no visible defects.

Abnormal findings
The presence of ST-segment depression, angina, and arrhythmias strongly suggests coronary artery disease (CAD). Persistent ST-segment depression generally indicates myocardial infarction. In contrast, transient ST-

segment depression indicates ischemia from CAD.

Cold spots usually indicate CAD but may result from sarcoidosis, myocardial fibrosis, cardiac contusion, attenuation due to soft tissue (for example, breast and diaphragm), apical cleft, and coronary spasm. The absence of cold spots in the presence of CAD may result from insignificant obstruction, single-vessel disease, or collateral circulation.

Interfering factors
- Failure to observe pretest restrictions
- Artifacts such as implants and electrodes (possible false-positive)
- Absence of cold spots with CAD (possible delay in imaging)

CARDIAC BLOOD POOL IMAGING

Cardiac blood pool imaging evaluates regional and global ventricular performance after I.V. injection of human serum albumin or red blood cells (RBCs) tagged with the isotope technetium-99m (^{99m}Tc) pertechnetate. In first-pass imaging, a scintillation camera records the radioactivity emitted by the isotope in its initial pass through the left ventricle. Higher counts of radioactivity occur during diastole because there is more blood in the ventricle; lower counts occur during systole as the blood is ejected. The portion of isotope ejected during each heartbeat can then be calculated to determine the ejection fraction; the presence and size of intracardiac shunts can also be determined.

Gated cardiac blood pool imaging, performed after first-pass imaging or as a separate test, has several forms;

however, most forms use signals from an electrocardiogram (ECG) to trigger the scintillation camera. In two-frame gated imaging, the camera records left ventricular end-systole and end-diastole for 500 to 1,000 cardiac cycles; superimposition of these gated images allows assessment of left ventricular contraction to find areas of hypokinesia or akinesia.

In multiple-gated acquisition (MUGA) scanning, the camera records 14 to 64 points of a single cardiac cycle, yielding sequential images that can be studied like motion picture films to evaluate regional wall motion and determine the ejection fraction and other indices of cardiac function. In the stress MUGA test, the same test is performed at rest and after exercise to detect changes in ejection fraction and cardiac output. In the nitro MUGA test, the scintillation camera records points in the cardiac cycle after the sublingual administration of nitroglycerin to assess its effect on ventricular function.

Blood pool imaging is more accurate and involves less risk to the patient than left ventriculography in assessing cardiac function.

Purpose
- To evaluate left ventricular function
- To detect aneurysms of the left ventricle and other motion abnormalities of the myocardial wall (areas of akinesia or hypokinesia)
- To detect intracardiac shunting
- To calculate ejection fraction, especially before certain chemotherapies

Patient preparation
- Explain to the patient that this test permits assessment of the heart's left ventricle.
- Describe the test, including who will perform it, where it will take place, and its expected duration.

• Tell him that he needn't restrict food or fluids before the test.

• Explain that he'll receive an I.V. injection of a radioactive tracer and that a detector positioned above his chest will record the circulation of this tracer through the heart.

• Reassure him that the tracer poses no radiation hazard and rarely produces adverse effects.

• Inform him that he may experience transient discomfort from the needle puncture, but that the imaging itself is painless.

• Instruct him to remain silent and motionless during imaging, unless otherwise instructed.

• Make sure the patient or a responsible family member has signed a consent form.

Procedure and posttest care

• The patient is placed in a supine position beneath the detector of a scintillation camera, and 15 to 20 millicuries of albumin or RBCs tagged with ^{99m}Tc pertechnetate are injected.

• For the next minute, the scintillation camera records the first pass of the isotope through the heart so that the aortic and mitral valves can be located.

• Then, using an ECG, the camera is gated for selected 60-millisecond intervals, representing end-systole and end-diastole, and 500 to 1,000 cardiac cycles are recorded on X-ray or Polaroid film.

• To observe septal and posterior wall motion, the patient may be assisted to modified left anterior oblique position; or he may be assisted to right anterior oblique position and given 0.4 mg of nitroglycerin sublingually. The scintillation camera then records additional gated images to evaluate abnormal contraction in the left ventricle.

• The patient may be asked to exercise as the scintillation camera records gated images.

Precautions

• Cardiac blood pool imaging is contraindicated during pregnancy.

Normal findings

Normally, the left ventricle contracts symmetrically, and the isotope appears evenly distributed in the scans. Normal ejection fraction is 55% to 65%.

Abnormal findings

Patients with coronary artery disease usually have asymmetrical blood distribution to the myocardium, which produces segmental abnormalities of ventricular wall motion; such abnormalities may also result from preexisting conditions, such as myocarditis. In contrast, patients with cardiomyopathies show globally reduced ejection fractions. In patients with left-to-right shunts, the recirculating radioisotope prolongs the downslope of the curve of scintigraphic data; early arrival of activity in the left ventricle or aorta signifies a right-to-left shunt.

Interfering factors

• None significant

MISCELLANEOUS TESTS

BONE SCAN

A bone scan involves imaging the skeleton by a scanning camera after I.V. injection of a radioactive tracer compound. The tracer of choice, radioactive technetium diphosphonate, collects in bone tissue in increased concentrations at sites of abnormal metabolism. When scanned, these sites appear as "hot spots" that are often detectable months before an X-ray can reveal any lesion. To promote early detection of lesions, this test may be performed with a gallium scan.

Purpose
• To detect or to rule out malignant bone lesions when radiographic findings are normal but cancer is confirmed or suspected
• To detect occult bone trauma due to pathologic fractures
• To monitor degenerative bone disorders
• To detect infection
• To evaluate unexplained bone pain

Patient preparation
• Describe the procedure to the patient. Explain that this test may detect skeletal abnormalities sooner than is possible with ordinary X-rays.
• Because the patient is required to drink 4 to 6 glasses of water or tea in the interval between injection of the tracer and the actual scanning, advise him not to drink large amounts of fluids before the test.
• Tell him who will perform the test and where and that he may have to assume various positions on a scanner table. Emphasize that he must keep still for the scan.
• Assure the patient that the scan itself, which takes about 1 hour, is painless and that the isotope, although radioactive, emits less radiation than a standard X-ray machine.
• Make sure the patient or a family member has signed a consent form.

• If a bone scan is ordered to diagnose cancer, evaluate the patient's emotional state and offer support.
• Administer prescribed analgesics.
• After the patient receives an I.V. injection of the tracer and imaging agent, encourage him to increase his intake of fluids for the next 1 to 3 hours to facilitate renal clearance of the circulating free tracer.

Equipment
Bone mineral tracer, 3-ml syringe, 21G needle, 70% alcohol or povidone-iodine solution, sterile sponge, tourniquet, scanning camera

Procedure and posttest care
• Instruct the patient to void immediately before the procedure; then position him on the scanner table.
• As the scanner head moves back and forth over the patient's body, it detects low-level radiation emitted by the skeleton and translates this into a film or paper chart, or both, to produce two-dimensional pictures of the area scanned.
• The scanner takes as many views as needed to cover the specified area. The patient may have to be repositioned several times during the test to obtain adequate views.
• Check the injection site for redness or swelling. If a hematoma develops, apply warm soaks.
• Don't schedule any other radionuclide tests for 24 to 48 hours.

Precautions
• To avoid exposing the fetus or infant to radiation, a bone scan is contraindicated during pregnancy or lactation.
• Allergic reactions to radionuclides may occur.

Normal findings

The tracer concentrates in bone tissue at sites of new bone formation or increased metabolism. The epiphyses of growing bone are normal sites of high concentration, or hot spots.

Abnormal findings

Although a bone scan demonstrates hot spots that identify sites of bone formation, it doesn't distinguish between normal and abnormal bone formation. But scan results can identify all types of bone malignancy, infection, fracture, and other disorders, if viewed in light of the patient's medical and surgical history, X-rays, and other laboratory tests.

Interfering factors

- Failure to observe pretest restrictions
- Distended bladder (possible obscuring of pelvic detail)
- Improper injection technique (possible seepage of tracer into muscle tissue, creating false hot spots)
- Antihypertensives (invalidate test results)

LIVER-SPLEEN SCANNING

In liver-spleen scanning, a gamma camera records the distribution of radioactivity within the liver and spleen after I.V. injection of a radioactive colloid. The colloid most commonly used, technetium sulfide-99m (^{99m}Tc), concentrates in the reticuloendothelial cells through phagocytosis. About 80% to 90% of the injected colloid is taken up by Kupffer's cells in the liver, 5% to 10% by the spleen, and 3% to 5% by

bone marrow. The gamma camera images either organ instantaneously without moving.

Although the indications for this test include the detection of focal disease, such as tumors, cysts, and abscesses, liver-spleen scanning demonstrates focal disease nonspecifically as a cold spot (a defect that fails to take up the colloid) and may fail to detect focal lesions smaller than ¾" (2 cm) in diameter. Although clinical signs and symptoms may aid diagnosis, liver-spleen scanning frequently requires confirmation by ultrasonography, computed tomography, gallium scanning, or biopsy.

Purpose

- To screen for hepatic metastases and hepatocellular disease, such as cirrhosis and hepatitis
- To detect focal disease, such as tumors, cysts, and abscesses, in the liver and spleen
- To demonstrate hepatomegaly or splenomegaly (in patients with palpable abdominal masses)
- To assess splenic infarcts
- To assess the condition of the liver and spleen after abdominal trauma

Patient preparation

- Explain to the patient that this procedure permits examination of the liver and spleen through scintigraphs or scans taken after I.V. injection of a radioactive substance.
- Inform him that he needn't restrict food or fluids before the test.
- Tell him who will perform the test, where it will take place, and that it takes about 1 hour.
- Explain that he may experience transient discomfort from the needle puncture.

IDENTIFYING LIVER INDENTATIONS IN NUCLEAR IMAGING

In nuclear imaging, normal indentations and impressions may be mistaken for focal lesions. These drawings of the liver — anterior view and posterior view — identify the contours and impressions that may be misread.

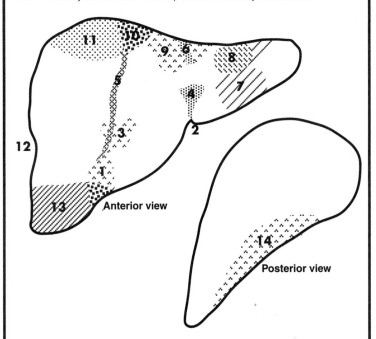

KEY:
1. Gallbladder fossa
2. Ligamentum teres and falciform ligament
3. Hilum, main branching of the portal vein
4. Pars umbilicalis portion, left portal vein
5. Variable stripe of lobar fissure between right and left lobes
6. Variable stripe of segmental fissure, left lobe
7. Thinning of left lobe
8. Impression of pectus excavatum
9. Cardiac impression
10. Hepatic veins and inferior vena cava
11. Shielding from right female breast
12. Harrison's groove or costal impression
13. Impression of hepatic flexure of colon
14. Right renal impression

- Make sure the patient isn't scheduled for more than one radionuclide scan on the same day.
- Assure him that the injection isn't dangerous because the test substance contains only trace amounts of radioactivity and allergic reactions to it are rare.
- Explain that the detector head of the gamma camera may touch his abdomen (if appropriate), and reassure him that this isn't dangerous.
- Advise him that he'll be asked to lie still and to breathe quietly during the procedure to ensure images of good quality; he may also be asked to hold his breath briefly. Explain that this technique helps to evaluate liver mobility and pliability.

Procedure and posttest care
- The ^{99m}Tc is injected I.V.; after 10 to 15 minutes, the patient's abdomen is scanned with the patient placed in supine, left and right lateral, left and right anterior oblique, and prone positions to ensure optimal visualization of the liver and spleen.
- The left anterior oblique position provides the best view of the spleen separate from the left lobe of the liver. With the patient supine, liver mobility and pliability may be evaluated by marking the costal margin and scanning as the patient breathes deeply (fixation suggests pathology).
- The scintigraphs are reviewed for clarity before the patient is allowed to leave. If necessary, additional views are obtained.
- Watch for anaphylactoid reactions (shortness of breath, chest tightness, itching, headache) or pyrogenic (fever-producing) reactions, which may result from a stabilizer, such as dextran or gelatin, added to ^{99m}Tc.

Precautions
- Liver-spleen scanning is usually contraindicated in children and during pregnancy and lactation.

Normal findings
Because the liver and spleen contain equal numbers of reticuloendothelial cells, both organs normally appear equally bright on the image. However, distribution of radioactive colloid is generally more uniform and homogeneous in the spleen than in the liver. The liver has various normal indentations and impressions, such as the gallbladder fossa and falciform ligament, that may mimic focal disease. (See *Identifying liver indentations in nuclear imaging.*)

Abnormal findings
Although liver-spleen scanning may fail to detect early hepatocellular disease, it shows characteristic, distinct patterns as such disease progresses. The most prominent sign of hepatocellular disease is a shift of the radioactive colloid that's caused by reduced hepatic blood flow and impaired function of Kupffer's cells. This inhibits distribution of the colloid in the liver, causing the liver to appear uniformly decreased or patchy. The spleen and bone marrow then take up the abnormally large amounts of the colloid unabsorbed by the liver, thus concentrating more radioactivity than the liver, and appear brighter on the scan. This same distribution pattern (colloid shift) also accompanies portal hypertension due to extrahepatic causes.

Hepatitis and cirrhosis are both associated with hepatomegaly and a colloid shift, but certain characteristics help distinguish them. In hepatitis, distribution of the colloid is usually uniformly decreased; in cirrhosis, it's patchy. Splenomegaly is typical in cirrhosis but not in hepatitis.

Metastasis to the liver or spleen may appear on the scan as a focal defect and requires biopsy to confirm the diagnosis. Liver metastasis usually originates in the GI or genitourinary tract, the breasts, or the lungs and is more common than metastasis to the spleen. After metastasis is confirmed, serial liver-spleen studies are useful in evaluating effectiveness of therapy.

Because cysts, abscesses, and tumors fail to take up the radioactive colloid, they appear on the scan as solitary or multiple focal defects. Hepatic cysts may appear as solitary defects; polycystic hepatic disease, as multiple defects. Splenic cysts are rarer than hepatic cysts and may have a parasitic or nonparasitic origin. Ultrasonography can confirm hepatic or splenic cysts.

Intrahepatic abscesses are usually pyogenic or amebic. Subphrenic abscesses, located beneath the diaphragm, may distort the dome of the right lobe. Splenic abscesses are characteristic in bacterial endocarditis. All abscesses require gallium scanning or ultrasonography to confirm diagnosis.

Benign hepatic tumors — such as hemangiomas, adenomas, and hamartomas — require confirming biopsy or flow studies. Primary malignant tumors, such as hepatomas, also require biopsy. Benign splenic tumors are rare and include hemangiomas, fibromas, myomas, and hamartomas. Primary malignant splenic tumors are also rare, except in lymphoreticular malignancies such as Hodgkin's disease. Splenic tumors also require biopsy to confirm diagnosis. Although focal disease usually inhibits uptake of radioactive colloid, both obstruction of the superior vena cava and Budd-Chiari syndrome cause markedly increased uptake.

A left upper quadrant mass may result from splenomegaly or, if the liver is grossly extended across the abdomen, from hepatomegaly. A right upper quadrant mass may result from hepatomegaly; a right lower quadrant mass may be a Riedel's lobe or a large dependent gallbladder. Splenic infarcts, often associated with bacterial endocarditis and massive splenomegaly, appear as peripheral defects, with decreased and irregular colloid distribution.

Scanning can assess hepatic injury after abdominal trauma. Intrahepatic hematoma appears as a focal defect; subcapsular hematoma, as a lentiform defect on the periphery of the liver; hepatic laceration, as a linear defect.

Scanning can also detect splenic injury after abdominal trauma. Splenic hematoma appears as a focal defect in or next to the spleen and may transect it. Subcapsular hematoma appears as a lentiform defect on the periphery of the spleen; splenic laceration appears as a linear defect.

Interfering factors
• Radionuclides administered in other studies on the same day (possible poor imaging)
• Patient's inability to remain still during the procedure

GALLIUM SCANNING

The gallium scan is a total-body scan used to assess certain neoplasms and inflammatory lesions that attract gallium. It's usually performed 24 to 48 hours after the I.V. injection of radioactive gallium (^{67}Ga) citrate; occasionally, it's performed 72 hours after the injection or, in acute inflammatory disease, after 4 to 6 hours.

Because gallium has an affinity for both benign and malignant neoplasms and inflammatory lesions, exact diagnosis requires additional confirming tests, such as ultrasonography and computerized tomography scanning. Also be aware that many neoplasms and a few inflammatory lesions may fail to demonstrate abnormal gallium activity.

Purpose

• To detect primary or metastatic neoplasms and inflammatory lesions when the site of the disease hasn't been clearly defined and when the patient's condition won't be jeopardized by the time required for the procedure
• To evaluate malignant lymphoma and identify recurrent tumors following chemotherapy or radiation therapy
• To clarify focal defects in the liver when liver-spleen scanning and ultrasonography prove inconclusive
• To evaluate bronchogenic carcinoma when sputum culture proves positive for malignancy but other tests are normal or when hydrothorax is present and bronchoscopy is contraindicated

Patient preparation

• Explain to the patient that this test helps detect abnormal or inflammatory tissue.
• Tell him he needn't restrict food or fluids before the test.
• Explain that the test requires a total body scan (usually performed 24 to 48 hours after the I.V. injection of radioactive gallium).
• Tell him who will perform the test, where it will take place, and that it takes 30 to 60 minutes.
• Warn him that he may experience transient discomfort from the needle

puncture during injection of the radioactive gallium. Reassure him, however, that the dosage is only slightly radioactive and isn't harmful.
• If a gamma scintillation camera is to be used, assure the patient that although the uptake probe and detector head may touch his skin, he'll experience no discomfort.
• If a rectilinear scanner is to be used, mention that it makes a soft, irregular clicking noise as it registers the radiation emissions.
• Make sure the patient or a responsible family member has signed a consent form.
• Administer a laxative, a cleansing enema, or both.

Procedure and posttest care

• The patient may be positioned erect or recumbent or in an appropriate combination of these positions, depending on his physical condition.
• Scans or scintigraphs of the patient are taken 24 to 48 hours after ^{67}Ga citrate injection, from anterior and posterior views and, occasionally, lateral views.
• If the initial gallium scan suggests bowel disease and additional scans are necessary, give the patient a cleansing enema before continuing the test.

Precautions

• This test should precede barium studies because barium retention may hinder visualization of gallium activity in the bowel.
• Gallium scanning is usually contraindicated in children and during pregnancy or lactation; however, it may be performed if the potential diagnostic benefit outweighs the risks of exposure to radiation.

Normal findings

Gallium activity is normally demonstrated in the liver, spleen, bones, and large bowel. Activity in the bowel results from mucosal uptake of gallium and fecal excretion of gallium.

Abnormal findings

Gallium scanning may reveal inflammatory lesions — discrete abscesses or diffuse infiltration. In pancreatic or perinephric abscess, gallium activity is relatively localized; in bacterial peritonitis, gallium activity is spread diffusely within the abdomen.

Abnormally high gallium accumulation is characteristic in inflammatory bowel diseases, such as ulcerative colitis and regional ileitis (Crohn's disease), and in carcinoma of the colon. However, because gallium normally accumulates in the colon, the detection of inflammatory and neoplastic diseases is sometimes difficult.

Abnormal gallium activity may be present in various sarcomas, Wilms' tumor, and neuroblastomas; carcinoma of the kidney, uterus, vagina, and stomach; and testicular tumors, such as seminoma, embryonal carcinoma, choriocarcinoma, and teratocarcinoma, which often metastasize via the lymphatic system. In Hodgkin's disease and malignant lymphoma, gallium scanning can demonstrate abnormal activity in one or more lymph nodes or in extranodal locations. However, gallium scanning supported by results of lymphangiography can gauge the extent of metastases more accurately than either test alone because neither test consistently identifies all neoplastic nodes.

After chemotherapy or radiation therapy, gallium scanning may be used to detect new or recurrent tumors. However, these forms of therapy tend to diminish tumor affinity for gallium without necessarily eliminating the tumor.

In the differential diagnosis of focal hepatic defects, abnormal gallium activity may help narrow the diagnostic possibilities. Gallium localizes in hepatomas, but not in pseudotumors; in abscesses, but not in pleural effusions; and in tumors, but not in cysts or hematomas.

In examining patients with suspected bronchogenic carcinoma, abnormal activity confirms the presence of tumor. However, because gallium also localizes in inflammatory pulmonary diseases, such as pneumonia and sarcoidosis, a chest X-ray should be performed to distinguish a tumor from an inflammatory lesion.

Interfering factors

- Hepatic and splenic intake (possible false-negative scans due to possible obscuring of abnormal para-aortic nodes in Hodgkin's disease)
- Stool accumulation in bowel (poor imaging of retroperitoneal space)
- Residual barium from other tests done 1 week before the scan (possible poor imaging)

RED BLOOD CELL SURVIVAL TIME

Normally, red blood cells (RBCs) are destroyed only when they reach senility. However, in hemolytic diseases, RBCs of all ages are randomly destroyed, resulting in anemia. The RBC survival time test measures the survival time of circulating RBCs and detects sites of abnormal RBC sequestration and destruction.

Survival time is measured by labeling a random sample of RBCs with radioactive chromium-51 sodium chromate (^{51}Cr). This labeled group of RBCs is then injected back into the patient. Serial blood samples measure the percent of labeled cells per unit volume over 3 to 4 weeks until 50% of the cells disappear (disappearance rate corresponds to destruction of a random cell population).

During the test period, a gamma camera scans the body for sites of abnormally high radioactivity, which indicate sites of excessive RBC sequestration and destruction. Other tests performed with the RBC survival time test may include spot-checks of the stool to detect GI blood loss; hematocrit; blood volume studies; and radionuclide iron uptake and clearance tests to aid differential diagnosis of anemia.

Purpose
• To help evaluate unexplained anemia, particularly hemolytic anemia
• To identify sites of abnormal RBC sequestration and destruction

Patient preparation
• Explain to the patient that this test helps identify the cause of his anemia.
• Advise him that he needn't restrict food or fluids.
• Explain that the test involves labeling a blood sample with a radioactive substance and requires regular blood samples at 3-day intervals for 3 to 4 weeks. Tell him who will perform the testing and where it will take place.
• Tell him that he may experience slight discomfort from the needle punctures. Reassure him that collecting each sample takes less than 3 minutes

and that the small amount of radioactive substance used is harmless.
• If stool collection is required to test for GI bleeding, teach the patient the proper collection technique.

Procedure and posttest care
• A 30-ml blood sample is drawn and mixed with 100 microcuries of ^{51}Cr for an adult (less for a child).
• After an incubation period, the mixture is injected I.V. into the patient. A blood sample is drawn 30 minutes after injection to determine blood and RBC volumes.
• A 6-ml sample is collected in a *green-top* tube after 24 hours; followup samples are collected at 3-day intervals for 3 to 4 weeks. (Intervals between samples may vary, depending on the laboratory.)
• To avoid error from physical decay of the ^{51}Cr, each sample is measured with a scintillation well counter on the day it's drawn.
• Radioactivity per milliliter of RBCs is calculated and the values are plotted to determine mean RBC survival time. Simultaneous gamma camera scans of the precordium, sacrum, liver, and spleen detect radioactivity at sites of excess RBC sequestration. A hematocrit test is done on a small portion of each blood sample to check for blood loss.
• At the end of the study, a sample is drawn to compare ending blood and RBC volumes with beginning volumes.
• If a hematoma develops at the venipuncture site, apply warm soaks.

Precautions
• This test is contraindicated during pregnancy because it exposes the fetus to radiation.
• Because excess blood loss can invalidate test results, this test is usually

contraindicated for a patient with active bleeding or poor clotting function. However, if the test is necessary for a patient with poor clotting function, observe the venipuncture sites carefully for signs of hemorrhage.

• The patient should not receive blood transfusions during the test period and should not have blood samples drawn for other tests.

Normal findings

Normal half-life for RBCs labeled with ^{51}Cr is 25 to 35 days. Normal gamma camera scans reveal slight radioactivity in the spleen, liver, and sometimes the bone marrow.

Abnormal findings

Decreased RBC survival time indicates a hemolytic disease, such as chronic lymphocytic leukemia, congenital nonspherocytic hemolytic anemia, hemoglobin C disease, hereditary spherocytosis, idiopathic acquired hemolytic anemia, paroxysmal nocturnal hemoglobinuria, elliptocytosis, pernicious anemia, sickle cell anemia, sickle cell hemoglobin C disease, or hemolytic-uremic syndrome. If hemolytic anemia is diagnosed, additional tests using cross-transfusion of labeled RBCs can determine whether anemia results from an intrinsic RBC defect or an extrinsic factor.

A gamma camera scan that detects a site of excess RBC sequestration provides direction for treatment. For example, abnormally high RBC sequestration in the spleen may require a splenectomy.

Interfering factors

• Dehydration, overhydration, or blood loss (possible invalidation of results due to changed circulating RBC volume)

• Blood transfusions during the test period (alters proportion of labeled RBCs to total RBCs)

RADIONUCLIDE RENAL IMAGING

Radionuclide renal imaging, which involves I.V. injection of a radionuclide followed by scintigraphy, provides a wealth of information for evaluating the kidneys. Observing the uptake concentration and transit of the radionuclide during this test allows assessment of renal blood flow, renal structure, and nephron and collecting system function. Depending on the patient's clinical presentation, this procedure may include dynamic scans to assess renal perfusion and function or static scans to assess structure.

The radioisotope injected depends on the specific information required and the examiner's preference. However, this procedure often includes double isotope technique to obtain a sequence of perfusion and function studies, followed by static images. This test may also be substituted for excretory urography in patients with hypersensitivity to contrast agents.

Purpose

• To detect and assess functional and structural renal abnormalities (such as lesions)

• To detect renovascular hypertension and acute and chronic renal disease (such as pyelonephritis and glomerulonephritis)

• To assess renal transplantation or renal injury due to trauma and obstruction of the urinary tract

Patient preparation

- Explain to the patient that this test permits evaluation of the structure, blood flow, and function of the kidneys.
- Tell him who will perform the test and where, and that it takes about 90 minutes. (If static scans are ordered, there will be a delay of several hours before the images are taken.)
- Inform him that he'll receive an injection of a radionuclide and that he may experience transient flushing and nausea.
- Emphasize that only a small amount of radionuclide is administered and that it's usually excreted within 24 hours.
- Tell him several series of films will be taken of his bladder.
- Make sure the patient or a responsible family member has signed a consent form.
- Make sure the patient isn't scheduled for other radionuclide scans on the same day as this test.
- If the patient receives antihypertensive medication, it may be withheld before the test.
- Women who are pregnant and young children may receive supersaturated solution of potassium iodide (SSKI) 1 to 3 hours before the test to block thyroid uptake of iodine.

Equipment

Computerized gamma scintillation camera, ^{99m}Tc-DTPA (technetium and diethylenetriaminepentaacetic acid) for perfusion study, ^{131}I-orthoiodohippurate (Hippuran) for function study, oscilloscope, magnetic tape, I.V. equipment

Procedure and posttest care

- The patient is commonly placed in a prone position so that posterior views may be obtained. If the test is being performed to evaluate transplantation, the patient is positioned supine for anterior views.
- Instruct the patient not change his position.
- A perfusion study (radionuclide angiography) is performed first to evaluate renal blood flow. The ^{99m}Tc-DTPA is administered I.V., and rapid-sequence photographs (one per second) are taken for 1 minute.
- Next, a function study is performed to measure the transit time of the radionuclide through the kidneys' functional units. After ^{131}I-orthoiodohippurate is administered I.V., images are obtained at a rate of one per minute for 20 minutes. Alternatively, this entire procedure can be recorded on computer-compatible magnetic tape and concurrent renogram curves plotted.
- Lasix 40 mg may be injected I.V. to evaluate an obstruction.
- Finally, static images are obtained 4 or more hours later, after the radionuclide has drained through the pelvicalyceal system.
- Instruct the patient to flush the toilet immediately after each voiding for 24 hours as a radiation precaution.

Normal findings

Because 25% of cardiac output goes directly to the kidneys, renal perfusion should be evident immediately following uptake of the ^{99m}Tc-DTPA in the abdominal aorta. Within 1 to 2 minutes, a normal pattern of renal circulation should appear. The radionuclide should delineate the kidneys simultaneously, symmetrically, and with equal intensity.

The ^{131}I-orthoiodohippurate administered for the function study rapidly outlines the kidneys — which should be normal in size, shape, and position — and also defines the collecting system and bladder. Maximum counts of the radionuclide in the kidneys occur within 5 minutes after injection (and within 1 minute of each other) and should fall to approximately one-third or less of the maximum counts in the same kidney within 25 minutes. Within this time, the function of both kidneys can be compared as the concentration of radionuclide shifts from the cortex to the pelvis and, finally, to the bladder.

Renal function is best evaluated by comparing these images to the renogram curves. Total function is considered normal when the effective renal plasma flow is 420 ml/minute or greater and the percentage of the dose excreted in the urine at 30 to 35 minutes is greater than 66%.

Abnormal findings

Images from the perfusion study can identify impeded renal circulation, such as that caused by trauma and renal artery stenosis or renal infarction. These conditions may occur in patients with renovascular hypertension and abdominal aortic disease. Because malignant renal tumors are usually vascular, these images can help differentiate tumors from cysts.

In evaluating a kidney transplant, abnormal perfusion may indicate obstruction of the vascular grafts. The function study can detect abnormalities of the collecting system and extravasation of the urine. Markedly decreased tubular function causes reduced radionuclide activity in the collecting system; outflow obstruction causes decreased radionuclide activity in the tubules, with increased activity in the collecting system. This test can also define the level of ureteral obstruction.

Static images can demonstrate lesions, congenital abnormalities, and traumatic injury. These images also detect space-occupying lesions within or surrounding the kidney, such as tumors, infarcts, and inflammatory masses (abscesses, for example); they can also identify congenital disorders, such as horseshoe kidney and polycystic kidney disease. They can define regions of infarction, rupture, or hemorrhage after trauma.

A lower-than-normal total concentration of the radionuclide, as opposed to focal defects, suggests a diffuse renal disorder, such as acute tubular necrosis, severe infection, or ischemia. In a patient who has had a kidney transplant, decreased radionuclide uptake generally indicates organ rejection. Failure of visualization may indicate congenital ectopia or aplasia.

Definitive diagnosis usually requires the combined analysis of static images, perfusion studies, and function studies.

Interfering factors

● Antihypertensives (possible masking of abnormalities)
● Scans of different organs performed on the same day (possible poor imaging)

HIDA SCAN

Also known as hepatobiliary imaging, cholescintigraphy, or gallbladder nuclear scanning, the HIDA scan obtains images of the hepatobiliary system to determine the patency of the cystic and common bile ducts through noninvasive scanning. The scanning is accomplished through injection of iminodiacetic acid analogues (IDAs) labeled with technetium-99m (^{99m}Tc). This test also evaluates gallbladder emptying.

Purpose

- To diagnose gallbladder disorders and determine degree of patency
- To diagnose acute and chronic cholecystitis
- To evaluate the patency of the biliary enteric bypass
- To assess obstructive jaundice in combination with radiography or ultrasonography

Patient preparation

- Explain to the patient that this test detects inflammation or obstruction of the gallbladder and its ducts.
- Tell him who will perform the test and where and that it takes about 90 minutes.
- Inform the patient that he'll receive an I.V. injection of a radionuclide. Tell him the needle insertion and the tourniquet may cause some discomfort.
- Explain that the radionuclide will be eliminated from the body within 6 to 24 hours.
- Inform the patient that repeat pictures may be taken up to 24 hours after the injection.
- Ask a female patient if she is pregnant.
- Ensure that the patient has no allergies to the media used, that he has fasted for 2 to 6 hours before the scan, and that he can comply with activity restriction during the scan.
- Ask the patient to remove all jewelry and metallic objects and to put on a gown and void before the test.
- Explain to the patient that sincalide may be given before the test to promote gallbladder contraction and emptying.

Procedure and posttest care

- Immediately after the radionuclide is injected I.V., the right quadrant of the abdomen is scanned while the patient is in a supine position; images are taken every 5 minutes for the first 30 minutes, then every 10 minutes for the next 30 minutes.
- Delayed views may be taken after 2, 4, and 24 hours if the gallbladder can't be visualized.
- If the gallbladder can't be visualized, morphine may also be given I.V. during the study to initiate spasms of Oddi's sphincter in an effort to move the radionuclide into the gallbladder.
- Monitor vital signs at baseline and every 15 to 30 minutes.
- Observe the patient carefully for up to 60 minutes after the study for a possible hypersensitivity reaction.
- Advise the patient to drink plenty of fluids, unless contraindicated, for 24 to 48 hours to eliminate the radionuclide from the body. Also tell him to flush the toilet immediately after each voiding and to wash his hands with soap and water.
- Rubber gloves should be worn by caregivers every time urine is discarded after the procedure. Gloves should be considered nuclear waste and disposed of appropriately.
- The patient may resume a regular diet after the test, unless contraindicated.

Precautions

- This test is generally contraindicated during pregnancy or lactation because it exposes the fetus or infant to radiation.
- Personnel involved should also be aware of the risks and precautions of this radioactive test.

Normal findings

A normal HIDA scan shows the gallbladder to be normal in size, shape, and function; cystic and common bile ducts are patent.

Abnormal findings

Images may demonstrate acute or chronic cholecystitis, or common bile duct obstruction.

Interfering factors

- Patient's inability to remain still during the procedure
- Failure to observe pretest restrictions
- Presence of barium in GI tract (possible poor imaging)
- Bilirubin levels $\geq$ 30 mg/dl (decreased hepatic uptake)
- Fasting more than 24 hours, total parenteral nutrition, or alcoholism (decreased hepatic uptake)

CHAPTER 15

Monitoring and Catheterization

FETAL MONITORING   666

666   External fetal monitoring   668   Internal fetal monitoring

NEUROLOGIC MONITORING   671

671   Electroencephalography   677   Electromyography
673   Evoked potential studies

CARDIAC MONITORING AND CATHETERIZATION   679

679   Electrocardiography   695   Impedance plethysmography
685   Exercise electrocardiography   696   Cardiac catheterization
689   Radiopharmaceutical myocardial 701   Pulmonary artery catheterization
         perfusion imaging   705   Electrophysiology studies
691   Ambulatory electrocardiography 707   Pulse oximetry
693   Signal-averaged
         electrocardiography

FETAL MONITORING

EXTERNAL FETAL MONITORING

In this noninvasive test, an electronic transducer and a cardiotachometer amplify and record fetal heart rate (FHR) while a pressure-sensitive transducer (tocodynamometer) records uterine contractions. Fetal monitoring records the baseline FHR (average FHR over two contraction cycles or 10 minutes), periodic fluctuations in the baseline FHR, and beat-to-beat heart rate variability. (See *Understanding fetal monitoring terminology*.) External fetal monitoring is also used during other tests of fetal health, notably the nonstress test and the contraction stress test (CST).

Purpose
● To measure FHR and the frequency of uterine contractions
● To evaluate antepartum and intrapartum fetal health during stress and nonstress situations
● To detect fetal distress
● To determine the necessity for internal fetal monitoring
● To assess uterofetoplacental physiology and adequacy of fetal oxygenation

Patient preparation
● Explain to the patient that this test assesses fetal health.
● Describe the procedure and answer all questions. Assure her that external fetal monitoring is painless and won't hurt the fetus or interfere with normal labor.

● Explain that she may have to restrict movement during baseline readings but that she may change position between the readings.
● Make sure the patient or a responsible family member has signed an informed consent form.

Equipment
Monitor, transducer, paper, ultrasound transmission jelly; elastic band, stockinette, or abdominal strap

Procedure and posttest care
● Place the patient in the semi-Fowler or left lateral position, with her abdomen exposed. Cover the ultrasound transducer receiver crystal with ultrasound transmission jelly.
● Palpate the patient's abdomen to identify the fetal chest area, locate the most distinct fetal heart sounds, and then secure the ultrasound transducer over this area with the elastic band, stockinette, or abdominal strap.
● Check the recording equipment for calibration, adequate paper, and alarm boundaries.
● During monitoring, check the elastic band, stockinette, or abdominal strap to ensure that the fit is comfortable yet tight enough to produce a good tracing.
● As labor progresses, reposition the pressure transducer as necessary so that it remains on the fundal portion of the uterus. You may have to reposition the ultrasound transducer as fetal or maternal position changes.
● Repeat antepartum monitoring weekly as long as indications, such as pregnancy over 42 weeks' gestation or any other high-risk pregnancy or fetal growth retardation, persist.
● If FHR patterns indicate distress, fetal oxygenation can often be improved by turning the mother on her side (preferably left) to alleviate supine hypoxia, administering oxygen to the

mother, or loading maternal fluids to increase placental perfusion. If the FHR returns to normal, labor may continue. If abnormal FHR patterns persist, cesarean birth may be required.

Antepartum monitoring with nonstress tests

● Tell the patient to hold the pressure transducer in her hand and to push it each time she feels the fetus move. Some monitoring systems document fetal movement without input from the mother.

● Monitor baseline FHR until you record two fetal movements that last longer than 15 seconds each and cause heart rate accelerations of more than 15 beats/minute from the baseline. If you can't obtain two FHR accelerations within 20 to 30 minutes, shake the patient's abdomen to stimulate the fetus, and repeat the test.

Antepartum monitoring with CST

● Induce contractions by oxytocin infusion or nipple stimulation (endogenous oxytocin).

● When administering oxytocin, infuse a dilute solution at a rate of 0.5 to 1.0 mU/minute, increasing the oxytocin rate until the patient experiences the desired contraction pattern.

● When using nipple stimulation, tell the patient to stimulate one nipple by hand until contractions begin. Some doctors recommend using a water-soluble jelly to prevent nipple damage. If a second contraction doesn't occur in 2 minutes, have her stimulate the nipple again. Stimulate both nipples if contractions don't occur in 15 minutes. Continue until the desired contraction pattern occurs.

● If no decelerations occur during three contractions, the patient may be discharged. Late decelerations during any of the contractions require notification of the doctor and further tests.

> ## UNDERSTANDING FETAL MONITORING TERMINOLOGY
>
> ● *Baseline fetal heart rate:* Average fetal heart rate (FHR) over two contraction cycles or 10 minutes
> ● *Baseline changes:* Fluctuations in FHR unrelated to uterine contractions
> ● *Periodic changes:* Fluctuations in FHR related to uterine contractions
> ● *Amplitude:* Difference in beats per minute between baseline readings and fluctuation in FHR
> ● *Recovery time:* Difference between the end of the contraction and the return to the baseline FHR
> ● *Acceleration:* Transient rise in FHR lasting longer than 15 seconds and associated with a uterine contraction
> ● *Deceleration:* Transient fall in FHR related to a uterine contraction
> ● *Lag time:* Difference between the peak of the contraction and the lowest point of deceleration

Intrapartum monitoring

● Secure the pressure transducer with an elastic band, a stockinette, or an abdominal strap over the area of greatest uterine electrical activity during contractions (usually the fundus).

● Adjust the machine to record 0 to 10 mm Hg pressure between palpable contractions.

● Reposition the ultrasound and pressure transducers as necessary to ensure continuous accurate readings. Review the tracings frequently for baseline abnormalities, periodic changes, variabil-

ity of changes, and uterine contraction abnormalities.
- Record maternal movement, administration of drugs, and procedures performed directly on the tracing to assist evaluation of changes in the tracing.
- Report abnormalities immediately.

Precautions
- During CST, watch for fetal distress with oxytocin infusion or nipple stimulation.

Normal findings

Normal baseline FHR ranges from 120 to 160 beats/minute, with a variability of 5 to 25 beats/minute. For the antepartum nonstress test, the fetus is considered healthy and should remain so for another week if two fetal movements causing a heart rate acceleration of more than 15 beats/minute from baseline FHR occur in a 20-minute period.

For the CST, the fetus is assumed to be healthy and should remain so for another week if three contractions occur during a 10-minute period, with no late decelerations.

Abnormal findings

Bradycardia (FHR < 120 beats/minute) may indicate fetal heart block, malposition, or hypoxia. Fetal bradycardia may also be drug-induced. Tachycardia (FHR > 160 beats/minute) may result from maternal fever, tachycardia, hyperthyroidism, or use of vagolytic drugs or narcotics; early fetal hypoxia; or fetal infection or arrhythmia.

Decreased variability (a fluctuation of < 5 beats/minute in the FHR) may be caused by fetal arrhythmia or heart block; fetal hypoxia, central nervous system malformation, or infections; or vagolytic drugs. FHR accelerations may result from early hypoxia. They

may precede or follow variable decelerations and may indicate that the fetus is in a breech position.

For the antepartum nonstress test, a positive result (< two accelerations of FHR that last longer than 15 seconds each, with a heart rate acceleration over 15 beats/minute) indicates an increased risk of perinatal morbidity and mortality and usually requires CST.

For the CST, persistent late decelerations during two or more contractions may indicate increased risk of fetal morbidity or mortality. Hyperstimulation (long or frequent uterine contractions) or suspicious results require biophysical profile assessment. If findings are unsatisfactory, cesarean birth may be indicated.

Interfering factors
- Gestational age
- Drugs that affect the sympathetic and parasympathetic nervous systems (possible low FHR)
- Certain fetal positions
- Excessive maternal or fetal activity (possible difficulty in recording uterine contractions or FHR)
- Maternal obesity (possible difficulty due to density of abdominal wall)
- Loose or dirty leads or transducer connections (possible production of artifacts)

INTERNAL FETAL MONITORING

Internal fetal monitoring is an invasive procedure that involves attaching an electrode to the fetal scalp to directly monitor fetal heart rate (FHR). A catheter introduced into the uterine cavity measures the frequency and pressure of uterine contractions. Internal monitoring is performed only during labor, after the membranes have ruptured and the cervix has dilated 1¼" (3 cm), with the fetal head lower than the −2 station and only if external monitoring provides inadequate data.

Internal monitoring provides more accurate information about fetal health than external monitoring and is especially useful in determining if cesarean delivery is necessary. The procedure carries minimal risks to the mother (perforated uterus and intrauterine infection) and fetus (scalp abscess and hematoma).

Purpose
• To monitor FHR, especially beat-to-beat variability (short-term variability)
• To measure the frequency and pressure of uterine contractions to assess the progress of labor
• To evaluate intrapartum fetal health
• To supplement or replace external fetal monitoring

Patient preparation
• Explain to the patient that this test accurately assesses fetal health and uterine activity and that it doesn't necessarily mean that there's a problem. Describe the procedure and answer all questions.
• Warn her that she may feel mild discomfort when the uterine catheter and scalp electrode are inserted.

Equipment
Sterile fetal scalp electrode and guide tube, intrauterine pressure catheter, catheter guide, pressure transducer, fetal heart monitor, elastic stockinette

Procedure and posttest care
Measuring FHR
• Place the patient in the dorsal lithotomy position, and prepare her perineal area for a vaginal examination, explaining each step of the procedure as it's performed by a doctor or certified nurse-midwife. As the procedure begins, ask the patient to breathe through her mouth and relax her abdominal muscles.
• After the vaginal examination, the fetal scalp is palpated and an appropriate site is identified. A plastic tube carrying the small electrode is introduced into the cervix, pressed firmly against the fetal scalp, and rotated clockwise to attach the electrode to the scalp. The electrode wire is tugged gently to ensure proper attachment and the tube is withdrawn.
• The electrode wire is connected to a recording device and then either attached to the mother's thigh or applied to her abdomen beneath the elastic stockinette.
• After the fetal scalp electrode is removed, apply antiseptic or antibiotic solution to the site.
Measuring uterine contractions
• Ask the patient to breathe deeply through her mouth and to relax her abdominal muscles.
• After the vagina has been examined and the presenting part of the fetus palpated, the catheter and catheter guide are inserted ⅜" to ¾" (1 to 2 cm) into the cervix, usually between the fetal head and the posterior cervix.
• The catheter is then gently advanced into the uterus until the black mark on the catheter is flush with the vulva. (The catheter guide should *never* be passed deeply into the uterus.)
• The guide is removed and the catheter is connected to a transducer that interprets intrauterine pressure.
Both procedures
• Watch for signs of fetal scalp abscess or maternal intrauterine infection.

NORMAL INTRAUTERINE PRESSURE READINGS
DURING LABOR

STAGE OF LABOR	FREQUENCY (number of contractions per 10 minutes)	BASELINE PRESSURE (mm Hg)	PRESSURE DURING CONTRACTION (mm Hg)
Prelabor	1 to 2	—	25 to 40
First stage	3 to 5	8 to 12	30 to 40 (or more)
Second stage	5	10 to 20	50 to 80

Precautions

• Internal fetal monitoring is contraindicated if there's uncertainty about the fetus's presenting part or a technical impediment to attaching the lead.

• This procedure is also contraindicated if the mother has cervical or vaginal herpes lesions.

• Make sure a low heart rate is actually the FHR; it's possible that the fetal cardiotachometer may be recording a maternal heart rate.

• If FHR patterns indicate fetal distress, fetal oxygenation often can be improved by loading maternal fluids to increase placental perfusion, turning the mother on her side (preferably left) to alleviate supine hypotension, and administering oxygen to the mother. If these measures return heart rate patterns to normal, labor may continue. If abnormal patterns persist, cesarean birth may be necessary.

• Make sure that the fetal scalp electrode and the uterine catheter are removed before cesarean delivery.

Reference values

Normal FHR ranges from 120 to 160 beats/minute, with a variability of 5 to 25 beats/minute. (See *Normal intrauterine pressure readings during labor.*)

Abnormal findings

Bradycardia (FHR < 120 beats/minute) may indicate fetal heart block, malposition, or hypoxia. Fetal bradycardia may also result from maternal ingestion of certain drugs, such as propranolol and narcotic analgesics.

Tachycardia (FHR > 160 beats/minute) may result from early fetal hypoxia, fetal infection or arrhythmia, prematurity, or maternal fever, tachycardia, hyperthyroidism, or use of vagolytic drugs.

Decreased variability (fluctuation of < 5 beats/minute from baseline) may result from fetal arrhythmia or heart block, hypoxia, central nervous system malformation, or infections, or from maternal use of narcotics or vagolytic drugs.

Early decelerations (slowing of FHR at the onset of a contraction with recovery to baseline within no more than 15 seconds after the contraction ends) are related to fetal head compression and usually ensure fetal health.

Late decelerations (slowing of FHR after a contraction begins, a lag time of more than 20 seconds, and a recovery time of more than 15 seconds) may be related to uteroplacental insufficiency, fetal hypoxia, or acidosis. Recurrent and persistently late decelerations with decreased variability usually indicate serious fetal distress, possibly resulting from conduction (spinal, caudal, or epidural) anesthesia or fetal hypoxia.

Variable decelerations (sudden precipitous drops in FHR unrelated to uterine contractions) are commonly related to cord compression. A severe drop in FHR (to < 70 beats/minute for more than 60 seconds) with a decrease in variability indicates fetal distress and may result in a compromised neonate. Poor beat-to-beat variability without periodic patterns may indicate fetal distress, requiring further evaluation, such as analysis of fetal blood gas levels.

Decreased intrauterine pressure during labor that's not progressing normally may require oxytocin stimulation. Elevated intrauterine pressure readings may indicate abruptio placentae or overstimulation from oxytocin, possibly resulting in fetal distress due to decreased placental perfusion.

Interfering factors
- Drugs that affect parasympathetic and sympathetic nervous systems
- Fetal position
- Gestational age

NEUROLOGIC MONITORING

ELECTROENCEPHALOG-RAPHY

In EEG, electrodes attached to areas of the patient's scalp record the brain's electrical activity and transmit this information to an electroencephalograph, which records the resulting brain waves on recording paper. The procedure may be performed in a special laboratory or by a portable unit at the bedside.

Purpose
- To determine the presence and type of seizure disorder
- To aid diagnosis of intracranial lesions, such as abscesses and tumors
- To evaluate the brain's electrical activity in metabolic disease, head injury, meningitis, encephalitis, mental retardation, and psychological disorders
- To evaluate brain death

Patient preparation
- Explain to the patient that this test records the brain's electrical activity.
- Describe the procedure to the patient and family members, and answer all questions.
- Tell him that he must forgo caffeine before the test; other than this, there are no food or fluid restrictions.
- Thoroughly wash and dry his hair to remove hair sprays, creams, and oils.
- Explain that during the test, he'll relax in a reclining chair or lie on a bed and that electrodes will be attached to his scalp with a special paste. Assure him that the electrodes won't shock him.
- If needle electrodes are used, explain that he'll feel a pricking sensation as they're inserted; however, flat electrodes are more commonly used.
- Do your best to allay the patient's fears because nervousness can affect brain wave patterns.
- Check his medication history for drugs that may interfere with test results, for example, anticonvulsants, antianxiety agents, sedative-hypnotics, and antidepressants. Withhold these medications for 24 to 48 hours before the test, as ordered by the doctor.

• A patient with a seizure disorder may require a "sleep EEG." In this case, keep the patient awake the night before the test, and administer a sedative (such as chloral hydrate) to help him sleep during the test.

• If the test is performed to confirm brain death, provide family members with emotional support.

Procedure and posttest care

• Position the patient on the bed or reclining chair. Reassure him as the electrodes are attached to his scalp.

• Before the recording procedure begins, instruct the patient to close his eyes, relax, and remain still.

• During the recording, observe the patient carefully; note blinking, swallowing, talking, or other movements, and record these findings on the tracing. These activities may cause artifacts on the tracing and be misinterpreted as abnormal tracing.

• The recording may be stopped at intervals to let the patient rest or reposition himself. This is important because restlessness and fatigue can alter brain wave patterns.

• After an initial baseline recording, the patient may be tested under various stress-producing conditions to elicit patterns not observable while he's at rest. For example, he may be asked to breathe deeply and rapidly for 3 minutes (hyperventilation), which may elicit brain wave patterns typical of seizure disorders or other abnormalities. This technique is commonly used to detect absence seizures. Also, photic stimulation tests central cerebral activity in response to bright light, accentuating abnormal activity in absence or myoclonic seizures.

• Review carefully the reinstatement of anticonvulsant medication or other drugs withheld before the test.

• Carefully observe the patient for seizure activity and provide a safe environment.

• Help the patient remove electrode paste from his hair.

• If the patient received a sedative before the test, take safety precautions, such as raising the bed's side rails.

Precautions

• Observe the patient carefully for seizure activity.

• If seizure activity occurs, record seizure patterns and be prepared to provide assistance. Have suction equipment and diazepam or lorazepam for I.V. injection readily available.

Normal findings

EEG records a portion of the brain's electrical activity as waves; some are irregular, whereas others demonstrate frequent patterns. Among the basic waveforms are the alpha, beta, theta, and delta rhythms.

Alpha waves occur at a frequency of 8 to 11 cycles/second in a regular rhythm. They're present only in the waking state when the patient's eyes are closed but he's mentally alert; usually, they disappear with visual activity or mental concentration. *Beta waves* (13 to 30 cycles/second) — generally associated with anxiety, depression, and use of sedatives — are seen most readily in the frontal and central regions of the brain. *Theta waves* (4 to 7 cycles/second) are most common in children and young adults and appear in the frontal and temporal regions. *Delta waves* (0.5 to 3.5 cycles/second) normally occur only in young children and during sleep.

Abnormal findings

Usually, about 100 pages of recordings are evaluated, with particular attention paid to basic waveforms, symmetry of cerebral activity, transient discharges, and responses to stimulation. A specific diagnosis depends on the patient's clinical status.

In seizure disorders, EEG patterns may identify the specific disorder. In *absence seizures,* the EEG shows spikes and waves at a frequency of 3 cycles/second. In *generalized tonic-clonic seizures*, it generally shows multiple, high-voltage, spiked waves in both hemispheres. In *complex partial seizures*, the EEG usually shows spiked waves in the affected temporal region. And in patients with *focal seizures*, it usually shows localized, spiked discharges.

In patients with intracranial lesions, such as tumors or abscesses, the EEG may show slow waves (usually delta waves but possibly unilateral beta waves). Vascular lesions, such as cerebral infarcts and intracranial hemorrhages, generally produce focal abnormalities in the injured area.

Generally, any condition that causes a diminishing level of consciousness alters the EEG pattern in proportion to the degree of consciousness lost. For example, in a patient with a metabolic disorder, an inflammatory process (such as meningitis or encephalitis), or increased intracranial pressure, the EEG shows generalized, diffuse, and slow brain waves.

Interfering factors
• Interference from extraneous electrical activity; head, body, eye, or tongue movement; or muscle contractions (possible production of excessive artifact)
• Noise in the environment (possible patient reactions)
• Hair spray and gel (possible faulty electrode contact with skin)
• Caffeine, anticonvulsants, barbiturates, antidepressants, hypnotics, and tranquilizers and other sedatives (possible masking of seizure activity)
• Acute drug intoxication or severe hypothermia resulting in loss of consciousness (flat EEG)

EVOKED POTENTIAL STUDIES

These tests evaluate the integrity of visual, somatosensory, and auditory nerve pathways by measuring evoked potentials — the brain's electrical response to stimulation of the sensory organs or peripheral nerves. Evoked potentials are recorded as electronic impulses by surface electrodes attached to the scalp and skin over various peripheral sensory nerves. A computer extracts these low-amplitude impulses from background brain wave activity and averages the signals from repeated stimuli. (See *Visual and somatosensory evoked potentials,* pages 674 and 675.)

Three types of responses are measured:
• *Visual evoked potentials,* produced by exposing the eye to a rapidly reversing checkerboard pattern, help evaluate demyelinating diseases, traumatic injury, and puzzling visual complaints.
• *Somatosensory evoked potentials,* produced by electrically stimulating a peripheral sensory nerve, help diagnose peripheral nerve disease and locate brain and spinal cord lesions.
• *Auditory brain stem evoked potentials,* produced by delivering clicks to the ear, help locate auditory lesions and evaluate brain stem integrity.

(Text continues on page 676.)

VISUAL AND SOMATOSENSORY EVOKED POTENTIALS

Visual (pattern-shift) evoked potentials: In this test, visual neural impulses are recorded as they travel along the pathway from the eye to the occipital cortex. Wave P100 is the most significant component of the resultant waveform. Normal P100 latency is about 100 msec after the application of a visual stimulus, as shown in the top diagram. Increased P100 latency, shown in the bottom diagram, is an abnormal finding, indicating a lesion along the visual pathway.

Normal tracing

Tracing in multiple sclerosis

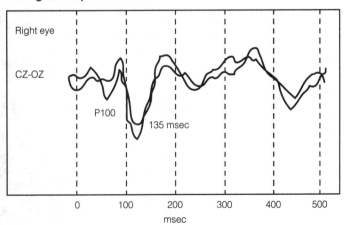

KEY: CZ = vertex; OZ = midocciput

VISUAL AND SOMATOSENSORY EVOKED POTENTIALS *(continued)*

Somatosensory evoked potentials: These tests measure the conduction time of an electrical impulse traveling along a somatosensory pathway to the cortex. Interwave latency is the most significant component of the resultant waveform. On the set of upper- and lower-limb tracings shown below, the top tracings represent normal interwave latencies; the bottom tracings, typical abnormal latencies found in a patient with multiple sclerosis. Because of the close correlation between waveforms and the anatomy of somatosensory pathways, such tracings allow precise location of lesions that produce conduction defects.

Upper limb

Normal tracing
FZ-Cc
N19
P22

0 5 10 15 20 25 30 35 40 45 50
msec

Tracing in muliple sclerosis
FZ-Cc
N19
P22

0 5 10 15 20 25 30 35 40 45 50
msec

Lower limb

Normal tracing
CZ-Cc
N27
P32

0 5 10 15 20 25 30 35 40 45 50
msec

Tracing in multiple sclerosis
CZ-Cc
N27
P32

0 5 10 15 20 25 30 35 40 45 50
msec

KEY: CZ = vertex; Cc = sensoparietal cortex contralateral to stimulated limb; FZ = midfrontal

Purpose
- To aid diagnosis of nervous system lesions and abnormalities
- To assess neurologic function
- To monitor comatose patients and patients under anesthesia
- To monitor spinal cord function during spinal cord surgery
- To evaluate neurologic function in infants whose sensory systems can't be adequately assessed

Patient preparation
- Tell the patient that this group of tests measures the electrical activity of his nervous system. Explain who will perform the test, where it will take place, and that it usually lasts 45 to 60 minutes.
- Tell him that he'll sit in a reclining chair or lie on a bed. If visual evoked potentials will be measured, electrodes will be attached to his scalp; if somatosensory evoked potentials will be measured, electrodes will be placed on his scalp, neck, lower back, wrist, knee, and ankle.
- Assure him that the electrodes won't hurt him. Encourage him to relax; tension can affect neurologic function and interfere with test results.
- Have him remove all jewelry and other metal objects.

Procedure and posttest care
- Position the patient in the reclining chair or on the bed and tell him to relax and remain still.

Visual evoked potentials
- Electrodes are attached to the patient's scalp at occipital, parietal, and vertex sites; a reference electrode is placed on the midfrontal area or ear.
- The patient is positioned 3' (1 m) from the pattern-shift stimulator.
- One eye is occluded, and the patient is instructed to fix his gaze on a dot in the center of the screen.

- A checkerboard pattern is projected and then rapidly reversed or shifted 100 times, once or twice per second.
- A computer amplifies and averages the brain's response to each stimulus, and the results are plotted as a waveform.
- The procedure is repeated for the other eye.

Somatosensory evoked potentials
- Electrodes are attached to the patient's skin over somatosensory pathways — typically the wrist, knee, and ankle — to stimulate peripheral nerves. Recording electrodes are placed on the scalp over the sensory cortex of the hemisphere opposite the limb to be stimulated. Additional electrodes may be placed at Erb's point (above the clavicle overlying the brachial plexus), at the second cervical vertebra, and over the lower lumbar vertebrae. Midfrontal or noncephalic electrodes are placed for reference.
- Painless electrical stimulation is delivered to the peripheral nerve through the electrode. The intensity is adjusted to produce a minor muscle response, such as a thumb twitch on median nerve stimulation at the wrist.
- Electrical stimuli are delivered 500 or more times at a rate of five per second.
- A computer measures and averages the time it takes for the electric current to reach the cortex; the results, expressed in milliseconds (msec), are recorded as waveforms.
- The test is repeated once to verify results; then the electrodes are repositioned and the entire procedure is repeated for the other side.

Normal findings
Visual evoked potentials
On the waveform, the most significant wave is P100, a positive wave appearing about 100 msec after the pattern-

shift stimulus is applied. The most clinically significant measurements are absolute P100 latency (the time between stimulus application and peaking of the P100 wave) and the difference between the P100 latencies of each eye. Because many physical and technical factors affect P100 latency, normal results vary greatly among laboratories and patients.

Somatosensory evoked potentials
Waveforms obtained vary, depending on locations of the stimulating and recording electrodes. The positive and negative peaks are labeled in sequence, based on normal time of appearance. For example, N19 is a negative peak normally recorded 19 msec after application of the stimulus. Each wave peak arises from a discrete location: N19 is generated mainly from the thalamus, P22 from the parietal sensory cortex, and so on. Interwave latencies (time between waves), rather than absolute latencies, are used as a basis for clinical interpretation. Latency differences between sides are significant.

Abnormal findings
Information from evoked potential studies is useful but insufficient to confirm a specific diagnosis. Test data must be interpreted in light of clinical information.

Visual evoked potentials
Generally, abnormal (extended) P100 latencies confined to one eye indicate a visual pathway lesion anterior to the optic chiasm. A lesion posterior to the optic chiasm usually doesn't produce abnormal P100 latencies. Because each eye projects to both occipital lobes, the unaffected pathway transmits sufficient impulses to produce a normal latency response. Bilateral abnormal P100 latencies have been found in patients with multiple sclerosis, optic neuritis,

retinopathies, amblyopia (although abnormal latencies don't correlate well with impaired visual acuity), spinocerebellar degeneration, adrenoleukodystrophy, sarcoidosis, Parkinson's disease, and Huntington's disease.

Somatosensory evoked potentials
Because somatosensory evoked potential components are assumed to be linked in series, an abnormal interwave latency indicates a conduction defect between the generators of the two peaks involved. This often allows precise location of a neurologic lesion. Abnormal upper-limb interwave latencies may indicate cervical spondylosis, intracerebral lesions, or sensorimotor neuropathies. Abnormalities in the lower limb demonstrate peripheral nerve and root lesions, such as those in Guillain-Barré syndrome, compressive myelopathies, multiple sclerosis, transverse myelitis, and traumatic spinal cord injury.

Interfering factors
- Interference from extraneous electrical equipment
- Noise in the environment (possible patient reactions)
- Incorrect electrode placement or equipment failure
- Patient tension, inability to relax, or failure to cooperate
- Poor patient vision
- Coolness of the patient's extremities

ELECTROMYOGRAPHY

This test records the electrical activity of selected skeletal muscle groups at rest and during voluntary contraction. It involves percutaneous insertion of a needle electrode into a muscle. The electrical discharge of the muscle is then measured by an oscilloscope. Nerve conduction time is often measured simultaneously.

Purpose
• To aid differentiation between primary muscle disorders, such as the muscular dystrophies, and secondary disorders
• To help assess diseases characterized by central neuronal degeneration, such as amyotrophic lateral sclerosis
• To aid diagnosis of neuromuscular disorders, such as myasthenia gravis

Patient preparation
• Explain to the patient that this test measures the electrical activity of his muscles.
• Tell him that there are usually no restrictions on food or fluids (in some cases, cigarettes, coffee, tea, and cola may be restricted for 2 to 3 hours before the test).
• Describe the test, including who will perform it, where it will take place, and its duration (1 hour).
• Tell him that he may wear a hospital gown or any comfortable clothing that permits access to the muscles to be tested.
• Advise him that a needle will be inserted into selected muscles and that he may experience mild discomfort. Reassure him that adverse effects and complications are rare.
• Make sure the patient or a responsible family member has signed an informed consent form.
• Check the patient's history for medications that may interfere with the results of the test, for example, cholinergics, anticholinergics, and skeletal muscle relaxants. If the patient is receiving such medications, note this on the test form.

Procedure and posttest care
• Position the patient on a stretcher or bed or in a chair, depending on the muscles to be tested. Position his arm or leg so that the muscle to be tested is at rest.
• Needle electrodes are quickly inserted and a metal plate is placed under the patient to serve as a reference electrode. Then the muscle's electrical signal (motor unit potential) is recorded during rest and contraction.
• The monitor display is photographed for a permanent record. Frequently, the leadwires of the recorder are attached to an audio amplifier so that the fluctuation of voltage within the muscle can be heard.
• If the patient experiences residual pain, apply warm compresses and administer prescribed analgesics.
• Resume administration of any medications withheld for the test.

Precautions
• Electromyography is contraindicated in patients with bleeding disorders.

Normal findings
At rest, a normal muscle exhibits minimal electrical activity. During voluntary contraction electrical activity increases markedly. A sustained contraction or one of increasing strength causes a rapid "train" of motor unit potentials that can be heard as a crescendo of sounds over the audio amplifier.

At the same time, the monitor displays a sequence of waveforms that vary in amplitude (height) and frequency. Waveforms that are close together indicate a high frequency, whereas waveforms that are far apart signify a low frequency.

Normal findings must be correlated with the patient's history and clinical features and with the results of other neurologic tests.

Abnormal findings

In primary muscle diseases such as muscular dystrophy, motor unit potentials are short (low amplitude), with frequent, irregular discharges. In disorders such as amyotrophic lateral sclerosis (as well as in peripheral nerve disorders), motor unit potentials are isolated and irregular but show increased amplitude and duration. In myasthenia gravis, motor unit potentials initially may be normal but progressively diminish in amplitude with continuing contractions. The interpreter distinguishes between waveforms that indicate a muscle disorder and those that indicate denervation.

Interfering factors

- Patient's inability to relax or comply with instructions
- Drugs affecting myoneural junctions, such as cholinergics, anticholinergics, and skeletal muscle relaxants
- Coolness of the patient's extremities

CARDIAC MONITORING AND CATHETERIZATION

ELECTROCARDIOGRAPHY

A common test for evaluating cardiac status, electrocardiography (ECG) graphically records the electric current (electrical potential) generated by the heart. This current radiates from the heart in all directions and, on reaching the skin, is measured by electrodes connected to an amplifier and strip chart recorder. The standard resting (scalar) ECG uses 5 electrodes to measure the electrical potential from 12 leads: the standard limb leads (I, II, III), the augmented limb leads (aV_R, aV_L, and aV_F), and the precordial, or chest, leads (V_1 through V_6).

Purpose

- To help identify primary conduction abnormalities, cardiac arrhythmias, cardiac hypertrophy, pericarditis, electrolyte imbalances, myocardial ischemia, and the site and extent of myocardial infarction (MI)
- To monitor recovery from MI
- To evaluate the effectiveness of cardiac medication (digitalis glycosides, antiarrhythmics, antihypertensives, and vasodilators)
- To assess pacemaker performance

Patient preparation

- Explain to the patient that this test evaluates the heart's electrical activity.
- Tell him that he needn't restrict food or fluids.
- Describe the test, including who will perform it, where it will take place, and its expected duration (5 to 10 minutes).
- Tell the patient that electrodes will be attached to his arms, legs, and chest and that the procedure is painless. Explain that during the test, he'll be asked to relax, lie still, and breathe normally.
- Advise him not to talk during the test because the sound of his voice may distort the ECG tracing.
- Check the patient's medication history for use of cardiac drugs, and note use of such drugs on the rhythm strip.

Equipment

Recording paper, disposable electrodes or reusable electrodes with suction bulbs, conductive gel, rubber straps, 4″ × 4″ gauze pads, moist cloth towel, sterile drape

Procedure and posttest care

• Place the patient in the supine position. If he can't tolerate lying flat, help him to assume the semi-Fowler position.

• Have him expose his chest, both ankles, and both wrists for electrode placement. If the patient is a woman, provide a chest drape until the chest leads are applied.

• Turn on the machine to warm up the stylus mechanism, and check the paper supply.

Multichannel ECG

• Place electrodes on the inner aspect of the wrists, the medial aspect of the lower legs, and the chest. If using disposable electrodes, remove the paper backing before positioning. For reusable electrodes, apply conductive gel and affix the electrodes with suction bulbs.

• Connect the leadwires after all electrodes are in place. Secure the limb electrodes with rubber straps, but avoid tightening them to prevent circulatory impairment and distortion on the recording.

• If frequent ECGs will be necessary, use a marking pen to indicate lead positions on the patient's chest to ensure consistent placement.

• Set the paper speed if required (usually 25 mm/second). Calibrate the machine by adjusting the sensitivity to normal and checking the quality and baseline position of the tracing. Press the START button, and record any required information (for example, patient's name and room number).

• The machine produces a printout showing all 12 leads simultaneously. Check to be sure that all leads are represented in the tracing. If not, determine which one has come loose, reattach it, and restart the tracing.

• Check for artifacts in the tracing, and be sure that the wave doesn't peak beyond the top edge of the recording grid. If it does, adjust the machine to bring the wave inside the boundaries.

• When the machine finishes the tracing, remove the electrodes and reposition the patient's gown and bed covers.

Single-channel ECG

• Apply either disposable or standard electrodes to the inner aspect of the wrists and medial aspect of the lower legs. Connect each leadwire to the corresponding electrode by inserting the wire prong into the terminal post and tightening the screw, if required.

• Set the paper speed if required (usually 25 mm/second), and calibrate the machine by adjusting the sensitivity to normal. Recalibrate the machine after running each lead to provide a consistent test standard.

• Turn the lead selector to I. Then mark the lead by writing "I" on the paper strip or by depressing the marking button on the machine (some machines do this automatically). Record for 3 to 6 seconds and then return the machine to the standby mode. Repeat this procedure for leads II, III, aV_R, aV_L, and aV_F.

• Determine proper placement for the chest electrodes. (If frequent ECGs are necessary, mark these spots on the patient's chest to ensure consistent placement.)

• Connect the pregelled disposable electrodes to the chest leadwire or to the suction bulb, apply gel to each of the six chest positions, and then firmly press the suction bulb to attach the chest lead to the V_1 position. Mark the strips as before.

• Turn the lead selector to V and record V_1 for 3 to 6 seconds. Return the lead selector to standby. Reposition the electrode and repeat the procedure for V_2 through V_6.

• After completing V_6, run a rhythm strip on lead II for at least 6 seconds.

Assess the quality of the tracings, and repeat any that are unclear.

• Disconnect the equipment, remove the electrodes, and wipe the gel from the patient with a moist cloth towel. Wash the gel from the electrodes and dry them thoroughly.

Both types

• Label each ECG strip with the patient's name and room number (if applicable), date and time of the procedure, and doctor's name. Note whether the ECG was performed during or on resolution of a chest pain episode.

• Disconnect the equipment. The electrode patches are usually left in place if the patient is having recurrent chest pain or if serial ECGs are ordered, as with the use of thrombolytics. If using suction cups, be sure to wash the conductive gel from the patient's skin.

Precautions

• The recording equipment and other nearby electrical equipment should be properly grounded to prevent electrical interference.

• Double-check color codes and lead markings to be sure connectors match.

• Make sure that the suction cups are firmly attached, and reattach electrodes if loose skin contact is suspected.

• Be sure the patient is quiet and motionless during the test because talking and movement distort the recordings.

• If the patient has a pacemaker in place, an ECG may be performed with or without a magnet. Indicate the presence of a pacemaker and whether or not a magnet is used. (Many pacemakers function only when the heartbeat falls below a preset rate; a magnet makes the pacemaker fire regularly, which permits evaluation of pacemaker performance.)

Normal findings

ECG tracings normally consist of three identifiable waveforms in each cardiac cycle: the P wave, the QRS complex, and the T wave. The P wave depicts atrial depolarization; the QRS complex, ventricular depolarization; and the T wave, ventricular repolarization.

The lead II waveform, known as the rhythm strip, depicts the heart's rhythm more clearly than any other waveform. In lead II, the normal P wave doesn't exceed 2.5 mm (0.25 mV) in height or last longer than 0.12 second. The PR interval, which includes the P wave plus the PR segment, persists for 0.12 to 0.2 second for heart rates above 60 beats/minute. The QT interval varies with the heart rate and lasts 0.4 to 0.52 second for heart rates above 60 beats/minute; the voltage of the R wave in the V_1 through V_6 leads doesn't exceed 27 mm. The total QRS complex lasts 0.06 to 0.1 second. (See *Normal ECG waveforms*, page 682.)

Abnormal findings

An abnormal ECG may show MI, right or left ventricular hypertrophy, arrhythmias, right or left bundle-branch block, ischemia, conduction defects or pericarditis, electrolyte abnormalities (such as hypokalemia), and the effects of cardioactive drugs. Sometimes an ECG may reveal abnormal waveforms only during angina episodes or during exercise. (See *Abnormal ECG waveforms*, pages 683 to 685.)

Interfering factors

• Strenuous exercise before the test

• Excessive chest hair (prevents good electrode contact)

• Improper placement of electrodes

• Reactions to medications

• Mechanical difficulties, such as ECG machine malfunction, faulty adherence

(Text continues on page 685.)

NORMAL ECG WAVEFORMS

Because each lead takes a different view of heart activity, it generates its own characteristic tracing. The traces shown here are representative of each of the 12 leads. Leads aV_R, V_1, V_2, V_3, and V_4 normally show strong negative deflections below the baseline. Negative deflections indicate that the current is flowing away from the positive electrode; positive deflections, that the current is flowing toward the positive electrode.

Lead I

Lead V₁

Lead II

Lead V₂

Lead III

Lead V₃

Lead aV_R

Lead V₄

Lead aV_F

Lead V₅

Lead aV_L

Lead V₆

ABNORMAL ECG WAVEFORMS

Premature ventricular contractions (PVCs) originate in an ectopic focus of the ventricular wall. They can be unifocal (having the same single focus), as shown in this tracing from lead V_1, or multifocal (arising from more than one ectopic focus). In PVCs, the P wave is absent and the QRS complex shows considerable distortion, usually deflecting in the opposite direction from the patient's normal QRS. The T wave also deflects in the opposite direction from the QRS complex, and the PVC usually precedes a compensatory pause. Some examples of abnormalities causing PVCs include electrolyte imbalances (especially hypokalemia), an old myocardial infarction (MI), hypoxia, and drug toxicity (digitalis glycosides, beta-adrenergics).

Premature ventricular contraction — Lead V_1

First-degree heart block, the most common conduction disturbance, occurs in healthy hearts as well as diseased hearts and usually is clinically insignificant. It's often characteristic in elderly patients with chronic degeneration of the cardiac conduction system, and it occasionally occurs in patients receiving digitalis glycosides or antiarrhythmic drugs, such as procainamide and quinidine. In children, first-degree heart block may be the earliest sign of acute rheumatic fever. In this lead V_1 tracing, the interval between the P wave and QRS complex (the PR interval) exceeds 0.20 second.

First-degree heart block — Lead V_1

Hypokalemia is a common electrolyte imbalance that's caused by low serum potassium levels and that affects the electrical activity of the myocardium. Mild hypokalemia may cause only muscle weakness, fatigue and, possibly, atrial or ventricular irritability; a severe imbalance causes pronounced muscle weakness, paralysis, atrial tachycardia with varying degrees of block, and PVCs that may progress to ventricular tachycardia and fibrillation.

(continued)

ABNORMAL ECG WAVEFORMS *(continued)*

Early signs of hypokalemia, as shown on this lead V_1 tracing, include prominent U waves, a prolonged QU interval, and flat or inverted T waves. Usually, T waves don't flatten or invert until potassium depletion becomes severe.

Hypokalemia — Lead V_1

MI produces typical ECG changes in several leads at once, enabling the doctor to accurately determine the location and extent of tissue damage. MI causes three changes: an inner zone of tissue necrosis, a surrounding zone of inflamed tissue, and an outer zone of ischemia (see diagram). As the infarction progresses, the first ECG change is an elevated ST segment, which indicates formation of an ischemic zone. Then the T wave begins to flatten and finally inverts and enlarged Q waves appear, indicating developing necrosis — a true infarction. (Abnormal Q waves should be larger than one small square on the chart — 0.04 second by 0.1 mV.) The T wave may stay inverted

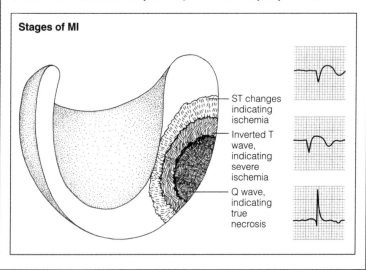

Stages of MI

ST changes indicating ischemia

Inverted T wave, indicating severe ischemia

Q wave, indicating true necrosis

ABNORMAL ECG WAVEFORMS *(continued)*

for the rest of the patient's life or it can revert to normal, whereas the deep Q wave remains as a permanent indicator of necrosis. The infarction can be located by studying the characteristic ST, T, and Q wave changes in various lead combinations. In the three tracings shown below, the ST-segment elevations in leads II, III, and aV_F indicate an infarction in the inferior (diaphragmatic) area of the heart.

ECG changes in an inferior MI

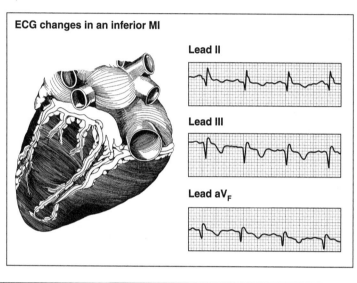

Lead II

Lead III

Lead aV_F

of electrode patches (for example, due to diaphoresis), and electromagnetic interference (production of artifact)
• Patient movement or muscle tremor

EXERCISE ELECTROCARDIOGRAPHY

Also referred to as a stress test, an exercise electrocardiogram (ECG) evaluates the heart's response to physical stress, providing important diagnostic

information that can't be obtained from a resting ECG alone.

An ECG and blood pressure readings are taken while the patient walks on a treadmill or pedals a stationary bicycle, and his response to a constant or an increasing workload is observed. Unless complications develop, the test continues until the patient reaches the target heart rate (determined by an established protocol) or experiences chest pain or fatigue. The patient who has recently had a myocardial infarction (MI) or coronary artery surgery may walk the treadmill at a slow pace to determine his activity tolerance before discharge.

Purpose
● To help diagnose the cause of chest pain or other possible cardiac pain
● To determine the functional capacity of the heart after surgery or MI
● To screen for asymptomatic coronary artery disease (CAD), particularly in men over age 35
● To help set limitations for an exercise program
● To identify arrhythmias that develop during physical exercise
● To evaluate the effectiveness of antiarrhythmic or antianginal therapy

Patient preparation
● Explain to the patient that this test records the heart's electrical activity and performance under stress.
● Instruct him not to eat, smoke, or drink alcoholic or caffeinated beverages for 3 hours before the test but to continue his prescribed drug regimen unless directed otherwise. When possible, digoxin should be withheld for 10 days before the test.
● Describe who will perform the test, where it will take place, and its expected duration.
● Tell him that the test will cause fatigue and that he'll be slightly breathless and sweaty, but assure him that the test poses few risks. He may, in fact, stop the test if he experiences fatigue or chest pain.
● Advise him to wear comfortable socks and shoes and loose, lightweight shorts or slacks. Men usually don't wear a shirt during the test, and women generally wear a bra and a lightweight short-sleeved blouse or a patient gown with a front closure.
● Explain that electrodes will be attached to several areas on his chest and, possibly, his back. Reassure him that he won't feel any current from the electrodes; however, they may itch slightly.
● Tell him that his blood pressure will be checked periodically throughout the procedure, and assure him that his heart rate will be monitored continuously.
● If the patient is scheduled for a multistage *treadmill test,* explain that the speed and incline of the treadmill will increase at predetermined intervals and that he'll be informed of each adjustment.
● If he's scheduled for a *bicycle ergometer test,* explain that the resistance he experiences in pedaling increases gradually as he tries to maintain a specific speed.
● Encourage him to report his feelings during the test. Tell him that his blood pressure and ECG will be monitored for 10 to 15 minutes after the test.
● Check the patient's history for a recent physical examination (within 1 week) and for baseline 12-lead ECG results.
● Be sure that the patient or a responsible family member has signed an informed consent form.

Procedure and posttest care
● The electrode sites are cleaned with an alcohol swab, and superficial epidermal cell layers and excess skin oils are removed with a gauze pad, fine sandpaper, or a dental burr. The electrode sites may need to be shaved if excessive hair is present.
● Chest electrodes are placed according to the lead system selected and are secured with adhesive tape or a rubber belt. The leadwire cable is placed over the patient's shoulder and the leadwire box is placed on his chest. The cable is secured by pinning it to the patient's clothing or taping it to his shoulder or back. Then the leadwires are connected to the chest electrodes.

- The monitor is started, and a stable baseline tracing is obtained. A baseline rhythm strip is checked for arrhythmias. A blood pressure reading is taken, and the patient is auscultated for the presence of S_3 or S_4 gallops or crackles.

- In a treadmill test, the treadmill is turned on to a slow speed, and the patient is shown how to step onto it and how to use the support railings to maintain balance but not support weight. Then the treadmill is turned off. The patient is instructed to step onto the treadmill, and it is turned on to slow speed until he gets used to walking on it.

- For a bicycle ergometer test, the patient is instructed to sit on the bicycle while the seat and handlebars are adjusted to comfortable positions. The patient is instructed not to grip the handlebars tightly but to use them only for maintaining balance and to pedal until he reaches the desired speed, as shown on the speedometer.

- In both tests, a monitor is observed continuously for changes in the heart's electrical activity. The rhythm strip is checked at preset intervals for arrhythmias, premature ventricular contractions (PVCs), ST-segment changes, and T-wave changes. The test level and the time elapsed in the test level are marked on each strip. Blood pressure is monitored at predetermined intervals, usually at the end of each test level, and changes in systolic readings are noted. Some common responses to maximal exercise are dizziness, light-headedness, leg fatigue, dyspnea, diaphoresis, and a slightly ataxic gait. If symptoms become severe, the test is stopped.

- Usually, testing stops when the patient reaches the target heart rate. As the treadmill speed slows, he may be instructed to continue walking for several minutes to allow for cooling down.

Then the treadmill is turned off, the patient is helped to a chair, and his blood pressure and ECG are monitored for 10 to 15 minutes or until the ECG returns to baseline.

- Auscultate for the presence of an S_3 or S_4 gallop. An S_4 gallop commonly develops after exercise because of increased blood flow volume and turbulence. An S_3 gallop is more significant than an S_4 gallop, indicating transient left ventricular dysfunction.

- Tell the patient that he may resume his usual diet.

- If any drugs were discontinued before the test, tell the patient that he may resume taking them.

- Remove electrodes and clean the electrode sites before the patient leaves.

Precautions

- Because an exercise ECG places considerable stress on the heart, it may be contraindicated in patients with ventricular aneurysm, dissecting aortic aneurysm, uncontrolled arrhythmias, pericarditis, myocarditis, severe anemia, uncontrolled hypertension, unstable angina, or heart failure.

- Stop the test immediately if the ECG shows three consecutive PVCs or any significant increase in ectopy, if systolic blood pressure falls below resting level, if heart rate falls to 10 beats/ minute below resting level, or if the patient becomes exhausted. Depending on the patient's condition, the test may be stopped if the ECG shows bundle-branch block, ST-segment depression that exceeds 1.5 mm, persistent ST-segment elevation, or frequent or complicated PVCs; if blood pressure fails to rise above resting level; if systolic pressure exceeds 220 mm Hg; or if the patient experiences angina.

EXERCISE ECG TRACINGS

These tracings are from an abnormal exercise electrocardiogram (ECG) obtained during a treadmill test performed on a patient who had just undergone a triple coronary artery bypass graft. The first tracing shows the heart at rest, with a blood pressure of 124/80 mm Hg. In the second tracing, the patient worked up to a 10% grade at 1.7 mph before experiencing angina at 2 minutes, 25 seconds. The tracing shows a depressed ST segment; heart rate was 85 beats/minute and blood pressure was 140/70 mm Hg. The third tracing shows the heart at rest 6 minutes after the test; blood pressure was 140/90 mm Hg.

Resting

Angina

Recovery

Normal findings

In a normal exercise ECG, the P and T waves, the QRS complex, and the ST segment change minimally and the patient attains the endurance levels predicted by his age and the appropriate exercise protocol. (See *Exercise ECG tracings.*)

Abnormal findings

Although criteria for judging test results vary, two findings strongly suggest an abnormality: a flat or downsloping ST-segment depression of 1 mm or more for at least 0.08 second after the junction of the QRS and ST segments (J point) and a markedly depressed J point, with an upsloping but depressed ST segment of 1.5 mm below the baseline 0.08 second after the J point. T-wave inversion also signifies ischemia. Initial ST-segment depression on the resting ECG must be further depressed by 1 mm during exercise to be considered abnormal. Arrhythmias and ectopic beats may indicate an abnormal response.

Hypotension resulting from exercise, ST-segment depression of 3 mm or more, downsloping ST segments, and ischemic ST segments appearing within the first 3 minutes of exercise and lasting 8 minutes into the posttest recovery period may indicate multivessel or left CAD. ST-segment elevation may indicate dyskinetic left ventricular wall motion or severe transmural ischemia.

The predictive value of this test for CAD varies with the patient's history and sex; false-negative and false-positive test results are common. To detect CAD accurately, thallium imaging and stress testing, exercise multiple-gated acquisition scanning, or coronary angiography may be necessary.

Interfering factors

- Failure to observe pretest restrictions
- Inability to exercise to the target heart rate due to fatigue or failure to cooperate
- Wolff-Parkinson-White syndrome (anomalous atrioventricular excitation), electrolyte imbalance, or use of a digitalis glycoside (possible false-positive)
- Left ventricular hypertrophy, such as congenital abnormalities, hypertension (possible interference with testing for ischemia)
- Smoking or consumption of alcohol or caffeinated drinks within 3 hours before the test (decreased patient tolerance)
- Digoxin (depressed ST segment)
- Vasodilators, antihypertensives, or beta blockers (may alter normal response to the test)

RADIOPHARMACEUTICAL MYOCARDIAL PERFUSION IMAGING

An imaging test also known as chemical stress imaging, radiopharmaceutical myocardial perfusion imaging is an alternative method of assessing coronary vessel function in patients who can't tolerate exercise electrocardiography (ECG).

In this test, I.V. infusion of a selected drug — for example, adenosine, dobutamine, or dipyridamole — is used to simulate the effects of exercise by increasing blood flow in the coronary arteries. Next, a radiopharmaceutical is injected I.V. to allow imaging that assists in evaluating the cardiac vessel's response to the drug-induced stress. Both resting and stress images are obtained to evaluate coronary perfusion.

Purpose
- To assess the presence and degree of coronary artery disease (CAD)
- To evaluate therapeutic procedures, such as bypass surgery or coronary angioplasty

Patient preparation
- Describe the test, including who will perform it and where it will take place.
- Tell the patient he'll need to arrive 1 hour before the test and that an I.V. line will be initiated before the test.
- If the patient will receive adenosine or dipyridamole, instruct him to avoid taking all theophylline medications for 24 to 36 hours and all caffeinated drinks for 12 hours before the test.
- If the patient will receive dobutamine, instruct him to withhold beta blockers for 48 hours before the test. Also tell him not to eat for 3 to 4 hours before the test, although he may have water. Instruct him to take his other medications as prescribed with sips of water.
- Tell the patient that a cardiologist, a nurse, an ECG technician, and a nuclear medicine technologist will be present for the medication infusion. Advise him that he'll be weighed first to determine the proper drug dose.
- Inform the patient that he may experience flushing, shortness of breath, dizziness, headache, chest pain, and increased heart rate during the infusion, but that these will end as soon as the infusion ends and that emergency equipment will be available, if needed.
- Make sure the patient or a responsible family member has signed an informed consent form.

Procedure and posttest care
- Place the patient on a bed or an examination table in the ECG or medical imaging department, and start an I.V. line.

- Apply 12 ECG leadwires to appropriate sites, and obtain baseline ECG and blood pressure readings.
- The selected chemical stress medication is infused and blood pressure, pulse, and cardiac rhythm are monitored continuously.
- Tell the patient to report the symptoms he's feeling.
- At the appropriate time, the selected radiopharmaceutical is injected.
- Depending on which radiopharmaceutical is used, the patient either undergoes imaging immediately or is instructed to return for imaging 45 minutes to 2 hours later. Resting imaging may be done before stress imaging or 3 to 4 hours afterward, depending on the radiopharmaceutical used.
- Tell the patient when he needs to return and whether he should continue to fast.
- Remove the I.V. line after the images are completed.
- When all scans are completed, allow the patient to resume his regular diet.

Precautions
- This test is usually contraindicated in pregnant women.
- The use of adenosine or dipyridamole is contraindicated in bronchospastic lung disease or asthma.

Normal findings
Imaging should reveal characteristic distribution of the radiopharmaceutical throughout the left ventrical and show no visible defects.

Abnormal findings
Cold spots are usually due to CAD but may result from myocardial fibrosis, attenuation due to soft tissue (for example, breasts and diaphragm), or coronary spasm. The absence of cold spots in the presence of CAD may result from insignificant artifact obstruc-

tion, single-vessel disease, or collateral circulation.

Interfering factors
• Systolic blood pressure greater than 200 mm Hg (forces a delay in the dobutamine stress test until blood pressure is under control)
• Cold spots due to artifacts, such as implants and electrodes
• Delayed imaging (may cause absence of cold spots in the presence of CAD)

AMBULATORY ELECTROCARDIOGRAPHY

Also called Holter monitoring, ambulatory electrocardiography (ECG) involves the continuous recording of heart activity over a 24-hour period as the patient follows his normal routine. During this period, the patient wears a small reel-to-reel or cassette tape recorder connected to electrodes placed on his chest and keeps a diary of his activities and any associated symptoms. After the recording period, the tape is analyzed by a computer and a doctor to correlate cardiac irregularities, such as arrhythmias and ST-segment changes, with the activities noted in the patient's diary.

Purpose
• To detect cardiac arrhythmias missed by an exercise or resting ECG
• To evaluate chest pain
• To evaluate cardiac status after acute myocardial infarction (MI) or pacemaker implantation
• To evaluate the effectiveness of antiarrhythmic drug therapy
• To assess and correlate dyspnea, central nervous system symptoms (such as

syncope and light-headedness), and palpitations with actual cardiac events and the patient's activities

Patient preparation
• Explain to the patient that this test helps determine how the heart responds to normal activity or, if appropriate, cardioactive medication. Tell him that electrodes will be attached to his chest and that his chest may be shaved.
• Explain that he'll wear a small tape recorder for 24 hours (for 5 to 7 days if a patient-activated monitor is being used), and show him how to position the recorder when he lies down.
• Encourage him to continue his routine activities during the monitoring period. Stress the importance of logging his usual activities (such as walking, climbing stairs, urinating, sleeping, and sexual activity), emotional upsets, physical symptoms (dizziness, palpitations, fatigue, chest pain, and syncope), and ingestion of medication; show the patient a sample diary.
• Tell him to wear loose-fitting clothing with front-buttoning tops during monitoring.
• Demonstrate the proper use of specific equipment, including how to mark the tape (if applicable) at the onset of symptoms.
• If a patient-activated monitor is being used, show the patient how to press the event button to activate the monitor if he experiences an unusual sensation. Instruct him not to tamper with the monitor or disconnect the leadwires or electrodes.
• Advise him to avoid magnets, metal detectors, high-voltage areas, and electric blankets. Show him how to check the recorder to make sure it's working properly. Instruct him how to troubleshoot problems if the monitor alarm sounds. Explain that if the monitor

light flashes, one of the electrodes may be loose and he should depress the center of each one. Tell him to notify you if one comes off.

• If the patient won't be returning to the office or hospital immediately after the monitoring period, show him how to remove and store the equipment. Remind him to bring the diary when he returns.

Procedure and posttest care

• Clean and gently abrade the electrode sites. Peel the backings from the electrodes and apply them to the correct sites, making sure to press the sides and center of each electrode firmly to ensure proper adhesion.

• Attach the electrode cable securely to the monitor.

• Position the monitor and case as the patient will wear it and then attach the leadwires to the electrodes.

• Make sure the recorder has a new or fully charged battery, insert the tape, and turn on the recorder.

• Test the electrode attachment circuit by connecting the recorder to a standard ECG machine. Watch for artifacts while the patient moves normally (stands, sits).

• After the testing period, remove all chest electrodes and clean the electrode sites.

Precautions

• To eliminate muscle artifact, make sure the lead cable is firmly plugged in. Check to ensure that electrodes aren't placed over large muscle masses, such as the pectorals.

Normal findings

When correlated with the patient's diary, the ECG pattern shows normal sinus rhythm with no significant arrhythmias or ST-segment changes.

Changes in heart rate normally occur during various activities.

Abnormal findings

Abnormalities of the heart detected by ambulatory ECG include premature ventricular contractions (PVCs), conduction defects, tachyarrhythmias, bradyarrhythmias, and brady-tachyarrhythmia syndrome. Arrhythmias may be associated with dyspnea and central nervous system symptoms, such as dizziness and syncope.

During recovery from an MI, this test can monitor for PVCs to determine the prognosis and effectiveness of drug therapy.

ST-T wave changes associated with ischemia may coincide with chest pain or increased patient activity. ST-segment changes associated with an acute MI require careful study because smoking, eating, postural changes, certain drugs, Wolff-Parkinson-White syndrome, bundle-branch block, myocarditis, myocardial hypertrophy, anemia, hypoxemia, and abnormal hemoglobin binding can produce a similar tracing on the ECG. Monitoring the MI patient for 1 to 3 days before discharge and again 4 to 6 weeks after discharge may detect ST-T wave changes associated with ischemia or arrhythmias; such information aids patient therapy and rehabilitation and refines the prognosis. Monitoring a patient with an artificial pacemaker may detect an arrhythmia, such as bradycardia, that the pacemaker fails to override.

Although ambulatory ECG correlates patient symptoms and ECG changes, it doesn't always identify the symptoms' causes. If initial monitoring proves inconclusive, the test may be repeated.

Interfering factors

- Electrode placement over muscle mass, poor electrode contact with skin, or other failure to correctly apply the electrodes (possible muscle or movement artifact)
- Patient's failure to carefully record daily activities and symptoms, to maintain his normal routine, or to turn on the monitor during symptoms (if using a patient-activated monitor)
- Physiologic variation in arrhythmia frequency and severity (possible failure to detect arrhythmia during 24-hour Holter monitoring)

SIGNAL-AVERAGED ELECTROCARDIOGRAPHY

Signal averaging is the amplification, averaging, and filtering of an electrocardiogram (ECG) signal that's recorded on the body surface by orthogonal leads. The recording detects high-frequency, low-amplitude cardiac electrical signals in the last part of the QRS complex and in the ST segment. In patients who have survived an acute myocardial infarction (MI), these distinctive signals, called late potentials, may represent delayed disorganized activity in abnormal areas of the myocardium at the interface of fibrous scar tissue and normal tissue. This activity can lead to life-threatening ventricular arrhythmias.

In this computerized procedure, each electrode lead input is amplified, its voltage measured or sampled at intervals of 1 msec or less, and each sample converted into a digital number. The ECG is thereby converted from an analogue voltage waveform into a series of digital numbers that are, in essence, a computer-readable ECG of 100 or more QRS complexes.

Purpose

- To detect late potentials and evaluate the risk of life-threatening arrhythmias

Patient preparation

- Explain to the patient that this test is used to evaluate the electrical activity of his heart and his potential for developing a life-threatening arrhythmia.
- Inform him that the test will be performed by a technician who has been specially trained to monitor recording and computerized equipment used to analyze the signal-averaged ECG.
- Describe the test, including who will perform it and where and its expected duration (about 30 minutes).
- Tell him that electrodes will be attached to his arms, legs, and chest and that the procedure is painless.
- Explain that during the test, he'll be asked to lie still and breathe normally. This is important because limb movement or the sound of his voice will distort the recording.
- Inform him that he needn't restrict food or fluids before the test.
- Record on the patient's chart any use of antiarrhythmics.

Equipment

Recording paper, disposable electrodes or reusable electrodes with suction bulbs, conductive gel, rubber straps, 4″ × 4″ gauze pads, moist cloth towel, sterile drape, computer equipment for analyzing the recorded ECG

Procedure and posttest care

- Place the patient in the supine position. If he can't tolerate lying flat, help him into the semi-Fowler position.

● Have him expose his chest, both ankles, and both wrists for electrode placement. If the patient is a woman, provide a chest drape until the chest leads are applied.

● The test is performed by a technician who is specially trained to operate the recording and computer equipment used in analyzing the signal-averaged ECG.

● The technician gathers the multiple inputs necessary for signal averaging from standard orthogonal bipolar X, Y, and Z leads over a series of ECG cycles. The average is taken over a large number of beats, typically 100 or more.

● After the test is completed, disconnect the equipment. If suction cups were used, be sure to wash the conductive gel from the patient's skin.

Precautions

● The recording equipment and other nearby electrical equipment should be properly grounded to prevent electrical interference.

● Tissue-electrode artifacts can be minimized by lightly sanding the skin with fine sandpaper (no. 220), wiping with alcohol, and using silver-silver chloride electrodes.

● Urge the patient to lie as quiet and motionless as possible to avoid signal distortion.

Normal findings

A QRS complex without low potentials is considered normal.

The areas of interest in the signal-averaged ECG are the following:

● duration of the filtered QRS complex (QRST), which indicates how long the completion of the QRS complex is delayed by late potentials

● amount of energy in the late potentials, as indicated by the root mean square (RMS) voltage in the terminal 40 msec of the QRS complex (RMS40)

● duration of the late potentials, as indicated by the duration of the low-amplitude signals of less than 40 µV in the terminal QRS region (LAS40).

The preceding values can be read either from the signal-averaged ECG itself or from the computer system.

Defining a late potential and scoring a signal-averaged ECG as normal or abnormal are highly dependent on technique. Representative criteria are that late potentials exist when the filtered QRS complex is longer than 114 msec, when there is less than 20 µV RMS of signal in the terminal 40 msec of the filtered QRS, or when the terminal portion of the filtered QRS remains below 40 µV for longer than 38 msec.

Abnormal findings

Identifying late potentials after the QRS complex indicates a risk for ventricular arrhythmias. Late potentials are most common and of greater prognostic value in patients who have sustained an MI. Those patients who don't have late potentials are at low risk for serious ventricular arrhythmias and sudden death. Although the predictive accuracy of a positive signal-averaged ECG is relatively low, it has been advocated as a screening test for patients who should undergo electrophysiologic testing.

Interfering factors

● Artifact from skeletal muscle movement (possible need to administer a muscle relaxant)

● Electromagnetic interference (possible need to shield and twist input cables to reduce noise)

● Poor tissue-electrode contact (production of artifact)

● Antiarrhythmic drugs

IMPEDANCE PLETHYSMOGRAPHY

Also called impedance phlebography, this reliable, widely used, noninvasive test measures venous flow in the limbs. Electrodes from a plethysmograph are applied to the patient's leg to record changes in electrical resistance (impedance) caused by blood volume variations that may result from respiration or venous occlusion.

Purpose
• To detect deep vein thrombosis (DVT) in the proximal deep veins of the leg
• To screen patients at high risk for thrombophlebitis
• To evaluate patients with suspected pulmonary embolism (because most pulmonary emboli are complications of DVT in the leg)

Equipment
Recording paper, disposable electrodes, pressure cuff, moist cloth towel

Patient preparation
• Explain to the patient that this test helps detect DVT.
• Inform him that he needn't restrict food, fluid, or medications before the test.
• Explain that the test requires that both legs be tested and that three to five tracings may be made for each leg.
• Tell him who will perform the test and where and that it takes 30 to 45 minutes.
• Assure him that the test is painless and safe.

• Emphasize that accurate testing requires that leg muscles be relaxed and breathing be normal. Reassure him that if he experiences pain that interferes with leg relaxation, a mild analgesic will be administered.
• Just before the test, instruct him to void and to put on a hospital gown.

Procedure and posttest care
• Place the patient in the supine position, elevating the leg to be tested 30 to 35 degrees. To promote venous drainage, place the calf above heart level.
• Ask him to flex his knee slightly and to rotate his hips by shifting weight to the same side as the leg being tested.
• After the electrodes have been loosely attached to the calf, the pressure cuff is wrapped snugly around the thigh.
• The pressure cuff is inflated to 45 to 60 cm H_2O, allowing full venous distention without interfering with arterial blood flow. Pressure is maintained for 45 seconds or until the tracing stabilizes. (In a patient with reduced arterial blood flow, pressure is maintained for 2 minutes or longer, after which the pressure cuff is rapidly deflated.)
• The strip chart tracing, which records the increase in venous volume after cuff inflation and the decrease in venous volume 3 seconds after deflation, is checked. Then the test is repeated for the other leg. If necessary, three to five tracings for each leg are obtained to confirm full venous filling and outflow; the tracing showing the greatest rise and fall in venous volume is used as the test result.
• If the result is ambiguous, the position of the patient's leg as well as cuff and electrode placement are checked.
• After the test, make sure the conductive gel is removed from the patient's skin.

Normal findings

Temporary venous occlusion normally produces a sharp rise in venous volume; release of the occlusion produces rapid venous outflow.

Abnormal findings

When clots in a major deep vein obstruct venous outflow, the pressure in the distal leg (calf) veins rises and these veins become distended. Such veins are unable to expand further when additional pressure is applied with an occlusive thigh cuff. Blockage of major deep veins also decreases the rate at which blood flows from the leg. If significant thrombi are present in a major deep vein of the lower leg (popliteal, femoral, or iliac), both calf vein filling and venous outflow rate are reduced. Note that this test is less sensitive for calf vein clots or partially occlusive thrombi because they are less likely to cause detectable obstruction in veins below the knee.

Interfering factors

• Decreased peripheral arterial blood flow due to shock, increased vasoconstriction, low cardiac output, or arterial occlusive disease
• Extrinsic venous compression, as from pelvic tumors, large hematomas, constricting clothing, or bandages
• Failure to breathe normally or to completely relax leg muscles due to pain
• Cold extremities due to cold room temperature
• Irregular respiratory pattern
• Muscle pain
• Patient's inability to tolerate the supine position with extremities elevated above the heart

CARDIAC CATHETERIZATION

This test involves passing a catheter into the right or left side of the heart. Catheterization can determine blood pressure and blood flow in the chambers of the heart, permit collection of blood samples, and record films of the heart's ventricles (contrast ventriculography) or arteries (coronary arteriography or angiography).

In catheterization of the left side of the heart, a catheter is inserted into an artery in the antecubital fossa or into the femoral artery through a puncture or cutdown procedure. Guided by fluoroscopy, the catheter is advanced retrograde through the aorta into the coronary artery orifices and left ventricle. Then, a contrast medium is injected into the ventricle, permitting radiographic visualization of the ventricle and coronary arteries and filming (cineangiography) of heart activity.

Catheterization of the left side of the heart assesses the patency of the coronary arteries, mitral and aortic valve function, and left ventricular function. It aids diagnosis of left ventricular enlargement, aortic stenosis and insufficiency, aortic root enlargement, mitral insufficiency, aneurysm, and intracardiac shunt.

In catheterization of the right side of the heart, the catheter is inserted into an antecubital vein or the femoral vein and is advanced through the inferior vena cava or right atrium into the right side of the heart and the pulmonary artery. Catheterization of the right side of the heart assesses tricuspid and pulmonic valve function and pulmonary artery pressures.

Purpose

- To evaluate valvular insufficiency or stenosis, septal defects, congenital anomalies, myocardial function and blood supply, and cardiac wall motion

Patient preparation

- Explain to the patient that this test evaluates the function of the heart and its vessels.
- Instruct him to restrict food and fluids for at least 6 hours before the test but to continue his prescribed drug regimen unless directed otherwise.
- Describe the test, including who will perform it, where it will take place, and its duration.
- Make sure the patient or a responsible family member has signed an informed consent form.
- Inform the patient that he may receive a mild sedative but will remain conscious during the procedure. He'll be strapped to a padded table, and the table may be tilted so that his heart can be examined from different angles.
- Warn him that the catheterization team will wear gloves, masks, and gowns to protect him from infection and that the changing X-ray plates and advancing film will make clacking noises.
- Inform him that he'll have an I.V. needle inserted in his arm to administer medication. Assure him that the electrocardiography (ECG) electrodes attached to his chest during the procedure will cause no discomfort.
- Tell him that the catheter will be inserted into an artery or a vein in his arm or leg; if the skin above the vessel is hairy, it'll be shaved and cleaned with an antiseptic.
- Explain that he'll experience a transient stinging sensation when a local anesthetic is injected to numb the incision site for catheter insertion, and he may experience pressure as the cath-

eter moves along the blood vessel. Assure him that these sensations are normal.

- Inform him that injection of a contrast medium through the catheter may produce a hot, flushing sensation or nausea that quickly passes; instruct him to follow directions to cough or breathe deeply.
- Explain that he'll be given medication if he experiences chest pain during the procedure and may also receive nitroglycerin periodically to dilate coronary vessels and aid visualization.
- Check the patient's history for hypersensitivity to shellfish, iodine, or the contrast media used in other diagnostic tests; notify the doctor of any hypersensitivities.
- If the patient is scheduled for catheterization of the right side of the heart, discontinue any anticoagulant therapy to reduce the risk of complications from venous bleeding. If he's scheduled for catheterization of the left side of the heart, begin or continue anticoagulant therapy to reduce the risk of arterial catheter-tip clotting.
- Just before the procedure, tell the patient to void and put on a hospital gown.

Procedure and posttest care

- The patient is placed in the supine position on a tilt-top table and secured by restraints. ECG leads are applied for continuous monitoring, and an I.V. line, if not already in place, is started with dextrose 5% in water or normal saline solution at a keep-vein-open rate.
- After a local anesthetic is injected at the catheterization site, a small incision or percutaneous puncture is made into the artery or vein, and the catheter is passed through the needle into the vessel; the catheter is guided to the cardiac chambers or coronary arteries using fluoroscopy.

• When the catheter is in place, the contrast medium is injected through it.
• The patient may be asked to cough or breathe deeply. Coughing helps counteract nausea or light-headedness caused by the contrast medium and can correct arrhythmias produced by its depressant effect on the myocardium; deep breathing can ease catheter placement into the pulmonary artery or the wedge position and moves the diaphragm downward, making the heart easier to visualize.
• During the procedure, the patient may be given nitroglycerin to eliminate catheter-induced spasm or measure its effect on the coronary arteries. Ergonovine maleate, a vasoconstrictor, may be administered to provoke coronary artery spasm (a risky but valuable test in Prinzmetal's angina).
• Monitor heart rate and rhythm, respiratory and pulse rates, and blood pressure frequently during the procedure.
• After completion of the procedure, the catheter is removed and pressure should be applied to the incision site for about 15 minutes either manually or with a mechanical compression device. An adhesive bandage or clear occlusive dressing should be applied to protect the site and permit visualization for detection of bleeding or hematoma formation.
• Monitor vital signs every 15 minutes for 1 hour after the procedure and then every hour until stable. If unstable, check every 5 minutes and notify the doctor.
• Observe the insertion site for a hematoma or blood loss. Additional compression may be necessary to control bleeding.
• Check the patient's color, skin temperature, and peripheral pulse below the puncture site every 15 minutes for 1 hour. Once the patient is stable, check every hour.
• Enforce bed rest for 8 hours. If the femoral route was used for catheter insertion, keep the patient's leg extended for 6 to 8 hours; if the antecubital fossa was used, keep the patient's arm extended for at least 3 hours.
• If medications were withheld before the test, check with the doctor about resuming administration.
• Administer prescribed analgesics.
• Unless the patient is scheduled for surgery, encourage intake of fluids high in potassium, such as orange juice, to counteract the diuretic effect of the contrast medium.
• Make sure a posttest ECG is scheduled to check for possible myocardial damage.

Precautions
• Coagulopathy, impaired renal function, and debilitation usually contraindicate catheterization of both sides of the heart. Unless a temporary pacemaker is inserted to counteract induced ventricular asystole, left bundle-branch block contraindicates catheterization of the right side of the heart.
• If the patient has valvular heart disease, prophylactic antimicrobial therapy may be indicated to guard against subacute bacterial endocarditis.

Normal findings
Cardiac catheterization should reveal no abnormalities of heart chamber size or configuration, wall motion or thickness, direction of blood flow, or valve motion; the coronary arteries should have a smooth and regular outline and vessels should be patent.

Cardiac catheterization provides information on pressures in the heart's chambers and vessels. Higher pressures than normal are clinically signifi-

Normal Pressure Curves

Chambers of right side of heart

Two pressure complexes are represented for each chamber. Complexes at far right in this diagram represent simultaneous recordings of pressures from the right atrium, right ventricle, and pulmonary artery.

Chambers of left side of heart

Overall pressure configurations are similar to those of the right side of the heart, but pressures in the left side of the heart are significantly higher because systemic flow resistance is much greater than pulmonary resistance.

KEY:
PA = Pulmonary artery
RV = Right ventricle
RA = Right atrium
a wave = Contraction
v wave = Passive filling
LV = Left ventricle

KEY:
LA = Left atrium
AscAo = Ascending aorta
1 = RV peak systolic pressure
2 = RV end-diastolic pressure
3 = PA peak systolic pressure
4 = PA dicrotic notch
5 = PA diastolic pressure

cant; lower pressures, except in shock, usually aren't significant. (See *Normal pressure curves,* above, and *Upper limits of normal pressures in cardiac chambers and great vessels in recumbent adults,* page 700.)

Cardiac catheterization also provides information for determining the ejection fraction, a comparison of the amount of blood ejected from the left ventricle during systole with the amount of blood remaining in the left ventricle at the end of diastole. A normal ejection fraction (60% to 70%) is a good indicator for successful cardiac surgery.

Abnormal findings

Common abnormalities confirmable by cardiac catheterization include coronary artery disease (CAD), myocardial incompetence, valvular heart disease, and septal defects.

In *CAD,* catheterization shows constriction of the lumen of the coronary arteries. Constriction greater than 70% is especially significant, particularly in proximal lesions. Narrowing of the left main coronary artery and occlusion or narrowing high in the left anterior descending artery are often indications for revascularization surgery. (This lesion responds best to coronary artery bypass grafting.)

UPPER LIMITS OF NORMAL PRESSURES IN CARDIAC
CHAMBERS AND GREAT VESSELS IN RECUMBENT ADULTS

CHAMBER OR VESSEL	PRESSURE (mm Hg)
Right atrium	6 (mean)
Right ventricle	30/6*
Pulmonary artery	30/12* (mean, 18)
Left atrium	12 (mean)
Left ventricle	140/12*
Ascending aorta	140/90* (mean, 105)
Pulmonary artery wedge	Almost identical (±1 to 2 mm Hg) to left atrial mean pressure

* Peak systolic and end-diastolic

Impaired wall motion can indicate *myocardial incompetence* from CAD, aneurysm, cardiomyopathy, or congenital anomalies. Comparing the size of the left ventricle in systole and diastole helps assess the efficiency of cardiac muscle contraction, segmental wall motion, chamber size, and ejection fraction. An ejection fraction under 35% generally increases the risk of complications and decreases the probability of successful surgery.

Valvular heart disease is indicated by a gradient, or difference in pressures, above and below a heart valve. For example, systolic pressure measurements on both sides of a stenotic aortic valve show a gradient across the valve. The higher the gradient, the greater the degree of stenosis. If left ventricular systolic pressure measures 200 mm Hg and aortic systolic pressure measures 120 mm Hg, the gradient across the valve is 80 mm Hg. Because these pressures should normally be equal during systole, when the aortic valve is open, a gradient of this magnitude indicates the need for corrective surgery. Incompetent valves can be visualized during ventriculography by watching retrograde flow of the contrast medium across the valve during systole.

Septal defects (both atrial and ventricular) can be confirmed by measuring blood oxygen content in both sides of the heart. Elevated blood oxygen levels on the right side indicate a left-to-right atrial or ventricular shunt; decreased oxygen levels on the left side indicate a right-to-left shunt.

Cardiac output can be measured by analyzing blood oxygen levels in the cardiac chambers. This may be accomplished by drawing blood from cardiac chambers or by injecting contrast medium into the venous circulation and measuring its concentration as it moves past a thermodilution catheter.

Interfering factors
- Allergy to iodine, shellfish, or contrast media
- Renal failure (hampering ability to receive contrast medium)
- Poor technique or equipment function
- Patient anxiety (increase in heart rate and cardiac chamber pressures)

PULMONARY ARTERY CATHETERIZATION

In this procedure, also known as Swan-Ganz catheterization, a balloon-tipped, flow-directed catheter is threaded through the right atrium to provide intermittent occlusion of the pulmonary artery (PA). PA catheterization permits measurement of both pulmonary artery pressure (PAP) and pulmonary artery wedge pressure (PAWP, also known as pulmonary capillary wedge pressure).

The PAWP reading accurately reflects left atrial pressure and left ventricular end-diastolic pressure, although the catheter itself never enters the left side of the heart. Obtaining this information is possible because the heart momentarily relaxes during diastole as it fills with blood from the pulmonary veins; at this instant, the pulmonary vasculature, left atrium, and left ventricle act as a single chamber, and all have identical pressures. Thus, changes in PAP and PAWP reflect changes in left ventricular filling pressure, permitting detection of left ventricular impairment.

The procedure is usually performed at bedside in an intensive care unit. The catheter is inserted through the cephalic vein in the antecubital fossa or the subclavian (sometimes femoral) vein. In addition to measuring atrial and PA pressures, this procedure evaluates pulmonary vascular resistance and tissue oxygenation, as indicated by mixed venous oxygen content. It should be performed cautiously in patients with left bundle-branch block or implanted pacemakers.

Purpose
- To help assess right and left ventricular function
- To diagnose, monitor, and treat myocardial infarction, cardiogenic shock, septic shock, pulmonary edema, fluid-related hypovolemia and hypotension, systolic murmur, unexplained sinus tachycardia, and various cardiac arrhythmias
- To monitor fluid status in patients with serious burns, renal disease, and noncardiogenic pulmonary edema after open-heart surgery
- To monitor the effects of cardiovascular drugs, such as nitroglycerin and nitroprusside

Patient preparation
- Explain to the patient that this test evaluates heart function and provides data necessary to determine appropriate therapy or manage fluid status.
- Tell him that he needn't restrict food or fluids before the test.
- Describe the test, including who will perform it and where.
- Tell him that he'll be conscious during catheterization and may experience transient discomfort from administration of the local anesthetic.
- Explain that catheter insertion takes about 30 minutes but that the catheter will remain in place, causing little or no discomfort, for 48 to 72 hours.
- Instruct him to report any discomfort immediately.

• Make sure the patient or a responsible family member has signed an informed consent form.

Equipment

Pressure cuff; balloon-tipped, flow-directed PA catheter; bag of heparinized normal saline solution (usually 500 ml of normal saline solution with 500 to 1,000 units of heparin, if ordered); alcohol sponges; medication-added label; pressure bag; pressure tubing with flush device and disposable transducer; I.V. pole with transducer mount; emergency resuscitation equipment; armboard (for antecubital insertion); lead aprons (if fluoroscope is used during insertion); sutures; 4″ × 4″ gauze pads or other dry occlusive dressing material; prepackaged introducer kit; dextrose 5% in water; shaving materials (optional).

If a prepackaged introducer kit is unavailable, obtain the following: an introducer (one size larger than the catheter), sterile tray containing instruments for procedure, masks, sterile gowns and gloves, povidone-iodine ointment, sutures, two 10-ml syringes, local anesthetic (1% to 2% lidocaine), one 5-ml syringe, 25G needle, 1″ and 3″ tape.

Procedure and posttest care

• Choose an appropriate flexible PA catheter. Catheters used in this test come in two- to five-lumen modes and in various lengths. One lumen contains the balloon and the balloon inflation valve.

• Before catheterization, set up the equipment according to the manufacturer's directions and the facility's protocol.

• If the insertion site is being prepared for a cutdown procedure, prepare the patient's skin and cover it with a sterile drape.

• Assist the patient to the supine position. For antecubital insertion, his arm is abducted with palm upward on an overbed table for support; for subclavian insertion, the patient is placed in the supine position with his head and shoulders slightly lower than his trunk to make the vein more accessible. If the patient can't tolerate the supine position, assist him to the semi-Fowler position. During the test, monitor all pressures with the patient in the same position.

• Check the catheter balloon for defects using sterile technique, and flush all ports to ensure patency.

• The catheter introducer is inserted into the vein percutaneously or by cutdown.

• Then, the catheter is inserted through the introducer and directed to the right atrium, and the catheter balloon is partially inflated so that venous flow carries the catheter tip through the right atrium and tricuspid valve into the right ventricle and the PA.

• Observe the monitor for characteristic waveform changes. Obtain a printout of each stage of catheter insertion.

• Instruct the patient to extend the appropriate arm (or leg, if the catheter is inserted into the femoral vein).

• As the catheter is passed into the chambers of the right side of the heart, observe the monitor screen for frequent premature ventricular contractions or tachycardia (including ventricular tachycardia), which may result from right ventricular catheter irritation. If irritation occurs, the catheter may be partially withdrawn or medication administered to suppress the arrhythmia or right bundle-branch block.

• A chest X-ray is obtained to verify catheter placement.

• To record the PAWP, carefully inflate the catheter balloon with the specified amount of air; the catheter tip will float into the wedge position, as indicated by an altered waveform on the monitor screen. If a PAWP waveform occurs with less than the recommended inflation volume, don't inflate the balloon further.

• After the balloon is inflated, record the PAWP. Then allow the balloon to deflate passively. This allows the catheter to float back into the PA. Observe the monitor screen for a PA waveform.

• Don't overinflate the balloon catheter. Overinflation could distend the PA, causing vessel rupture.

• If the balloon can't be fully deflated after recording the PAWP, don't re-inflate it unless the doctor is present; balloon rupture may cause a life-threatening air embolism. Check all connections for air leaks that may have prevented balloon inflation, particularly if the patient is confused or uncooperative.

• When the catheter's correct positioning and function are established, it's sutured to the skin. Antimicrobial ointment and an airtight dressing are applied to the insertion site.

• Set alarms on the electrocardiogram (ECG) and pressure monitors.

• Monitor vital signs.

• Document PAP waveforms at the beginning of each shift, and monitor them frequently throughout each shift and with changes in treatment. Check PAWP and cardiac output, as ordered.

• Take routine aseptic precautions to prevent infection.

• When the catheter is no longer needed, the dressing is removed and the catheter slowly withdrawn after ensuring that the balloon is deflated. The ECG is monitored for arrhythmias. In some facilities, the doctor is required to remove the catheter.

• After the catheter is withdrawn, the catheter tip is often sent for analysis.

• Apply a sterile dressing over the catheter introducer.

• Observe the site for signs of infection, such as redness, swelling, and discharge.

• Watch for complications, such as pulmonary emboli, PA perforation, heart murmurs, thrombi, and arrhythmias.

Precautions

• Before obtaining a PAWP reading, flush the monitoring system and recalibrate the system per your facility's protocol.

• After obtaining a PAWP, make sure the balloon is completely deflated.

• Maintain 300 mm Hg of pressure in the pressure bag to permit fluid flow of 3 to 6 ml/hour. Instruct the patient to extend the appropriate arm (or leg, if the catheter is inserted in the femoral vein).

• If a damped waveform occurs, the catheter may need to be adjusted. Pulmonary infarct may occur if the catheter is allowed to remain in a wedged position.

• Make sure stopcocks are properly positioned and connections are secure. Loose connections may introduce air into the system or cause blood backup, leakage of deoxygenated blood, or inaccurate pressure readings.

• Be sure the lumen hubs are properly identified to serve the appropriate catheter ports.

• The proximal port of the PA catheter is used to transduce a central venous pressure (CVP) waveform, measure thermodilution cardiac output, and administer I.V. fluids.

● The PA catheter's proximal port can be used for blood sampling. Before sample collection, about 2½ times the catheter's dead-space volume must be withdrawn.

● The distal port is used to transduce a PA waveform and obtain intermittent PAWP. The distal port is also used to measure mixed venous blood gases.

● Infusions shouldn't be administered through the distal port due to the risk of damage to the PA.

● Some PA catheters have an infusion port that can be used to administer fluids into the right atrium or right ventricle.

● If the catheter has not been sutured to the skin, tape it securely to prevent dislodgment.

● If the patient shows signs of sepsis, treat the catheter as the source of infection, and send it for culture when removed.

Reference values

Normal pressures are as follows:
● right atrial CVP: 2 to 8 mm Hg
● systolic PAP: 15 to 28 mm Hg
● diastolic PAP: 5 to 16 mm Hg
● PAWP: 6 to 15 mm Hg
● cardiac output: 3 to 6 L/minute.

Abnormal findings

An abnormally high right atrial pressure can indicate pulmonary disease, failure of the right side of the heart, fluid overload, cardiac tamponade, tricuspid stenosis and insufficiency, or pulmonary hypertension.

Elevated right ventricular pressure can result from pulmonary hypertension, pulmonary valvular stenosis,

right-sided heart failure, pericardial effusion, constrictive pericarditis, chronic heart failure, or ventricular septal defects.

An abnormally high PAP is characteristic in increased pulmonary blood flow, as occurs in a left-to-right shunt secondary to atrial or ventricular septal defect; increased PA resistance, as occurs in pulmonary hypertension or mitral stenosis; chronic obstructive pulmonary disease; pulmonary edema or embolus; and left ventricular failure from any cause. PA systolic pressure is the same as right ventricular systolic pressure. PA diastolic pressure is the same as left atrial pressure, except in patients with severe pulmonary disease causing pulmonary hypertension; in such patients, catheterization is still important diagnostically.

Elevated PAWP can result from left ventricular failure, mitral stenosis and insufficiency, cardiac tamponade, or cardiac insufficiency; depressed PAWP can result from hypovolemia.

Interfering factors

● Malfunctioning monitoring and recording devices, loose connections, clot formation at the catheter tip, air in the fluid column, or a ruptured balloon

● Mechanical ventilation with positive pressure, causing increased intrathoracic pressure (increase in catheter pressure)

● Incorrect catheter placement, causing excessive movement called catheter fling (damped pressure tracing)

● Migration of the catheter against a vessel wall (possible constant occlusion, or wedging, of the PA)

● Extreme patient agitation

ELECTROPHYSIOLOGY STUDIES

Intracardiac electrocardiogram (ECG) recording and stimulation studies have revolutionized the diagnosis and treatment of severe arrhythmias. Electrophysiologic testing is important for evaluating unexplained syncope. The location and severity of atrioventricular (AV) conduction disturbances and sinus node dysfunction can be assessed in symptomatic patients in whom diagnostic information can't be obtained by ambulatory monitoring.

Purpose
• To evaluate recurrent syncope of possible cardiac origin when ambulatory ECG is inconclusive
• To evaluate the efficacy of pharmacotherapy in survivors of aborted sudden death and in other patients with symptomatic or life-threatening ventricular arrhythmias
• To differentiate supraventricular from ventricular arrhythmias
• To evaluate therapy in patients with accessory AV pathways
• To evaluate patients for antitachycardia pacing devices and surgical or catheter ablation procedures

Patient preparation
• Explain to the patient that this test will help evaluate his heart's electrical activity.
• Tell him not to eat or drink anything for at least 6 hours before the test.
• Instruct him to continue his prescribed drug regimen unless his doctor tells him otherwise. Usually, antiarrhythmic drugs will be discontinued before the test because they can interfere with the induction of the arrhythmia.
• Describe the test, including who will perform it, where it will take place, and its duration (3 to 4 hours).
• Inform the patient that he'll be given a mild sedative but will remain conscious during the test.
• Explain that the doctors and nurses will wear gloves, masks, and gowns to protect him from infection.
• Inform him that an I.V. needle will be inserted in his arm to administer medication. Assure him that the ECG electrodes attached to his chest during the test will cause no discomfort.
• Tell him that a catheter will be inserted into an artery or a vein in his groin or arm. If the skin at the site is hairy, it will be shaved and cleaned with an antiseptic.
• Explain that he'll experience a stinging sensation when a local anesthetic is injected to numb the incision site for catheter insertion, and he may experience pressure as the catheter moves along the blood vessel. Assure him that these feelings are normal.
• Inform the patient that during the test, the doctor will attempt to induce an arrhythmia and, if successful, will administer medication to identify which antiarrhythmics stop the arrhythmia. If the medication is unsuccessful, the arrhythmia will be converted by defibrillation.
• Make sure the patient or a responsible family member has signed an informed consent form.
• Just before the procedure, ask the patient to void and to put on a hospital gown.

Procedure and posttest care
• The patient is placed in the supine position on a padded table.

- ECG leads are applied for continuous monitoring. If not already in place, an I.V. line is started and dextrose 5% in water or normal saline solution is administered at a keep-vein-open rate.
- After a local anesthetic is injected at the catheterization site, a small incision or percutaneous puncture is made and the catheter is passed through the needle into the vessel. The catheter is guided to the cardiac chambers using fluoroscopy.
- When the catheter is in place, it can record electrical activity in different areas of the heart and can be used to pace the heart and induce arrhythmias.
- When an arrhythmia is induced, the arrhythmia pathway can be mapped.
- Monitor the patient's vital signs frequently during the test, noting especially a drop in blood pressure during an arrhythmia.
- After completion of the procedure, the catheter is removed and pressure is applied to the incision site for about 15 minutes either manually or with a mechanical compression device. An adhesive bandage or clear occlusive dressing is applied to protect the site and permit visualization for detection of bleeding or hematoma formation.
- Monitor vital signs every 15 minutes for 1 hour after the procedure and then every hour until stable. If unstable, check every 5 minutes and notify the doctor.
- Monitor the patient's heart rhythm closely, and notify the doctor of any arrhythmias that occur.
- Observe the insertion site for hematoma and blood loss. Additional compression of the site may be necessary to control bleeding.
- Check the patient's color, skin temperature, and peripheral pulse below the puncture site every 15 minutes for

1 hour. Once the patient is stable, check every hour for 8 to 12 hours.
- Enforce bed rest for 8 hours. If the femoral route was used for catheter insertion, keep the patient's leg extended for 6 to 8 hours. If the antecubital fossa was used, keep the patient's arm extended for at least 3 hours.
- If medications were withheld before the test, check with the doctor about resuming them.
- Administer prescribed analgesics or antianxiety agents.
- Make sure a posttest ECG is scheduled to check for possible myocardial damage.

Precautions

- Antiarrhythmics should be stopped before the test because they'll interfere with the induction of an arrhythmia.
- Coagulopathies should be corrected before testing because of the potential for bleeding at the catheter insertion site.

Normal findings

If ventricular tachycardia is inducible, antiarrhythmics are started and the patient is restudied with therapeutic drug levels to assess their efficacy in arrhythmia suppression. Placement of an implantable cardioverter-defibrillator (ICD) device is occasionally necessary for patients with poorly controlled, inducible malignant arrhythmias.

The presence of accessory AV pathways allows for rapid conduction of atrial impulses to the ventricles, resulting in "preexcitation." Premature beats may trigger AV reciprocating tachycardias or atrial fibrillation or flutter that can result in extremely fast ventricular rates, eventually resulting in ventricular fibrillation. Electrophysiologic testing can identify the particular arrhythmia and the location of the abnormal pathway. The focus from which the arrhythmia has originated can then be ablated using the electrophysiology catheter. Electrophysiology catheters that are used for ablation are steerable, can deliver radiofrequency energy, and can be used to record the temperature of the tissue being ablated.

Abnormal findings

Many patients who survive an episode of sudden death haven't sustained an infarction and won't have an inducible arrhythmia. Those patients who do have an inducible arrhythmia may not have an identifiable focus that can be ablated. ICD placement in such patients won't prevent the arrhythmia but can treat it when it occurs.

Interfering factors

• Antiarrhythmics (unless testing is to evaluate efficacy)
• Patient's inability to tolerate the procedure

PULSE OXIMETRY

Pulse oximetry is a continuous noninvasive study of arterial blood oxygen saturation (SaO_2) using a clip or probe attached to a sensor site (usually earlobe or fingertip). The percentage expressed is the ratio of oxygen to hemoglobin.

Purpose

• To monitor oxygenation of the tissues and organs perioperatively and during an acute illness
• To monitor oxygenation in patients with higher oxygen needs (such those on a ventilator or those receiving a high percentage of oxygen) or when weaning from an oxygen source
• To monitor oxygen saturation during activities to determine patient tolerance
• To determine effectiveness of bronchodilators
• To monitor oxygenation during testing for sleep apnea

Patient preparation

• Explain to the patient that this test assesses oxygen content in the hemoglobin. Describe the procedure and answer all questions.
• Explain who will perform the test and where and its duration.
• Make sure that the patient has no false fingernails or nail polish.
• Explain to the patient that the area where the clip or probe is attached must be massaged to increase blood flow.

Procedure and posttest care

• Place the probe or clip over the finger or other intended sensor site so that the light beams and sensors are opposite each other.
• Turn on the monitor and ensure that it accurately detects the patient's pulse and reads the percentage of oxygen.
• If the monitor is to remain on continuously, ensure that the skin remains intact under the probe or clip and that the circulation is adequate. Select alternate sensor sites if the skin doesn't remain intact.
• After the test is performed, remove the probe and clean it with alcohol.

Precautions

• Closely observe the monitor and report decreasing or abnormal SaO_2 levels.

Normal findings
SaO_2 levels are normally greater than 95%.

Abnormal findings
Hypoxemia with levels less than 95% indicate impaired cardiopulmonary function or abnormal gas exchange.

Interfering factors
• Movement of the finger, ear, or alternate sensor site
• Improper placement of the probe or clip
• Anemic conditions, vasoconstriction, certain medications (such as vasopressors), hypotension, vessel obstruction, nail polish or false fingernails, administrations of lipid emulsions

CHAPTER 16

Special Function Tests

EYES AND VISION			710
710	Visual acuity tests	712	Ophthalmoscopy
711	Slit-lamp examination	715	Corneal staining

EARS AND HEARING			716
716	Otoscopy	722	Screening tests for vestibular
717	Tuning fork tests		and cerebellar dysfunction
719	Pure tone audiometry		

GASTROINTESTINAL FUNCTION			723
723	Esophageal acidity test	725	Acid perfusion test

RENAL FUNCTION			726
726	Uroflometry	731	External sphincter
728	Cystometry		electromyography

MISCELLANEOUS TESTS			733
733	Tensilon test	741	D-Xylose absorption
735	Cold stimulation test for	742	Dexamethasone suppression test
	Raynaud's syndrome	743	Sleep studies
736	Pulmonary function tests		

EYES AND VISION

VISUAL ACUITY TESTS

A visual acuity test evaluates the patient's ability to distinguish the form and detail of an object. In this test, the patient is asked to read letters on a standardized visual chart, commonly called the Snellen chart, from a distance of 20′ (6 m). Charts showing the letter E in various positions and sizes are used for young children and other people who can't read. The smaller the symbol the patient can identify, the sharper his visual acuity. A patient's near (reading) vision may be tested as well, using a standardized chart such as the Jaeger card (a card with print in graded sizes).

The Snellen test should be performed on all patients with eye complaints. Near-vision test is routine for those complaining of eyestrain or reading difficulty and for everyone over age 40. Results serve as a baseline for treatments, follow-up examinations, and referrals.

Purpose
- To test distance and near visual acuity
- To identify refractive errors in vision

Patient preparation
- Tell the patient that these tests evaluate distant and near vision.
- Explain that the tests take only a few minutes. If he wears glasses, tell him to bring them to the examination.

Equipment
Standardized eye charts, including the Snellen or E chart and Jaeger card; occlusion supplies, including a handheld occluder and disposable tissues for insertion between the patient's eyes and glasses; disposable eye patches; standard 20′ (6-m) room or equipment to simulate correct distance (mirrors or chart with proportionately reduced letters)

Procedure and posttest care
Distance visual acuity
- Have the patient sit 20′ away from the eye chart. If he's wearing glasses, tell him to remove them so his uncorrected vision can be tested first.
- Begin with the right eye unless vision in the left eye is known to be more acute. Have the patient occlude the left eye; then ask him to read the smallest line of letters he can see on the chart. Encourage him to try to read lines he can't see clearly because intelligent guesses usually indicate that the patient can recognize some of the symbols' details.
- Record the number of the smallest line the patient can read. This number is expressed as a fraction. The numerator is the distance between the patient and the chart; the denominator is the distance from which a patient with normal vision can read the line. The greater the denominator, the poorer the vision.
- If the patient makes an error on a line, record the results with a minus number. For example, if the patient reads the 20/40 line but makes one error, record his vision as $20/40 - 1$. If the patient reads the 20/40 line and one symbol on the next line, record his vision as 20/40+1.
- Have the patient occlude the right eye, and repeat the test for the left eye. To minimize recall, use a different set of symbols or have the patient read the lines backward.
- If the patient wears glasses, test his corrected vision using the same procedure. If he normally wears glasses but doesn't have them with him, note this on the test results.

- In recording the patient's responses, indicate which eye was tested and whether it was tested with or without corrective lenses.
- If the patient can't read the largest letter on the chart, further testing is necessary.

Near visual acuity
- Have the patient remove his glasses and occlude the left eye. Ask him to read the Jaeger card at his customary reading distance. Both eyes are tested with and without corrective lenses.
- In reporting near visual acuity, specify both the size of the smallest print legible to the patient and the nearest distance at which reading is possible.

Normal findings
Most charts for distance visual acuity are read at 20′ (6 m). If the patient's vision is normal, results are expressed as 20/20, which means that the smallest symbol he can identify at 20′ is the same symbol a patient with normal vision can identify from the same distance.

If the patient can read the 20/20 line on the Snellen chart, he has normal distance visual acuity. If the denominator is more than 20 (for example, 40), his visual acuity is less than normal. In this case, it means he reads at 20′ what a person with normal vision can read at 40′ (12 m). A person with visual acuity of 20/200 in the better corrected eye is considered legally blind. Similarly, if the denominator is less than 20, the patient's distance visual acuity is better than normal. For example, 20/15 vision means that the patient can read at 20′ what a person with normal visual acuity can see at 15′ (4.5 m).

Normal near visual acuity is usually recorded as 14/14 because standard testing charts, such as the Jaeger card, are generally held 14″ (35 cm) from the patient's eyes. Decreased near visual acuity is indicated by a larger denominator. For example, 14/20 near vision means that the patient can read at 14″ what a person with normal vision can read at 20″ (50 cm).

Normal or better-than-normal visual acuity doesn't necessarily indicate normal vision. For example, a visual field defect may be present if the patient consistently misses the letters on one side of all the lines. A field defect is present if the patient states that one or more of the letters disappear or become illegible when he is looking at a nearby letter. Such findings indicate the need for further visual field testing, such as the Amsler grid test and the tangent screen examination.

Abnormal findings
Patients with less-than-normal visual acuity require further testing, including refraction and a complete ophthalmologic examination, to determine whether visual loss is due to injury, disease, or a need for corrective lenses.

Interfering factors
- Patient's failure to bring glasses to the examination
- Glasses improperly prescribed or outdated in their degree of correction (possible to have better visual acuity without them)
- Patient's inability to cooperate

SLIT-LAMP EXAMINATION

The slit lamp is an instrument equipped with a special lighting system and a binocular microscope that allows an ophthalmologist to visualize in detail the anterior segment of the eye, including the eyelids, eyelashes, conjunctiva, sclera, cornea, tear film, anterior chamber, iris, crystalline lens, and vitreous face. To evaluate normally transparent or near-transparent ocular fluids and tissues, the size, shape, intensity, and depth of the light source as well as the magnification of the microscope may be altered. If abnormalities are noted, special devices are attached to the slit lamp to allow more detailed investigation.

Purpose
● To detect and evaluate abnormalities of anterior segment tissues and structures

Patient preparation
● Explain to the patient that this examination evaluates the front portion of the eyes. Tell him that the test takes 5 to 10 minutes and requires that he remain still. Reassure him that the examination is painless.
● If he wears contact lenses, tell him to remove them for the test, unless the test is being performed to evaluate the fit of the lens.
● If the test calls for dilating eyedrops, check the patient's history for adverse reactions to mydriatics or for the presence of narrow-angle glaucoma before administering the drops. Dilating eyedrops aren't used in routine eye examinations; however, some diseases require pupillary dilation before slit-lamp examination.

Procedure and posttest care
● Seat the patient in the examining chair. Have him place both feet on the floor and position his chin on the rest and his forehead against the bar. Dim the lights in the room.
● The ophthalmologist examines the patient's eyes starting with the lids and lashes and progressing to the vitreous face, altering light and magnification as necessary. In some cases, a special camera can be attached to the slit lamp to photograph portions of the eye.

● If dilating drops were instilled, tell the patient that his near vision will be blurred for up to 2 hours.

Precautions
● Don't instill mydriatic drops into the eyes of a patient who has had a hypersensitivity reaction to them or who has angle-closure glaucoma.

Normal findings
Slit-lamp examination should reveal no abnormalities of anterior segment tissues and structures.

Abnormal findings
Slit-lamp examination may detect pathologic conditions, such as corneal abrasions and ulcers, lens opacities, iritis, and conjunctivitis, as well as irregularly shaped corneas. A parchment-like consistency of the lid skin, with redness, minor swelling, and moderate itching, may indicate a hypersensitivity reaction. If a corneal abrasion or ulcer is detected, a fluorescein stain may be applied to allow better viewing of the area. If a tearing deficiency is suspected, the ophthalmologist may examine the eye after applying a fluorescein or rose bengal stain; he may also perform the Schirmer tearing test. Some abnormal findings may indicate impending disorders. For example, early-stage lens opacities may signal the development of cataracts.

Interfering factor
● Patient's inability to cooperate

OPHTHALMOSCOPY

Ophthalmoscopy allows magnified examination of the vascular and nerve tissue of the fundus, including the optic disk, retinal vessels, macula, and retina. This test is conducted with either a direct or indirect ophthalmo-scope — one of the most important diagnostic tools in ophthalmology. Generally, examiners use the direct ophthalmoscope, a small, handheld instrument consisting of a light source, viewing device, a reflecting device to channel light into the patient's eyes, and spherical lenses to correct refractive error of the patient or examiner. If a slit lamp isn't available, the examiner may also use the ophthalmoscope to examine the patient's cornea, iris, and lens.

If an abnormality of the retina is suspected, further testing, such as fluorescein angiography, may be necessary. (See *Fluorescein angiography*.)

Purpose
• To detect and evaluate eye disorders as well as ocular manifestations of systemic disease

Patient preparation
• Explain to the patient that this test permits examination of the back of the eye.
• Describe the test, who will perform it, where it will take place, and its duration (usually less than 5 minutes).
• Advise him that eyedrops may be used to dilate the pupils for a clearer examination, but reassure him that he'll experience no discomfort during the test.
• When using eyedrops, check the patient's history for previous use of dilating eyedrops, indications of possible hypersensitivity, and angle-closure glaucoma.

Procedure and posttest care
• Routine examination of the ocular media and fundus is usually conducted without dilating the pupil if there is sufficient light in the ophthalmoscope and room lighting is subdued. If indicated, two instillations of mydriatic

> ## FLUORESCEIN ANGIOGRAPHY
>
> This special diagnostic test is used to visualize and photograph the vascular structures of the eye. A fluorescein angiogram may be used to rule out retinal disease or follow the progression of retinal disorders.
>
> A fundus camera system rapidly photographs the retina after an I.V. injection of sodium fluorescein dye. The dye enters the arteries of the eye and gives a clear view of the vasculature. Then the angiogram is carefully examined to detect the precise location of abnormalities, such as leakage from diabetic retinopathy and age-related macular degeneration.

eyedrops are usually necessary to achieve maximum dilation.
• Have the patient sit upright in the examination chair. Dim the room lights to keep irregular reflections from interfering with the examination.
• The examiner sits about 2′ (60 cm) away from the patient and slightly to his right. The examination begins with the patient's right eye. The ophthalmoscope is held in the right hand in front of the examiner's right eye. A small adjustment near the forefinger allows him to select different lenses quickly.
• The patient is told to look straight ahead at a specific object 20′ (6 m) away, for example, a large symbol on a standardized vision chart, for the duration of the examination.
• Remaining on the patient's right side, the examiner moves forward until he is within 6″ (15 cm) of the patient. At this point, he directs the light beam into the pupil and looks for the red reflex (red reflection from the fundus), which is

visible without magnification. Then he focuses on the optic disk, noting its size, shape, and color.

• Next, the examiner looks for a white central depression in the optic disk — the physiologic cup — and observes the retinal vessels that emerge from the disk.

• Finally, the examiner focuses on the macula — a yellowish depression slightly below the center of the optic disk — and its center, the fovea.

• This procedure is then repeated for the left eye.

Precautions

• Don't administer dilating eyedrops to a patient who has a history of hypersensitivity reactions to them or who has angle-closure glaucoma.

• Make sure the patient maintains fixation throughout the procedure.

Normal findings

With the beam of light from the ophthalmoscope directed into the patient's pupil, the red reflex should be visible through the aperture. The slightly oval optic disk lies to the nasal side of the fundus center. Although its color varies widely, it's usually pink, with darker edges at its nasal border. The physiologic cup, a pale depression in the center of the optic disk, varies widely in size; it tends to be larger in patients with myopia and smaller in those with hyperopia.

The semitransparent retina surrounds the optic disk. Branching out from the disk are the retinal vessels, including venules and the slightly smaller arterioles. Vessel diameter progressively decreases with distance from the optic disk. Retinal arterioles generally have a medium red color; venules appear dark red or blue.

The macula is the most darkly pigmented area of the retina. In its center lies a small, even darker spot — the fovea. A tiny light reflex can be seen at the center of the fovea, caused by reflection of the ophthalmoscopic light from the concave inner surface of the area.

Abnormal findings

An absent or a diminished red reflex may be due to gross corneal lesions, dense opacities of the aqueous or vitreous (such as from blood after hemorrhage), cataracts, or detached retina. A cloudy vitreous that obscures the fundus may be caused by inflammatory disease of the optic disk, retina, or uvea. Fundal lesions should be sketched or photographed for further study.

Optic neuritis causes the optic disk to become elevated and more vascular; small hemorrhages may also occur. Optic nerve atrophy causes the disk to appear white. Papilledema, which may result from increased intracranial pressure, causes abnormal elevation of the disk, blurring of disk margins, engorged vessels, and hemorrhages.

In glaucoma, the physiologic cup may appear enlarged and gray, with white edges. A milky-white retina characterizes the acute phase of a central retinal artery occlusion; the fovea, in contrast to the ischemic macula, appears as a bright red spot. Central retinal vein occlusion is marked by widespread retinal hemorrhaging, patches of white exudate, and disk elevation.

Retinal detachments appear as gray elevated areas, possibly with areas of red vascular choroid exposed by retinal tears. A choroidal tumor appears as a dark lesion.

The integrity of retinal vessels is commonly evaluated to aid diagnosis of systemic disease. Hypertension, for example, causes vasospasm, sclerosis, and eventual occlusion of retinal arterioles, leading to retinal edema and hemorrhage and papilledema. Diabetes mellitus may be complicated by retinal fibroses, patches of white exudate, and microaneurysms. Other systemic disorders present similar findings.

Interpretation of ophthalmoscopic findings depends largely on the examiner's knowledge and experience because an abnormality can arise from several sources. After an ophthalmoscopic evaluation, referral for complete medical evaluation may be necessary.

Interfering factors

• Room not sufficiently dark, inadequate light source, or other condition improper for examination
• Patient's inability to cooperate
• Conditions prohibiting a good view of the fundus, such as insufficient dilation, dense cataracts, cloudy media, and gross nystagmus

CORNEAL STAINING

Corneal staining with fluorescein dye allows a detailed view of the anterior part of the eye that can't ordinarily be seen during slit-lamp examination. A special attachment is used during the slit-lamp examination to enhance visualization.

Purpose

• To detect the depth and pattern of injuries to the corneal surface of the eye
• To diagnose corneal injuries

Patient preparation

• Describe the procedure to the patient. Explain that this test evaluates the eye surface, is painless, and takes about 15 minutes.
• Tell the patient who will perform the test and where.
• Ask the patient for a detailed history of the eye injury and symptoms associated with the injury.

• Ask him to remove glasses or contact lenses before the test.

Procedure and posttest care

• Seat the patient in the examination chair.
• Stain his eye surface with the fluorescein dye by touching the tip of the fluorescein strip to the lower conjunctival sac.
• Ask the patient to close his eye to help spread the dye over the corneal surface.
• Have him sit properly in the examination chair with his forehead placed against the bar apparatus.
• Instruct him to look straight ahead while his eyes are examined with the slit lamp.
• Defects are recorded while the eye is being examined with a bright light.
• Inform the patient that any blurring of vision will gradually disappear within 2 hours.

Precautions

• Monitor the patient for any allergic reaction to the fluorescein dye.
• Because the dye used in this test causes blurred vision, ensure that the patient has a responsible person to drive him home.

Normal findings

The normal cornea is convex in shape and has a smooth, shiny appearance. No scratches or indentations are noted.

Abnormal findings

Abnormal findings include corneal scratches, abrasions, ulcerations, and keratitis.

Interfering factors

• Patient's inability to remain still during the examination
• Allergy to the fluorescein dye

OTOSCOPY

Otoscopy is the direct visualization of the external auditory canal and the tympanic membrane through an otoscope. It's a basic part of physical examination of the ear and should be performed before other auditory or vestibular tests. Otoscopy indirectly provides information about the eustachian tube and the middle ear cavity.

Purpose
• To detect foreign bodies, cerumen, or stenosis in the external canal
• To detect external or middle ear pathology, such as infection or tympanic membrane perforation

Patient preparation
• Describe the procedure to the patient, and explain that this test permits visualization of the ear canal and eardrum.
• Reassure him that the examination is usually painless and takes less than 5 minutes to perform.
• Tell him that his ear will be pulled upward and backward to straighten the canal, to facilitate insertion of the otoscope.

Procedure and posttest care
• When assembling the otoscope, test the lamp and be sure to attach the largest speculum that fits comfortably into the patient's ear.
• With the patient seated, tilt his head slightly away from you so that the ear to be examined is pointed upward.
• Pull the auricle up and back (pull downward if the patient is under age 3); insert the otoscope gently into the ear canal with a downward and forward motion. If insertion is difficult, replace the speculum with a smaller one.
• Look through the lens, and gently advance the speculum until you see the tympanic membrane. Obtain as full a view as possible, and note redness, swelling, lesions, discharge, foreign bodies, and scaling in the canal. Check the tympanic membrane for color, scarring, contours, and perforation.
• Locate the malleus, partially visible through the translucent tympanic membrane. Examine the membrane itself and the surrounding fibrous rim (annulus).

Precautions
• The otoscope should be advanced slowly and gently through the medial portion of the ear canal to avoid irritation of the canal lining, especially if an infection is suspected.
• Continuing to insert an otoscope against resistance may cause perforation of the tympanic membrane.

Normal findings
The normal tympanic membrane is thin, translucent, shiny, and slightly concave. It appears as a pearl gray or pale pink disk that reflects light in its inferior portion. The short process, manubrium mallei, and umbo should be visible but not prominent.

Abnormal findings
Scarring, discoloration, or retraction or bulging of the tympanic membrane indicates a pathologic condition. (See *Common abnormalities of the tympanic membrane.*) Movement of the tympanic membrane in tandem with respiration suggests abnormal patency of the eustachian tube.

COMMON ABNORMALITIES OF THE TYMPANIC MEMBRANE

ABNORMAL FINDINGS	USUAL CAUSE
Bright red color	Inflammation (otitis media)
Yellowish color	Pus or serum behind the tympanic membrane (acute or chronic otitis media)
Fluid behind tympanic membrane	Serous fluid in middle ear (serous otitis media)
Absent light reflection	Bulging tympanic membrane (acute otitis media)
Absent or diminishing landmarks	Thickened tympanic membrane (chronic otitis media, otitis externa, or tympanosclerosis)
Oval dark areas	Perforated or scarred tympanic membrane (otitis media or trauma)
Prominent malleus	Retracted tympanic membrane (nonfunctional eustachian tube)
Reduced mobility	Stiffened middle ear system (serous otitis media or, less frequently, middle ear adhesions)

Interfering factors
• Obstruction of the ear canal by cerumen or foreign matter
• Recumbent position during otoscopy (possible masking of serous otitis media)

TUNING FORK TESTS

The Weber, Rinne, and Schwabach tuning fork tests are quick, valuable screening tools for detecting hearing loss and obtaining preliminary information as to its type. The Weber test determines whether a patient lateralizes the tone of the tuning fork to one ear. The Rinne test compares air and bone conduction in both ears. The Schwabach test compares the patient's bone conduction response with that of the examiner, who is assumed to have normal hearing.

Test results are most reliable when a low-frequency tuning fork is used; results aren't definitive because they depend on subjective factors, such as the examiner's ability to strike the fork with equal force each time and the patient's ability to report audible tones correctly.

Results of the Weber test may be misleading, and the Rinne test frequently doesn't detect a mild conductive hearing loss (10 to 35 dB). Thus, abnormal test results require confirmation by pure tone audiometry.

Purpose
• To screen for or confirm hearing loss
• To help distinguish conductive from sensorineural hearing loss

Patient preparation
● Describe the procedure to the patient, and explain that these tests help detect and assess hearing loss. Tell him who will conduct the tests, and reassure him that they're painless and take only a few minutes.
● Explain that concentration and prompt responses are essential for accurate testing. Have the patient use hand signals to indicate whether a tone is louder in his right ear or left ear and when he stops hearing the tone.
● Inform him that tuning fork tests aren't definitive and that further testing may be necessary to confirm abnormal results.

Procedure and posttest care
● Using a low-frequency tuning fork (256 or 512 Hz), practice achieving a consistent tone by gently striking a prong against your elbow or the heel of your hand, by stroking the prongs upward, or by pinching them together.
● When performing each test, be careful to strike the tuning fork with equal force. Hold the fork at its base to allow the prongs to vibrate freely. Record the name of the test, the result, and the vibrating frequency of the tuning fork.
Weber test
● Vibrate the fork and place its base on the midline of the patient's skull at the forehead.
● Ask the patient if the tone is louder in his left ear or his right ear or is equally loud in both. Describe the results as Weber left, Weber right, or Weber midline, according to his response.
Rinne test
● Test bone conduction by holding the tuning fork between your thumb and index finger and placing the base of the vibrating fork against the patient's mastoid process.
● Test air conduction by moving the vibrating prongs next to (not touching) the external ear. Ask the patient which

location has the louder or longer sound. Repeat the procedure for the other ear.
● Record results as Rinne-positive if the air-conducted sound is heard louder or longer, or Rinne-negative if the bone-conducted sound is heard louder or longer.
Schwabach test
● Holding the tuning fork between thumb and index finger, place the base of the vibrating tuning fork against the patient's left mastoid process and ask if he hears the tone. If he does, immediately place the tuning fork on your left mastoid process and listen for the tone.
● Alternate the tuning fork between the patient's left mastoid process and your own until one of you stops hearing the sound. Record the length of time the patient continues to hear it.
● Repeat the procedure on the right mastoid process.
All tests
● Refer the patient for further audiologic testing if the tuning fork tests suggest a hearing loss.

Normal findings
A patient with normal hearing will respond to the Weber test by hearing the same tone equally loudly in both ears (Weber midline result); to the Rinne test by hearing the air-conducted tone louder or longer than the bone-conducted tone (Rinne-positive result); and to the Schwabach test by hearing the tone for the same duration as the examiner.

Abnormal findings
In the Weber test, lateralization of the tone to one ear suggests a conductive loss on that side or a sensorineural loss on the other side. Lateralization results if the tone is louder in one ear (Stenger effect) or reaches one ear sooner (phase effect). If one ear has a sensorineural loss, the Stenger effect causes

lateralization to the unaffected ear; if one ear has a conductive loss, either the Stenger or phase effect produces lateralization to that ear. If a patient's hearing loss is unilateral, the Weber test may suggest the type of loss. If a patient's hearing loss is bilateral, this test may help to identify the ear with the better bone conduction.

In the Rinne test, hearing the bone-conducted tone louder or longer than the air-conducted tone indicates a conductive loss. In unilateral hearing loss, the tone may be heard louder when conducted by bone, but in the opposite ear; this is a false-negative Rinne test result. A sensorineural loss is indicated when the sound is heard louder by air conduction.

In the Schwabach test, hearing the tone longer than the examiner hears it suggests a conductive loss; conversely, a shorter duration indicates a sensorineural loss. A conductive loss attenuates (decreases the energy of) air-conducted sound in a room with ambient noise, enabling patients with this type of loss to hear bone-conducted sound longer than the examiner can hear such sound.

If the patient has abnormal results on retesting, pure tone audiometry is indicated to confirm hearing loss and determine its type and severity.

Interfering factors
• Failure to strike the tuning fork with equal force or to hold it correctly during the procedure
• Striking the tuning fork on a hard surface rather than on the elbow or knee
• Failure to use either the 512-Hz frequency tuning fork or the more sensitive 256-Hz tuning fork
• Inaccurate patient response due to poor understanding of his task
• Undetected hearing loss in the examiner

PURE TONE AUDIOMETRY

This test, performed with an audiometer, provides a record of the thresholds (the lowest intensity levels) at which a patient can hear a set of test tones introduced through earphones or a bone conduction (sound) vibrator. The energy of these pure tones is concentrated at discrete frequencies. The octave frequencies between 125 and 8,000 Hz are used to obtain air conduction thresholds; frequencies between 250 and 4,000 Hz are used to obtain bone conduction thresholds.

Comparison of air and bone conduction thresholds can suggest a conductive, sensorineural, or mixed hearing loss but doesn't indicate the cause of the loss; further audiologic and vestibular tests and X-rays may be needed. Pure tone audiometry results may also suggest a need to consult an audiologist for evaluation of communication difficulties. (See *Interpreting pure tone audiograms,* page 720.)

Pure tone audiometry is indicated for any patient who requires quantitative hearing assessment. There are no contraindications; however, results depend on the patient's cooperation. Acoustic emission test results may provide additional information.

Purpose
• To determine the presence, type, and degree of hearing loss
• To assess communication abilities and rehabilitation needs

Patient preparation
• Describe the procedure to the patient, and explain that this test determines the presence and degree of hear-

INTERPRETING PURE TONE AUDIOGRAMS

Sensorineural hearing loss depresses both air (circles) and bone (arrows) conduction thresholds to about the same degree. No matter how sound vibrations reach the inner ear, they must be transmitted to higher neural centers through the sensorineural system.

Conductive hearing loss, produced by interference with the conductive mechanism, depresses air conduction thresholds but generally doesn't affect bone thresholds.

Mixed hearing loss involves abnormal air and bone conduction thresholds. Air conduction thresholds demonstrate a greater loss due to a conductive lesion.

ing loss. Explain who will perform the test and where.
• Tell him that each ear will be tested, beginning with the ear with the better hearing acuity. Explain that he'll hear tones at various intensities and that he should signal (or press the response button) each time he hears the tone.

Emphasize that he should respond even if the tone is faint.
• Just before the test, ask the patient to remove any jewelry or apparel that obstructs proper earphone placement.
• Postpone the test if the patient has been exposed to loud noises (loud enough to cause tinnitus or make

face-to-face communication difficult) within the past 16 hours.

Equipment
Otoscope, calibrated audiometer with earphones, and bone conduction vibrator. Note that the test environment must be quiet; a sound-treated room is recommended.

Procedure and posttest care
• The patient's ear canal is checked with the otoscope for impacted cerumen.

• The examiner presses a finger on the auricle and then the tragus to rule out possible closure of the ear canal under pressure from the earphones. If the canal tends to close, a stiff-walled plastic tube is carefully inserted into the canal. This modification is recorded on the audiogram.

• The earphones are positioned properly and the headband is tightened.

• A test tone is presented to the patient's better ear.

Air conduction testing
• A 1,000-Hz tone is presented to the patient's better ear. The intensity of the tone is decreased in 10-dB steps until the patient fails to respond. Then intensity is increased in 5-dB steps until he hears the tone again. Sequences of 10-dB decrements and 5-dB increments are repeated until the patient responds to at least two of three presentations at a single level. The threshold level is the lowest decibel level at which the response rate is at least 50%.

• Using this procedure, tones are presented to the better ear in this order: 1,000 Hz, 2,000 Hz, 4,000 Hz, 8,000 Hz, 1,000 Hz, 500 Hz, and 250 Hz.

• After testing the better ear, the other ear is tested.

Bone conduction testing
• The earphones are removed and the vibrator is placed on the mastoid process of the better ear (the auricle shouldn't touch the vibrator).

• Ascending and descending tones are presented, as in air conduction testing, using 250, 500, 1,000, 2,000, and 4,000 Hz.

Both tests
• Refer the patient to an audiologist if test results are inconsistent or are confounded by possible crossover.

Precautions
• Any modifications of standard testing procedure — such as inserting a plastic tube to prevent ear canal collapse — must be recorded on the audiogram.

Normal findings
The normal range of hearing sensitivity is 0 to 25 dB for adults and 0 to 15 dB for children. Normal test results don't rule out a hearing disorder; a mild middle ear infection or other disorder may exist without interfering with auditory function.

Abnormal findings
The pure tone average, the average of pure tone air conduction thresholds obtained at 500, 1,000, and 2,000 Hz, quantifies the degree of hearing loss. When these three thresholds vary widely, the mean of the best two — the Fletcher average — indicates the degree of hearing loss.

The relation between threshold responses for air and bone conduction tones determines the type of hearing loss. In *sensorineural hearing loss,* both thresholds are depressed; in *conductive hearing loss,* air thresholds are depressed, but bone thresholds are unchanged; and in *mixed hearing loss,* both thresholds are abnormal, with air conduction more depressed than bone conduction. (See *Relating pure tone average to hearing loss and speech audibility,* page 722.)

RELATING PURE TONE AVERAGE TO HEARING LOSS AND SPEECH AUDIBILITY

PURE TONE AVERAGE (dB)	DEGREE OF HEARING LOSS	SPEECH AUDIBILITY
0 to 25	Normal limits	No significant difficulty
26 to 40	Mild	Difficulty with faint or distant speech
41 to 55	Moderate	Difficulty with conversational speech
56 to 70	Moderately severe	Speech must be loud; difficulty with group conversation
71 to 90	Severe	Difficulty with loud speech; understands only shouted or amplified speech
91+	Profound	May not understand amplified speech

Interfering factors

• Impacted cerumen or a closed ear canal (possible 35- to 40-dB artifactual conductive hearing loss)

• Patient's confusion of vibrotactile with auditory sensation or tinnitus with the signal (invalid results)

• Cracked or poorly fitting earphones (low-frequency leakage and false-high thresholds)

• Uncalibrated audiometer or background noise (possible invalidation)

• Presenting extraneous cues to the patient, such as a rhythmic pattern of test tones or hand movement near the attenuator dial (possible invalidation)

• Patient uncooperative or inattentive (possible invalidation)

SCREENING TESTS FOR VESTIBULAR AND CEREBELLAR DYSFUNCTION

A patient who reports disequilibrium, dizziness, or nystagmus may undergo screening tests for vestibular or cerebellar dysfunction. These tests evaluate balance and coordination as the patient performs various maneuvers with eyes open and closed. Abnormal results suggest the need for further evaluation.

Purpose

• To help identify vestibular or cerebellar disorders that affect the entire body (balance tests)

• To help identify vestibular or cerebellar disorders that affect the arms (coordination tests)

Patient preparation

• Explain to the patient that these tests help identify neurologic dysfunction and that some evaluate his sense of balance.

• Describe the tests, including who will perform them and where and their duration.

• Reassure him that he's in no danger of falling during the test.

• Assess the patient's general physical condition, which will influence his ability to perform the maneuvers.

• Check the patient's history for use of drugs that affect the central nervous system (CNS) and for recent alcohol consumption.

Procedure and posttest care
To assess balance
Ask the patient to perform as many of the following test maneuvers as possible, and observe for a tendency to sway or fall.

- Have him stand with his feet together, arms at his sides, and eyes open for 20 seconds. Tell him to maintain this position for another 20 seconds with eyes closed.
- Have the patient stand on one foot for 5 seconds and then on the other foot for 5 seconds; instruct him to repeat the procedure with eyes closed.
- Tell him to stand heel to toe for 20 seconds with eyes opened and then to maintain the same position with eyes closed for another 20 seconds.
- Instruct him to walk forward and backward in a straight line, heel to toe, first with eyes open and then with eyes closed.

To assess coordination
- With the patient seated and facing you, hold out your index finger at his shoulder level.
- Tell him to touch your finger with his right index finger.
- Then tell him to lower his arm and close his eyes. Have him touch your finger again.
- The patient then repeats the entire maneuver using his left index finger.
- Failure to perform this maneuver rapidly and accurately is called past-pointing. Observe the degree and direction of past-pointing.

Precautions
- Any of these tests may be contraindicated if the patient is physically incapable of performing some or all of the required maneuvers.
- When assessing balance, the examiner should stand close to the patient to catch him if he falls. If the patient is

tall or heavy, someone should assist the examiner.

Normal findings
During tests for balance, a healthy person maintains his balance with eyes open and closed. When testing coordination, a healthy person touches the examiner's finger with eyes open and closed; past-pointing does not occur.

Abnormal findings
A peripheral vestibular lesion can cause swaying or falling in the direction opposite to the nystagmus when the patient's eyes are closed; a cerebellar lesion causes swaying or falling when eyes are open or closed.

A labyrinthine disorder can lead to past-pointing in the direction opposite to the nystagmus when the patient's eyes are closed; a cerebellar lesion can lead to past-pointing when eyes are open or closed; a lateralized lesion can lead to past-pointing with the arm on the affected side only.

Interfering factors
- Alcohol or drugs that affect the CNS, such as stimulants, antianxiety agents, sedatives, and medications to relieve vertigo

GASTROINTESTINAL FUNCTION

ESOPHAGEAL ACIDITY TEST

This test evaluates the competence of the lower esophageal sphincter — the major barrier to reflux — by measuring intraesophageal pH with an electrode attached to a manometric catheter.

Purpose
• To evaluate competence of the lower esophageal sphincter
• To evaluate gastric reflux in patients who complain of persistent heartburn with or without regurgitation

Patient preparation
• Explain to the patient that this test evaluates the function of the sphincter between the esophagus and stomach. Tell him to fast and avoid smoking after midnight before the test.
• Describe the test, including who will perform it and where and its duration (about 45 minutes).
• Tell him that a tube will be passed through his mouth into his stomach and that he may experience slight discomfort, a desire to cough, or a gagging sensation.
• Just before the test, check the patient's pulse rate and blood pressure, and instruct him to void.
• Withhold antacids, anticholinergics, cholinergics, adrenergic blockers, alcohol, corticosteroids, cimetidine, and reserpine for 24 hours before the test. If they must be continued, note this on the laboratory slip.

Procedure and posttest care
• After the patient is placed in the high Fowler position, the catheter with electrode is introduced into his mouth.
• The patient is instructed to swallow when the electrode reaches the back of his throat.
• Using a manometer, the examiner locates the lower esophageal sphincter. The catheter is raised 3/4″ (2 cm). The patient is told to perform Valsalva's maneuver or lift his legs to stimulate reflux. After he does so, intraesophageal pH is measured.

• If the pH is normal, the catheter is passed into the patient's stomach. A prescribed acid solution is instilled over 3 minutes. Then the catheter is raised 3/4″ above the sphincter. Again, the patient is asked to perform Valsalva's maneuver or lift his legs and intraesophageal pH is measured.
• After the test, tell the patient he may resume his usual diet and restart any medications withheld for the test.
• Provide lozenges if the patient complains of a sore throat.

Precautions
• During insertion, the electrode may enter the trachea instead of the esophagus. If the patient develops cyanosis or paroxysms of coughing, move the electrode immediately.
• Observe the patient closely during intubation because arrhythmias may develop.
• Clamp the catheter before removing it to prevent aspiration of fluid into the lungs.

Reference values
The pH of the esophagus normally exceeds 5.0.

Abnormal findings
An intraesophageal pH of 1.5 to 2 indicates gastric acid reflux resulting from incompetence of the lower esophageal sphincter. Persistent reflux leads to chronic reflux esophagitis. Additional studies, such as barium swallow and esophagogastroduodenoscopy, are necessary to diagnose and determine the extent of esophagitis.

Interfering factors
• Failure to adhere to pretest restrictions
• Antacids, anticholinergics, and cimetidine (possible lowering of intraesophageal pH because of decrease in gastric secretions or acidity)

• Alcohol, cholinergics, reserpine, adrenergic blockers, and corticosteroids (possible elevation of intraesophageal pH because of reflux from a relaxed lower esophageal sphincter or an increase in gastric secretions)

ACID PERFUSION TEST

Also called the Bernstein test, this procedure helps to distinguish pain caused by esophagitis (burning epigastric or retrosternal pain that radiates to the back or arms) from pain caused by angina pectoris or other disorders. It requires perfusion of saline and acidic solutions into the esophagus through a nasogastric (NG) tube.

Purpose
• To distinguish chest pains caused by esophagitis from those caused by cardiac disorders

Patient preparation
• Tell the patient that this test helps determine the cause of chest pain.
• Explain the following restrictions: no antacids for 24 hours before the test and no food, fluids, or smoking for 12 hours before the test.
• Describe the test, including who will perform it and where and its duration.
• Explain that the test involves passing a tube through his nose into the esophagus and that he may experience some discomfort, a desire to cough, or a gagging sensation during intubation.
• Tell him that liquid is slowly perfused through the tube into the esophagus and that he should immediately report any pain or burning during perfusion.
• Just before the test, check the patient's pulse rate and blood pressure.

Ask him if he's experiencing any chest pain and, if so, to describe it.

Procedure and posttest care
• After the patient is seated, insert an NG tube that has been marked 12″ (30 cm) from the tip into his stomach. Attach a 20-ml syringe to the tube and aspirate stomach contents. Withdraw the tube into the esophagus (to the 12″ mark).
• Hang labeled containers of normal saline solution and a prescribed acidic solution on an I.V. pole behind the patient; then connect the NG tube to I.V. tubing.
• Open the line from the normal saline solution, and infuse it at a rate of 60 to 120 drops/minute. Continue perfusion for 5 to 10 minutes.
• Ask the patient if he's experiencing any discomfort and record his response.
• Without the patient's knowledge, close the line from the normal saline solution and open the line from the acidic solution. Infuse the acidic solution into the esophagus at the same rate used for the saline solution. Continue perfusion for 30 minutes.
• Ask the patient again if he's experiencing any discomfort, and record his response.
• If the patient experiences discomfort, close the line from the acidic solution immediately and open the line from the normal saline solution. Continue to perfuse this solution until the discomfort subsides.
• Unless perfusion of the acidic solution is to be repeated, the NG tube is withdrawn.
• If the patient complains of pain or burning, administer an antacid. If he complains of a sore throat, provide soothing lozenges or an ice collar.
• Tell him that he may resume his usual diet and any medications withheld for the test.

Precautions

• The acid perfusion test is contraindicated in patients with esophageal varices, heart failure, acute myocardial infarction, or other cardiac disorders.
• During intubation, make sure the tube enters the esophagus and not the trachea. Withdraw the tube immediately if the patient develops cyanosis or paroxysmal coughing.
• Assess the patient's pulse rate and rhythm to detect any arrhythmias that may develop.
• Clamp the tube before removing it to prevent aspiration of fluid into the lungs.

Normal findings

Absence of pain or burning during perfusion of either solution indicates a healthy esophageal mucosa.

Abnormal findings

In patients with esophagitis, the acidic solution causes pain or burning, and the normal saline solution should produce no adverse effects. Occasionally, both solutions cause pain in patients with esophagitis, but they may cause no pain in patients with asymptomatic esophagitis.

Interfering factor

• Failure to adhere to pretest restrictions

RENAL FUNCTION

UROFLOMETRY

This simple, noninvasive test uses a uroflometer to detect and evaluate dysfunctional voiding patterns. The uroflometer, contained in a funnel into

which the patient voids, measures flow rate (volume of urine voided per second), continuous flow (time of measurable flow), and intermittent flow (total voiding time, including any interruptions).

Types of uroflometers include rotary disc, electromagnetic, spectrophotometric, and gravimetric systems. The gravimetric system, which weighs urine as it's voided and plots the weight against time, is the simplest to use.

Purpose

• To evaluate lower urinary tract function
• To demonstrate bladder outlet obstruction

Patient preparation

• Explain to the patient that this test evaluates his pattern of urination. Advise him not to urinate for several hours before the test and to increase fluid intake so he'll have a full bladder and a strong urge to void.
• Describe the test, including who will perform it and where and its duration.
• Instruct him to remain still while voiding during the test to help ensure accurate results. Assure him that he'll have complete privacy during the test.
• Discontinue drugs that may affect bladder and sphincter tone, such as urinary spasmolytics and anticholinergics.

Equipment

Commode chair with funnel containing a uroflometer or beaker to hold urine, transducer, start and flow cables, data recording module

Procedure and posttest care

• Check cable connections before the test.
• Remind the patient not to strain while voiding.

• Ask a male patient to void while standing and a female patient to void while sitting.

• The patient pushes the start button on the commode chair, counts for 5 seconds (1 one-thousand, 2 one-thousand, and so on), and voids. When finished, he counts for 5 seconds and pushes the button again. The volume of urine voided is then recorded and plotted as a curve over the time of voiding. The patient's position and the route of fluid intake (oral or I.V.) are noted.

• Instruct the patient to resume any medications discontinued for the test.

Precautions

• The transducer must be level, and the beaker must be centered beneath the funnel.

• The beaker must be large enough to hold all urine; overflow can invalidate results and damage the transducer.

Reference values

Flow rate varies according to the patient's age and sex and the volume of urine voided. The chart below lists minimum volumes needed to obtain adequate recordings.

AGE	MINIMUM VOLUME (ml)	MALE (ml/sec)	FEMALE (ml/sec)
4 to 7	100	10	10
8 to 13	100	12	15
14 to 45	200	21	18
46 to 65	200	12	15
66 to 80	200	9	10

Abnormal findings

Increased flow rate indicates reduced urethral resistance, possibly associated with external sphincter dysfunction. (See *Characteristic uroflow curves.*) A high peak on the curve plotted over the

CHARACTERISTIC UROFLOW CURVES

Normal curve

Normal peak with hesitancy may result from the patient's embarrassment or advanced age.

High peak flow over short voiding time may indicate incontinence.

Many peaks over normal voiding time indicate abdominal straining and detrusor muscle weakness.

Low peak with long voiding time and urethral dribbling indicates obstruction.

voiding time indicates decreased outflow resistance, possibly due to stress incontinence. Decreased flow rate indicates outflow obstruction or hypotonia of the detrusor muscle. More than one distinct peak in a normal curve indicates abdominal straining, possibly due to pushing against an obstruction to empty the bladder.

Interfering factors
• Drugs that affect bladder and sphincter tone, such as urinary spasmolytics and anticholinergics
• Strong drafts (possible effect on transducer function)
• Patient movement while seating on the commode chair (possible inaccuracy of flow recording)
• Presence of toilet tissue in the beaker (invalidation)
• Straining to void

CYSTOMETRY

Cystometry assesses the bladder's neuromuscular function by measuring efficiency of the detrusor muscle reflex, intravesical pressure and capacity, and the bladder's reaction to thermal stimulation. Because results from cystometry can be ambiguous, they're typically supported by results of other tests, such as cystourethrography, excretory urography, and voiding cystourethrography. (See *Normal and abnormal cystometry findings.*)

Purpose
• To evaluate detrusor muscle function and tonicity
• To help determine the cause of bladder dysfunction
• To detect the cause of involuntary bladder contractions in an unstable bladder

Patient preparation
• Explain to the patient that this test evaluates bladder function.

• Tell him that he needn't restrict food or fluid before the test.
• Describe the procedure, including who will perform it and where and its duration (about 40 minutes unless additional tests are ordered).
• Tell him that he'll feel a strong urge to void during the test and may feel embarrassed or uncomfortable. Provide reassurance.
• Make sure that the patient or a responsible family member has signed an informed consent form.
• Check the patient's medication history for drugs that may affect test results, such as antihistamines.
• Just before the procedure, tell the patient to urinate.

Equipment
Four-channel gas cystometer, set of catheters

Procedure and posttest care
• Place the patient in the supine position on the examination table.
• A catheter is passed into the bladder to measure residual urine level. Any difficulty with insertion of the catheter may reflect meatal or urethral obstruction.
• To test the patient's response to thermal sensation, 30 ml of room-temperature physiologic saline solution or sterile water is instilled into the bladder. Then an equal volume of warm (110° to 115° F [43.3° to 46.1° C]) fluid is instilled into the bladder. The patient is asked to report his sensations, such as the need to void, nausea, flushing, discomfort, and a feeling of warmth.
• After the fluid is drained from the patient's bladder, the catheter is connected to the cystometer, and normal saline solution, sterile water, or gas (usually carbon dioxide) is slowly introduced into the bladder. The flow of gas is adjusted automatically to the

Normal and Abnormal Cystometry Findings

Because cystometry assesses micturition and vesical function, it can aid diagnosis of neurogenic bladder dysfunction. The five main types of neurogenic bladder, as presented in the following chart, result from lesions of the central or peripheral nervous system. Uninhibited neurogenic bladder results from a lesion to the upper motor neuron and causes frequent, often uncontrollable micturition in the presence of even a small amount of urine. A complete upper motor neuron lesion characterizes reflex neurogenic bladder and causes total loss of conscious sensation and vesical control.

FEATURE OR RESPONSE	NORMAL BLADDER FUNCTION	UNINHIBITED NEUROGENIC BLADDER (mildly spastic, incomplete upper motor neuron lesion)	REFLEX NEUROGENIC BLADDER (completely spastic, complete upper motor neuron lesion)
Micturition			
Start	+	+/0	0
Stop	+	0	0
Residual urine	0	0	+
Vesical sensation	+	+	0
First urge to void	150 to 200 ml	E (<150 ml)	0
Bladder capacity	400 to 500 ml	↓	↓
Bladder contractions	0	+	+
Intravesical pressure	L	↑	↑
Bulbocavernosus reflex	+	+	↑
Saddle sensation	+	+	0
Bethanechol test (exaggerated response)	0	+	0
Ice water test	+	+	+
Anal reflex	+	+	+
Heat sensation and pain	+	+	0

KEY

+ = Present/Positive
0 = Absent/Negative
↑ = Increased

↓ = Decreased
V = Variable
E = Early

D = Delayed
L = Low

(continued)

NORMAL AND ABNORMAL CYSTOMETRY FINDINGS *(continued)*

In autonomous neurogenic bladder, a lower motor neuron lesion produces a flaccid bladder that fills without contracting. The patient can't perceive bladder fullness or initiate and maintain urination without applying external pressure. Lower motor neuron lesions can cause sensory or motor paralysis of the bladder. In sensory paralysis, the patient experiences chronic urine retention because he can't perceive bladder fullness. In motor paralysis, the patient has full sensation but can't initiate or control urination.

FEATURE OR RESPONSE	AUTONOMOUS NEUROGENIC BLADDER (flaccid, incomplete lower motor neuron lesion)	SENSORY PARALYTIC BLADDER (lower motor neuron lesion)	MOTOR PARALYTIC BLADDER (lower motor neuron lesion)
Micturition			
Start	0	+	0
Stop	0	+	0
Residual urine	+	+	++
Vesical sensation	0	0	+
First urge to void	0	D	+
Bladder capacity	↑	↑ (<1,000 ml)	V
Bladder contractions	0	0	0
Intravesical pressure	↓	↓	L
Bulbocavernosus reflex	0	+/↓/0	+
Saddle sensation	0	V	+
Bethanechol test (exaggerated response)	+	+	0
Ice water test	0	0	0
Anal reflex	0	V	V
Heat sensation and pain	0	0	+

KEY
+ = Present/Positive   ↓ = Decreased   D = Delayed
0 = Absent/Negative   V = Variable   L = Low
↑ = Increased   E = Early

desired reading (100 ml/minute) by a four-channel cystometer.

• The patient is asked to indicate when he *first* feels an urge to void and then when he feels he *must* urinate. The related pressure and volume are automatically plotted on the graph.

• When the bladder reaches its full capacity, the patient is asked to urinate so that the maximal intravesical voiding pressure can be recorded. The patient's bladder is then drained and, if no additional tests are required, the catheter is removed.

• Administer a sitz bath or warm tub bath if the patient experiences discomfort after the test.

• Measure fluid intake and urine output for 24 hours. Watch for hematuria that persists after the third voiding and for signs of sepsis (such as fever or chills).

Precautions

• Cystometry is contraindicated in patients with acute urinary tract infections because uninhibited contractions may cause erroneous readings and the test may lead to pyelonephritis and septic shock.

• Tell the patient not to strain at voiding; it can cause ambiguous cystometric readings.

• If the patient has a spinal cord injury that has caused motor impairment, transport him on a stretcher so that the test can be performed without transferring him to the examination table.

Findings

For characteristic findings, see the accompanying chart.

Interfering factors

• Failure to follow instructions because of misunderstanding or embarrassment

• Inability to urinate in the supine position

• Concurrent use of drugs, such as antihistamines (possible interference with bladder function)

• Cystometry performed within 6 to 8 weeks after surgery for spinal cord injury (inconclusive results)

EXTERNAL SPHINCTER ELECTROMYOGRAPHY

This procedure measures electrical activity of the external urinary sphincter using needle electrodes inserted in perineal or periurethral tissues, electrodes in an anal plug, or skin electrodes. Skin electrodes are the most common method used.

Incontinence is the primary indication for external sphincter electromyography. Often, the test is done with cystometry and voiding urethrography as part of a full urodynamic study.

Purpose

• To assess neuromuscular function of the external urinary sphincter

• To assess the functional balance between bladder and sphincter muscle activity

Patient preparation

• Explain to the patient that this test will determine how well his bladder and sphincter muscles work together.

• Describe the test, including who will perform it and where and its duration.

• If skin electrodes are used, describe their placement and explain the preparatory procedure, which may include shaving a small area.

• If needle electrodes are used, describe their placement and explain that the discomfort is equivalent to an intramuscular injection. Assure him that he'll feel discomfort only during insertion. Explain that wires connect the needles to the recorder but pose no danger of electric shock. If the patient is a woman, tell her that she may notice slight bleeding at the first voiding.

● If an anal plug is used, tell the patient that only the tip of the plug will be inserted into the rectum and that he may feel fullness but no discomfort.

● Check the patient's history for use of cholinergic or anticholinergic drugs and note such use.

Equipment
Electromyograph and recorder; skin, needle, or anal plug electrodes; ground plate; electrode paste; tape; antiseptic solution such as povidone-iodine; preparatory tray if shaving is necessary.

Procedure and posttest care
● Place the patient in the lithotomy position for electrode placement. After placement, he may lie in the supine position. Record the patient's position, type of electrode and measuring equipment used, and any other tests done at the same time.

● Electrode paste is applied to the ground plate, which is taped to the thigh and grounded. The electrodes are positioned and connected to electrode adapters.

● When using skin electrodes, clean the skin with antiseptic solution and then dry the area. If necessary, shave a small area to optimize electrode contact. Apply electrode paste and tape the electrodes in place. For women, electrodes are placed in the periurethral area; for men, in the perineal area beneath the scrotum.

● To position needle electrodes on a male patient, a gloved finger is inserted in the rectum. The needles and

wires are inserted through the perineal skin toward the apex of the prostate. Needle positions are 3:00 and 9:00. The needles are withdrawn, and the wires are held in place and then taped to the thigh.

● To position needle electrodes on a female patient, the labia are spread, and the needles and wires inserted periurethrally at the 2:00 and 10:00 positions. The needles are withdrawn and the wires taped to the thigh.

● When using anal plug electrodes, the plug is lubricated and the patient is asked to breathe slowly and deeply and to relax the anal sphincter to accommodate the plug by bearing down.

● After electrode placement, the adapters are inserted in the preamplifier and recording starts. The patient is asked to alternately relax and tighten the sphincter.

● When sufficient data have been recorded, the patient is asked to bear down and exhale while the anal plug and needle electrodes are removed. Remove skin electrodes gently to avoid pulling hair and tender skin.

● Clean and dry the area before the patient dresses.

● In some urodynamic laboratories, cystometrography is done with electromyography for a thorough evaluation of detrusor and sphincter coordination.

● For women, watch for and report hematuria after the first voiding if needle electrodes were used.

● Watch for and report symptoms of mild urethral irritation, such as dysuria, hematuria, and urinary frequency.

● Advise the patient to take a warm sitz bath, and encourage him to drink 2 to 3 L of fluids daily, unless contraindicated.

Precautions
- Insert the needles quickly to minimize discomfort.
- The ground plate should be properly applied and anchored; wires should be taped securely to prevent artifacts.

Normal findings
The electromyogram shows increased muscle activity when the patient tightens the external urinary sphincter and decreased muscle activity when he relaxes it. If electromyography and cystometrography are performed simultaneously, a comparison of results shows that muscle activity of the normal sphincter increases as the bladder fills. During voiding and bladder contraction, muscle activity decreases as the sphincter relaxes. This comparison is important in assessing external sphincter efficiency and functional balance between bladder and sphincter muscle activity.

Abnormal findings
Failure of the sphincter to relax or increased muscle activity during voiding demonstrates detrusor–external sphincter dyssynergia. Confirmation of such muscle activity by electromyography may indicate neurogenic bladder, spinal cord injury, multiple sclerosis, Parkinson's disease, or stress incontinence.

Interfering factors
- Patient movement (possible distortion)
- Effect of anticholinergic or cholinergic drugs on detrusor and sphincter activity
- Improperly placed and anchored electrodes

TENSILON TEST

This test involves careful observation of the patient after I.V. administration of Tensilon (edrophonium chloride), a rapid, short-acting anticholinesterase that improves muscle strength by increasing muscle response to nerve impulses.

Purpose
- To aid diagnosis of myasthenia gravis (results of other procedures, including electromyography, may supplement Tensilon test findings)
- To aid in differentiation between myasthenic and cholinergic crises
- To monitor oral anticholinesterase therapy

Patient preparation
- Explain to the patient that this test helps determine the cause of muscle weakness.
- Describe the test, including who will perform it and where and its duration (15 to 30 minutes).
- Don't describe the exact response that will be evaluated; foreknowledge can affect the test's objectivity.
- Explain to the patient that a small tube will be inserted into a vein in his arm and that a drug will be administered periodically. He'll be asked to make repetitive muscle movements and his reactions will be observed. To ensure accuracy, the test may be repeated several times.
- Advise him that Tensilon may produce some unpleasant adverse effects,

but reassure him that someone will be with him at all times and that any reactions will quickly disappear.

● Check the patient's history for medications that affect muscle function, anticholinesterase therapy, drug hypersensitivities, and respiratory disease. Withhold medications. If the patient is receiving anticholinesterase therapy, note this on the requisition slip; include the time of the most recent dose.

Equipment

Standard: 10 mg Tensilon, 0.4 mg atropine (may be prescribed for patients with respiratory distress), one tuberculin and one 3-ml syringe, I.V. infusion set, 50-ml bag of I.V. solution (dextrose 5% in water [D_5W] or normal saline solution), tape, tourniquet, alcohol swabs

Emergency: 0.5 to 1.0 mg atropine I.V. for cholinergic crisis, 0.5 to 2.0 mg neostigmine methylsulfate I.V. for myasthenic crisis (may be repeated up to a total of 5 mg), extra tuberculin and 3-ml syringes (for atropine or neostigmine injections), resuscitation equipment, including a tracheotomy tray

Procedure and posttest care

● Begin an I.V. infusion of D_5W or normal saline solution.

● When performing the test on an adult patient suspected of having myasthenia gravis, 2 mg of Tensilon are administered initially. Before the rest of the dose is administered, the doctor may want to fatigue the muscles by asking the patient to perform various exercises, such as looking up until ptosis develops, counting to 100 until his voice diminishes, or holding his arms above his shoulders until they drop. When the muscles are fatigued, the remaining 8 mg of Tensilon are administered over 30 seconds.

● The test may begin with a placebo injection to evaluate the patient's muscle response more accurately. The placebo isn't necessary if cranial muscles are being tested because cranial strength can't be simulated voluntarily.

● After Tensilon is administered, the patient is asked to perform repetitive muscle movements, such as opening and closing his eyes and crossing and uncrossing his legs. Closely observe the patient for improved muscle strength. If muscle strength doesn't improve within 3 to 5 minutes, the test may be repeated.

● To differentiate between myasthenic crisis and cholinergic crisis, 1 to 2 mg of Tensilon is infused. After infusion, continually monitor the patient's vital signs. Watch closely for respiratory distress, and be prepared to provide respiratory assistance.

● If muscle strength doesn't improve, more Tensilon is infused cautiously, 1 mg at a time up to a maximum of 5 mg, and the patient is observed for distress.

● Neostigmine is administered immediately if the test demonstrates myasthenic crisis; atropine is administered for cholinergic crisis.

● To evaluate oral anticholinesterase therapy, 2 mg of Tensilon is infused 1 hour after the patient's last dose of the anticholinesterase. The patient is observed carefully for adverse effects and muscle response.

● After Tensilon administration, the I.V. line is kept open at a rate of 20 ml/hour until all the patient's responses have been evaluated.

● When the test is complete, discontinue the I.V., and check the patient's vital signs.

● Check the puncture site for hematoma, excessive bleeding, and swelling.

● Tell the patient to resume any medications withheld for the test.

Precautions
• Because of the systemic adverse reactions Tensilon may produce, this test may be contraindicated in patients with hypotension, bradycardia, apnea, and mechanical obstruction of the intestine or urinary tract.
• Patients with respiratory ailments such as asthma should receive atropine during the test to minimize adverse reactions to Tensilon.
• Stay with the patient during the test, and observe him closely for adverse reactions.
• Keep resuscitation equipment handy in case of respiratory failure.

Normal findings
People who don't have myasthenia gravis usually develop fasciculation in response to Tensilon. The doctor must interpret the responses carefully to distinguish a normal person from one with myasthenia gravis.

Abnormal findings
If the patient has myasthenia gravis, muscle strength should improve promptly after administration of Tensilon. The degree of improvement depends on the muscle group being tested; improvement is usually obvious within 30 seconds. Although the maximum benefit lasts only several minutes, lingering effects may persist — up to 2 hours in a patient receiving prednisone, for example. All patients with myasthenia gravis show improved muscle strength in this test; some patients respond slightly and the test may need to be repeated to confirm the diagnosis.

The test may yield inconsistent results if myasthenia gravis affects only ocular muscles, as in mild or early forms of the disorder. It may produce a positive response in motor neuron disease and in some neuropathies and myopathies. The response is usually less dramatic and less consistent than in myasthenia gravis.

Patients in myasthenic crisis show brief improvement in muscle strength after Tensilon administration. Patients in cholinergic crisis (anticholinesterase overdose) may experience exaggerated muscle weakness. If Tensilon increases the patient's muscle strength without increasing adverse effects, oral anticholinesterase therapy can be increased. If Tensilon decreases muscle strength in a person with severe adverse reactions, therapy should be reduced. If the test shows no change in muscle strength and only mild adverse effects occur, therapy should remain the same.

Interfering factors
• Prednisone (possible delay of Tensilon's effect on muscle strength)
• Quinidine and anticholinergics (inhibit the action of Tensilon)
• Procainamide and muscle relaxants (inhibit normal muscle response)

COLD STIMULATION TEST FOR RAYNAUD'S SYNDROME

This test demonstrates Raynaud's syndrome by recording temperature changes in the patient's fingers before and after submersion in ice water. Note that digital blood pressure recording or examination of the arteries in the arm and palmar arch should precede this test to rule out arterial occlusive disease.

Purpose
• To detect Raynaud's syndrome, an arteriospastic disorder characterized by intense vasospasm of the small cuta-

neous arteries and arterioles of the hands after exposure to cold or stress

Patient preparation
• Explain to the patient that this test detects vascular disorders.
• Tell him that he needn't restrict food or fluids for the test.
• Describe the test, including who will perform it and where and how long it will take.
• Explain that he may experience discomfort when his hands are briefly immersed in ice water.
• Have him remove his watch and other jewelry, and encourage him to relax.

Procedure and posttest care
• To minimize extraneous environmental stimuli, make sure the test room is neither too warm nor too cold.
• Tape a thermistor to each of the patient's fingers and record the temperature.
• Have the patient submerge his hands in an ice-water bath for 20 seconds.
• When he removes his hands from the water, record the temperature of his fingers immediately and every 5 minutes thereafter until it returns to the baseline temperature.

Precautions
• The cold stimulation test is contraindicated in patients with gangrenous fingers or open, infected wounds.

Normal findings
Normally, digital temperature returns to baseline levels within 15 minutes.

Abnormal findings
If digital temperature takes longer than 20 minutes to return to the baseline level, Raynaud's syndrome is indicated. Its benign form, Raynaud's disease, requires no specific treatment and has no serious sequelae. Its more serious

form, Raynaud's phenomenon, is associated with connective tissue disorders that may not be clinically apparent for several years, such as scleroderma, systemic lupus erythematosus, and rheumatoid arthritis. Distinguishing between Raynaud's phenomenon and Raynaud's disease is difficult.

Interfering factor
• Excessively warm or cold test environment

PULMONARY FUNCTION TESTS

Pulmonary function tests (volume and capacity tests) are a series of measurements that evaluate ventilatory function through spirometric measurements; they're performed on patients with suspected pulmonary dysfunction.

Of the seven tests used to determine volume, tidal volume (V_T) and expiratory reserve volume (ERV) are direct spirographic measurements; minute volume (MV), carbon dioxide response, inspiratory reserve volume (IRV), and residual volume (RV) are calculated from the results of other pulmonary function tests; and thoracic gas volume (TGV) is calculated from body plethysmography.

Of the pulmonary capacity tests, vital capacity (VC), inspiratory capacity (IC), functional residual capacity (FRC), total lung capacity (TLC), and forced expiratory flow (FEF) may be measured directly or calculated from the results of other tests. Forced vital capacity (FVC), flow-volume curve, forced expiratory volume (FEV), peak expiratory flow rate (PEFR), and maximal voluntary ventilation (MVV) are direct spirographic measurements. Diffusing capacity for carbon monoxide (DL_{co}) is calculated from the amount of carbon monoxide exhaled. (See *Interpreting pulmonary function tests,* pages 738 to 740.)

Purpose
- To determine the cause of dyspnea
- To assess the effectiveness of specific therapeutic regimens
- To determine whether a functional abnormality is obstructive or restrictive
- To measure pulmonary dysfunction
- To evaluate a patient before surgery

Patient preparation
- Explain to the patient that these tests evaluate pulmonary function. Instruct him to eat only a light meal before the tests and not to smoke for 4 to 6 hours before the tests.
- Describe the tests and equipment. Explain who will perform the tests and where and their duration.
- Describe the operation of a spirometer.
- Advise him that the accuracy of the tests depends on his cooperation.
- Assure him that the procedures are painless and that he'll be able to rest between tests.
- Inform the laboratory if the patient is taking an analgesic that depresses respiration.
- Withhold bronchodilators and intermittent positive-pressure breathing therapy.
- Just before the test, tell the patient to void and to loosen tight clothing. If he wears dentures, tell him to wear them during the test to help form a seal around the mouthpiece.

Equipment
For direct spirography: spirometer, recording paper, nose clip, mouthpiece

For body plethysmography: body plethysmograph, mouthpiece, transducer

Procedure and posttest care
- When measuring *tidal volume,* tell the patient to breathe normally into the mouthpiece 10 times.
- When measuring *expiratory reserve volume,* tell the patient to breathe normally for several breaths and then to exhale as completely as possible.
- When measuring *vital capacity,* tell the patient to inhale as deeply as possible and to exhale into the mouthpiece as completely as possible. This procedure is repeated three times, and the test result showing the largest volume is used.
- When measuring *inspiratory capacity,* tell the patient to breathe normally for several breaths and then to inhale as deeply as possible.
- When measuring *functional residual capacity,* tell the patient to breathe normally into a spirometer that contains a known concentration of an insoluble gas (usually helium or nitrogen) in a known volume of air. After a few breaths, the concentrations of gas in the spirometer and in the lungs reach equilibrium. Then the point of equilibrium and the concentration of gas in the spirometer are recorded.
- When measuring *thoracic gas volume,* the patient is put in an airtight box (or *body plethysmograph*) and told to breathe through a tube connected to a transducer. At end-expiration, the tube is occluded, the patient is told to pant, and changes in intrathoracic and plethysmographic pressures are measured. The results are used to calculate total TGV and FRC.
- When measuring *forced vital capacity* and *forced expiratory volume,* tell the patient to inhale as slowly and deeply as possible and then exhale into

(Text continues on page 740.)

INTERPRETING PULMONARY FUNCTION TESTS

PULMONARY FUNCTION TEST	METHOD OF CALCULATION	IMPLICATIONS
Tidal volume (V_T): amount of air inhaled or exhaled during normal breathing	Determine the spirographic measurement for 10 breaths and then divide by 10.	Decreased V_T may indicate restrictive disease and requires further testing, such as full pulmonary function studies or chest X-rays.
Minute volume (MV): total amount of air expired per minute	Multiply V_T by the respiratory rate.	Normal MV can occur in emphysema; decreased MV may indicate other diseases, such as pulmonary edema. Increased MV can occur with acidosis, increased CO_2, decreased Pao_2, exercise, and low compliance states.
CO_2 response: increase or decrease in MV after breathing various CO_2 concentrations	Calculate by plotting changes in MV against increasing inspired CO_2 concentrations.	Reduced CO_2 response may occur in emphysema, myxedema, obesity, hypoventilation syndrome, and sleep apnea.
Inspiratory reserve volume (IRV): amount of air inspired over above-normal inspiration	Subtract V_T from inspiratory capacity	Abnormal IRV alone doesn't indicate respiratory dysfunction; IRV decreases during normal exercise.
Expiratory reserve volume (ERV): amount of air exhaled after normal expiration	Direct spirographic measurement	ERV varies, even in healthy people, but usually decreases in the obese.
Residual volume (RV): amount of air remaining in the lungs after forced expiration	Subtract ERV from functional residual capacity (FRC).	RV > 35% of TLC after maximal expiratory effort may indicate obstructive disease.
Vital capacity (VC): total volume of air that can be exhaled after maximum inspiration	Direct spirographic measurement, or add V_T, IRV, and ERV.	Normal or increased VC with decreased flow rates may indicate any condition that causes a reduction in functional pulmonary tissue, such as pulmonary edema. Decreased VC with normal or increased flow rates may indicate decreased respiratory effort resulting from neuromuscular disease, drug overdose, or head injury; decreased thoracic expansion; or limited movement of the diaphragm.

INTERPRETING PULMONARY FUNCTION TESTS *(continued)*

PULMONARY FUNCTION TEST	METHOD OF CALCULATION	IMPLICATIONS
Inspiratory capacity (IC): amount of air that can be inhaled after normal expiration	Direct spirographic measurement, or add IRV and V_T.	Decreased IC indicates restrictive disease.
Thoracic gas volume (TGV): total volume of gas in lungs from both ventilated and non-ventilated airways	Body plethysmography	Increased TGV indicates air trapping, which may result from obstructive disease.
Functional residual capacity (FRC): amount of air remaining in lungs after normal expiration	Nitrogen washout, helium dilution technique, or add ERV and RV.	Increased FRC indicates overdistention of lungs, which may result from obstructive pulmonary disease.
Total lung capacity (TLC): total volume of the lungs when maximally inflated	Add V_T, IRV, ERV, and RV; or FRC and IC; or VC and RV.	Low TLC indicates restrictive disease; high TLC indicates overdistended lungs caused by obstructive disease.
Forced vital capacity (FVC): amount of air exhaled forcefully and quickly after maximum inspiration	Direct spirographic measurement; expressed as a percentage of the total volume of gas exhaled	Decreased FVC indicates flow resistance in respiratory system from obstructive disease such as chronic bronchitis or from restrictive disease such as pulmonary fibrosis.
Flow-volume curve (also called flow-volume loop): greatest rate of flow (V_{max}) during FVC maneuvers versus lung volume change	Direct spirographic measurement at 1-second intervals; calculated from flow rates (expressed in liters/second) and lung volume changes (expressed in liters) during maximal inspiratory and expiratory maneuvers	Decreased flow rates at all volumes during expiration indicate obstructive disease of the small airways, such as emphysema. A plateau of expiratory flow near TLC, a plateau of inspiratory flow at mid-VC, and a square wave pattern through most of VC indicate obstructive disease of large airways. Normal or increased PEFR, decreased flow with decreasing lung volumes, and markedly decreased VC indicate restrictive disease.
Forced expiratory volume (FEV): volume of air expired in the 1st, 2nd, or 3rd second of FVC maneuver	Direct spirographic measurement; expressed as percentage of FVC	Decreased FEV_1 and increased FEV_2 and FEV_3 may indicate obstructive disease; decreased or normal FEV_1 may indicate restrictive disease.

(continued)

INTERPRETING PULMONARY FUNCTION TESTS *(continued)*

PULMONARY FUNCTION TEST	METHOD OF CALCULATION	IMPLICATIONS
Forced expiratory flow (FEF): average rate of flow during middle half of FVC	Calculated from the flow rate and the time needed for expiration of middle 50% of FVC	Low FEF (25% to 75%) indicates obstructive disease of the small and medium-sized airways.
Peak expiratory flow rate (PEFR): V_{max} during forced expiration	Calculated from flow-volume curve or by direct spirographic measurement, using a pneumotachometer or electronic tachometer with a transducer to convert flow to electrical output display	Decreased PEFR may indicate a mechanical problem, such as upper airway obstruction, or obstructive disease. PEFR is usually normal in restrictive disease but decreases in severe cases. Because PEFR is effort-dependent, it's also low in a person who has poor expiratory effort or doesn't understand the procedure.
Maximal voluntary ventilation (MVV), also called maximum breathing capacity: greatest volume of air breathed per unit of time	Direct spirographic measurement	Decreased MVV may indicate obstructive disease; normal or decreased MVV may indicate restrictive disease such as myasthenia gravis.
Diffusing capacity for carbon monoxide (DL_{CO}): milliliters of carbon monoxide diffused per minute across the alveolo-capillary membrane	Calculated from analysis of amount of carbon monoxide exhaled compared with amount inhaled	Decreased DL_{CO} due to a thickened alveolocapillary membrane occurs in interstitial pulmonary diseases, such as pulmonary fibrosis, asbestosis, and sarcoidosis; DL_{CO} is reduced in emphysema because of the loss of alveolocapillary membrane.

the mouthpiece as quickly and completely as possible. This procedure is repeated three times, and the largest volume is recorded. The volume of air expired at 1 second (FEV_1), at 2 seconds (FEV_2), and at 3 seconds (FEV_3) during all three repetitions is also recorded.

• When measuring *maximal voluntary ventilation,* tell the patient to breathe into the mouthpiece as quickly and deeply as possible for 15 seconds.

• When measuring *diffusing capacity for carbon monoxide,* the patient inhales a gas mixture with a low concentration of carbon monoxide and then holds his breath for 10 seconds before exhaling.

• After the tests, tell the patient to resume his usual diet and daily activities as well as any medications withheld for the test.

Precautions
- Pulmonary function tests are contra-indicated in patients with acute coronary insufficiency, angina, or recent myocardial infarction.
- Watch for respiratory distress, changes in pulse rate and blood pressure, and coughing or bronchospasm.

Reference values
Normal values are predicted for each patient based on age, height, weight, and sex and are expressed as a percentage. Usually, results are considered abnormal if they're less than 80% of these values.

The following reference values can be calculated at bedside with a portable spirometer: V_T, 5 to 7 ml/kg of body weight; ERV, 25% of VC; IC, 75% of VC; FEV_1, 83% of VC (after 1 second); FEV_2, 94% of VC (after 2 seconds); and FEV_3, 97% of VC (after 3 seconds).

Abnormal findings
See the accompanying chart.

Interfering factors
- Hypoxia, metabolic disturbances, or lack of patient cooperation
- Pregnancy or gastric distention (possible displacement of lung volume)
- Narcotic analgesic or sedative (possible decrease in inspiratory and expiratory forces)
- Bronchodilators (possible temporary improvement in pulmonary function)

D-XYLOSE ABSORPTION

This test evaluates patients with symptoms of malabsorption, such as weight loss and generalized malnutrition, weakness, and diarrhea. D-Xylose is a pentose sugar that's absorbed in the small intestine without the aid of pancreatic enzymes, passes through the liver without being metabolized, and is excreted in the urine. Because of its absorption in the small intestine without digestion, measurement of D-xylose in the urine and blood indicates the absorptive capacity of the small intestine.

Purpose
- To aid differential diagnosis of malabsorption
- To determine the cause of malabsorption syndrome

Patient preparation
- Tell the patient that this test helps evaluate digestive function by analyzing blood samples and urine specimens after ingestion of a sugar solution.
- Explain that he must fast overnight before the test and that he'll have to fast and remain in bed during the test.
- Explain that several blood samples will be taken; tell him who will perform the venipunctures and when.
- Advise him that he may experience some discomfort from the needle punctures and the tourniquet but that collecting each sample takes less than 3 minutes.
- Inform him that all his urine will be collected for 5 or 24 hours.
- Withhold medications that alter test results, such as aspirin and indomethacin. Record any medications the patient is taking on the laboratory slip.

Procedure and posttest care
- Perform a venipuncture to obtain a fasting blood sample. Collect a first-voided morning urine specimen. Label these specimens, and send them to the laboratory immediately to serve as a baseline.

- Give the patient 25 g of D-xylose dissolved in 8 oz (240 ml) of water, followed by an additional 8 oz of water. If the patient is a child, administer 0.5 g of D-xylose per pound of body weight, up to 25 g. Record the time of D-xylose ingestion.
- For an adult, draw a blood sample 2 hours after D-xylose ingestion; for a child, 1 hour after ingestion. Collect the sample in a 10-ml *red-top* tube. Occasionally, a 5-hour sample may be drawn to support the findings of the 1- or 2-hour sample.
- Collect and pool all urine during the 5 or 24 hours after D-xylose ingestion.
- If a hematoma develops at the venipuncture site, apply warm soaks.
- Observe the patient for abdominal discomfort or mild diarrhea caused by D-xylose ingestion.
- Tell him that he may resume his usual diet and any medications withheld for the test.

Precautions

- The patient must have adequate renal function for the absorption and excretion of D-xylose.
- Handle the sample gently to prevent hemolysis.
- Tell the patient not to contaminate the urine specimens with toilet tissue or stool.
- Be sure to collect all urine and refrigerate the specimen during the collection period.
- Because patients age 65 and older and those with borderline or elevated creatinine levels tend to have low 5-hour urine levels but normal 24-hour levels, the doctor will have to establish the length of the collection period. At the end of the collection period, send the urine specimen to the laboratory immediately.
- Maintain bed rest and withhold food and fluids (other than D-xylose) throughout the test period.

Reference values

Normal values are as follows:
- Children: blood concentration > 30 mg/dl in 1 hour; urine, 16% to 33% of ingested D-xylose excreted in 5 hours
- Adults: blood concentration 25 to 40 mg/dl in 2 hours; urine, > 4 g excreted in 5 hours

Abnormal findings

Depressed blood and urine D-xylose levels most commonly result from malabsorption disorders that affect the proximal small intestine, such as sprue and celiac disease. Depressed levels may also result from regional enteritis involving the jejunum, Whipple's disease, multiple jejunal diverticula, myxedema, diabetic neuropathic diarrhea, rheumatoid arthritis, alcoholism, severe heart failure, and ascites.

Interfering factors

- Failure to adhere to pretest restrictions
- Aspirin (decreased D-xylose excretion by the kidneys)
- Indomethacin (decreased intestinal D-xylose absorption)
- Failure to obtain a complete urine specimen or to collect blood samples at designated times
- Intestinal overgrowth of bacteria, renal insufficiency, or renal retention of urine (possible drop in urine levels)

DEXAMETHASONE SUPPRESSION TEST

This test requires administration of dexamethasone, an oral steroid. Dexamethasone suppresses levels of circulating adrenal steroid hormones in normal people but fails to suppress them in patients with Cushing's syndrome and some forms of clinical depression.

Purpose
- To diagnose Cushing's syndrome
- To aid diagnosis of clinical depression

Patient preparation
- Explain the purpose of the test.
- Inform the patient that the test requires two blood samples drawn after administration of dexamethasone. Tell him who will perform the venipuncture and when and that he may experience transient discomfort from the needle puncture and the tourniquet.
- Restrict food and fluids for 10 to 12 hours before the test.
- Many medications, including corticosteroids, oral contraceptives, lithium, methadone, aspirin, diuretics, morphine, and monoamine oxidase (MAO) inhibitors, can affect the accuracy of test results. If possible, don't administer any of these medications for 24 to 48 hours before the test.

Procedure and posttest care
- On the first day, give the patient 1 mg of dexamethasone at 11 p.m. On the next day, collect blood samples at 4 p.m. and 11 p.m. More frequent sampling may increase the likelihood of measuring a nonsuppressed cortisol peak.
- If a hematoma develops at the venipuncture site, apply warm soaks.

Reference values
A cortisol level of 5 µg/dl (140 nmol/L) or greater indicates failure of dexamethasone suppression.

Abnormal findings
A normal test result doesn't rule out major depression, but an abnormal result strengthens a clinically based diagnosis. Failure of suppression occurs in patients with Cushing's syndrome, severe stress, and depression that's likely to respond to treatment with antidepressants.

Interfering factors
- Diabetes mellitus, pregnancy, and severe stress, such as trauma, severe weight loss, dehydration, and acute alcohol withdrawal (possible false-positive)
- Certain drugs, particularly barbiturates or phenytoin, within 3 weeks of the test (possible false-positive)
- Caffeine consumed after midnight the night before the test (possible false-positive)
- Failure to withhold corticosteroids, oral contraceptives, lithium, methadone, aspirin, diuretics, morphine, or MAO inhibitors before the test

SLEEP STUDIES

Also known as polysomnography, sleep studies are tests used to help in the differential diagnosis of sleep-disordered breathing. Several parameters are evaluated for the patient being tested for sleep disorder; these include cardiac rate and rhythm, chest and abdominal wall movement, nasal and oral airflow, oxygen saturation, muscle activity, retinal function, and brain activity during the sleep phase.

Purpose
- To diagnose breathing disorders in persons with a history of excessive snoring, narcolepsy, excessive daytime sleepiness, insomnia, cardiac rhythm disorders, and restless leg spasms

Patient preparation

• Explain the purpose of the test to the patient and have him maintain normal sleep schedules so that he's neither deprived of sleep nor overrested.

• Inform the patient that sleep studies are usually scheduled for the evening and night hours, usually 10 p.m. to 6 a.m, and take place in a designated sleep laboratory.

• Explain to him that he should abstain from caffeinated products and naps for 2 to 3 days before the test.

• Tell him that he may bathe or shower before the test.

Procedure and posttest care

• Electrodes are secured to the patient's skin, depending on the type of monitoring being used.

• Ensure the patient's comfort and tell him that normal body movements won't interfere with the electrodes.

• The lights are turned off and the EEG monitored for a baseline reading before the patient falls asleep.

• Ensure that the recording and video equipment record the sleep events as they occur.

• Monitoring of the patient during sleep continues until the test is completed.

Precautions

• For the patient with known sleep apnea, split-night studies may be ordered. These include monitoring the patient for the first half of the night, then using continuous positive airway pressure or nasal ventilation to open the obstructed airway during the second half of the night.

• Monitor the patient for respiratory distress.

Normal findings

A normal sleep study shows a respiratory disturbance index (or apnea-hypopnea index) of fewer than 5 to 10 episodes per study period and normal electrocardiogram (cardiac rate and rhythm), impedance (chest and abdominal wall motion), airway (nasal and oral airflow), arterial oxygen saturation (oximetry), leg electromyogram (for muscle activity), electro-oculogram (for retinal function), and EEG (for brain activity).

Abnormal findings

Abnormal recordings reveal obstructive sleep apnea syndrome. Abnormal movement during sleep indicates a seizure or movement disorder.

Interfering factors

• Electrophysiologic artifacts, defective electrodes, diaphoresis, environmental noises

• Patient's inability to fall asleep

APPENDICES AND INDEX

APPENDIX A
NORMAL LABORATORY TEST VALUES

APPENDIX B
NORMAL AND ABNORMAL SERUM DRUG LEVELS

APPENDIX C
ILLUSTRATED GUIDE TO HOME TESTING

Normal Laboratory Test Values

HEMATOLOGY

Activated partial thromboplastin time
21 to 35 seconds

Bleeding time
Template: 3 to 6 minutes
Ivy: 3 to 6 minutes
Duke: 1 to 3 minutes

Clot retraction
50%

Erythrocyte sedimentation rate
Males: 0 to 15 mm/hour
Females: 0 to 20 mm/hour

Fibrin split products
Screening assay: < 10 µg/ml
Quantitative assay: < 3 µg/ml

Fibrinogen, plasma
175 to 350 mg/dl

Hematocrit
Males: 42% to 52%
Females: 36% to 48%

Hemoglobin, total
Males: 14 to 17.4 g/dl
Females: 12 to 16 g/dl

Platelet aggregation
3 to 5 minutes

Platelet count
140,000 to 400,000/µl

Prothrombin time
11 to 13 seconds; INR for patients on warfarin therapy, 2 to 2.5 (those with prosthetic heart valve, 3 to 4.5)

Red blood cell count
Males: 4.5 to 5.5 million/ml venous blood
Females: 4 to 5 million/ml venous blood

Red cell indices
Mean corpuscular volume: 82 to 98 µm³
Mean corpuscular hemoglobin: 26 to 34 pg/cell
Mean corpuscular hemoglobin concentration: 31 to 37 g/dl

Reticulocyte count
0.5% to 2.5% of total red blood cell count

Thrombin time, plasma
7 to 12 seconds

White blood cell differential, blood
Neutrophils: 50% to 60%
Lymphocytes: 25% to 40%
Monocytes: 3% to 7%
Eosinophils: up to 3%
Basophils: up to 1%

BLOOD CHEMISTRY

Acid phosphatase, serum
0 to 3.7 ng/ml

Alanine aminotransferase
Adults: 7 to 56 U/L
Children: 10 to 35 U/L

Amylase, serum
≥ *18 years:* 35 to 115 U/L

Arterial blood gases
pH: 7.35 to 7.45
$Paco_2$: 35 to 45 mm Hg
Pao_2: 75 to 100 mm Hg
HCO_3^-: 22 to 26 mEq/L
Sao_2: 94% to 100%

Aspartate aminotransferase
Adults: 5 to 40 U/L

Bilirubin, serum
Adults, total: 0.2 to 1 mg/dl
Neonates, total: 1 to 10 mg/dl
Neonates, unconjugated indirect: 0.2 to 0.8 mg/dl

Blood urea nitrogen
8 to 20 mg/dl

Calcium, serum (atomic absorption)
Males ≥ *22 years:* 8.9 to 10.1 mg/dl
Females ≥ *19 years:* 8.9 to 10.1 mg/dl

Carbon dioxide, total, blood
23 to 30 mEq/L

Cholesterol, total, serum
Adults: 140 to 199 mg/dl (desirable)

C-reactive protein, serum
Negative or < 0.8 mg/dl

Creatine, serum
Males: 0.2 to 0.6 mg/dl
Females: 0.6 to 1 mg/dl

Creatine kinase, isoenzymes
CK-BB: none
CK-MB: 0 to 7 U/L
CK-MM: 5 to 7 U/L

Creatinine, serum
Adults: 0.6 to 1.3 mg/dl

Free thyroxine, serum
0.7 to 2 ng/dl

Free triiodothyronine
2.3 to 4.2 pmol/L

Glucose, plasma, fasting
65 to 110 mg/dl

Glucose, plasma, 2-hour postprandial
65 to 139 mg/dl

Iron, serum
Males: 50 to 150 μg/dl
Females: 35 to 145 μg/dl

Lactate dehydrogenase
Total: 94 to 257 U/L in adults, 108 to 540 U/L in children
LD_1: 17.5% to 28.3%
LD_2: 30.4% to 36.4%
LD_3: 19.2% to 24.8%
LD_4: 9.6% to 15.6%
LD_5: 5.5% to 12.7%

Lactic acid, blood
Venous blood: 0.5 to 2.2 mEq/L
Arterial blood: 0.5 to 1.6 mEq/L

Lipase
56 to 239 U/L

Lipoproteins, serum
HDL cholesterol:
–*Males:* 37 to 70 mg/dl
–*Females:* 40 to 84 mg/dl
LDL cholesterol: < 130 mg/dl

Magnesium, serum
1.7 to 2.1 mEq/L
Atomic absorption: 1.7 to 2.1 mg/dl

Phosphates, serum
1.8 to 2.6 mEq/L
Atomic absorption: 2.5 to 4.5 mg/dl

Potassium, serum
3.8 to 5.5 mEq/L

Protein, serum
Total: 6.3 to 7.9 g/dl
Albumin fraction: 3.4 to 4.8 g/dl
Alpha$_1$-globulin: 0.1 to 0.4 g/dl
Alpha$_2$-globulin: 0.5 to 1.1 g/dl
Beta globulin: 0.6 to 1.2 g/dl
Gamma globulin: 0.7 to 1.7 g/dl

Sodium, serum
135 to 145 mEq/L

Thyroxine, total, serum
5 to 12.5 μg/dl

Triglycerides, serum
Males > 20 years: 40 to 160 mg/dl
Females > 20 years: 35 to 135 mg/dl

Uric acid, serum
Males: 3.5 to 7.2 mg/dl
Females: 2.6 to 6 mg/dl

URINE CHEMISTRY

Amylase, urine
10 to 80 U/hour

Bence Jones protein, urine
Negative

Bilirubin, urine
Negative

Calcium, urine
Males: 25 to 300 mg/24 hours
Females: 20 to 275 mg/24 hours

Chloride, urine
140 to 250 mEq/L

Creatinine, urine
Males: 0.8 to 1.8 g/24 hours
Females: 0.6 to 1.6 g/24 hours

Glucose, urine
Negative

17-Hydroxycorticosteroids, urine
Males: 3 to 10 mg/24 hours
Females: 2 to 6 mg/24 hours

17-Ketogenic steroids, urine
Males: 5 to 24 mg/24 hours
Females: 5 to 15 mg/24 hours

Ketones, urine
Negative

17-Ketosteroids, urine
Males: 6 to 21 mg/24 hours
Females: 4 to 17 mg/24 hours

Protein, urine
Males: 0 to 150 mg/24 hours
Females: 27 to 93 mg/24 hours

Red blood cells, urine
0 to 3 per high-power field

Sodium, urine
40 to 220 mEq/L/24 hours

Sodium chloride, urine
140 to 250 mEq/L

Urinalysis, routine
Color: straw
Appearance: clear
Specific gravity: 1.005 to 1.035
pH: 4.5 to 8
Epithelial cells: few
Casts: occasional hyaline casts
Crystals: present

Urine osmolality
24-hour urine: 300 to 900 mOsm/kg
Random urine: 50 to 1,400 mOsm/kg

Urobilinogen, urine
< 4 mg/24 hours

Vanillylmandelic acid, urine
< 8 mg/24 hours

White blood cell count, urine
0 to 4 per high-power field

MISCELLANEOUS

Cerebrospinal fluid
Pressure: 50 to 180 mm H_2O
Appearance: clear, colorless
Gram stain: no organisms

Lupus erythematosus cell preparation
Negative

Occult blood, fecal
≤ 2 mg total Hb/g feces

Rheumatoid factor, serum
Negative

Venereal Disease Research Laboratory, serum
Negative

Normal and Abnormal Serum Drug Levels

DRUG NAME AND THERAPEUTIC VALUE*	PURPOSE OF TEST	SIGNIFICANCE OF ABNORMAL VALUE
Acetaminophen < 50 mcg/ml	Monitoring for overdose	• Increased value (≥120 mcg/ml) signifies overdose. • Decreased value shows that drug has little therapeutic effect.
Amikacin Peak: 20 to 25 mcg/ml Trough: 5 to 10 mcg/ml	Monitoring drug therapy	• Adjust time or amount of dose or both.
Amitriptyline 75 to 200 ng/ml	Monitoring drug therapy	• Decreased value shows that drug has little therapeutic effect. • Higher levels may signify toxicity.
Digoxin 0.5 to 2 ng/ml	Monitoring drug therapy	• Increased value (≥ 3 ng/ml) may signify toxicity. • Decreased value shows that drug may have decreased therapeutic effect.
Ethanol 0 (legal limit for blood alcohol level for drivers varies from state to state)	Detecting ethanol in bloodstream (degree of alcohol in blood correlates to level of intoxication)	• Value > 300 mcg/ml suggests alcohol ingestion. • Value > 3,000 mcg/ml depresses respirations and can be considered lethal.
Ethosuximide 40 to 75 mcg/ml	Monitoring drug therapy	• Increased value (≥ 100 mcg/ml) may signify toxicity. • Decreased value shows that drug may have decreased therapeutic effect.
Ethylene glycol 0	Monitoring for overdose	• Increased value (≥ 2 mEq/L) may signify toxicity. • Value > 20 mEq/L is considered lethal.

These values are for adults.

DRUG NAME AND THERAPEUTIC VALUE*	PURPOSE OF TEST	SIGNIFICANCE OF ABNORMAL VALUE
Gentamycin Peak: 4 to 8 mcg/ml Trough: 1 to 2 mcg/ml	Monitoring drug therapy	• Adjust time or amount of dose or both.
Lidocaine 2 to 5 mcg/ml	Monitoring drug therapy and evaluating toxicity	• Increased value (≥ 6 mcg/ml) may signify toxicity. • Decreased value shows that drug may have decreased therapeutic effect.
Lithium Trough: 0.8 to 1.2 mEq/L	Monitoring drug therapy and evaluating toxicity	• Increased value (trough > 1.5 mEq/L) may signify toxicity. • Decreased value shows that drug may have decreased therapeutic effect.
Methotrexate < 10 micromol 24 hr postdose < 1 micromol 48 hr postdose < 0.2 micromol 72 hr post-dose	Monitoring drug therapy	• Adjust time or amount of dose or both.
Nitroprusside (thiocyanate level) 4 to 20 mcg/dl	Evaluating toxicity	• Increased value (≥ 60 mcg/ml) may signify toxicity. • Decreased value shows that drug may have decreased therapeutic effect.
Nortriptyline 50 to 150 ng/ml	Monitoring drug therapy	• Decreased value shows that drug has little therapeutic effect. • Increased levels can cause depression.
Phenobarbital 1 to 5 mcg/ml	Monitoring drug therapy, evaluating toxicity, and evaluating for possible abuse	• Increased value (≥ 10 mcg/ml) may signify toxicity; 30 to 40 mcg/ml is used to reduce intracranial pressure but requires artificial respiratory support. • Decreased value shows that drug may have decreased therapeutic effect.
Phenytoin Plasma: 10 to 20 mcg/ml	Monitoring drug therapy and evaluating toxicity	• Increased value (> 30 mcg/ml) may signify toxicity. • Decreased value shows that drug may have decreased therapeutic effect.

(continued)

These values are for adults.

DRUG NAME AND THERAPEUTIC VALUE*	PURPOSE OF TEST	SIGNIFICANCE OF ABNORMAL VALUE
Procainamide 4 to 8 mcg/ml	Monitoring drug therapy and evaluating toxicity	• Increased value (> 16 mcg/ml) may signify toxicity. • Decreased value shows that drug may have decreased therapeutic effect.
Propafenone 0.5 to 2 mcg/ml	Monitoring drug therapy	• Adjust time or amount of dose or both.
Quinidine 2 to 5 mcg/ml	Monitoring drug therapy and evaluating toxicity	• Increased value (≥ 7 mcg/ml) may signify toxicity. • Decreased value shows that drug may have decreased therapeutic effect.
Salicylate 2 to 20 mg/dl	Monitoring drug therapy and evaluating toxicity	• Increased value (≥ 50 mg/dl) may signify toxicity. • Decreased value shows that drug may have decreased therapeutic effect.
Theophylline 10 to 20 mcg/ml	Monitoring drug therapy and evaluating toxicity	• Increased value (≥ 20 mcg/ml) may signify toxicity. • Decreased value shows that drug may have decreased therapeutic effect.
Tobramycin Peak: 4 to 8 mcg/ml Trough: 1 to 2 mcg/ml	Monitoring drug therapy	• Adjust time or amount of dose or both.
Valproic acid Trough: > 40 mcg/ml	Monitoring drug therapy	• Increased value (≥ 120 mcg/ml) may signify toxicity. Adverse effects may occur at levels > 125 mcg/ml. • Decreased value shows that drug may have decreased therapeutic effect.
Vancomycin Peak: 20 to 40 mcg/ml Trough: 5 to 10 mcg/ml	Monitoring drug therapy	• Increased value (≥ 400 ng/ml) may signify toxicity. • Decreased value shows that drug may have decreased therapeutic effect.
Verapamil 50 to 200 ng/ml	Monitoring drug therapy	• Increased value (peak ≥ 400 ng/ml) may signify toxicity. • Decreased value shows that drug may have decreased therapeutic effect.

These values are for adults.

Illustrated Guide to Home Testing

In recent years, the number of diagnostic tests that people can perform themselves at home has greatly increased. The teaching aids on the following pages describe how to accurately perform several of the newest and most common home tests, including tests for blood cholesterol levels, pacemaker function, and the presence of human immunodeficiency virus.

When you review these tests with your patient, be sure to:
• stress the importance of following the manufacturer's instructions exactly
• explain unfamiliar terms
• review any special forms that the patient must complete, such as the diary needed when using a Holter monitor
• discuss how to follow up on test results.

TESTING YOUR BLOOD GLUCOSE LEVEL

Dear Patient:
Testing your blood glucose levels daily will tell you whether your diabetes is under control. Follow these steps to learn how to obtain blood for testing and how to perform the test.

Getting ready
1. Begin by assembling the necessary equipment: your glucose meter, a lancet, an alcohol pad, gauze pads, and a vial with reagent strips.
2. Remove a reagent strip from the vial. Then replace the cap, making sure that it's tight.
3. Turn on the glucose meter and, if necessary, calibrate the machine according to the manufacturer's instructions. Then wait for the display window to show that the meter is ready for the blood sample.

Obtaining blood
1. Wash your hands thoroughly and dry them. Choose a site on the end or side of any fingertip. To enhance blood flow, hold your finger under warm water for a minute or two.
2. Hold your hand below your heart, and press the blood toward the fingertip you plan to pierce by squeezing that fingertip with the thumb of the same hand. Wipe the designated fingertip with an alcohol pad, and dry it with a gauze pad. Then place your fingertip (with your thumb still pressed against it) on a firm surface such as a table.

3. Twist off the lancet's protective cap. Then grasp the lancet and quickly pierce your fingertip just to the side of the finger pad, where you have more blood vessels and fewer nerve endings.
4. Next, push the sharp end of the lancet into the protective cap to avoid accidental sticks. Place the device in a sharps container (a coffee can or a 2-L plastic soda bottle).
5. Remove your thumb from your fingertip to permit blood flow. Then gently press your finger until you get a large, hanging drop of blood.

Testing blood
1. When the display window indicates that the meter is ready, touch the drop of blood to the reagent strip at the indicated spot, and insert the strip into the glucose meter. In most cases, the drop of blood will automatically start the meter's timer. Apply pressure to the puncture site with a dry gauze pad to stop the bleeding.
2. After the meter has finished the test, you can read the results from the display window. The meter will automatically store the date, time, and results of the test.

COLLECTING A URINE SPECIMEN: FOR MALES

Dear Patient:
Your doctor wants you to have your urine tested. A urine test can tell whether you have an infection or too much or too little of certain substances in your body. To make sure that test results are accurate, your urine shouldn't contain "outside germs" from your hands or penis.

Follow these directions carefully. Read them through to the end before collecting the specimen.

1. Wash your hands thoroughly. Open the package of disposable wipes that the nurse gave you, and place it on a clean, dry surface nearby.

2. Remove the lid from the specimen cup and place it flat side down. Do not touch the inside of the cup or lid.

4. Urinate a small amount into the toilet. After 1 or 2 seconds, catch about 1 ounce (30 milliliters) of urine in the specimen cup.

3. Prepare to urinate. (If you're uncircumcised, first pull back your foreskin.) Using a disposable wipe, clean the head of your penis from the urethral opening toward you (as shown at the top of the next column). Then discard the used wipe.

The nurse will tell you how far to fill the cup. As a rule, you'll fill it about one-fourth or more full.

Don't allow the cup to touch your penis at any time. When you're done, place the lid on the cup and return it to the nurse.

Note: Don't drink a lot of water before the test. This could affect the accuracy of the test results.

COLLECTING A URINE SPECIMEN: FOR FEMALES

Dear Patient:
Your doctor has asked you to provide a urine specimen for testing. The specimen can tell whether you have an infection or too much or too little of certain substances in your body.

To make sure that the test results are accurate, your urine shouldn't contain "outside germs" from your hands, labia, or urethral opening.

Follow the instructions below carefully. Read them through to the end before collecting your specimen.

1. Wash your hands thoroughly. Open the package of disposable wipes that the nurse gave you, and place it on a clean, dry, surface nearby.

2. Remove the lid from the specimen cup and place it flat side down. Do not touch the inside of the cup or lid.

3. Sit as far back on the toilet as possible. Spread your labia apart with one hand (as shown), keeping the folds separated for the rest of the procedure.

4. Using the disposable wipes, clean the area between the labia and around the urethra thoroughly from front to back (as shown). Use a new wipe for each stroke. Discard the used wipes.

5. Urinate a small amount into the toilet. After 1 or 2 seconds, hold the specimen cup below your urine stream (as shown) and catch about 1 ounce (30 milliliters) of urine in the cup. Don't allow the cup to touch your skin at any time.

6. Place the lid on the cup and return it to the nurse.
Note: Don't drink a lot of water before the test. This could affect the accuracy of the test results.

TESTING YOUR URINE FOR KETONES

Dear Patient:

If your urine contains waste chemicals, called ketones, your blood sugar level may be too high.

You should test your urine for ketones when your blood sugar level rises above 240 mg/dl or when you're ill. Even a minor illness can dramatically affect your blood sugar levels.

Your doctor will probably recommend testing every 4 hours until your blood sugar levels have stabilized or until your illness is over. To test your urine for ketones, follow these steps:

1. First, gather a clean container (such as a small plastic cup), a bottle of reagent strips, and a wristwatch or a clock with a second hand.

2. Collect a urine specimen in the container.

3. Remove one reagent strip from the bottle and replace the cap. Hold the strip so that the test blocks face up, but don't touch the blocks (as shown).

4. Dip the end of the strip with the test blocks into the urine for about 2 seconds. Then remove the strip and shake off excess urine. (Or you can perform the test while you urinate by simply holding the strip under the urine stream for about 2 seconds.)

5. Now hold the reagent strip horizontally and immediately begin timing (as shown), following the manufacturer's directions.

6. After waiting the recommended time, compare the ketone test block with the ketone color chart on the bottle label (as shown).

7. Keep a record of your tests, listing the date, time, results, and any other pertinent information. Call the doctor if your urine is positive for ketones.

TESTING FOR BLOOD IN YOUR STOOL

Dear Patient:
A home fecal occult blood test is an easy, inexpensive way to detect blood in your stool. For accurate results, follow the directions given by the nurse or doctor, read the instructions included with the test kit, and review these guidelines.

How to get ready
Don't eat red meat or raw fruits or vegetables for 3 days before you take the test and during the test period. Also avoid diet supplements containing iron or vitamin C and painkillers containing aspirin or ibuprofen (such as Advil and Nuprin) for the same time period. All of these substances can affect test results.

Increase your intake of high-fiber foods, such as whole grain breads and cereals. Your doctor may also ask you to eat popcorn or nuts.

How to perform the test
1. Make sure all your supplies are in one place. They may include your test cards (or slides), a chemical developer, a wooden applicator, and a watch with a second hand.
2. Obtain a stool sample. You can do this by laying a long sheet of clear plastic wrap across the toilet bowl to catch the stool, or by removing stool from the bowl. Flush the remaining stool down the toilet.

Use the applicator to smear a thin film of the sample onto the slot marked "A" on the front of the test card. Smear a thin film of a second sample from a *different area of the same stool* onto the slot marked "B" on the same side of the card.

1. Collect small stool specimen on applicator. Apply thin smear in box A.

2. Reuse applicator to obtain another sample from a different part of the stool. Apply thin smear in box B.

3. Close cover. Place slide away from heat and light. Return slide to doctor.

3. *If the doctor or a lab will be analyzing the test samples,* close slots A and B, put your name and the date on the test kit, and return the card (or slide) to the doctor or lab as soon as possible.

If you're doing the test yourself, turn the card over and open the back window. Apply 2 drops of the chemical developer to the paper covering each sample. Wait 1 minute; then read the results.

If either slot has a bluish tint, the test results are positive for blood in the stool. *If neither slot looks blue,* the test results are normal. Write down the results. Discard the used applicator and wash your hands thoroughly.
4. Repeat the test on your next two bowel movements. Report the results of all of the tests to the doctor. Even if only one of the six test results is positive, the doctor may recommend other tests.

USING A HOLTER MONITOR

Dear Patient:

Your doctor has ordered you to wear a Holter monitor for 24 hours. It works like a continuous electrocardiogram (ECG) by recording any irregular heartbeats you may have. The information from this recording will help your doctor determine if abnormal heartbeats are causing your symptoms, such as chest pain or discomfort, dizziness, or weakness. If you're taking a heart medication, the Holter monitor can also help your doctor evaluate how well the medication is working.

The monitor has adhesive patches (called *leads*) that the nurse will attach to your skin. She'll also show you how to wear the monitor on a belt or over your shoulder. If one of the leads becomes loose, secure it with a piece of tape.

While wearing the monitor, you can perform most of your usual activities. You'll even wear it to bed.

Practice these safety measures while wearing the Holter monitor:

• Don't get the monitor wet — don't shower, bathe, or swim with it on.

• Avoid high-voltage areas, strong magnetic fields, and microwave ovens.

While you're wearing the monitor, you'll write down your activities and feelings. This diary will help your doctor establish a connection between your monitor tracing and your activities and feelings. Jot down the time of day when you perform any activity, such as taking medication, eating, drinking, moving your bowels, urinating, engaging in sexual activity, exercising, and sleeping, or experience any strong emotions, such as anger or fear. (See the sample entries below.)

If your monitor has an event button, the nurse will show you how to press it in case you experience anything unusual, such as a sudden, rapid heartbeat.

DAY	TIME	ACTIVITY	FEELINGS
Tuesday	10:30 am	Rode from hospital in car	Legs tired, some shortness of breath
	11:30 am	Watched TV in living room	Comfortable
	12:15 pm	Ate lunch, took Inderal	Indigestion
	1:30 pm	Walked next door to see neighbor	Shortness of breath
	2:45 pm	Walked home	Very tired, legs hurt
	3:00 - 4:00pm	Urinated, took nap	Comfortable
	5:30 pm	Ate dinner, slowly	Comfortable
	7:20 pm	Had bowel movement	Shortness of breath
	9:00 pm	Watched TV - drank 1 beer	Heart beating fast for about one minute, no pain
	11:00 pm	Took Inderal, urinated, went to bed	Tired
Wednesday	8:15 am	Awoke, urinated, washed face and arms	Very tired, rapid heart beat for about 30 seconds
	10:30 am	Returned to hospital	Felt better

CHECKING YOUR PACEMAKER BY TELEPHONE

Dear Patient:

Your doctor wants to check your pacemaker regularly by telephone. Doing this helps him monitor how well the pacemaker is working and the strength of the battery while you stay at home. Here's how to use your pacemaker's transmitter.

Insert the battery

Before using your transmitter for the first time, remove the battery cover and insert the battery supplied by the manufacturer. You'll need to replace the battery every 2 to 3 months, according to the manufacturer's instructions.

Set up the transmitter

When you're ready, take the transmitter out of its case. Also remove the electrode cable from the case, and plug the cable into the jack on the transmitter.

Place the electrodes on your fingers or on your wrists. Then turn on the transmitter and listen for the tones indicating that the power is on.

Phone in your electrocardiogram

Dial the telephone number of your doctor's office or the pacemaker clinic, and listen for instructions.

When directed, place the telephone handset in the pacemaker transmitter. Stay still (for up to 60 seconds) to minimize interference with the signals from your heart.

Wait for further instructions. For example, the doctor may ask you to use a special magnet that's in the transmitter's case. To do so, simply hold the magnet over the pacemaker and transmit your electrocardiogram as before.

When you finish transmitting, take off the electrodes and turn off the transmitter. Place the equipment in the storage case until the next time you use it.

Transmitter — — ON-OFF button

— Cable jack

— Wrist electrode

— Finger electrode

CHECKING YOUR BLOOD CHOLESTEROL LEVEL

Dear Patient:

Testing your blood cholesterol level can tell you whether you're at risk for heart disease. If you take cholesterol-lowering medication or are on a low-cholesterol diet, testing your blood cholesterol level will help you determine if your cholesterol is under control. If you have any questions about test results or the risk factors associated with heart disease, always consult your doctor.

Follow these steps to learn how to obtain a blood sample and how to perform the test. Remember, because cholesterol levels can change from day to day and can be affected by stress, weight loss, illness, or pregnancy, one cholesterol reading may not be final.

Getting ready

1. Begin by assembling the necessary equipment included in the packet: the test device, the test result chart, and a lancet, plus an alcohol pad and gauze pads.
2. Read the instructions thoroughly.

Obtaining blood

1. Wash your hands thoroughly and dry them. Choose a site on the end or side of any fingertip. To enhance blood flow, hold your finger under warm water for a minute or two.
2. Hold your hand below your heart, and press the blood toward the fingertip you plan to pierce by squeezing that fingertip with the thumb of the same hand. Wipe the designated fingertip with an alcohol pad, and dry it with a gauze pad. Place your fingertip (with your thumb still pressed against it) on a firm surface such as a table.
3. Twist off the lancet's protective cap. Then grasp the lancet and

quickly pierce your fingertip just to the side of the finger pad, where you have more blood vessels and fewer nerve endings.
4. Push the sharp end of the lancet into the protective cap to avoid accidental sticks. Place the device in a sharps container (such as a coffee can or a 2-L plastic soda bottle).
5. Remove your thumb from your fingertip to permit blood flow. Apply gentle pressure to your finger until you get a large, hanging drop of blood.
6. Point your finger down directly over the blood well, and place the hanging drop of blood into the blood well, making sure that you fill the black circle completely. Then wait at least 2 but no more than 4 minutes. Press the puncture site with a dry gauze pad to stop the bleeding.

Reading the results

When the display windows indicate that the test is complete, read the results. Compare the reading on the testing device with the chart included in the packet for your cholesterol level. Remember to inform your doctor about the results.

Performing a Home Ovulation Test

Dear Patient:
A home ovulation test helps you determine the best time to try to become pregnant. It works by monitoring the amount of luteinizing hormone (LH) that's found in your urine.

Normally, during each menstrual cycle, levels of this hormone rise suddenly (LH surge), causing an egg to be released from the ovary 24 to 36 hours later. The release of the egg is known as ovulation. Ovulation normally occurs once a month, about 2 weeks before your period, and lasts about 24 hours. This is your most fertile period — the only time each month that you can become pregnant.

Follow these directions to test your urine for the presence of LH and to determine when you're most likely to become pregnant. To know when to begin testing, you'll need to know the length of your menstrual cycle. Count from the beginning of one period to the beginning of the next period. (Count the first day of bleeding as day 1). Use the chart below to determine when to begin testing.

Length of cycle	Start test this many days after your last period begins	Length of cycle	Start test this many days after your last period begins
21	5	31	14
22	5	32	15
23	6	33	16
24	7	34	17
25	8	34	18
26	9	36	19
27	10	37	20
28	11	38	21
29	12	39	22
30	13	40	23

Getting ready
1. Read the instructions thoroughly before you perform the test. This test can be performed any time of the day or night but should be performed at the same time each day.

Note: Don't urinate for at least 4 hours before taking this test, and don't drink a lot of liquids for several hours before testing.
2. Remove the test stick from the package and remove the cap.

Performing the test
1. Sit on the toilet. Direct the absorbent tip of the test stick downward and directly into your urine stream for at least 5 seconds or until it's thoroughly wet. *Don't urinate on the windows of the stick.* You can also urinate into a clean, dry cup or container and dip the test stick (absorbent tip only) into the urine for at least 5 seconds.
2. Lay the test stick on a clean, dry, flat surface.

Reading the results
1. Wait at least 5 minutes to read the results. When the test is finished, a line will appear in the small window (control window).
2. *If there is no line in the large rectangular window (test window) or if the line is lighter than the line in the small rectangular window,* you haven't begun your LH surge. You should continue with daily testing.
3. *If you see one line in the large window that is similar to or darker than the line in the small window* (as shown at right), you've detected an LH surge. This means that you should ovulate within the next 24 to 36 hours.

Positive

Once you've determined that you're about to ovulate, you know you're at the start of the most fertile time of your cycle.

PERFORMING A HOME PREGNANCY TEST

Dear Patient:

A home pregnancy test will detect a hormone in your urine that your body produces only if you are pregnant. The test can detect this hormone — human chorionic gonadotropin (hCG) — as early as 1 day after you miss your period. If you have been pregnant or had a miscarriage within the last 8 weeks or if you are taking a medication that contains hCG or that's used in combination with hCG, the test may produce a false-positive result. In any case, *always* consult your doctor before and after taking this test.

Follow these steps to learn how to perform the test.

Getting ready

1. Read the instructions thoroughly before you perform the test. This test can be performed any time of the day or night — it doesn't need to be done first thing in the morning.

2. Remove the test stick from the package and slide the clear splash guard back to expose the absorbent tip.

Performing the test

1. Straddle the toilet and hold the test stick by the thumb grip.

2. Direct the absorbent tip downward and directly into your urine stream (as shown at the top of the next column) for at least 5 seconds or until it's thoroughly wet. *Don't urinate on the windows of the stick.*

3. You can also urinate into a clean, dry cup or container and dip the test stick (absorbent tip only) into the urine for at least 5 seconds.

4. Lay the test stick on a clean, dry, flat surface.

Reading the results

1. Wait at least 3 minutes to read the results. When the test is finished, a line will appear in the small rectangular window (control window).

2. *If you see one line in the round and rectangular windows* (test window), as shown at right, the test has indicated that you are pregnant. You should consult your doctor as soon as possible to discuss your pregnancy.

3. *If the only visible line is in the control (rectangular) window*, the test has indicated that you are not pregnant. You can perform a repeat test with a new test kit if your period doesn't start within a week.

Note: If results appear in the round window but not in the rectangular control window, don't read the results because they may be inaccurate. Call the toll-free number located on the test box or package insert.

PERFORMING A HOME HIV TEST

Dear Patient:

Human immunodeficiency virus (HIV) is a virus that attacks your immune system and causes acquired immunodeficiency syndrome (AIDS). By testing your blood, you can determine if you've been infected with HIV. Remember that even if you've been exposed to the HIV virus, it may not become evident in your blood for 6 months. If you have any questions about your test results or the risk factors associated with HIV, *always* consult a doctor.

Follow these steps to learn how to obtain a blood sample and how to perform the test.

Getting ready

1. Begin by assembling the necessary equipment included in the packet: a lancet, a test card with your personal identification number (to receive the confidential and anonymous test results), and the envelope in which to send the test card to the laboratory. Also gather an alcohol pad and gauze pads.

2. Read the instructions thoroughly before you stick your finger. Remove the personal identification card from the bottom of the test card, and place it in a safe place.

Obtaining blood

1. Wash your hands thoroughly and dry them. Choose a site on the end or side of any fingertip. To enhance blood flow, hold your finger under warm water for a minute or two.

2. Hold your hand below your heart, and press the blood toward the finger-

tip you plan to pierce by squeezing that fingertip with the thumb of the same hand. Wipe the designated fingertip with an alcohol pad, and dry it with a gauze pad. Place your fingertip (with your thumb still pressed against it) on a firm surface such as a table.

3. Twist off the lancet's protective cap. Then grasp the lancet and quickly pierce your fingertip just to the side of the finger pad, where you have more blood vessels and fewer nerve endings.

4. Push the sharp end of the lancet into the protective cap to avoid accidental sticks.

---

5. Remove your thumb from your fingertip to permit blood flow. Then apply gentle pressure to your finger until you get a large, hanging drop of blood.

6. Point your finger down directly over the three circles on the test card (as shown at right). Completely fill each circle with blood from your finger.
7. Place any used lancets in the containers attached to the mailing card. Slip the test card in the postage-paid mailer, seal the mailer, and send it to the address printed on the front. Save the part of the card that lists the toll-free number to call for results.

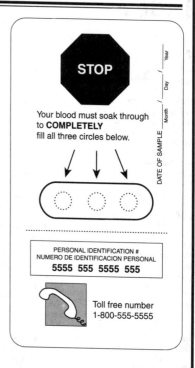

STOP

Your blood must soak through to **COMPLETELY** fill all three circles below.

DATE OF SAMPLE

Month / Day / Year

PERSONAL IDENTIFICATION #
NUMERO DE IDENTIFICACION PERSONAL
5555 555 5555 555

Toll free number
1-800-555-5555

Obtaining the results

In about 1 week, call the toll-free number on the identification card. Give your identification number to the person who answers, and wait for the results. *If your test is positive for HIV,* a specially trained counselor will advise you what to do next and will tell you about HIV and AIDS organizations nationwide. *If your test results are nega-* *tive for HIV,* the trained counselor will advise you how to maintain your negative HIV status.

Remember, a negative test result doesn't necessarily mean you're free from HIV infection. It may simply mean that the antibodies are not yet present in your blood. To be certain, repeat the test with a new package in 6 months.

Index

A

AAT. *See* Alpha$_1$-antitrypsin.
Abdominal aorta, ultrasonography of, **523-524**
Abdominal aortic aneurysm, 2
  ultrasonography of, 523-524
Abdominal aortic disease, renal imaging in, 660-662
Abdominal pain, upper, cholangiography in, 574-576
Abdominal trauma
  arteriography in, 580-583
  CT scan in, 621-623
  liver-spleen scanning in, 653, 655-656
  peritoneal fluid analysis in, 390-393
  ultrasonography in, 526-530
ABG. *See* Arterial blood gases.
ABO blood typing, **255-256**
Abruptio placentae, 2
  FSP levels in, 120-121
  pelvic ultrasonography in, 532-533
ACE. *See* Angiotensin-converting enzyme.
Acetaminophen, serum levels of, 748
Acetest tablet, 372
Acetylcholine receptor antibodies, **287-288**
Achalasia, 562-567
AChR. *See* Acetylcholine receptor antibodies.
Acid-base disorders, 130t, 131
Acidified serum lysis test, **275-276**
Acid mucopolysaccharides, **373-374**
Acidosis, urinalysis in, 321-324
Acid perfusion test, **725-726**
Acid phosphatase, **155-156,** 746
ACP. *See* Acid phosphatase.
Acquired immunodeficiency states, 265, 267
Acquired immunodeficiency syndrome, 3
  Candida antibody in, 306-307
  CMV in, 456
  HIV antibodies in, 299-300
Acromegaly
  growth hormone suppression test and, 200-201
  hGH levels in, 199
  LH levels in, 205-207
  skull radiography in, 539-540

ACTH. *See* Adrenocorticotropic hormone.
Activated clotting time, **115-116**
Activated partial thromboplastin time, **113-114,** 476
ACT. *See* Activated clotting time.
AcuTect, DVT diagnosis by, 561
Acute hepatitis, 148
  AFP levels in, 314-315
  vitamin B$_{12}$ levels in, 246-247
Acute infections, TORCH test in, 315-316
Acute intermittent porphyria, 163
Acute renal failure, 3
  renal angiography in, 596-598
  sodium and chloride urine tests in, 376-377
Acute tubular necrosis, 4
  renal imaging in, 660-662
  urinalysis in, 321-324
Addison's disease, 135
  ADH levels in, 212-213
  corticotropin levels in, 197
  cortisol levels in, 225-227
  HLA test in, 276-277
  17-KGS urine levels in, 346
  17-KS urine levels in, 343-345
  magnesium levels in, 135
  17-OHCS urine levels in, 342-343
  potassium levels in, 137
  rapid ACTH levels in, 198
  renin levels in, 158
  urine tests in, 376-377, 334-335
Adenocarcinoma
  barium enema in, 567-570
  breast biopsy in, 469
  arteriography in, 580-583
  ultrasonography in, 526-528
  CT scan of pancreas in, 623-625
Adenofibroma, breast biopsy in, 469
Adenomas
  arteriography in, 580-583
  scanning in, 653, 655-656
ADH. *See* Antidiuretic hormone.
Adrenal adenoma
  17-KGS urine levels in, 346
  17-KS urine levels in, 343-345
Adrenal cancer, 337-339
  17-KGS urine levels in, 346
  17-KS urine levels in, 343-345
  17-OHCS urine levels in, 342-343
Adrenal disorders, 4
  corticotropin levels in, 196-197
  cortisol levels in, 225-227

Adrenal disorders *(continued)*
  free cortisol levels in, 335-336
  glycosuria in, 369-372
  insulin tolerance test in, 201-202
  pregnanediol levels in, 350-351
  rapid corticotropin levels in, 198
  sodium and chloride in, 376-377
  sweat test findings in, 433-435
  ultrasonography in, 533-535
  urine estrogen levels in, 337-339
Adrenal hormones, **224-231**
Adrenal hyperplasia, congenital
  estrogen levels in, 235-237
  17-KGS urine levels in, 346
  17-KS urine levels in, 343-345
  male, testosterone levels in, 238-240
  urine pregnanetriol levels in, 341-342
Adrenal medulla function, VMA urine levels in, 347-348
Adrenal medullary tumor, catecholamine levels in, 227-228
Adrenal tumor. *See also* Adrenal medullary tumor.
  free cortisol levels in, 335-336
  KUB in, 583-584
  nephrotomography in, 584-587
  renal CT scan in, 636-638
Adrenocortical function
  17-KGS urine levels in, 346
  17-OHCS urine levels in, 342-343
Adrenocortical hyperplasia
  progesterone levels in, 237-238
  urine aldosterone levels in, 334-335
  urine estrogen levels in, 337-339
Adrenocorticotropic hormone, **196-197,** 201-202
Adrenoleukodystrophy, evoked potential in, 676-677
AFP. *See* Alpha-fetoprotein.
AIDS. *See* Acquired immunodeficiency syndrome.
AIP. *See* Acute intermittent porphyria.
Alanine aminotransferase, **148-149,** 746
Alcoholic hepatitis, 148
  ALT levels in, 148-149
  AST levels in, 146-148
Alcoholic polymyopathy, 363

Boldface page numbers indicate major entries; i refers to an illustration; t refers to a table.

764

Alcoholism, 5
  chronic, folic acid levels in,
    249-250
  D-xylose absorption in, 741-742
  urine amylase levels in, 329-330
Aldosterone
  serum, **224-225**
  urine, **334-335**
Aldosteronism
  serum aldosterone levels in,
    224-225
  sodium and chloride urine tests in,
    376-377
  urine aldosterone levels in,
    334-335
  urine potassium levels in, 377-378
Alkaline phosphatase, **149-150**
Alkaptonuria, urinalysis in, 321-324
Allergens, RAST test of, 275
Allergic reactions, WBC differential
  in, 103-107
Allografts, rapidly rejecting, comple-
  ment assays in, 273-275
Alpha₁-antitrypsin, **145-146**
Alpha-fetoprotein, **314-315**
Alpha-PGH. *See* Alpha-subunit of
  pituitary glycoprotein hor-
  mones.
Alpha-subunit of pituitary glycopro-
  tein hormones, **213-214**
ALP. *See* Alkaline phosphatase.
ALT. *See* Alanine aminotransferase.
Alzheimer's disease, 5, 425-427
Ambiguous genitalia, sex chromatin
  tests in, 402-403
Amblyopia, evoked potential in,
  676-677
Amebiasis, 5
  sputum examination for, 384-385
  stool examination for, 399-401
Amenorrhea
  FSH levels in, 204-205
  LH levels in, 205-207
  pregnanediol urine levels in,
    350-351
  progesterone levels in, 237-238
  prolactin levels in, 207-209
  sex chromatin tests in, 402-403
  urine estrogen levels in, 337-339
Amikacin, serum levels of, 748
Amino acid disorders, 353, 354-356,
  355t
Amino acid screening, **353-356**,
  354-355t
Aminoacidurias, 353, 356
Amitriptyline, serum levels of, 748
AML. *See* Amylase.
Amniocentesis, 409-414, 532-533
Amniotic fluid analysis, **409-414**,
  412t
AMPs. *See* Acid mucopolysaccha-
  rides.
Amsler grid test, 710-711

Amylase, **153-154, 329-330**, 746,
  747
Amyloid infiltration, renal biopsy in,
  485-486, 488
Amyloidosis, 5
  bone marrow aspiration and biop-
    sy in, 478
  KUB in, 583-584
  synovial membrane biopsy in,
    478-479
  urinalysis in, 321-324
  urine protein levels in, 351-352
Amyotrophic lateral sclerosis, 5-6
  electromyography in, 677-679
Anaerobic specimen collector, 448i
Anal abscess, 499-501
Anal fissure, 6 , 501-504
Anal fistulas and polyps, 501-504
ANAs. *See* Antinuclear antibodies.
Androgenic arrhenoblastoma, 17-KS
  urine levels in, 343-345
Androstenedione, **229-230**
Anemia. *See also* Hemolytic anemia
  and Megaloblastic anemia.
  EGD in, 496-499
  EPO levels in, 230
  Hb levels in, 92-93
  HCT levels in, 86-87
  RBC levels in, 85-86
  RBC survival time in, 658-660
  red cell indices in, 88t
  reticulocyte count in, 89-90
  vitamin C levels in, 247-248
Anesthesia, evoked potential in,
  676-677
Aneurysm
  cerebral angiography in, 540-542
  KUB in, 583-584
  left ventricular, cardiac blood pool
    imaging in, 650-651
Aneurysm of the eye, fluorescein
  angiography in, 546-548
ANF. *See* Plasma atrial natriuretic
  factor.
Angina
  ECG in, 679, 681
  imaging in, 649-650
  technetium pyrophosphate scan-
    ning in, 646-647
Angiodysplasia, arteriography in,
  580-583
Angioma, arteriography in, 580-583
Angiosarcoma, biopsy in, 467
Angiotensin-converting enzyme,
  165-166
Anion gap, **139-141**
Ankle-arm pressure index, 521
Ankle-brachial index, 521
Ankylosing spondylitis, 6
  vertebral radiography in, 607-608
Anovulation, pregnanediol urine
  levels in, 350-351
Antegrade pyelography, **592-594**

Anthrax, 7
Antibody response, 295t
Antibody screening test, **261-262**
Anticholinesterase therapy, Tensilon
  test in, 733-735
Anticoagulation therapy, INR values
  in, 125-126
Antidiuretic hormone, **212-213**
Anti-double-stranded DNA antibod-
  ies, **289-290**
Anti-insulin antibody, **288-289**
Antimitochondrial antibodies,
  280-281
Antinuclear antibodies, **277-279,**
  278t
Antipernicious anemia factor,
  246-247, 246
Anti-smooth-muscle antibodies,
  281-282
Antistreptolysin-O test, **301-302**
Antitachycardia pacing, 705-707
Antithyroid antibodies, **282**
Aortic aneurysm
  cardiac catheterization in,
    696-701
  chest radiography of, 549-550t
  thoracic CT scan in, 632-634
  transesophageal echocardiography
    in, 517-519
Aortic dissection, echocardiography
  in, 517-519
Aortic insufficiency, 7
  cardiac catheterization in,
    696-701
  echocardiography in, 514-517
Aortic root enlargement, cardiac
  catheterization in, 696-701
Aortic stenosis, 7
  cardiac catheterization in,
    696-701
  Doppler ultrasonography in,
    519-522
Aortic valve function, cardiac
  catheterization in, 696-701
API. *See* Ankle-arm pressure index.
Aplastic anemia, 7-8
  bone marrow aspiration and biop-
    sy in, 474
  fecal urobilinogen in, 398-399
Aplitest, 316-318
Appendicitis, 8
  acute, barium enema in, 567-570
  peritoneal fluid analysis in,
    390-393
  WBC count in, 102-103
APTT. *See* Activated partial throm-
  boplastin time.
Arachnoiditis, 542-545
Argentaffinomas. *See* Carcinoid
  tumor.
Arginine test, **202-204**
Arrhythmias
  electrocardiography in, 693-694
  imaging in, 649-650

ARSA. *See* Arylsulfatase A.
Arterial blood gases, **129-132,** 746
Arterial ischemia index, 521
Arterial occlusion, 8, 519-522
Arterial stenosis, Doppler ultrasonography in, 519-522
Arterial trauma, Doppler ultrasonography in, 519-522
Arteriovenous malformation, angiography in, 540-542
Arteriovenous shunts, 546-548
Arthritis
   synovial fluid analysis in, 427-429
   vertebral radiography in, 607-608
Arthrocentesis, synovial fluid aspiration for analysis, 427-429
Arthrography, **609-611**
Arthroscopy, **508-512,** 509i
Arylsulfatase A, **330-331**
Ascites
   CT scan of pancreas in, 623-625
   D-xylose absorption in, 741-742
   peritoneal fluid analysis in, 390-393
Ascorbic acid. *See* Vitamin C.
Aspartate aminotransferase, 142, **146-148,** 746
Aspergillosis, 8, 491-493
Asthma, 8-9
   ABG levels in, 131
   chest radiography in, 549-550t
   intrinsic, anti-smooth-muscle antibodies in, 281-282
Astrocytomas
   CT scan in, 616-618
   myelography in, 542-545
AST. *See* Aspartate aminotransferase.
Ataxia-telangiectasia, 9, 314-315
Atelectasis, 9
   chest radiography in, 548, 549-550t, 551
Atherosclerosis, 549-550t
Atrial tumor, 514-517
Atrionatriuretic peptides, **231**
Atriopeptins, **231**
Atrioventricular conduction disturbance, 707
Atrophic pyelonephritis, 583-584
Auditory lesions, evoked potential in, 673, 674-675i, 676-677
Australia antigen, **291-292**
Autoantibodies, **277-290**
Autoimmune disease
   ANAs in, 277-279
   ENAs in, 279-280
   Raji cell assay in, 273

B

Bacteremia, 446-447
Bacteria and fungi, **301-310**
Bacterial endocarditis, 514-517, 653, 655-656
Bacterial infections, 478-479

Bacterial meningitis antigen, **307-308**
Bacterial peritonitis, gallium scanning in, 656-658
Bacterial skin infections, skin biopsy in, 484-485
Balance tests, screening tests and, 722-723
Barium enema, lower GI examination and, **567-570**
Barium swallow (esophagography), **562-564**
Bartter's syndrome, 158
Basal cell carcinoma, 11, 484-485
Basal gastric secretion test, **387-389**
Basophils, 104, 105, 746
ß-thalassemia, 94t
Bence Jones protein, 352, 353, 747
Benign prostatic hyperplasia, 11
   cystourethrography in, 601-602
   prostate gland biopsy in, 469, 471
Benzene toxicity, 363-365
Bernard-Soulier syndrome
   platelet aggregation test in, 111-113
   platelet count in, 108-110
Bernstein test, **725-726**
ß-hydroxybutyrate, **190-191**
Bile duct carcinoma, 26, 577-580
Biliary enteric bypass, 662-664
Biliary tract
   cancer
      AFP levels in, 314-315
      cholangiography in, 574-576
   disease, cholecystography in, 572-574
   infection, duodenal contents culture and, 451-452
   obstruction
      pregnanediol levels in, 350-351
      ultrasonography of, **524-526**
Bilirubin, 367t, 747
   serum, **182-183**
   urine, **366-368**
Biofield test, 605
Bladder cancer, 11
   prostate gland biopsy in, 471
   urine ARSA levels in, 330-331
Bladder disorders
   cystourethrography in, 601-602
   retrograde cystography in, 588-590
Bladder infection, urine culture and, 438-439
Bladder outlet obstruction
   ultrasonography in, 533-535
   uroflowmetry test in, 726-728
Bleeding tendencies, APTT levels in, 113-114
Bleeding time, **107-108,** 746
Blood chemistry tests, **127-194**
Blood cholesterol, home test for, 759i
Blood culture, **446-447**

Blood dyscrasias, urinalysis in, 321-324
Blood glucose home test, 752i
Blood supply, cardiac catheterization in, 696-701
Blood in stool, home test for, 756i
Blood transfusion
   ABO blood typing in, 255-256
   antibody screening test in, 261-262
   crossmatching in, 258-260
   multiple, urine hemosiderin levels in, 381-382
   reactions to, 11-12
      direct antiglobulin test in, 260-261
      leukoagglutinin test in, 262-263
   RH typing in, 256-257
Blood urea nitrogen, **180-181,** 746
Body section roentgenography, **554-555**
Bone disorders
   biopsy in, **472-474**
   bone densitometry in, 608-609
   bone scan in, 651-653
   DEXA scan in, **608-609**
   hydroxyproline levels in, 357-358
Bone marrow aplasia, 275-276
Bone marrow aspiration and biopsy, **474-475, 477-478,** 476-477t
Bone marrow composition, skeletal MRI scan in, 629-630
Bone marrow failure, parvovirus B-19 antibody in, 300-301
Bone pain, evaluation of, 651-653
Bone scan, **651-653**
Bone tumor, 12
   bone biopsy in, 472-473
   bone marrow aspiration and biopsy in, 477
   skeletal CT scan in, 628-629
   skeletal MRI scan in, 629-630
Brain abscess, 12, 421-425
Brain death
   EEG recording in, 671-673
   Doppler studies in, 535-536
Brain lesions, evoked potential in, 673, 674-675i, 676-677
Brain stem integrity, evoked potential in, 673, 674-675i, 676-677
Brain tumor, CSF analysis in, 421-425
Breast biopsy, **467-469**
Breast cancer, 12
   BRCA testing in, 468
   biopsy in, 467-469, 482-484
   calcitonin levels in, 221-222
   CEA levels in, 313-314
   fibrinogen levels in, 119-120
   hCG urine levels in, 340-341
   mammography in, 604-606

Breast cysts, mammography in, 604-606
Bronchial obstruction
  bronchography in, 555-557
  fluoroscopy test in, 553-554
Bronchiectasis, 12, 555-557
Bronchitis, 13
  chest radiography in, 549-550t
  sputum culture and, 444-446
Bronchogenic carcinoma
  bronchoscopy and, 491-493
  gallium scanning in, 656-658
  lung ventilation scan in, 645-646
  mediastinoscopy in, 494
Bronchogenic cyst, chest radiography of, 549-550t
Bronchography, **555-557**
Bronchoscopy, **491-493**
Brucellosis, 13, 302-304
BUN. *See* Blood urea nitrogen.

C

CA 19-9 antigen, 313
CAD. *See* Coronary artery disease.
Calcium, 132-133, 379t, 746, 747
Calcium and phosphates, urine test, **378-379**
cAMP. *See* Cyclic adenosine monophosphate.
Cancer. *See specific type.*
Candida antibody, **306-307**
Capillary fragility test, **110-111**
Carbohydrates, **184-194**
Carbon monoxide poisoning, 101
Carbon tetrachloride toxicity, urine porphyrin levels in, 363-365
Carcinoembryonic antigen, **313-314**
Carcinoid tumor
  5-HIAA urine levels in, 349-350
  arteriography in, 580-583
Carcinoma. *See specific type.*
Cardiac abnormalities, cardiac radiography in, 558-560
Cardiac arrhythmias
  ECG test in, 679, 681, 683i
  Holter monitoring in, 691-693
  PA catheterization in, 701-704
  sleep studies in, 743-744
Cardiac catheterization, **696-701**
  normal pressure curves in, 699i
  pressures in recumbent adults in, 700t
Cardiac contusion, Persantine-thallium imaging in, 649-650
Cardiac disease. *See also* Heart failure *and* Myocardial infarction.
  cardiac radiography in, 558-560
  chest radiography of, 548, 549-550t, 551
  concentration and dilution tests in, 327-328
  imaging in, 647-648, 649-650

Cardiac enzymes and proteins, **141-145**
Cardiac monitoring and catheterization, **679-708**
Cardiac output, cardiac catheterization in, 696-701
Cardiac therapy, radiopharmaceutical myocardial perfusion imaging in, 689-691
Cardiac tumor, echocardiography in, 517-519
Cardiac volume, ANF levels in, 231
Cardiac wall motion, cardiac catheterization in, 696-701
Cardiolipin antibodies, **283-284**
Cardiolipin antibody syndrome, 283-284
Cardiomyopathy
  cardiac blood pool imaging in, 650-651
  echocardiography in, 514-517
  MRI scan in, 634-636
Cardiovascular drugs, PA catheterization and, 701-704
Cardiovascular system
  cardiac blood pool imaging in, **650-651**
  cardiac radiography in, **558-562**
  nuclear scans in, **646-651**
  Persantine-thallium imaging in, 649-650
  technetium pyrophosphate scanning in, 646-647
  thallium imaging in, 647-648
  ultrasonography of, **514-524**
Cartilaginous abnormalities, arthroscopy in, 609-611
Catecholamines, **336-337**
Catheter ablation procedures, electrophysiology studies in, 705-707
CBC. *See* Complete blood count.
CEA. *See* Carcinoembryonic antigen.
Celiac arteriography, **580-583**
Celiac disease, 14
  D-xylose absorption in, 741-742
  HLA test in, 276-277
  Raji cell assay in, 273
  vitamin A levels in, 244-245
  vitamin B$_{12}$ levels in, 245-246
  vitamin D$_3$ levels in, 248-249
Celiac sprue, 465
Cellular function, **264-269**
Central nervous system disorders
  CSF analysis in, 421-425
  glycosuria in, 369-372
  manganese levels in, 250-251
  tryptophan challenge test in, 374-375
  urine porphyrin levels in, 363-365
  vitamin B$_{12}$ levels in, 246-247
Cerebellar tumor, 618-621
Cerebral abscess, 618-621

Cerebral angiography, **540-542**
Cerebral anomalies, congenital, CT scan in, 616-618
Cerebral atrophy, 616-618
Cerebral blood flow, 535-536
Cerebral edema
  CT scan in, 616-618
  MRI scan in, 618-621
Cerebral hemorrhage, 618-621
Cerebral infarction, 616-618
Cerebral tumor, CT scan in, 616-618
Cerebral vasospasm, 535-536
Cerebrospinal fluid analysis, **421-425**, 423-424t, 747
Cerebrovascular abnormalities, 540-542
Ceruloplasmin, **175**
Cervical cancer
  biopsy in, **471-472**
  colposcopy in, 505-506
  Pap test for, 414-416
Cervical disk syndrome, 607-608
Cervical dysplasia, biopsy in, 472
Cervical spondylosis
  CT scan of spine in, 625-627
  evoked potential in, 676-677
Charcot's disease, vertebral radiography in, 607-608
Chelation therapy, urine copper levels in, 380-381
Chemical stress imaging, **689-691**
Chemstrip K, 372
Chest lesions, 554-555
Chest pain
  acid perfusion test and, 725-726
  Holter monitoring of, 691-693
Chest radiography, **548-558**, 549-550t
Chest tomography, **554-555**
Chest trauma, closed, pericardial fluid analysis in, 429-433
Chlamydia, culture for, **457-458**
Chloride, serum, **133-134**
Cholangiocellular carcinoma, liver biopsy in, 467
Cholangitis, ERCP in, 577-580
Cholecalciferol, **248-249**. *See also* Vitamin D$_3$.
Cholecystitis
  cholecystography in, 572-574
  HIDA scan in, 662-664
  ultrasonography in, 524-526
Cholelithiasis, 16
  cholangiography in, 574-576
  duodenal contents culture and, 451-452
  ultrasonography in, 524-526
Cholescintigraphy, **662-664**
Cholinesterase, **159-160**
Chondromalacia patellae, arthroscopy in, 609-611
Choriocarcinoma, 16
  hCG urine levels in, 340-341
  hPL levels in, 241-242

Chorionic villi sampling, 410-411i
Chromosomal abnormalities
  chromosome analysis in, 403-408
  features of, 404-405t
  sex chromatin tests in, 402-403
Chromosome analysis, **403-408**,
  407-408t
Chronic obstructive pulmonary disease, lung ventilation scan
  in, 645-646
Cirrhosis, 17, 148
  ADH levels in, 212-213
  alcoholic
    AFP levels in, 314-315
    FSP levels in, 120-121
    zinc levels in, 251-252
  ALP levels in, 150
  antimitochondrial antibodies in,
    280-281
  arteriography in, 580-583
  biliary
    ERCP in, 577-580
    urine copper levels in, 380-381
  CEA levels in, 313-314
  cholangiography in, 574-576
  cholinesterase levels in, 159-160
  cold agglutinins in, 285-286
  complement assays in, 273-275
  cryptogenic, antimitochondrial
    antibodies in, 280-281
  estrogen levels in, 235-237
  fecal urobilinogen in, 398-399
  5'NT levels in, 152-153
  INR values in, 125-126
  liver biopsy in, 467
  liver-spleen scanning in, 653,
    655-656
  liver ultrasonography in, 526-528
  peritoneal fluid analysis in,
    390-393
  plasma ammonia levels in,
    179-180
  primary biliary, anti-smooth-mus-
    cle antibodies in, 281-282
  Raji cell assay in, 273
  renin levels in, 158
  urine aldosterone levels in,
    334-335
  urine amylase levels in, 329-330
  urine porphyrin levels in, 363-365
  urobilinogen test in, 368
  vitamin B_{12} levels in, 246-247
CK. *See* Creatine kinase.
Clinical depression, dexamethasone
  suppression test in, 742-743
Clinistix, 370
Clinitest, 369-370
Clot retraction, normal values in,
  746
Clotting factors. *See specific factors.*
CMV. *See* Cytomegalovirus.
CNS. *See* Central nervous system
  disorders.
Coagulation, **113-126**

Cobalt, critical trace element of, 246
Coccidioidomycosis, 18, 478-479
Coccidiosis, biopsy in, 465
Cold agglutinin disease
  cold agglutinins in, 285-286
  idiopathic, cold agglutinins in,
    285-286
Cold agglutinins, **285-286**
Cold spot myocardial imaging,
  647-648
Collagen disorders
  urinalysis in, 321-324
  urine uric acid levels in, 360
Collagen vascular disease
  ANAs in, 277-279
  pleural biopsy in, 461-462
Colon, splenic flexure of, 549-550t
Colon cancer
  gallium scanning in, 656-658
  urine ARSA levels in, 330-331
Colonic strictures, 499-501
Colonoscopy, **499-501**
Colorectal cancer, 18
  barium enema in, 567-570
  CEA levels in, 313-314
  fecal occult blood test in, 395-397
  urine ARSA levels in, 330-331
Colposcopy, **505-506**
  cervical biopsy in, 471
Comatose patient, evoked potential
  in, 673, 674-675i, 676-677
Common bile duct obstruction
  HIDA scan in, 662-664
  oral cholecystography in, 572-574
  urobilinogen test in, 368
Complement assays, **273-275**
Complete blood count, **85-86**
Computed tomography scan,
  615-638
  GI system, 621-625
  intracranial, 616-618
  liver and biliary tract, **621-623**
  miscellaneous tests, 631-638
  musculoskeletal system, **625-630**
  neurologic system, **616-621**
  orbital, **631-632**
  pancreatic, **623-625**
  renal, **636-638**
  skeletal, **628-629**
  spinal, **625-627**
  thoracic, **632-634**
Computer tomography laser mammography, 605
Concentration and dilution tests,
  327-328
Conduction abnormalities
  ECG test in, 679, 681
  Holter monitoring in, 691-693
Condylar disease, arthroscopy examination in, 508-512
Congenital anomalies
  cardiac catheterization in,
    696-701
  echocardiography in, 517-519

Congenital anomalies *(continued)*
  excretory urography in, 594-596
  KUB in, 583-584
  lower urinary tract, cystoureth-
    rography in, 601-602
  radiography in, 539-540,
    607-608
  retrograde urethrography in,
    587-588
Congenital coagulation deficiencies,
  APTT levels in, 113-114
Congenital heart disease
  echocardiography in, 514-519
  FSP levels in, 120-121
  MRI scan in, 634-636
Congenital hypothyroidism, screen-
  ing test for, 219-221
Congenital infection, 315-316
Congenital malformation, 606-607
Congenital microphthalmia, radiog-
  raphy in, 545-546
Congenital vertebral disorder, radi-
  ography in, 607-608
Conjunctivitis, 18, 297
Connecting-peptide assay, 233
Connective tissue disorder, cold stim-
  ulation test in, 735-736
Conn's syndrome. *See* Aldosteronism.
Contraction stress test, **420-421**
  external fetal monitoring in,
    666-668
Coordination tests, 722-723
COPD. *See* Chronic obstructive
  pulmonary disease.
Copper urine test, **380-381**
Copper reduction test, **369-370**
Corneal abrasion, 19, 711-712
Corneal lesion, 711-715
Corneal staining, **715**
Coronary artery disease, 19
  cardiac blood pool imaging in,
    650-651
  cardiac catheterization in,
    696-701
  cholesterol levels in, 168
  ECG stress test in, 685-686, 689
  echocardiography in, 514-517
    lipoprotein-cholesterol frac-
      tionation in, 169-170
  Persantine-thallium imaging in,
    649-650
  radiopharmaceutical myocardial
    perfusion imaging in,
    689-691
  thallium imaging, stress imaging
    in, 647-648
  triglyceride levels in, 166-167
Coronary perfusion, 689-691
Cor pulmonale, 18, 549-550t
Corticotropin. *See* Adrenocorticotropic hormone.
Cosyntropin test, **197-199**
C-peptide. *See* Connecting-peptide
  assay.

C-reactive protein, serum, 746
Creatine, serum, 746
Creatine kinase, 141, 142, 746
Creatinine, 181, 358, 746, 747
Creatinine clearance, **359-360**
Cretinism
    17-KGS urine levels in, 346
    17-KS urine levels in, 343-345
Crohn's disease, 19
    colonoscopy in, 499-501
    gallium scanning in, 656-658
    Raji cell assay in, 273
    urine oxalate levels in, 382
Crossmatching, **258-260**
Cryoglobulinemia
    cryoglobulins in, 286-287
    heterophil antibody tests in,
        292-294
Cryoglobulins, **286-287**
CSF. *See* Cerebrospinal fluid analysis.
CST. *See* Contraction stress test.
CTLM. *See* Computer tomography
    laser mammography.
CT scan. *See* Computed tomography
    scan.
Cultures, **437-458**
Cushing's disease
    cortisol levels in, 225-227
    urine potassium levels in, 377-378
Cushing's syndrome, 19-20, 132
    ACTH levels in, 196-197
    calcium levels in, 133
    carbon dioxide content in, 132
    cortisol levels in, 225-227
    dexamethasone suppression test
        in, 742-743
    free cortisol levels in, 335-336
    17-KGS urine levels in, 346
    17-OHCS urine levels in, 342-343
    serum potassium levels in, 138
    urinalysis in, 321-324
CVS. *See* Chorionic villi sampling.
Cyanocobalamin, **246-247**
Cyclic adenosine monophosphate,
    332-334
Cyst, paranasal sinus radiography of,
    552t
Cystic fibrosis, 20
    sweat test findings in, 433-435
    vitamin D₃ levels in, 248-249
Cystic fibrosis of the pancreas
    vitamin A levels in, 244-245
Cystic tumor, 583-584
Cystitis, urinalysis in, 321-324
Cystocele, 601-602
Cystometry, **728-731**, 729-730t
Cystosarcoma, breast biopsy in, 469
Cytomegalovirus
    rapid monoclonal test in, 456
    TORCH test in, 315-316
Cytomegalovirus antibody screen,
    298-299

Cytomegalovirus infection, 20
    cold agglutinins in, 285-286
    lower respiratory tract infection,
        RSV antibodies in, 296

D

δ-aminolevulinic acid, **365-366**
D-dimer, **124-125**
Decreased renal blood flow, 327-328
Deep vein thrombosis
    AcuTect test in, 561
    impedance plethysmography in,
        695-696
    ultrasonography in, 519-522
    venography in, 560-562
Dehydration
    creatinine clearance in, 359-360
    sodium and chloride urine tests in,
        376-377
Dementia. *See* Alzheimer's disease.
Demyelinating disease
    evoked potential in, 673,
        674-675i, 676-677
    MRI scan in, 618-621
Dermal lesion, generalized, HSV an-
    tibodies in, 297
Dermatitis herpetiformis, HLA test
    in, 276-277
Detrusor-external sphincter dysyner-
    gia, 731-733
Detrusor muscle function, cystome-
    try test in, 728, 731
DEXA. *See* Dual energy X-ray ab-
    sorptiometry.
Dexamethasone suppression test,
    742-743
Diabetes
    Candida antibody in, 306-307
    complement assays in, 273-275
    KUB in, 583-584
Diabetes insipidus, 20, 321-324
Diabetes mellitus, 21
    ß-hydroxybutyrate levels in, 190
    fasting blood sugar levels in,
        184-186
    glycosuria in, 369-372
    glycosylated hemoglobin levels in,
        191
    hGH levels in, 199-200
    hPL levels in, 241-242
    insulin levels in, 232-233
    ketonuria in, 372-373
    ophthalmoscopy in, 712-715
    phospholipid levels in, 168-169
    routine urinalysis in, 321-324
    urine oxalate levels in, 382
Diabetic acidosis, 376-377
Diabetic ketoacidosis
    ß-hydroxybutyrate levels in, 190
    ketone test in, 372-373
    urine sodium and chloride tests in,
        376-377

Diabetic neuropathic diarrhea,
    D-xylose absorption in,
        741-742
Diaphoresis, 376-377
Diastix, 370
DIC. *See* Disseminated intravascular
    coagulation.
Digoxin, serum levels of, 748
Diphtheria, 21, 441-442
Direct antiglobulin test, **260-261**
Direct Coombs'test, **260-261**
Direct laryngoscopy, **490-491**
Disequilibrium, screening tests for,
    722-723
Disseminated intravascular coagula-
    tion, 21
    bleeding time in, 107-108
    capillary fragility test in, 110-111
    D-dimer values in, 124-125
    FSP levels in, 120-121
    INR values in, 125-126
    plasminogen levels in, 122-123
    platelet count in, 108-110
    thrombin time in, 118-119
Disseminated lupus erythematosus,
    485-486, 488
Diverticula
    barium swallow in, 562-564
    bladder or urethra, cysto-
        urethrography in, 601-602
    bleeding, arteriography in,
        580-583
    upper GI and small-bowel series
        in, 564-567
    urethrography in, 587-588
Diverticular disease, colonoscopy in,
    21, 499-501
Diverticulitis, barium enema in,
    567-570
Dizziness, screening for 722-723
Doppler ultrasonography, **519-522**,
    520i
Down syndrome, 21-22
    amniotic fluid analysis in,
        409-414
Drug reactions, 273
Dual energy X-ray absorptiometry,
    609-611
Duodenal contents culture, **451-452**
Duodenal infection, duodenal con-
    tents culture and, 451-452
Duodenal lesion, 570-572
Duodenal papilla carcinoma, ERCP
    in, 577-580
Duodenal parasites, test for, **393-395**
Duodenal ulcer
    EGD in, 496-499
    gastric acid stimulation test in,
        389-390
    gastric secretion test in, 387-389
    H. pylori antibody in, 309-310
    peritoneal fluid analysis in,
        390-393

Duodenal ulcer *(continued)*
    upper GI and small-bowel series, 564-567
DVT. *See* Deep vein thrombosis.
Dwarfism, hGH levels in, 199-200
D-xylose absorption, **741-742**
Dysautonomia, 336-337
Dysentery, stool culture in, 439-441
Dysfunctional uterine bleeding, 22
    vaginal ultrasonography in, 536
Dysphagia, EGD in, 496-499
Dyspnea, 736-737, 740-741

E

Ear infection, otoscopy in, 716-717
Ears and hearing, 716-723
EBV. *See* Epstein-Barr virus.
ECG. *See* Electrocardiography.
Echocardiography, **514-517**
    M-mode, 514, 515i, 516-517
    two-dimensional (cross sectional), 514, 516-517
Eclampsia
    17-OHCS urine levels in, 342-343
    plasminogen levels in, 122-123
    urinalysis in, 321-324
Ectopic corticotropin production, 335-336
Ectopic renal lobe, nephrotomography in, 584-587
Edematous disorder, urine aldosterone levels in, 334-335
EGD. *See* Esophagogastroduodenoscopy.
Ejection fraction, cardiac blood pool imaging in, 650-651
Electrocardiography, **679-681**, **685**
    ambulatory, **691-693**
    waveforms in, 682i, 683-685i
Electroencephalography, **671-673**
Electrolyte imbalances, ECG test in, 679, 681
Electrolytes, **132-141**
Electromyography, **677-679**
Electrophysiology studies, **705-707**
Emphysema, 22, 131, 145-146
    AAT levels in, 145-146
    ABG levels in, 131
    chest radiography in, 549-550t
    lung ventilation scan in, 645-646
Empyema, 56, 495-495
ENA. *See* Extractable nuclear antigen antibodies.
Encephalitis, 22-23
    EEG recording in, 671-673
    HSV antibodies in, 297
    HSV culture in, 455-457
Endocarditis, 23, 517-519
Endocrine disorders
    calcium levels in, 132
    urine hydroxyproline levels in, 357-358
Endometriosis, 23, 507-508

Endoscopic biopsy of GI tract, 464
Endoscopic cholangiopancreatography, **577-580**
Endoscopic ultrasound, **504-505**
Enterovirus, stool culture in, 439-441
Eosinophilic enteritis, small-bowel biopsy in, 465
Eosinophils, 105, 746, 104
Ependymomas, myelography in, 542-545
Epidural hematomas, CT scan in, 616-618
Epigastric pain, EGD in, 496-499
EPO. *See* Erythropoietin.
Epstein-Barr virus, antibodies, **294-296**
    HSV culture in, 455-457
ERCP. *See* Endoscopic cholangiopancreatography.
Erythema infectiosum, parvovirus B-19 antibody in, 300-301
Erythroblastosis fetalis, 24. *See also* Hemolytic disease of the newborn.
    amniotic fluid analysis in, 409-414
    bleeding time in, 107-108
    hCG urine levels in, 340-341
    osmotic fragility in, 90-91
Erythrocyte count, **85-86**
Erythrocyte indices, **87-88**, 746
Erythrocyte sedimentation rate, **88-89**, 746
Erythropoietin, **230**
Esophageal acidity test, **723-725**
Esophageal lesions, 24, 25-26, 74, 504-505
Esophageal spasm, barium swallow in, 562-564
Esophageal sphincter, lower, esophageal acidity test of, 723-725
Esophageal stenosis, EGD in, 496-499
Esophageal stricture, upper GI and small-bowel series in, 564-567
Esophageal tumor, upper GI and small-bowel series in, 564-567
Esophagitis
    EGD in, 496-499
    esophageal acidity test in, 723-725
Esophagogastroduodenoscopy, **496-499**
ESR. *See* Erythrocyte sedimentation rate.
Estrogens, **235-237**
Estrogen therapy, urine copper levels in, 380-381
Ethanol serum levels, 748

Ethosuximide serum levels, 748
Ethylene glycol serum levels, 748
Ethylene glycol ingestion
    urinalysis in, 321-324
    urine oxalate levels, 382
Euglobulin lysis time, **123-124**
EUS. *See* Endoscopic ultrasound.
Evoked potential, **673**, **676-677**, 674-675i
Ewing's sarcoma, 473
Excretory urography, **594-596**
Exercise electrocardiography stress test, **685-689**, 688i
Exophthalmos, 25
    orbital CT scan in, 631-632
    TSI in, 282-283
External sphincter dysfunction
    electromyography in, **731-733**
    uroflowmetry test in, 726-728
Extractable nuclear antigen antibodies, **279-280**
Extrarenal infection, urine lysozyme levels in, 331-332
Extrasynovial disease, arthroscopy in, 508-512
Extrinsic factor, **246-247**, 246
Extrinsic tumor, renal venography in, 598-601
Eye disorders, **710-715**, 712-715
    orbital CT scan in, 631-632
    radiography in, **545-546**

F

Factor I deficiency, 108, 115
Factor II deficiency, 108, 115-117
Factor V deficiency, 108, 114-117
Factor VII deficiency, 108, 111, 114, 116, 117
Factor VIII deficiency, 108, 115, 117, 118
Factor IX deficiency, 108, 115, 117, 118
Factor X deficiency, 114-117
Factor XI deficiency, 108, 115, 117, 118
Factor XII deficiency, 115, 117, 118
Familial hyperlipoproteinemias, 171t-172t
Fanconi's syndrome, 25
    glycosuria in, 369-372
    urinalysis in, 321-324
    urine uric acid levels in, 360
Fasting plasma glucose, **184-186**, 747
Febrile agglutination tests, **302-304**
Fecaliths, KUB in, 583-584
Fecal lipids, **397-398**
Fecal occult blood test, **395-397**, 747
Fecal urobilinogen, **398-399**
Ferritin, **100-101**
Fetal abnormalities, 532-533, 536
Fetal adrenal insufficiency, placental estriol levels in, 339-340

Fetal congenital anomalies, urine estriol levels in, 339-340
Fetal hemoglobin, **93-94**, 94t
Fetal loss, parvovirus B-19 antibody in, 300-301
Fetal-maternal erythrocyte distribution, **257-258**
Fetal maturity, amniotic fluid analysis in, 409-414
Fetal monitoring, **666-671**
Fetal status
external monitoring of, 666-668
internal monitoring of, 668-671
pelvic ultrasonography in, 532-533
urine levels of placental estriol in, 339-340
Fetoplacental status, 337-340
Fibrinogen, plasma, 746
Fibrinogen deficiency, plasma thrombin time in, 118-119
Fibrinolysis, secondary, D-dimer values in, 124-125
Fibrinolytic disorders, 122-124
Fibrin split products, **120-121**, 746
Fibrocystic disease, breast biopsy in, 469
Fibroma, bone biopsy in, 473
Fibrosis, 17, 549-550t
Flow study, **602-604**
Fluid-electrolyte imbalance, sodium and chloride urine tests in, 376-377
Fluid-related hypovolemia, PA catheterization in, 701-704
Fluorescein angiography, **546-548**, 713
Fluorescein stain in visual exam, 712
Fluorescent treponemal antibody absorption test, **311-312**
Fluoroscopy, **553-554**
Focal hepatic defects, CT of liver and biliary tract, 621-623
Folacin, **249-250**
Folate, **249-250**
Folate deficiency, small-bowel biopsy in, 465
Folic acid, **249-250**
Folic acid deficiency, 87-88, 249-250
Follicle-stimulating hormone, **204-205**
Forbes-Albright syndrome. *See* Galactorrhea.
Fractionated erythrocyte porphyrins, **183-184**
Fracture
clavicle, 549-550t
jaw, 21
leg, 8
orbit, 631-632
Free cortisol, urine, **335-336**
Free thyroxine, **218-219**, 746
Free triiodothyronine, **218-219**, 746
FSP. *See* Fibrin split products.

FT₃. *See* Free triiodothyronine.
FT₄. *See* Free thyroxine.
FTA-ABS test. *See* Fluorescent treponemal antibody absorption test.
Fungal infection, test methods for, 305-306t
Fungal serology, **304**, 305-306t, **306**
Fungal skin infection, skin biopsy in, 484-485
Funicular degeneration, vitamin B₁₂ levels in, 246-247
Furunculosis, 26

G

G6PD. *See* Glucose-6-phosphate dehydrogenase.
Galactorrhea, prolactin levels in, 26, 207-209
Galactose-1-phosphate uridyl transferase, **164-165**
Galactosemia, 26, 164-165
Gallbladder, 390-393, **524-526**
Gallbladder carcinoma, 26, 524-526
Gallbladder disorders
cholecystography in, 572-574
HIDA scan in, 662-664
nuclear scanning, **662-664**
polyp, ultrasonography of, 524-526
tumor, oral cholecystography in, 572-574
urine amylase levels in, 329-330
Gallium scanning, **656-658**
Gallstones, 524-526, 572-574
Gamma glutamyl transferase, **151-152**
Gamma glutamyl transpeptidase, **151-152**
Ganglioneuroma
catecholamine levels in, 336-337
HVA urine levels in, 348-349
VMA urine levels in, 347-348
Gangrene, WBC count in, 102-103
Gastric acid stimulation test, **389-390**
Gastric adenocarcinomas, hCG levels in, 240-241
Gastric cancer, hCG urine levels in, 340-341
Gastric carcinoma, 27, 387-390
Gastric culture, **449-451**
Gastric reflex, esophageal acidity test in, 723-725
Gastric ulcer, 234, 580-583
Gastrin, **233-234**
Gastrinomas. *See* Zollinger-Ellison syndrome.
Gastritis, 27
EGD in, 496-499
gastric culture in, 449-451
Helicobacter pylori in, 449-451
Helicobacter pylori antigen in, 309-310

Gastroenteritis, 27, 567-570
Gastroesophageal reflux disease
barium swallow in, 562-564
EGD in, 496-499
Gastrointestinal bleeding
arteriography in, 580-583
EGD in, 496-499
fecal occult blood test in, 395-397
sites and causes of, 396i
Gastrointestinal function, **723-726**
Gastrointestinal lesions
colonoscopy in, 499-501
EUS examination in, 504-505
Gastrointestinal organ cancer, CEA levels in, 313-314
Gastrointestinal system
biopsy of, **463-467**
CT scanning of, **621-625**
endoscopic biopsy of, 464
endoscopic tests of, **496-505**
radiography of, **562-583**
specimen tests of, **387-402**
ultrasonography of, **524-531**
Gastrointestinal tumor
EGD in, 496-499
upper GI and small-bowel series in, 564-567
Gaucher's disease, 27, 165-166
ACE levels in, 165-166
General cultures, **438-452**
Genital cultures, **453-455**
Genital herpes, 27, 311-312
Genital lesions, HSV antibodies in, 297
Genitourinary system, radiography of, **583-604**
Genitourinary tract infection, 50
urinalysis in, 321-324
Gentamicin serum levels, 749
GERD. *See* Gastroesophageal reflux disease.
Germ cell tumor, AFP levels in, 314-315
GGT. *See* Gamma glutamyl transferase.
Giant-cell tumor, bone biopsy in, 473
Giardiasis, 28
duodenal parasites in, 393-395
small-bowel biopsy in, 465
stool examination in, 399-401
Gigantism, 199-201
Gingivostomatitis, HSV culture in, 455-457
GI system. *See* Gastrointestinal system.
Glaucoma, 28, 712-715
Glioblastomas, CT scan in, 616-618
Gliomas, CT scan in, 631-632
Globulins, FTA-ABS test in, 311-312
Glomerular filtration, urine creatinine levels in, 358
Glomerular function
renal biopsy in, 485-486, 488
urine magnesium levels in, 379-380

Glomerular permeability, increased, urine protein levels in, 351-351
Glomerulonephritis
  acute
    creatinine clearance in, 359-360
    hemoglobinuria in, 361-362
    renal biopsy in, 485-486, 488
    urinalysis in, 321-324
    urine protein levels in, 351-352
  acute poststreptococcal, complement assays in, 273-275
  chronic, 16-17
    creatinine clearance in, 359-360
    renal biopsy in, 485-486, 488
    urinalysis in, 321-324
    urine protein levels in, 351-352
    urine uric acid levels in, 360
  end-stage
    glycosuria in, 369-372
    KUB in, 583-584
  membranoproliferative
    plasma fibrinogen levels in, 119-120
    renal imaging in, 660-662
    ultrasonography in, 533-535
    urinalysis in, 321-324
Glomerulosclerosis, 321-324, 360
Glucocorticoid deficiency, insulin levels in, 232-233
Glucose, plasma, 187i, 747
Glucose-6-phosphate dehydrogenase, **160-161**
Glucose loading test, **200-201**
Glucose oxidase test, **370-372**
Glycogen storage disease, 27-28
Glycosuria, 321-324, 369-370
Glycosylated hemoglobin, **191**
Goiter, 29, 209, 642t
Gonadal dysfunction
  17-KS urine levels in, 343-345
  testosterone levels in, 238-240
Gonadal hormones, **235-240**
Gonorrhea, 29, **453-455**, 454i
Gout, 29
  fractionated erythrocyte porphyrin levels in, 183-184
  PSP test in, 325-327
  synovial fluid analysis in, 427-429
  synovial membrane biopsy in, 478-479
  uric acid levels in, 360
Granuloma
  bone marrow aspiration and biopsy in, 474-475, 478
  chest tomography in, 554-555
Granulomatous colitis, barium enema in, 567-570
Granulomatous disease, 17
  cholangiography in, 574-576
  liver biopsy in, 465, 467
  synovial membrane biopsy in, 478-479

Graves' disease. *See also* Hyperthyroidism.
  antithyroid antibodies in, 282
  CT scan in, 631-632
  HLA test in, 276-277
  RAIU test in, 640-641
  T_3 levels in, 215-216
  thyrotoxicosis and, 210
  TRH in, 210
  TSI in, 282-283
Group A beta-hemolytic streptococci, throat culture in, 441-442
Growth hormone, **199-200**
  insulin tolerance test of, 201-202
Growth hormone stimulation test. *See* Arginine test.
Growth hormone suppression test, **200-201**
Growth retardation
  arginine test in, 202-203
  hGH levels in, 199-200
Guillain-Barré syndrome, 30
  evoked potential in, 676-677
Guthrie screening test, **178-179**
Gynecologic laparoscopy, **506-508**
Gynecomastia, androstenedione levels in, 229-230

H

Haemophilus influenzae infection, 30
Hamartoma, liver-spleen scanning in, 653, 655-656
Ham test, **275-276**
Hand-Schüller-Christian disease, ADH levels in, 212-213
Haptoglobin, serum, **175-176**
Hashimoto's thyroiditis
  antithyroid antibodies in, 282
  HLA test in, 276-277
  RAIU test in, 640-641
  thyroid biopsy in, 479-481
HBD. *See* Hydroxybutyric dehydrogenase.
HBsAG. *See* Hepatitis B surface antigen.
Hb F. *See* Hemoglobin F.
Hb H. *See* Hemoglobin H. disease.
Hb M. *See* Methemoglobin.
HCG-secreting tumor, hCG urine levels in, 340-341
HCG. *See* Human chorionic gonadotropin.
HDL. *See* High-density lipoproteins.
HDN. *See* Hemolytic disease of the newborn.
Head injury, EEG in, 671-673
Hearing loss, 30
  pure tone audiometry in, 719-722
  tuning fork tests in, 717-719
Heart chamber measurement, echocardiography in, 514-517

Heart failure, 30
  ANF levels in, 231
  chest radiography in, 549-550t
  creatinine clearance in, 359-360
  D-xylose absorption in, 741-742
  echocardiography in, 514-517
  PSP test in, 325-327
  sodium and chloride urine tests in, 376-377
  urinalysis in, 321-324
  urine aldosterone levels in, 334-335
Heart function after surgery, ECG stress test for, 685-686, 689
Heavy metal poisoning
  glycosuria in, 369-372
  urinalysis in, 321-324
Heavy metal toxicity, urine porphyrin levels in, 363-365
Heinz bodies, **97-98**
Helicobacter pylori antibody test, 309-310
Hemangiomas
  fluorescein angiography in, 546-548
  liver-spleen scanning in, 653, 655-656
  orbital CT scan in, 631-632
Hematemesis, EGD in, 496-499
Hematocrit, **86-87**, 746
Hematologic disorder, urobilinogen test in, 368
Hematoma, 540-542, 580-583
Hematuria, 321-325
Hemochromatosis, 30
  siderocyte stain in, 99
  synovial membrane biopsy in, 478-479
  TIBC levels in, 98-100
  urine hemosiderin levels in, 381-382
Hemoglobin, **92-101**
  total, 746
  type and distribution, 94t
  urine, **361-362**, 362
Hemoglobin C disease, 94t, 658-660
Hemoglobin electrophoresis, **94-95**
Hemoglobin F, **93-94**
Hemoglobin H disease, 94t
Hemoglobin S test, **95-96**
Hemoglobinuria, 361-362
Hemolysis, haptoglobin levels in, 176
Hemolytic anemia. *See also* Anemia.
  antibody screening test in, 261-262
  antithyroid antibodies in, 282
  cold agglutinins in, 285-286
  direct antiglobulin test in, 260-261
  ferritin levels in, 100-101
  G6PD levels in, 160-161
  HAM test in, 275-276
  Heinz bodies in, 97-98
  hemoglobinuria, 361-362

Hemolytic anemia *(continued)*
PK levels in, 161
RBC survival time test in, 658-660
siderocyte stain in, 99
zinc levels in, 251-252
Hemolytic disease
RBC survival time test in, 658-660
urinalysis in, 321-324
Hemolytic disease of the newborn, 260-261. *See also* Erythroblastosis fetalis.
antibody screening test in, 261-262
direct antiglobulin test in, 260-261
Hemolytic disorder, fecal urobilinogen in, 398-399
Hemolytic jaundice, urobilinogen test in, 368
Hemolyticuremic syndrome, RBC survival time test in, 658-660
Hemophilia, 30
HBsAG in, 291-292
Hemoptysis, bronchography in, 555-557
Hemorrhage
esophageal, arteriography in, 580-583
intracranial
CSF analysis in, 421-425
CT scan in, 616-618
Hemorrhagic disorder, urinalysis in, 321-324
Hemorrhagic gastritis, arteriography in, 580-583
Hemorrhoids, 30-31, 501-504
Hemosiderin, urine, **381-382**
Hemothorax, 31
Hepatic abscess, 329-330, 621-623
Hepatic cancer
δ-aminolevulinic acid levels in, 365-366
hCG urine levels in, 340-341
Hepatic cyst, CT scan of liver and biliary tract, 621-623
Hepatic disease
acute, 146-148
ALP levels in, 149-150
ALT levels in, 148-149
ammonia levels in, 179-180
AST levels in, 146-148
benign, CEA levels in, 313-314
bilirubin levels in, 182-183
bleeding time in, 107-108
cholesterol levels in, 167-168
chronic, ANAs in, 277-279
δ-aminolevulinic acid levels in, 365-366
estrogen levels in, 235-237
ferritin levels in, 100-101
fibrinogen levels in, 119-120
free cortisol levels in, 335-336
GGT levels in, 151-152
glycosuria in, 369-372

Hepatic disease *(continued)*
insulin levels in, 232-233
LAP levels in, 150-151
plasminogen levels in, 122-123
primary, pregnanediol urine levels in, 350-351
prothrombin time in, 118-119
PSP test in, 325-327
PT time in, 114-115
TBG levels in, 216-217
urine estrogen levels in, 337-339
urobilinogen test in, 368
viral, RF in, 284-285
vitamin B_{12} levels in, 246-247
vitamin D_3 levels in, 248-249
Hepatic enzymes and proteins, **145-153**
Hepatic hematoma, 526-528, 621-623
Hepatic metastasis
liver-spleen scanning in, 653, 655-656
liver ultrasonography of, 526-528
percutaneous liver biopsy in, 467
Hepatic parenchymal disease, percutaneous liver biopsy in, 465
Hepatic tumor, liver ultrasonography of, 526-528
Hepatitis. *See also* Hepatic disease *and specific type.*
acute viral, anti-smooth-muscle antibodies in, 281-282
ADH levels in, 212-213
cholangiography in, 574-576
cholinesterase levels in, 159-160
chronic,148
antimitochondrial antibodies in, 280-281
anti-smooth-muscle antibodies, 281-282
B_{12} levels in, 246-247
copper levels in, 380-381
chronic autoimmune, HLA test in, 276-277
δ-aminolevulinic acid levels in, 365-366
fecal urobilinogen in, 398-399
INR values in, 125-126
liver biopsy in, 467
liver-spleen scan in, 653, 655-656
urine amylase levels in, 329-330
urine porphyrin levels in, 363-365
urobilinogen test in, 368
VDRL test in, 310-311
viral, HGsAG in, 291-292
vitamin A levels in, 244-245
WBC count in, 102-103
Hepatitis-associated antigen, **291-292**
Hepatitis B screen for blood donors, HBsAG in, 291-292
Hepatitis B surface antigen, **291-292**

Hepatobiliary disease
fecal urobilinogen in, 398-399
vitamin D_3 levels in, 248-249
Hepatobiliary imaging, **662-664**
Hepatocellular carcinoma
AFP levels in, 314-315
liver biopsy in, 467
Hepatocellular disease
haptoglobin levels in, 175-176
liver-spleen scan in, 653, 655-656
liver ultrasonography of, 526-528
Hepatoma
AFP levels in, 314-315
hPL levels in, 241-242
Hepatomegaly
liver-spleen scan in, 653, 655-656
liver ultrasonography in, 526-528
Hercept test, 313
Herniated disk, 31
CT scan of spine in, 625-627
myelography in, 542-545
Herpes simplex antibodies, TORCH test in, 315-316
Herpes simplex virus, 32
culture for, **455-457**
HSV antibodies in, **297**
Heterophil antibody tests, **292-294**
Hexosaminidase A and B, 162-163
hGH. *See* Growth hormone.
5-HIAA. *See* 5-Hydroxyindoleacetic acid.
Hiatal hernia, 32
arteriography in, 580-583
barium swallow in, 562-564
EGD in, 496-499
upper GI and small-bowel series in, 564-567
HIDA scan, **662-664**
High-density lipoproteins, 169-170
Hirschsprung's disease, 32
Histocompatibility typing, 265, 267, 276-277
Histoplasmosis, 32, 494
HIV. *See* Human immunodeficiency virus antibody.
HLA. *See* Human leukocyte antigen test.
Hodgkin's disease, 32
bleeding time in, 107-108
ferritin levels in, 100-101
gallium scanning in, 656-658
HBsAG in, 291-292
liver-spleen scanning in, 653, 655-656
lymphangiography in, 611-614
lymph node biopsy in, 481-482
mediastinoscopy in, 494
staging of, bone marrow aspiration and biopsy in, 474
thoracic CT scan in, 632-634
upper GI and small-bowel series in, 564-567
urine porphyrin levels in, 363-365

Holter monitoring, **691-693**, 757i
Home testing, illustrated guide to, **751-763**
Homovanillic acid test, **348-349**
Homozygous hemoglobin S, 94t
Hookworm disease, 32-33
  duodenal parasites in, 393-395
  sputum examination for ova and parasites, 384-385
Hormones, serum, **195-242**
Hormones, urine, **334-436**
Hot spot myocardial imaging, **646-647**
HPFH. *See* Fetal hemoglobin.
HPL. *See* Human placental lactogen.
HSV. *See* Herpes simplex virus.
Human chorionic gonadotropin
  serum levels of, **240-241**
  urine levels of, **340-341**
Human chorionic gonadotropin–secreting tumor, hCG urine levels in, 340-341
Human chorionic somatomammotropin, **241-242**
Human growth hormone deficiency
  arginine test in, 203
  insulin tolerance test in, 201
Human growth hormone stimulation test, **202-204**
Human herpesvirus-6, HSV culture in, 455-457
Human immunodeficiency virus, home test for, 762-763i
Human immunodeficiency virus antibody, **299-300**
Human leukocyte antigen test, **276-277**
Human placental lactogen, human chorionic somatomammotropin and, 241-242
Humoral function, **269-277**
Huntington's disease, 33, 676-677
HVA. *See* Homovanillic acid test.
Hydatid disease, sputum examination for, 384-385
Hydatidiform mole, 33
  hCG levels in, 240-241
  hCG urine levels in, 340-341
  hPL levels in, 241-242
  urine pregnanediol in, 350-351
Hydrocephalus, 33, 540-542, 616-618
Hydronephrosis, 33
  antegrade pyelography in, 592-594
  excretory urography in, 594-596
  KUB in, 583-584
  ultrasonography in, 533-535
  urinalysis in, 321-324
Hydrops fetalis, parvovirus B-19 antibody in, 300-301
Hydrosalpinx, vaginal ultrasonography in, 536
Hydroxybutyric dehydrogenase, 142

17-hydroxycorticosteroids, **342-343**, 747
5-hydroxyindoleacetic acid, **349-350**
Hydroxyproline, **357-358**
Hyperbilirubinemia syndrome, urobilinogen test in, 368
Hypercalcemia, 133
  urinalysis in, 321-324
  vitamin D_3 levels in, 248-249
Hyperchloremia, 134
Hypercholesterolemia, vitamin A levels in, 244-245
Hyperestrogenism, female, urine estrogens in, 337-339
Hyperinsulinemia, insulin levels in, 232-233
Hyperkalemia, 137
  urine potassium levels in, 377-378
Hyperlipidemia, 166-167, 244-245
Hyperlipoproteinemia, 34, 170-173
Hypermagnesemia, 135
Hypernatremia, 139
Hyperoxaluria, 382
Hyperparathyroidism, 34-35, 133
  PTH levels in, 222-223, 223i
  urine calcium and phosphorus levels in, 379t
Hyperplasia, ACTH levels in, 197
Hypertension, 35
  capillary fragility test in, 110-111
  catecholamine levels in, 227-228, 336-337
  17-OHCS urine levels in, 342-343
Hypertensive disorder, urine aldosterone levels in, 334-335
Hypertensive retinopathy, fluorescein angiography in, 546-548
Hyperthyroidism, 35
  cholesterol levels in, 168
  congenital, neonatal thyroid-stimulating hormone in, 210-212
  folic acid levels in, 249-250
  FT_3 and FT_4 levels in, 218-219
  17-OHCS urine levels in, 342-343
  RAIU test in, 640-641
  recurrence of, TSI in, 282-283
  T_3 levels in, 215-216
  T_3 uptake levels in, 217-218
  T_4 levels in, 214-215
  thyroid biopsy in, 479-481
  thyroid imaging results in, 642t
  vitamin B_{12} levels in, 246-247
Hypertonia, Whitaker test in, 602-604
Hypertonic bladder, retrograde cystography in, 588-590
Hypertrophic anal papilla, proctosigmoidoscopy in, 501-504
Hypertrophy, compensatory, KUB in, 583-584
Hypochloremic metabolic alkalosis, 134
Hypocholesterolemia, 168

Hypochromic microcytic anemia, tryptophan challenge test in, 374-375
Hypofunctioning adenoma, thyroid imaging results in, 642t
Hypogammaglobulinemia
  complement assays in, 273-275
  X-linked infantile, 82
Hypoglycemia, 35
  anti-insulin antibody test in, 288-289
  ß-hydroxybutyrate levels in, 190
  C-peptide assay levels in, 233
  glucagon levels in, 235
  insulin levels in, 232-233
Hypogonadism, 35
  estrogen levels in, 235-237
  FSH levels in, 204-205
  LH levels in, 207
  testosterone levels in, 238-240
Hypokalemia, 138, 158, 377-378
Hypolipoproteinemia, lipoprotein phenotyping in, 170-173
Hypomagnesemia, 135
Hyponatremia, 139
Hypoparathyroidism, 35-36, 133, 379t
Hypophosphatemia, 136
Hypopituitarism, 36
  estrogen levels in, 235-237
  17-OHCS urine levels in, 342-343
Hypoplasia, congenital, KUB in, 583-584
Hypoplastic anemia, 7-8
  bone marrow aspiration and biopsy in, 474
  reticulocyte count in, 89-90
Hypotension, PA catheterization in, 701-704
Hypothalamic dysfunction, prolactin levels in, 207-209
Hypothalamic tumor, 199-200, 212-213
Hypothyroid goiter, thyroid imaging in, 642t
Hypothyroidism, 36
  ADH levels in, 212-213
  cholesterol levels in, 168
  congenital
    screening test for, **219-221**
    T_4 levels in, 219-221
  FT_4 and FT_3 levels in, 218-219
  phospholipid levels in, 168-169
  prolactin levels in, 207-209
  RAIU test in, 640-641
  T_3 levels in, 215-216
  T_3 uptake levels in, 217-218
  T_4 levels in, 214-215
  TBG levels in, 216-217
  thyroid imaging in, 642t
  TSH levels in, 209-212
Hypotonic bladder, retrograde cystography in, 588-590

Boldface page numbers indicate major entries; i refers to an illustration; t refers to a table.

Hypotonic duodenography, **570-572**
Hypovolemic shock, 36
Hysterosalpingography, **606-607**

I

ICD. *See* Implantable cardioverter–defibrillator.
Ichthyosis, vitamin A levels in, 244-245
ICP. *See* Intracranial pressure, increased.
Idiopathic cyclic edema, urine aldosterone levels in, 334-335
Idiopathic venous thrombosis, protein C deficiency in, 123
IgA. *See* Immunoglobulin A.
IgE. *See* Immunoglobulin E.
IgG. *See* Immunoglobulin G.
IgM. *See* Immunoglobulin M.
Ileal resection, urine oxalate levels in, 382
Ileitis, zinc levels in, 251-252
Immune complex assays, **271-272**
 lymphocyte assays in, 264-265, 267
Immunoglobulin A, **269**, 270t, **271**
 deficiency, 37
Immunoglobulin E, RAST in, 275
Immunoglobulin G, **269**, 270t, **271**
Immunoglobulin M, **269**, 270t, **271**
Immunohematology, **255-263**
Immunologic tests, **253-318**
Impaired renal perfusion, urine creatinine levels in, 358
Impaired tubular reabsorption, urinalysis in, 321-324
Impaired wall motion, cardiac catheterization in, 696-701
Impedance plethysmography, **695-696**
Impedance phlebography, **695-696**
Implantable cardioverter-defibrillator device, 705-707
Incontinence, urinary, cystourethrography in, 601-602
Indirect Coombs'test, **261-262**
Infantile autism, 37
Infarct avid imaging, **646-647**
Infection
 bone scan in detection of, 651-653
 hemoglobinuria, 361-362
 urine vitamin C levels in, 375-376
 viral, microbial, and parasitic, Raji cell assay in, 273
Infectious bowel disease, 499-504
Infectious gastroenteritis, small-bowel biopsy in, 465
Infertility, female, 38
 estrogen levels in, 235-237
 FSH levels in, 204-205
 hysterosalpingography in, 606-607
 LH levels in, 205-207
 prolactin levels in, 207-209
 vaginal ultrasonography in, 536

Infertility, male, semen analysis for, 38, 417-420
Inflammatory bowel disease
 CEA levels in, 313-314
 cholecystography in, 572-574
 colonoscopy in, 499-501
 proctosigmoidoscopy in, 501-504
Inflammatory masses, renal angiography in, 596-598
Influenza, 38
 capillary fragility test in, 110-111
 cold agglutinins in, 285-286
 RF in, 284-285
 WBC count in, 102-103
INR. *See* International normalized ratio.
Insect bites and stings, 38-39
Insomnia, sleep studies in, 743-744
Insulin, **232-233**
Insulin allergy, anti-insulin antibody test in, 288-289
Insulin resistance, anti-insulin antibody test in, 288-289
Insulin tolerance test, **201-202**
Intermittent porphyria, TBG levels in, 216-217
International normalized ratio, **125-126**
Interstitial pulmonary disease, bronchoscopy in, 491-493
Intervertebral disk disorders, radiography in, 607-608
Intestinal obstruction, 39, 329-330
Intestinal parasitic infection, stool examination in, 399-401
Intracardiac masses, cardiac MRI scan in, 634-636
Intracardiac shunt, 650-651, 696-701
Intracardiac thrombi, echocardiography in, 517-519
Intracerebral lesions, evoked potential in, 676-677
Intracranial abnormalities, CT scan in, 616-618
Intracranial hemorrhage
 CT scan in, 616-618
 ECG recording in, 671-673
Intracranial lesions
 CT scan in, 616-618
 EEG recording in, 671-673
 MRI scan in, 618-621
 orbital CT scan in, 631-632
Intracranial pressure, increased
 angiography in, 540-542
 EEG recording in, 671-673
 radiography in, 539-540
 urinalysis in, 321-324
Intraductal carcinoma or papilloma, breast biopsy in, 469
Intraepithelial neoplasia, cervical biopsy in, 472
Intrahepatic abscesses, liver-spleen scanning in, 653, 655-656

Intrahepatic hematomas, CT of liver and biliary tract, 621-623
Intraluminal bacterial overgrowth, small-bowel biopsy in, 465
Intraocular foreign bodies, orbital radiography of, 545-546
Intraorbital foreign bodies, orbital radiography of, 545-546
Intrapartum infections, TORCH test in, 315-316
Intrarenal calcifications, renal angiography in, 596-598
Intrarenal reflux, antegrade pyelography, 592-594
Intraspinal tumor, vertebral radiography in, 607-608
Intrauterine infection, HSV antibodies in, 297
Intravascular hemolysis, urine protein levels in, 351-352
Intravenous pyelography. *See* Excretory urography.
Intussusception, 39-40, 567-570
Iodine deficiency, 40
Iron, serum, 747
Iron deficiency, ferritin levels in, 100-101
Iron deficiency anemia, 40
 bone marrow aspiration and biopsy in, 478
 osmotic fragility in, 90-91
 red cell indices in, 87-88
 reticulocyte count in, 89-90
Iron and total iron-binding capacity, **98-100**
Irritable bowel syndrome, 40
Irritable colon, barium enema in, 567-570

J

Jaundice, 280-281, 366-368, 526-528
Jejunal ulcer, basal gastric secretion test in, 387-389
Joint abnormalities
 arthrography in, 609-611
 skeletal CT scan in, 628-629
 synovial fluid analysis in, 427-429
Joint arthralgia, parvovirus B-19 antibody in, 300-301
Joint surgery, arthroscopy and, 508-512
Junctional tachycardia, 40
Juvenile angiofibroma, 40

K

Keratitis, 40-41, 297, 455-457
Keratosis follicularis, vitamin A levels in, 244-245
Keto-Diastix, 372
17-Ketogenic steroids, **346**
Ketones, urine, 747, 755i

Ketones and mucopolysaccharides, **369-374**
Ketone test, **372-373**
Ketonuria, ketone test for, 372-373
17-Ketosteroids, **343-345,** 344-345, 747
Kidney abnormalities
  KUB in, 583-584
  ultrasonography in, 533-535
Kidney cancer, 41, 119-120, 656-658
Kidney enlargement, renal angiography in, 596-598
Kidney evaluation, KUB in, 583-584
Kidney transplantation
  renal CT scan in, 636-638
  renal ultrasonography in, 533-535
  urine lysozyme levels in, 331-332
Kidney tumor, EPO levels in, 230
Kidney-ureter-bladder radiography, **583-584**
Klinefelter syndrome, 41, 404-405t
Klippel-Feil syndrome, vertebral radiography in, 607-608
17-KS. *See* 17-ketosteroids
KUB. *See* Kidney-ureter-bladder radiography.
Kyphosis, 41, 549-550t, 607-608

L

Labor, 668-671, 670t
Labyrinthitis, 41
Lactate dehydrogenase, **143-145,** 746
  levels in myocardial infarction, 144
  levels in pulmonary infarction, anemias, hepatic disease, 144
Lactic acid, blood, 747
Lactic acid and pyruvic acid, **193-194**
Lactic acidosis, lactic acid and pyruvic acid levels in, 193-194
Laminography, **554-555**
LAP. *See* Leucine aminopeptidase.
Laryngeal cancer, 41
  laryngoscopy and, 490-491
Laryngeal foreign bodies, laryngoscopy removal of, 490-491
Laryngeal lesions and polyps, laryngoscopy and, 490-491
Laryngeal strictures, laryngoscopy and, 490-491
Larynx, congenital abnormalities, laryngoscopy in, 490-491
Lassa fever, 41
Late potentials, signal-averaged ECG in, 693-694
LD. *See* Lactate dehydrogenase.
LDL. *See* Low-density lipoproteins.
LE. *See* Lupus erythematosus.
Lead poisoning
  δ-aminolevulinic acid levels in, 365-366
  urinalysis in, 321-324

Left bundle-branch block, ECG test in, 679, 681
Left ventricular enlargement, cardiac catheterization in, 696-701
Left ventricular function
  cardiac blood pool imaging in, 650-651
  cardiac catheterization in, 696-701
  PA catheterization in, 701-704
Leiomyoma, arteriography in, 580-583
Lens opacities, slit-lamp examination in, 711-712
Leprosy, 42, 165
  ACE levels in, 165
  VDRL test in, 310-311
Leucine aminopeptidase, **150-151**
Leukemia, 3, 17. *See also* Myeloid leukemia *and* Myelomonocytic leukemia.
  bleeding time in, 107-108
  bone marrow aspiration and biopsy in, 474, 477, 478
  ferritin levels in, 100-101
  HBsAG in, 291-292
  myelogenous, platelet count in, 108-110
  RBC survival time in, 658-660
  TdT test in, 267-269
  urine lysozyme levels in, 331-332
  WBC count in, 102-103
  WBC differential in, 103-107
  zinc levels in, 251-252
Leukoagglutinin test, **262-263**
Leukocyte count, **102-103**
Leukopenia, folic acid levels in, 249-250
LH. *See* Plasma luteinizing hormone.
Lidocaine serum levels, 749
Ligament injuries, arthroscopy and, 508-512
Ligament tears of joints, arthrography in, 609-611
Lipase, **154-155,** 746
Lipids and lipoproteins, **166-173**
Lipoprotein-cholesterol fractionation, **169-170**
Lipoprotein phenotyping, **170-173**
Lipoproteins, 171-172, 746
Lithium serum levels, 749
Liver
  malignant tumor, anti-smooth-muscle antibodies in, 281-282
  ultrasonography of, **526-528**
Liver cancer, 42
  percutaneous biopsy in, 465
  urine amylase levels in, 329-330
Liver disease, urinalysis in, 321-324
Liver failure, urinalysis in, 321-324

Liver-spleen scanning, 653, 654i, **655-656**
Lobular carcinoma, breast biopsy in, 469
Long-acting thyroid stimulator, **282-283**
LOOP. *See* Loop electrosurgical excision procedure.
Loop electrosurgical excision procedure, cone biopsy in, 471
Lordosis, radiography in, 607-608
Loss of functional nephrons, concentration and dilution tests in, 327-328
Low-density lipoproteins, 169-170
Lower GI bleeding, colonoscopy in, 499-501
Lower GI carcinoma, arteriography in, 580-583
Lower GI examination, **567-570**
Lower limb venography, **560-562**
Lower urinary tract function, 43
  uroflowmetry test in, 726-728
Low-salt diet, sodium and chloride urine tests in, 376-377
Lumbar stenosis, CT scan of spine in, 625-627
Lung abscess, 43
  sputum culture and, 444-446
Lung biopsy, **460-461**
Lung cancer, 43, 197
  CEA levels in, 313-314
  oat cell, lung biopsy in, 460-461
  plasma calcitonin levels in, 221-222
  plasma fibrinogen levels in, 119-120
  squamous cell, lung biopsy in, 460-461
  staging, mediastinoscopy in, 494
Lung expansion and contraction, fluoroscopy test in, 553-554
Lung perfusion scan, **643-644**
Lung ventilation scan, **645-646**
Lupus erythematosus, 43
  cardiolipin antibody test in, 283-284
Lupus erythematosus cell preparation, 747
Lupus nephritis, urinalysis in, 321-324
Luteinizing tumor
  progesterone levels in, 237-238
  testosterone levels in, 238-240
Lymphangiectasia, small-bowel biopsy in, 465
Lymphangiography, **611-614**
Lymphatic leukemia
  chronic, biopsy in, 481-482
  during radiotherapy, urine uric acid levels in, 360
Lymphedema, lymphangiography in, 611-614

Lymph node biopsy, **481-482**, 483
Lymph node enlargement, thoracic CT scan in, 632-634
Lymph nodes, metastatic, lymphangiography in, 611-614
Lymphocyte marker assays, 266t
Lymphocytes
  influence of disease on, 106
  values for, 104 , 746
Lymphocyte transformation tests, **265, 267**
Lymphocytic proliferative diseases T- and B-lymphocyte assays in, 264-265
Lymphography. See Lymphangiography.
Lymphoma
  bone marrow aspiration and biopsy in, 475, 478
  cold agglutinins in, 285-286
  CT scan in, 631-632
  hPL levels in, 241-242
  KUB in, 583-584
  peritoneal fluid analysis in, 390-393
  prostate gland biopsy in, 471
  small-bowel biopsy in, 465
  staging of, 611-614
  TdT test in, 267-269
Lymphoreticular cancer, cold agglutinins in, 285-286
Lymphosarcoma, 360, 564-567
Lysozyme, **331-332**

M

Magnesium, 746
  deficiency, 379-380
  serum, **134-135**
  urine, **379-380**
Magnetic resonance imaging, **615-638**
  cardiac, **634-636**
  intracranial, **618-621**, 620
  miscellaneous tests in, **631-638**
Malabsorption
  D-xylose absorption in, 741-742
  urine vitamin C levels in, 375-376
Malabsorption syndrome
  duodenal parasites in, 393-395
  D-xylose absorption in, 741-742
Malaria, 44
  cold agglutinins in, 285-286
  hemoglobinuria in, 361-362
  urinalysis in, 321-324
  VDRL test in, 310-311
Malignant bone lesion, bone scan in, 651-653
Malignant GI lesion, colonoscopy in, 499-501
Malignant hypertension
  aldosterone levels in, 334-335
  urinalysis in, 321-324

Malignant lesion, chest tomography in, 554-555
Malignant lymphoma, 44
  gallium scanning in, 656-658
  lymphangiography in, 611-614
Malignant melanoma, 44, 484-485
Malignant neoplasm
  orbital radiography of, 545-546
  paranasal sinus radiography in, 551-553, 552t
  proctosigmoidoscopy in, 501-504
Malignant renal tumor, radionuclide renal imaging in, 660-662
Malignant stomach tumor, upper GI and small-bowel series in, 564-567
Malignant tumor of GI tract, EGD in, 496-499
Mallory-Weiss syndrome, 44
  arteriography in, 580-583
  EGD in, 496-499
Malnutrition
  small-bowel biopsy in, 465
  urine vitamin C levels in, 375-376
Mammary duct ectasia, breast biopsy in, 469
Mammary fat necrosis, breast biopsy in, 469
Mammography, **604-606**
  alternatives to, 605
Manganese, **250-251**
Mantoux test, 316-318
Maple syrup disease, urinalysis in, 321-324
Marasmic kwashiorkor, vitamin A levels in, 244-245
Measles
  capillary fragility test in, 110-111
  WBC count in, 102-103
Meconium ileus, sweat test findings in, 433-435
Medial meniscal lacerations, arthrography in, 609-611
Mediastinal abnormalities, radiography in, 548, 549-550t, 551
Mediastinal masses, CT scan in, 632-634
Mediastinitis, radiography of, 549-550t
Mediastinoscopy, **494**
Medullary or circumscribed carcinoma, breast biopsy in, 469
Megaloblastic anemia
  folic acid levels in, 245-246, 249-250
  vitamin B$_{12}$ levels in, 245-146, 249-250
Melanoma
  hCG urine levels in, 340-341
  sentinel lymph node biopsy in, 482-483
Melena, EGD in, 496-499

Mellituria, copper reduction test in, 369-370
Meningioma
  CT scan in, 616-618, 625-627, 631-632
  myelography in, 542-545
  orbital, radiography of, 545-546
  skull radiography in, 539-540
  sphenoid ridge, radiography of, 545-546
Meningitis, 45
  bacterial meningitis antigen in, 307-308
  CSF analysis in, 421-425
  EEG recording in, 671-673
  WBC count in, 102-103
Meningocele, CT scan of spine in, 625-627
Meniscal disorders, arthroscopy in, 508-512
Menkes' syndrome, ceruloplasmin levels in, 175
Menopause, 45
  estrogen levels in, 235-237
  LH levels in, 205-207
Menstrual abnormalities, pregnanediol urine levels in, 350-351
Mental retardation, EEG recording in, 671-673
Mesenteric arteriography, **580-583**
Metabolic acidosis, 45-46, 130t
  ABG findings in, 130t
  anion gap levels in, 139-140
  total carbon dioxide levels in, 132
Metabolic alkalosis, 46, 130t
  ABG findings in, 130t
  hypochloremic, sodium and chloride urine tests in, 376-377
  total carbon dioxide level in, 132
  urinalysis in, 321-324
Metabolic disorders, urine estrogen levels in, 337-339
Metabolic vertebral disorders, radiography in, 607-608
Metabolites, urine, **341-351**
Metachromatic leukodystrophy, urine ARSA levels in, 330-331
Metastasis, Raji cell assay in, 273
Metastatic bone tumor
  bone marrow aspiration and biopsy in, 474
  MRI scanning in, 629-630
  urine hydroxyproline levels in, 357-358
Metastatic carcinoma
  orbital CT scan in, 631-632
  urine calcium and phosphorus levels in, 379t
Metastatic disease, ADH levels in, 212-213
Metastatic neoplasms
  chest radiography of, 549-550t
  gallium scanning in, 656-658

Metastatic neoplasms *(continued)*
liver ultrasonography of, 526-528
myelography in, 542-545
MetHb. *See* Methemoglobin.
Methemoglobin, **101**
Methemoglobinemia, Hb M levels in, 101
Methotrexate, serum levels of, 749
MI. *See* Myocardial infarction.
Microaneurysms of eye, fluorescein angiography in, 546-548
Middle ear pathology, 716-717
Milk-alkali syndrome, urine calcium and phosphorus levels in, 379t
Minerals, urine test, **376-382**
Mitral insufficiency, 46, 696-701
Mitral stenosis, 46, 514-517
Mitral valve function, cardiac catheterization in, 696-701
Mitral valve prolapse, echocardiography in, 514-517
Monitoring and catheterization, **665-708**
Monitoring cerebral function, current techniques for, 620
Monocytes
influence of disease on, 106
values for, 104 , 746
Mononucleosis, 37-38
ALP levels in, 150
ALT levels in, 148
ANAs in, 277-279
anti-smooth-muscle antibodies, 281-282
AST levels in, 148
bone marrow aspiration and biopsy in, 478
cold agglutinins in, 285-286
haptoglobin levels in, 176
heterophil antibody in, 292-294
lymph node biopsy in, 481-482
monospot test for, 293
RF in, 284-285
VDRL test in, 310-311
WBC count in, 102-103
MonoVacc test, 316-318
Motion abnormalities, myocardial wall, cardiac blood pool imaging in, 650-651
Motion mode echocardiography, 514, 515, **516-517**
Motion sickness, 46
MRI. *See* Magnetic resonance imaging.
Mucocele, paranasal sinus radiography in, 552t
Mucopolysaccharidosis, acid mucopolysaccharides test in, 373-374
Multiple endocrine neoplasia, 46
VMA urine levels in, 347-348

Multiple jejunal diverticula, D-xylose absorption in, 741-742
Multiple myeloma, 46-47
bone biopsy in, 473
cold agglutinins in, 285-286
complement assays in, 273-275
ESR levels in, 88-89
hCG urine levels in, 340-341
KUB in, 583-584
PSP test in, 325-327
urinalysis in, 321-324
urine Bence Jones levels in, 353
urine calcium and phosphorus levels in, 379t
urine protein levels in, 351-352
urine uric acid levels in, 360
Multiple sclerosis, 47
evoked potential in, 674-675i, 676-677
external sphincter electromyography in, 731-733
MRI scan in, 618-621
Mumps, 47, 329-330
Muscle disease, urine myoglobin in, 362-363
Muscular dystrophy, 47
catecholamine levels in, 336-337
electromyography in, 677-679
Musculoskeletal system
CT scanning of, 625-629
MRI scanning of, 629-630
radiography of, **607-611**
Myasthenia gravis, 47
acetylcholine receptor antibodies in, 287-288
catecholamine levels in, 336-337
electromyography in, 677-679
HLA test in, 276-277
Tensilon test in, 733-735
Mycobacterial infections, gastric culture in, 449-451
Mycosis fungoides, 47, 304-306
Myeloblastic leukemia, urine lysozyme levels in, 331-332
Myelocele, CT scan in, 625-627
Myelocytic leukemia, vitamin B$_{12}$ levels in, 246-247
Myelofibrosis, bone marrow aspiration and biopsy in, 475
Myelography, **542-545**
Myeloid leukemia
urine ARSA levels in, 330-331
urine lysozyme levels in, 331-332
urine uric acid levels in, 360
Myelomonocytic leukemia, urine lysozyme levels in, 331-332
Myocardial fibrosis, Persantine-thallium imaging in, 649-650
Myocardial function, cardiac catheterization in, 696-701
Myocardial hypertrophy, Holter monitoring in, 691-693

Myocardial infarction, 48, 141-145
AAT levels in, 146
ALT levels in, 148
AST levels in, 146-148
CK levels in, 141-143
complement assays in, 273-275
ECG test in, 679, 681
FSP levels in, 120-121
GGT levels in, 152
Holter monitoring in, 691-693
LD levels in, 143-145
MRI scan in, 634-636
myoglobin levels in, 145
PA catheterization in, 701-704
pericardial fluid analysis in, 429-433
Persantine-thallium imaging in, 649-650
post, exercise electrocardiography stress test in, 685-686, 689
technetium pyrophosphate scanning in, 646-647
thallium imaging in, 647-648
urine myoglobin in, 362-363
WBC count in, 102-103
zinc levels in, 251-252
Myocardial ischemia
ECG test in, 679, 681
Holter monitoring in, 691-693
Myocardial scarring and perfusion, thallium imaging in, 647-648
Myocarditis, 48
cardiac blood pool imaging in, 650-651
Holter monitoring in, 691-693
Myoglobin, **145, 362-363**
Myoglobinuria, 363
Myxedema
D-xylose absorption in, 741-742
idiopathic, antithyroid antibodies, 282
17-KS urine levels in, 343-345
17-OHCS urine levels in, 342-343
Myxedema, thyroid imaging in, 642t

N

Narcolepsy, sleep studies in, 743-744
Nasopharyngeal culture, **442-443**
Near visual acuity, 710-711
Necrotizing enterocolitis, 49
Neonatal infections, HSV antibodies in, 297
Neonatal septicemia, gastric culture in, 449-451
Neonatal thyroid-stimulating hormone, **210-212**
Neoplasm
arteriography in, 580-583
chest radiography of, 549-550t
CT of liver and biliary tract, 621-623

Neoplasm *(continued)*
pericardial fluid analysis in, 429-433
pleural biopsy in, 461-462
retrograde ureteropyelography in, 590-592
skull radiography in, 539-540
Neoplastic disease, D-dimer values in, 124-125
Neovascularization, fluorescein angiography in, 546-548
Nephritis
urine calcium and phosphorus levels in, 379t
vitamin A levels in, 244-245
Nephrogenic diabetes insipidus
ADH levels in, 212-213
urinalysis in, 321-324
Nephrolithiasis, 321-324
Nephropathies, toxic, 351-352
Nephrosclerosis, 359-360
Nephrosis
glycosuria in, 369-372
17-KS urine levels in, 343-345
urinalysis in, 321-324
urine calcium and phosphorus levels in, 379t
Nephrotic syndrome, 49
aldosterone levels in, 334-335
cholesterol levels in, 168
phospholipid levels in, 168-169
triglyceride levels in, 166-167
urinalysis in, 321-324
urine copper levels in, 380-381
urine lysozyme levels in, 331-332
urine protein levels in, 351-352
Nephrotomography, **584-587**, 586t
Nervous system abnormalities, evoked potential in, 673, 674-675i, 676-677
Neuroblastoma
catecholamine levels in, 336-337
gallium scanning in, 656-658
HVA urine levels in, 348-349
VMA urine levels in, 347-348
Neurofibroma, myelography in, 542-545
Neurogenic bladder, 49-50
external sphincter electromyography in, 731-733
retrograde cystography in, 588-590
voiding cystourethrography in, 601-602
Whitaker test in, 602-604
Neurogenic bladder function, cystometry test in, 728, 731
Neurologic function, evoked potential in, 673, 674-675i, 676-677
Neurologic monitoring, **671-673**

Neurologic system
CT scanning in, **616-618**
MRI scanning in, **618-621**
radiography in, **539-545**
Neurosyphilis, CSF analysis in, 421-425
Neutrophils, 104, 105, 746
Nezelof syndrome, 50
Night blindness, vitamin A levels in, 244-245
Nitroprusside serum levels, 749
Nonobstructive jaundice
cholangiography in, 574-576
CT scan in, 621-623
ultrasonography in, 524-526
Nonseminiferous testicular tumor, AFP levels in, 314-315
Nonstress test, external fetal monitoring in, 666-668
Nonsyphilitic treponemal diseases, VDRL test in, 310-311
Nonsyphilitic treponemata, heterophil antibody tests in, 292-294
Nontoxic nodular goiter, thyroid biopsy in, 479-481
Nontrophoblastic tumor, hPL levels in, 241-242
Nonviral hepatitis, 50
Nortriptyline, serum levels of, 749
5'NT. *See* 5'-Nucleotidase.
Nuclear medicine scans, **639-664**
5'-Nucleotidase, **152-153**
Nystagmus, 50, 722-723

O

Oat cell carcinoma of the lungs. *See also* Lung cancer.
ACTH levels in, 197
calcitonin levels in, 221-222
Obesity, 50
Candida antibody in, 306-307
free cortisol levels in, 335-336
Obstructive jaundice
cholangiography in, 574-576
complement assays in, 273-275
CT scan of liver and biliary tract in, 621-623
ERCP in, 577-580
HIDA scan in, 662-664
ultrasonography in, 524-526
urobilinogen test in, 368
vitamin A levels in, 244-245
Obstructive sleep apnea syndrome, sleep studies in, 743-744
17-OHCS. *See* 17-hydroxycorticosteroids.
One-stage factor assay, **116-118**
Ophthalmoscopy, **712-715**
Optic disorders, orbital radiography of, 545-546
Optic nerve atrophy, ophthalmoscopy in, 712-715

Optic neuritis, 676-677, 712-715
Oral cholecystography, **572-574**
Oral glucose tolerance test, **188-190**
Oral lactose tolerance test, **191-192**
Orbital disorders
CT scan of, 631-632
radiography in, 545-546
Orbital radiography, **545-546**
Organ-specific biopsies, **479-488**
Organ transplantation
CMV antibody screen in, 298-299
parvovirus antibody in, 300-301
Orthostatic proteinuria, 321-324
Osgood-Schlatter disease, 51
Osmotic fragility, **90-91**
Osteoarthritis, 51
synovial fluid analysis in, 427-429
vertebral radiography in, 607-608
Osteoblastic metastasis, orbital radiography of, 545-546
Osteoblastoma, bone biopsy in, 473
Osteochondral fracture, arthroscopy in, 609-611
Osteochondritis dissecans, arthroscopy in, 609-611
Osteochondroma, bone biopsy in, 473
Osteoid osteoma, bone biopsy in, 473
Osteomalacia, 248-249, 379t
Osteomyelitis, 51, 539-540
Osteoporosis, 51
bone densitometry in, 608-609
other diagnostic tools, 609
vertebral radiography in, 607-608
Osteosarcoma, bone biopsy in, 473
Otoscopy, **716-717**
Outlet obstruction, retrograde urethrography in, 587-588
Ovarian agenesis, urine estrogen levels in, 337-339
Ovarian cancer, 52
CEA levels in, 313-314
hCG urine levels in, 240-241, 340-341
laparoscopy in, 506-508
metastatic, urine pregnanediol in, 350-351
urine estrogen levels in, 337-339
Ovarian cysts, 52
laparoscopy in, 506-508
progesterone levels in, 237-238
Ovarian function
estrogen levels in, 337-339
pregnanediol levels in, 350-351
Ovarian masses, ultrasonography in, 536
Ovary, lutein cell tumor of, 17-KS urine levels in, 343-345
Ovulation
LH secretion peaks at, 206i, 207
home testing for, 760i
Oxalate, urine, **382**

Oxygenation, pulse oximetry in, 707-708

Oxytocin challenge test, **420-421**

PQ

PA. *See* Pulmonary artery catheterization.

Pacemaker performance,
ECG test in, 679, 681
home testing for, 758i

Paget's disease, 52, 133
ALP levels in, 150
breast biopsy in, 469
calcium levels in, 133
orbital radiography of, 545-546
skull radiography in, 539-540
urine calcium and phosphorus levels in, 379t
urine hydroxyproline levels in, 357-358
vertebral radiography in, 607-608

Pancreas
anatomic abnormalities, ultrasonography of, 530-531
normal CT scan of, 624i
ultrasonography of, 530-531

Pancreatic abscess, gallium scanning in, 656-658

Pancreatic cancer, 52-53
AFP levels in, 314-315
cholangiography in, 574-576
CT scan in, 621-625
ERCP in, 577-580
fibrinogen levels in, 119-120
hCG levels in, 240-241, 340-341
hypotonic duodenography in, 570-572
ultrasonography in, 530-531
upper GI and small-bowel series in, 564-567
urine amylase levels in, 329-330

Pancreatic cysts, ERCP in, 577-580

Pancreatic duct obstruction, urine amylase levels in, 329-330

Pancreatic enzymes, **153-155**

Pancreatic fibrosis, 577-580

Pancreatic and gastric hormones, **232-235**

Pancreatic insufficiency, 382

Pancreatic lesions, 504-505

Pancreatic pseudocysts, 623-625

Pancreatitis
acute, 133, 152
amylase levels in, 329-330
CT scan in, 623-625
17-OHCS levels in, 342-343
alcoholic, CEA levels in, 313-314
AML levels in, 154
biliary system ultrasonography of, 524-526
calcium levels in, 133
cholesterol levels in, 168

Pancreatitis *(continued)*
chronic
CT scan in, 623-625
ERCP in, 577-580
hypotonic duodenography in, 570-572
plasma glucagon levels in, 235
urine amylase levels in, 329-330
CT scan of pancreas in, 623-625
GGT levels in, 152
glucagon levels in, 235
lipase levels in, 154-155
magnesium levels in, 135
MetHb, levels in, 101
peritoneal fluid analysis in, 390-393
phospholipid levels in, 168-169
ultrasonography in, 530-531
upper GI and small-bowel series in, 564-567
urine amylase levels in, 329-330
vitamin D_3 levels in, 248-249

Panhypopituitarism
17-KGS urine levels in, 346
17-KS urine levels in, 343-345
progesterone levels in, 238-240

PAP. *See* Papanicolaou test; Pulmonary artery pressure measurement.

Papanicolaou test, **414-416**

Papillary stenosis, 577-580

Papilla of Vater carcinoma, cholangiography in, 574-576

Papilledema, fluorescein angiography in, 546-548

Paracardiac masses, cardiac MRI scan in, 634-636

Paragonimiasis, sputum examination in, 384-385

Paranasal sinus disease, 551-553

Paranasal sinus radiography, **551-553, 552t**

Parasitic infection
of bladder, urinalysis in, 321-324
parasite test for, 393-395
peritoneal fluid analysis in, 390-393
pulmonary, sputum examination of, 384-385
WBC differential in, 103-107

Parathyroid function
tubular reabsorption of phosphate test in, 328-329
urine levels in, 332-334

Parathyroid hormone, **214-223**, 223i

Parenchymal pulmonary disease, biopsy in, 460-461

Parkinson's disease, 53
evoked potential in, 676-677
external sphincter electromyography in, 731-733

Paroxysmal nocturnal hemoglobinuria
Ham test in, 275-276
hemoglobinuria in, 361-362
hemosiderin levels in, 381-382

Parvovirus B-19 antibody, **300-301**

Parvovirus B-19 aplastic crisis, 300-301

Patellar disease, arthroscopy in, 508-512

Paternity testing, 276-277

Pathogen detection, lymphocyte transformation tests in, 265, 267

Pathologic fracture, bone scan in, 651-653

PAWP. *See* Pulmonary artery wedge pressure.

Pedal-brachial index, 521

Pelvic disease, ultrasonography in, 532-533

Pelvic inflammatory disease, 53
laparoscopy in, 507-508

Pelvic ultrasonography, **532-533**

Peptic ulcer, 53
arteriography in, 580-583
EGD in, 496-499
gastric culture and, 449-451
Helicobacter pylori in, 449-451

Percutaneous liver biopsy, **465-467**

Percutaneous renal biopsy, **485-488**

Percutaneous transhepatic cholangiography, **574-576**

Perforated intestine, peritoneal fluid analysis in, 390-393

Perforated ulcer, 329-330, 549-550t

Pericardial disease, cardiac MRI scan in, 634-636

Pericardial effusion
echocardiography in, 514-517
pericardial fluid analysis in, 429-433

Pericardial fluid analysis, **429-433**

Pericardiocentesis, 429-433, 430i

Pericarditis, 54
ECG test in, 679, 681
pericardial fluid analysis in, 429-433

Perineal hypospadias, retrograde urethrography in, 587-588

Perinephric abscess
gallium scanning in, 656-658
retrograde ureteropyelography in, 590-592

Perinephric inflammation, retrograde ureteropyelography in, 590-592

Peripheral artery disease, Doppler ultrasonography in, 519-522

Peripheral nerve disease, evoked potential in, 673, 674-675i, 676-677

Peripheral vascular disease, cold agglutinins in, 285-286

Peritoneal fluid analysis, **390-393,**
    392t
Peritonitis, 54, 390-393
Peritubal adhesions, hysterosalpin-
    gography in, 606-607
Pernicious anemia, 54
    bone marrow aspiration and
        biopsy in, 474
    fecal urobilinogen in, 398-399
    gastric acid stimulation test in,
        389-390
    gastrin levels in, 234
    gastric secretion test in, 387-389
    hemosiderin levels in, 381-382
    RBC survival time test, 658-660
    reticulocyte count in, 89-90
    siderocyte stain in, 99
    urine uric acid levels in, 360
Persantine-thallium imaging,
    649-650
PET. *See* Positron emission tomogra-
    phy.
Pharyngeal muscular disorders, bari-
    um swallow in, 562-564
Pharyngitis, 54, 441-442
Phenobarbital serum levels, 749
Phenolsulfonphthalein excretion test,
    325-327
Phenylalanine screening, **178-179**
Phenylketonuria, 54, 178-179,
    321-324
Phenytoin serum levels, 749
Pheochromocytoma, 54-55. *See also*
    Adrenal medullary tumor.
    catecholamine levels in, 336-337
    glucagon levels in, 235
    hPL levels in, 241-242
    HVA urine levels in, 348-349
    urinalysis in, 321-324
    VMA urine levels in, 347-348
Phlebography, **560-562**
Phosphates, **135-136,** 746
Phospholipids, **168-169**
Phosphorus imbalance, 55, 379t
Photosensitivity reaction, 55
Phrenic nerve paresis, chest radiogra-
    phy of, 549-550t
PID. *See* Pelvic inflammatory
    disease.
Pigmented villonodular synovitis,
    synovial membrane biopsy
    in, 478-479
Pigments, **182-184, 361-369**
Pinworms, collection of, 400
Pituitary diabetes insipidus, ADH
    levels in, 212-213
Pituitary dysfunction
    concentration and dilution tests
        in, 327-328
    hGH levels in, 199
    insulin tolerance test in, 201-202
    prolactin levels in, 207-209
    urine estrogen levels in, 337-339

Pituitary hormones, **196-214**
Pituitary tumor, 55
    ADH levels in, 212-213
    alpha-PGH levels in, 213-214
    arginine test in, 203
    free cortisol levels in, 335-336
    hGH levels in, 199
    17-OHCS urine levels in, 342-343
    orbital radiography of, 545-546
    prolactin levels in, 207-209
    skull radiography in, 539-540
Pityriasis rosea, 55
PK. *See* Pyruvate kinase.
PKU. *See* Phenylketonuria.
Placenta, trophoblastic neoplasm of,
    hCG levels in, 240-241
Placental estriol, **339-340**
Placental function during pregnancy
    estrogen levels in, 237-238
    hPL levels in, 241-242
    urine estriol levels in, 339-340
    urine pregnanediol levels in,
        350-351
Placental hormones, **240-242**
Placenta previa, 55, 532-533
Planigraphy, **554-555**
Plasma amino acid screening,
    177-178
Plasma ammonia, **179-180**
Plasma atrial natriuretic factor, **231**
Plasma calcitonin, **221-222**
Plasma catecholamines, **227-228**
Plasma cortisol, **225-227**
Plasma fibrinogen, **119-120**
Plasma glucagon, 235
Plasma luteinizing hormone,
    205-207, 207i
Plasma plasminogen, **122-123**
Plasma progesterone, **237-238**
Plasma renin activity, **157-159**
Plasma thrombin time, **118-119**
Platelet activity, **107-113**
Platelet aggregation, **111-113,** 746
Platelet function disorder, 56
Platelet count, 107-108, 746
Pleural biopsy, **461-462**
Pleural effusion, 56
    CT scan in, 623-625,632-634
    radiography in, 549-550t
    thoracentesis for, 385-387
    thoracoscopy in, 495-496
Pleural fluid analysis, **385-387**
Pleurisy, 56, 549-550t
Pneumocystis carinii pneumonia, 56
    bronchoscopy in, 490-493
Pneumonia, 56
    cold agglutinins in, 285-286
    HSV antibodies in, 297
    lung ventilation scan in, 645-646
    plasma fibrinogen levels in,
        119-120
    radiography in, 548, 549-550t,
        551
    sputum culture and, 444-446

Pneumonitis
    lung perfusion scan in, 643-644
    sputum examination for ova and
        parasites, 384-385
Pneumothorax, 56
    radiography of, 548, 549-550t,
        551
PNH. *See* Paroxysmal nocturnal
    hemoglobinuria.
Polyarteritis nodosa, urinalysis in,
    321-324
Polycystic disease, KUB in, 583-584
Polycystic kidney disease, 57
    creatinine clearance in, 359-360
    CT scan in, 636-638
    excretory urography in, 594-596
    radionuclide imaging in, 660-662
    urinalysis in, 321-324
    urine creatinine levels in, 358
Polycystic ovary syndrome. *See* Stein-
    Leventhal syndrome.
Polycythemia, 57
    EPO levels in, 230
    ESR levels in, 88-89
    Hb levels in, 92-93
    HCT levels in, 86-87
    RBC levels in, 85-86
Polycythemia vera, 57
    capillary fragility in, 110-111
    platelet aggregation in, 111-113
    platelet count in, 108-110
    urine lysozyme levels in, 331-332
    urine uric acid levels in, 360
Polyps
    barium enema in, 567-570
    colonoscopy in, 499-501
    sinus radiography in, 552t
Polysomes, 404-405t
Polysomnography, **743-744**
Pontine tumor, MRI in, 618-621
Porphyria, 57-58
    urine porphyrin levels in,
        363-365, 364t, 366
Porphyrins, urine, **363-365,** 364t
Portal hypertension
    arteriography in, 580-583
    liver-spleen scan in, 653, 655-656
Positron emission tomography
    of brain, 618
    of heart, 635t
Posterolateral sclerosis, vitamin
    B_{12} levels in, 246-247
Postmenopausal bleeding, vaginal
    ultrasonography in, 536
Postmenopausal women, FSH levels
    in, 204-205
Postoperative cholangiography,
    576-577
Postpartum pituitary infarction,
    prolactin levels in, 209
Poststreptococcal glomerulonephri-
    tis, antistreptolysin-O test,
    301-302

Potassium, 736
  serum, **137-138**
  urine, **377-378**
Pott's disease. *See* Tuberculosis.
Precocious puberty, 58
  estrogen levels in, 235-237
  FSH levels in, 204-205
  testosterone levels in, 238-240
Preeclampsia
  FSP levels in, 120-121
  plasma plasminogen levels in, 122-123
  pregnanediol urine levels in, 350-351
  urine levels of placental estriol, 339-340
Pregnancy, 58
  abnormal, vaginal ultrasonography in, 536
  anomalies of, AFP levels in, 314-315
  antibody screening test in, 261-262
  Candida antibody in, 306-307
  carotene levels in, 244-245
  cold agglutinins in, 285-286
  CST in, 420-421
  CVS testing in, 410
  detection of, hCG urine levels in, 340-341
  early, hCG levels in, 240-241
  ectopic, laparoscopy in, 507-508
  ectopic, hCG levels in, 22, 240-241, 340-341
  ectopic, ultrasonography in, 536
  ESR levels in, 88-89
  fetal-maternal blood transfer, detection of, 257-258
  folic acid levels in, 249-250
  FTA-ABS test in, 311-312
  glycosuria in, 369-372
  high risk, urine levels of placental estriol in, 339-340
  17-KS urine levels in, 343-345
  late, D-dimer values in, 124-125
  multiple
    hCG levels in, 240-241, 340-341
    placental estriol levels in, 339-340
  pelvic ultrasonography in, 532-533
  placental location
    D-dimer values in, 124-125
    ultrasonography in, 536
    vitamin C levels in, 247-248
  premature rupture of membranes in, **59**
  Rh immune globulin injection in, 256-258, 261-262
  Rh isoimmunization during, placental estriol levels in, 339-340

Pregnancy *(continued)*
  urine aldosterone levels in, 334-335
  urine estriol levels in, 339-340
  vaginal ultrasonography in, 536
  vitamin B_{12} levels in, 246-247
  vitamin C levels in, 247-258
Pregnancy, home testing for, 761i
Pregnanediol, **350-351**
Pregnanetriol, **341-342**
Premature labor, 59, 236
Premature ventricular contractions, Holter monitoring in, 691-693
Pressure study, **602-604**
Primary aldosteronism, 135
  chloride levels in, 134
  magnesium levels in, 135
  renin levels in, 158
  total carbon dioxide levels in, 132
Primary bone tumor, skeletal MRI scanning in, 629-630
Primary hyperparathyroidism, tubular reabsorption of phosphate in, 328-329
Primary hypogonadism. *See* Turner's syndrome.
Primary hypothyroidism, TSH levels in, 209-212
Procainamide, serum levels of, 750
Proctosigmoidoscopy, **501-504**
Prolactin, **207-209**
Propafenone, serum levels of, 750
Prostate cancer, 59, 155
  ACP levels in, 155-156
  plasma fibrinogen in, 119-120
  prostate gland biopsy in, 469-471
Prostate gland biopsy, **469-471**
Prostate-specific antigen, **156-157**
Prostatitis, 59-60, 471
Prostatovesiculitis, urinalysis in, 321-324
Protein, serum and urine values, 747
Protein C, **123**
Protein-calorie malnutrition, 60
Protein electrophoresis, **173-175,** 174i
Protein levels, abnormal, implications of, 174i
Proteins, urine, **351-352**
Proteins and protein metabolites, **173-182, 351-368**
Prothrombin time, **114-115,** 746
Proximal tubular function, urine lysozyme levels in, 331-332
PSA. *See* Prostate-specific antigen.
Pseudocysts, ERCP in, 577-580
Pseudogout, 427-429, 478-479
Pseudohypoparathyroidism, urine levels in, 332-334
Pseudotumor, renal angiography in, 596-598

PSP. *See* Phenolsulfonphthalein excretion test.
PT. *See* Prothrombin time.
Pteroylglutamic acid, **249-250**
PTH. *See* Parathyroid hormone.
Pulmonary abscess, 549-550t
Pulmonary angiography, **557-558**
Pulmonary arteriography, **557-558**
Pulmonary artery catheterization, **701-704**
Pulmonary artery pressures, cardiac catheterization in, 696-701
Pulmonary artery pressure measurement, 701-704
Pulmonary artery wedge pressure, 701-704
Pulmonary disease
  bronchography in, 555-557
  chest radiography in, 548, 549-550t, 551
  fluoroscopy test in, 553-554
  pulmonary function tests in, 736-737, 740-741
Pulmonary edema, 61, 701-704
Pulmonary embolism, 61
  angiography in, 557-558
  cold agglutinins in, 285-286
  D-dimer values in, 124-125
  FSP levels in, 120-121
  impedance plethysmography in, 695-696
  lung perfusion scan in, 643-644
  lung ventilation scan in, 645-646
Pulmonary function tests, **736-737,** 738-740t, **740-741**
Pulmonary hypertension, 61
Pulmonary infarction, 61
Pulmonary infection, bronchoscopy diagnosis of, 491-493
Pulmonary lesions
  bronchography in, 555-557
  chest radiography of, 548, 549-550t, 551
  lung biopsy in, 460-461
Pulmonary vascular abnormalities, angiography in, 557-558
Pulmonary volume tests, **736-737,** 738-740t, **740-741**
Pulmonic valve function, cardiac catheterization in, 696-701
Pulse oximetry, **707-708**
Pure tone audiometry, 719-722
  interpretation of, 720i
  speech audibility and, 722t
Purified Protein Derivative test, 316-318
Purpura fulminans, protein C deficiency in, 123
Purpura senilis, capillary fragility in, 110-111
PVC. *See* Premature ventricular contractions.

Pyelonephritis
acute
ultrasonography in, 533-535
urine lysozyme levels in,
331-332
bilateral chronic
creatinine clearance in,
359-360
urine creatinine levels in, 358
chronic
renal angiography in, 596-598
urine protein levels in, 351-352
excretory urography in, 594-596
hemoglobinuria in, 361-362
renal angiography in, 596-598
renal biopsy in, 485-486, 488
renal imaging in, 660-662
urinalysis in, 321-324
Pyelonephrosis, antegrade pyelography in, 592-594
Pyloric stenosis, EGD in, 496-499
Pyogenic infection, urinalysis in,
321-324
Pyrexia, urinalysis in, 321-324
Pyridoxin deficiency, urine oxalate
levels in, 382
Pyruvate kinase, **161-162**

R

Radiation enteritis, small-bowel
biopsy in, 465
Radioactive iodine uptake test,
640-641
Radioallergosorbent test, **275**
Radionuclide renal imaging,
660-663
Radionuclide thyroid imaging,
641-643
Radiopharmaceutical myocardial
perfusion imaging, **689-691**
RAIU. See Radioactive iodine uptake
test.
Raji cell assay, **273**
Rape victim, semen collection from,
417-420
Rapid corticotropin test, **197-199**
RAST. See Radioallergosorbent test.
Raynaud-like vascular symptoms,
cryoglobulins in, 286-287
Raynaud's syndrome, cold stimulation test for, **735-736**
RBC count. See Red blood cell count.
Rectal disorders
proctosigmoidoscopy in, 501-504
prostate gland biopsy in, 471
urine ARSA levels in, 330-331
Red blood cell count, **85-86**, 142i
serum, normal values in, 746
urine, normal values in, 747
Red blood cell survival time test,
658-669
Red cell indices, **87-88**, 746

Regional enteritis
jejunum, D-xylose absorption,
741-742
upper GI and small-bowel series
in, 564-567
Reiter's disease, synovial membrane
biopsy in, 478-479
Renal angiography, **596-598**
Renal anomalies, congenital, renal
CT scan in, 636-638
Renal artery obstruction, creatinine
clearance in, 359-360
Renal artery stenosis
radionuclide renal imaging in,
660-662
renal angiography in, 596-598
Renal calculi, 63
excretory urography in, 594-596
renal CT scan in, 636-638
routine urinalysis in, 321-324
Renal cancer
creatinine clearance in, 359-360
hemoglobinuria in, 361-362
nephrotomography in, 584-587
percutaneous renal biopsy in,
485-486, 488
renal angiography in, 596-598
renal CT scan in, 636-638
renal venography in, 598-601
retrograde ureteropyelography in,
590-592
Renal collecting system, retrograde
ureteropyelography in,
590-592
Renal disorders
advanced, urinalysis in, 321-324
angiography in, 596-598
biopsy in, 485-486, 488
BUN levels in, 180-181
capillary fragility test in, 110-111
creatinine levels in, 181
CT scan in, 636-638
excretory urography in, 594-596
ferritin levels in, 100-101
fractionated erythrocyte porphyrin levels in, 183-184
FSP levels in, 120-121
GGT levels in, 152
nephrotomography in, 584-587,
586t
PA catheterization in, 701-704
radionuclide imaging in, 660-662
retrograde ureteropyelography in,
590-592
sodium and chloride urine tests in,
376-377
urinalysis in, 321-324
urine amylase levels in, 329-330
urine protein levels in, 351-352
urine vitamin C levels in, 375-376
venography in, 598-601

Renal failure, 17
angiography in, 596-598
magnesium levels in, 135
renin levels in, 158
sweat test findings in, 433-435
urine potassium levels in, 377-378
zinc levels in, 251-252
Renal function, **726-733**
creatinine clearance in, 359-360
urine creatinine levels in, 358
Renal hormones, **224-231**
Renal hypertension, urinalysis in,
321-324
Renal hypertrophy, ultrasonography
in, 533-535
Renal impairment
concentration and dilution tests
in, 327-328
urine lysozyme levels in, 331-332
Renal insufficiency
creatinine clearance in, 359-360
hyperoxaluria in, 382
urine calcium and phosphorus
levels in, 379t
Renal obstruction
CT scan in, 636-638
Whitaker test in, 602-604
Renal plasma flow, PSP test in,
325-327
Renal transplantation
angiography in, 596-598
radionuclide imaging in, 660-662
rejection, FSP levels in, 120-121
ultrasonography in, 533-535
Renal trauma
angiography in, 596-598
urinalysis in, 321-324
Renal tuberculosis
creatinine clearance in, 359-360
excretory urography in, 594-596
urinalysis in, 321-324
Renal tubular acidosis, 63
urine calcium and phosphorus
levels in, 379t
urine potassium levels in, 377-378
Renal tubular degeneration, urinalysis in, 321-324
Renal tubular function, concentration and dilution tests,
327-328
Renal ultrasonography, **533-535**
Renal vascular disease
PSP test in, 325-327
urinalysis in, 321-324
Renal vein thrombosis, 63
biopsy in, 485-486, 488
urinalysis in, 321-324
venography in, 598-601
Renal venography, **598-601**
Renovascular hypertension, 63
excretory urography in, 594-596
radionuclide renal imaging in,
660-662

Renovascular hypertension
(continued)
renal angiography in, 596-598
renal venography in, 598-601
Reproductive system
biopsy tests in, **467-472**
endoscopy tests in, **505-508**
radiography of, **604-607**
specimen tests in, **402-421**
Respiratory acidosis, 63, 130t
ABG findings in, 130t
total carbon dioxide levels in, 132
Respiratory alkalosis, 63, 130t
ABG findings in, 130t
total carbon dioxide content in, 132
urinalysis in, 321-324
Respiratory distress syndrome, 64
Respiratory syncytial virus, 64, **296**
Respiratory system, **460-462**
endoscopy tests in, **490-496**
nuclear medicine scans in, **643-644**
radiography of, **548-558**
specimen tests in, **384-387**
Restless leg spasms, sleep studies in, 743-744
Reticulocyte count, **89-90**, 746
Retinal circulation, fluorescein angiography in, 546-548
Retinal detachment, 64, 712-715
Retinal edema, fluorescein angiography in, 546-548
Retinoblastoma, radiography of, 545-546
Retinopathy
evoked potential in, 676-677
fluorescein angiography in, 546-548
Retrograde cystography, **588-590**
Retrograde ureteropyelography, **590-592**
Retrograde urethrography, **587-588**
Retroperitoneal fibrosis, renal venography in, 598-601
RF. *See* Rheumatoid factor.
Rhesus factor typing, 256-257
Rheumatic fever, 65
acute, complement assays in, 273-275
antistreptolysin-O test in, 301-302
echocardiography in, 514-517
ESR levels in, 88-89
synovial fluid analysis in, 427-429
Rheumatoid arthritis, 65
antistreptolysin-O test in, 301-302
antithyroid antibodies in, 282
complement assays in, 273-275
D-xylose absorption in, 741-742
ESR levels in, 88-89

Rheumatoid arthritis *(continued)*
immune complex assays in, 271-272
juvenile, 65
lymph node biopsy in, 481-482
RF test in, 284-285
synovial membrane biopsy in, 478-479
TIBC levels in, 98-100
urine copper levels in, 380-381
VDRL test in, 310-311
vertebral radiography in, 607-608
zinc levels in, 251-252
Rheumatoid disease, pericardial fluid analysis in, 429-433
Rheumatoid factor, **284-285**, 747
RhIG. *See* Rh immune globulin.
Rh immune globulin, 256-257
Rib fracture, chest radiography of, 549-550t
Riboflavin, **245**
Rickets, vitamin D_3 levels in, 248-249
Rickettsial infections. *See* Rocky Mountain spotted fever.
Right atrial pressure, PA catheterization in, 701-704
Right bundle-branch block, ECG test in, 679, 681
Right ventricular function, PA catheterization in, 701-704
Rinne test, 717-719
Rocky Mountain spotted fever, 65
febrile agglutination tests in, 302-304
Rotator cuff tears, arthroscopy in, 609-611
Rotavirus gastroenteritis, stool examination for, 401-402
RSV. *See* Respiratory syncytial virus.
Rubella, 66
rubella antibodies in, 290-291
TORCH test in, 315-316
WBC count in, 102-103
Rubella, antibodies, **290-291**
Ruptured disk, 542-545, 607-608

S

Sahara Clinical Bone Sonometer, 609
SalEst test, 236
Salicylate, serum drug levels of, 750
Salicylate intoxication
INR values in, 125-126
urine potassium levels in, 377-378
Salicylate toxicity, sodium and chloride urine tests in, 376-377
Salivary duct obstruction, urine amylase levels in, 329-330
Salivary gland disorders, urine amylase levels in, 329-330
Salt-losing nephritis, sodium and chloride urine tests in, 376-377

Salt-losing syndrome, urine aldosterone levels in, 334-335
Sarcoidosis, 66, 165
ACE levels in, 165-166
ADH levels in, 212-213
evoked potentials in, 676-677
lung ventilation scan in, 645-646
mediastinoscopy in, 494
Persantine-thallium imaging in, 649-650
synovial membrane biopsy in, 478-479
urine calcium and phosphorus levels in, 379t
vitamin D_3 levels in, 248-249
Sarcoma, breast biopsy in, 469
Scarlatina, cold agglutinins in, 285-286
Scarlet fever, 66 , 110-111, 442-443
Schönlein-Henoch purpura, bleeding time in, 107-108
Schwabach test, 717-719
Scleroderma
ANAs in, 277-279
cold agglutinins in, 285-286
Scoliosis, 66-67
chest radiography of, 549-550t
vertebral radiography in, 607-608
Scurvy
capillary fragility in, 110-111
urinalysis in, 321-324
urine vitamin C levels in, 375-376
vitamin C levels in, 247-248
Seizure disorder
EEG recording in, 671-673
sleep studies in, 743-744
Semen analysis, **417-420**
Sensorimotor neuropathies, evoked potential in, 676-677
Sentinel lymph node biopsy, **482-484**
Septal defects, cardiac catheterization in, 696-701
Septicemia, 444-447
Septic shock, 67, 701-704
Serum enzyme and isoenzyme levels after MI, 142i, **329-334**
Serum sickness, acute, complement assays in, 273-275
Sex chromatin tests, **402-403**
Sex chromosome anomalies, 404-405t
Sexual development, abnormal, sex chromatin tests in, 402-403
Sexual precocity, male, testosterone levels in, 238-240
Sheehan's syndrome. *See* Postpartum pituitary infarction.
Shock, 321-324, 359-360
Shoulder abnormalities, arthroscopy in, 609-611
SIADH. *See* Syndrome of inappropriate antidiuretic hormone.

Sickle cell anemia, 68
ESR levels in, 88-89
fecal urobilinogen in, 398-399
hemoglobin electrophoresis in, 94, 96
hemoglobin levels in, 94-95
osmotic fragility in, 90-91
Raji cell assay in, 273
red blood cell survival time in, 658-660
urinalysis in, 321-324
zinc levels in, 251-252
Sickle cell disease, 94t
Sickle cell test, **95-96**
Sickle cell trait, 94-96
Sideroblastic anemia, bone marrow aspiration and biopsy in, 478
Siderocyte stain, 99
Sigmoid torsion, barium enema in, 567-570
Sigmoid volvulus, barium enema in, 567-570
Signal-averaged electrocardiography, **693-694**
Sinusitis, 69, 552t
Sinus tachycardia, 68-69, 701-704
Sjögren's syndrome, 69
ENAs in, 279-280
HLA test in, 276-277
Skeletal muscle trauma, myoglobinuria in, 363
Skeletal system
biopsy tests in, **472-479**
endoscopy tests in, **508-512**
radiography of, **607-611**
Skin biopsy, **484-485**
Skull radiography, **539-540**
SLE. See Systemic lupus erythematosus.
Sleep studies, **743-744**
Slit-lamp examination, **711-712**
Small-bowel biopsy, **464-465**
Small-bowel malabsorption syndrome, folic acid levels in, 249-250
Sodium, 746, 747
serum, **138-139**
urine, 139
Sodium and chloride, urine tests, **376-377**, 747
Soft-tissue tumor
skeletal CT scan in, 628-629
skeletal MRI scan in, 629-630
Soluble amyloid beta protein precursor, **425-427**
Somatotropin test, **199-200**
Soundscan 2000, 609
Special enzymes, **155-166**
Spherocytic anemia, congenital, siderocyte stain in, 99
Spherocytosis, hereditary, osmotic fragility in, 90-91

Spina bifida
amniotic fluid analysis in, 409-414
CT scan in, 625-627
Spinal abnormalities, CT scan in, 625-627
Spinal abscess, myelography in, 542-545
Spinal cord diseases, MRI scan in, 629-630
Spinal cord injury, external sphincter electromyography in, 731-733
Spinal cord lesions
CT scan in, 625-627
evoked potential in, 673, 674-675i, 676-677
Spinal fractures, chest radiography of, 549-550t
Spinal neoplasm, 70
Spinal nerve root injury, myelography in, 542-545
Spinal stenosis, myelography in, 542-545
Spinal tumor, CT scan in, 625-627
Spinocerebellar degeneration, evoked potential in, 676-677
Spleen, ultrasonography of, **528-530**
Spleen injury, acute, urine amylase levels in, 329-330
Splenic abscesses, liver-spleen scanning in, 653, 655-656
Splenic cysts, ultrasonography of, 528-530
Splenic infarcts, liver-spleen scanning in, 653, 655-656
Splenic metastasis, liver-spleen scanning in, 653, 655-656
Splenomegaly
liver-spleen scanning in, 653, 655-656
ultrasonography of, 528-530
Spondylolisthesis, vertebral radiography in, 607-608
Sprue, D-xylose absorption in, 741-742
Sputum culture, **444-446**
Sputum examination for ova and parasites, **384-385**
Squamous cell carcinoma, 70
skin biopsy in, 484-485
Staghorn calculus, KUB in, 583-584
Staphylococcemia, cold agglutinins in, 285-286
Starvation, 372-373, 377-378
Steatorrhea, 379t, 397-398
Stein-Leventhal syndrome
androstenedione levels in, 229-230
FSH levels in, 204-205
17-KS urine levels in, 343-345
LH levels in, 205-207
urine estrogen levels in, 337-339

Stenosis, cardiac catheterization in, 696-701
Stomach, gas distention of, chest radiography of, 549-550t
Stomach cancer
AFP levels in, 314-315
fibrinogen levels in, 119-120
gallium scanning in, 656-658
gastrin levels in, 234
Stomach ulcer, upper GI and small-bowel series in, 564-567
Stomatitis, 70
Stool culture, **439-441**
Stool examination for ova and parasites, **399-401**
Stool examination for rotavirus antigen, 401-402
Stratigraphy, **554-555**
Streptococcal infection, antistreptolysin-O test in, 301-302
Stress incontinence
electromyography in, 731-733
uroflowmetry test in, 726-728
Stress test, **685-687**, 688i, 689
Strictures, EGD and, 496-499
Strongyloidiasis, 70
duodenal parasites in, 393-395
sputum examination for ova and parasites, 384-385
Subacute bacterial endocarditis, routine urinalysis in, 321-324
Subacute granulomatous thyroiditis, thyroid biopsy in, 479-481
Subcapsular hematomas, CT of liver and biliary tract, 621-623
Subdural hematoma
chronic, skull radiography in, 539-540
CT scan in, 616-618, 631-632
Subluxations, 21
Subphrenic abscess, ultrasonography of, 528-530
Sudden death episode, electrophysiology studies in, 705-707
Sudden infant death syndrome, 71
Sugars, ketones, and mucopolysaccharides, **369-374**
Superficial thromboses, Doppler ultrasonography in, 519-522
Supraventricular arrhythmias, electrophysiology studies in, 705-707
Surgical ablation procedures, electrophysiology studies in, 705-707
Swan-Ganz catheterization, **701-704**
Sweat test, **433-435**
Syncope, electrophysiology studies in, 705-707
Syndrome of inappropriate antidiuretic hormone, ADH levels in, 71, 212-213

Synovial abnormalities, arthroscopy in, 609-611

Synovial cancer, synovial membrane biopsy in, 478-479

Synovial cysts, arthrography in, 609-611

Synovial disease, arthroscopy in, 508-512

Synovial fluid analysis, **427-429**

Synovial membrane biopsy, **478-479**

Synovial tumor, biopsy in, 478-479

Syphilis, 71
  ADH levels in, 212-213
  congenital, cold agglutinins in, 285-286
  FTA-ABS test in, 311-312
  heterophil antibody tests, 292-294
  RF in, 284-285
  VDRL test in, 310-311

Syringomyelia, myelography in, 542-545

Systemic infection
  Candida antibody in, 306-307
  HSV antibodies in, 297

Systemic lupus erythematosus, 145
  anti-double-stranded DNA antibodies in, 289-290
  antinuclear antibodies in, 277-279
  antithyroid antibodies, 282
  complement assays in, 273-275
  ENAs in, 279-280
  FTA-ABS test in, 311-312
  heterophil antibodies in, 292-294
  HLA test in, 276-277
  immune complex assays in, 271-272
  myoglobin levels in, 145
  pericardial fluid analysis in, 429-433
  RF in, 284-285
  synovial fluid analysis in, 427-429
  synovial membrane biopsy in, 478-479

Systolic murmur, PA catheterization in, 701-704

T

T₃. *See* Triiodothyronine.

T₄. *See* Thyroxine.

T- and B-lymphocyte assays, **264-265**

Tay-Sachs disease, 71, 162

TBG. *See* Thyroxine-binding globulin.

Technetium pyrophosphate scanning, **646-647**

TEE. *See* Transesophageal echocardiography.

Telescoping of the bowel, barium enema in, 567-570

Tensilon test, **733-735**

Tension pneumothorax, chest radiography of, 549-550t

Terminal deoxynucleotidyl transferase test, **267-269**

Testicular cancer, 71-72
  gallium scanning in, 656-658
  hCG urine levels in, 340-341
  17-KS urine levels in, 343-345
  urine estrogen levels in, 337-339

Testicular torsion, 72

Testosterone levels, luteinizing tumor, 238-240

Tetanus, 72

Tetralogy of Fallot, 72

Thalassemia, 72
  bone marrow aspiration and biopsy in, 478
  fecal urobilinogen in, 398-399
  Hb levels in, 94-95
  Heinz bodies in, 97-98
  osmotic fragility in, 90-91
  red cell indices in, 87-88
  siderocyte stain in, 99

Thallium imaging, **647-648**

Thallium scintigraphy, **647-648**

Theca cell tumor, pregnanediol urine levels in, 350-351

Theophylline, serum levels of, 750

Thiocyanate, serum levels of, 749

Thoracentesis. *See* Pleural effusion.

Thoracoscopy, **495-496**

Throat culture, **441-442**

Thrombasthenia, 110-113

Thrombin clotting time, **118-119**

Thrombin time, plasma, 746

Thrombocytopathia, bleeding time in, 107-108

Thrombocytopenia, 73
  bleeding time in, 107-108
  bone marrow aspiration and biopsy in, 474
  capillary fragility test in, 110-111
  cardiolipin antibody test in, 283-284
  folic acid levels in, 249-250
  platelet count in, 108-110

Thrombocytosis, platelet count in, 108-110

Thromboembolism, protein C deficiency in, 123

Thrombophlebitis, 73, 695-696

Thrombosis
  cerebral angiography in, 540-542
  D-dimer values in, 124-125
  FSP levels in, 120-121
  spontaneous, cardiolipin antibody test in, 283-284

Thrush, throat culture and, 441-442

Thymus, radiography of, 549-550t

Thyrocalcitonin, **221-222** *See also* Plasma calcitonin.

Thyroid, scans of, **640-641**

Thyroid adenomas, ultrasonography of, 531-532

Thyroid and parathyroid hormones, **214-223**

Thyroid biopsy, **479-481**

Thyroid cancer, 73
  biopsy in, 479-481
  imaging results in, 642t
  TSH levels in, 209-212
  ultrasonography in, 531-532

Thyroid cysts, ultrasonography of, 531-532

Thyroid disorders
  glycosuria in, 369-372
  hGH levels in, 199
  RAIU test in, 640-641
  thyroid biopsy in, 479-481
  thyroid imaging results in, 642t

Thyroid function, 640-643

Thyroid gland, 549-550t, 641-643

Thyroiditis, 73
  complement assays in, 273-275
  subacute, RAIU test in, 640-641

Thyroid medullary carcinoma, thyrocalcitonin levels in, 221-222

Thyroid-stimulating hormone, **209-212**

Thyroid-stimulating immunoglobulin, **282-283**

Thyroid suppressive therapy, ultrasonography in, 531-532

Thyroid ultrasonography, **531-532**

Thyrotoxicosis, TSI in, 282-283

Thyrotoxicosis. *See* Graves' disease.

Thyrotropin-releasing hormone, 209-212

Thyrotropin. *See* Thyroid-stimulating hormone.

Thyroxine, **214-215**, 746

Thyroxine-binding globulin, **216-217**

TIBC. *See* Iron and total iron-binding capacity.

Tine test, 316-318

Tobramycin, abnormal, normal serum drug levels of, 750

Tonsillitis, 73
  cold agglutinins in, 285-286
  WBC count in, 102-103

TORCH test, **315-316**

Torticollis, 73-74, 607-608

Total carbon dioxide content, **131-132**, 746

Total cholesterol, **167-168**, 746

Total fasting hemoglobin, **191**

Total hemoglobin, **92-93**

Total parenteral nutrition
  glycosuria in, 369-372
  ketonuria in, 372-373

Tourniquet test, **110-111**

Toxemia of pregnancy, urine aldosterone levels in, 334-335

Toxic nodular goiter, thyroid imaging tests in, 642t

Toxic renal tubular disease, glycosuria in, 369-372

Toxoplasmosis, 74, 315-316
Trace elements, **250-252**
Transcranial Doppler studies, **535-536**
Transesophageal echocardiography, **517-519**
Transferrin, **176-177**
Transfusion reaction, hemoglobinuria in, 361-362
Transient aplastic anemia, parvovirus B-19 antibody in, 300-301
Transplant recipients, CMV in, 456
Transverse myelitis, evoked potential in, 676-677
Traumatic injury, evoked potential in, 673, 676-677
Traumatic spinal cord injury, evoked potential in, 676-677
Treponema pallidum, tests for, 312
TRH. *See* Thyrotropin-releasing hormone.
Trichinosis, 75
Trichomoniasis, 75, 435-436
Trichuriasis, 75
Tricuspid insufficiency, 75
Tricuspid stenosis, 75
Tricuspid valve function, cardiac catheterization in, 696-701
Trigeminal neuralgia, 76
Triglycerides, **166-167**, 747
Triiodothyronine, **215-216**
Triiodothyronine toxicosis
FT$_4$ and FT$_3$ levels in, 218-219
T$_3$ levels in, 215-216
Triiodothyronine uptake, **217-218**
Tropical sprue, small-bowel biopsy in, 463, 465
Trypanosomiasis, cold agglutinins in, 285-286
Tryptophan challenge test, **374-375**
TSH. *See* Thyroid-stimulating hormone.
TSI. *See* Thyroid-stimulating immunoglobulin.
Tubal abnormalities, hysterosalpingography in, 606-607
Tubercle bacillus infection, tuberculin skin tests in, 316-318
Tuberculin skin tests, **316-318.** *See also specific test.*
Tuberculosis, 76
ADH levels in, 212-213
bronchoscopy in, 491-493
chest radiography of, 549-550t
ESR levels in, 88-89
extrapulmonary, 25
gastric culture in, 449-451
hemoglobinuria in, 361-362
lung ventilation scan in, 645-646
percutaneous liver biopsy in, 467
pericardial fluid analysis in, 429-433

Tuberculosis *(continued)*
peritoneal fluid analysis in, 390-393
pleural biopsy in, 461-462
prostate gland biopsy in, 471
RF in, 284-285
sputum culture in, 444-446
synovial fluid analysis in, 427-442
synovial membrane biopsy in, 478-479
thoracic CT scan in, 632-634
tuberculin skin tests for, 316-318
vertebral radiography in, 607-608
Tuberculosis, kidney, 331-332
Tubo-ovarian abscess, vaginal ultrasonography in, 536
Tubular epithelial damage, 327-328
Tubular function
PSP test in, 325-327
renal biopsy in, 485-486, 488
Tubular reabsorption of phosphate test, **328-329**
Tularemia, 76, 302-304
Tuning fork tests, **717-719**
Turner's syndrome
estrogen levels in, 235-237
features of, 404-405t
FSH levels in, 204-205
LH levels in, 205-207
Tympanic membrane abnormalities, 716-717, 717t
Typhoid fever
stool culture in, 439-441
WBC count in, 102-103
Typhus, 76, 302-304

U

Ulcerative bowel disease
colonoscopy in, 499-501
proctosigmoidoscopy in, 501-504
Ulcerative colitis, 76
barium enema in, 567-570
complement assays in, 273-275
gallium scanning in, 656-658
Raji cell assay in, 273
Ultrasonography
of cardiovascular system, **514-524**
of GI system, **524-531**
Unstable hemoglobin, **96-97**
Heinz bodies in, 97-98
Upper GI and small-bowel series, **564-567**
Upper respiratory tract pathogens, nasopharyngeal culture, 442-443
Ureter abnormalities, KUB in, 583-584
Ureteral calculi, excretory urography in, 594-596
Ureteral obstruction, radionuclide renal imaging in, 660-662

Ureterocele, voiding cystourethrography in, 601-602
Ureteropyelography, obstruction in, 591i
Urethral disorders
retrograde urethrography in, 587-588
voiding cystourethrography in, 601-602
Urethritis, urinalysis in, 321-324
Uric acid, 746
serum, **181-182**
urine, **360**
Urinalysis, 747
routine, **321-324**
Urinary calculi, **324-325**
Urinary incontinence, external sphincter electromyography in, 731-733
Urinary stones, **324-325**
Urinary system trauma, excretory urography in, 594-596
Urinary tract brush biopsy, 486
Urinary tract disease, excretory urography in, 594-596
Urinary tract infection
retrograde cystography in, 588-590
routine urinalysis in, 321-324
urine culture in, 438-439
urine protein levels in, 351-352
voiding cystourethrography in, 601-602
Urinary tract obstruction
PSP test in, 325-327
ultrasonography in, 533-535
urine creatinine levels in, 358
Urine blood pigments, bedside testing for, 362
Urine culture, **438-439**
Urine estrogens, **337-339**
Urine ketones, home testing for, 755i
Urine osmolality, 747
Urine specimen, home testing for
females, 754i
males, 753i
Urine tests, **319-382**
Urobilinogen, 367t, **368**, 747
Uroflowmetry, **726-728**, 727i
Urogenital secretions, for trichomonads, **435-436**
Uroporphyrinogen I synthase, **163-164**
Uterine disorders, hysterosalpingography in, 606-607
Uterine cancer, 76
gallium scanning in, 656-658
Uterine contractions, fetal monitoring of, 666-671
Uterine injuries, hysterosalpingography in, 606-607
UTI. *See* Urinary tract infection.

V

Vaginal cancer, 77, 656-658
Vaginal ultrasonography, **536**
Vaginitis, urinalysis in, 321-324
Valproic acid, serum levels of, 750
Valvular abnormalities, echocardiography in, 514-517
Valvular disease, transesophageal echocardiography in, 517-519
Valvular heart disease, cardiac catheterization in, 696-701
Valvular repairs, transesophageal echocardiography in, 517-519
Vancomycin, serum levels of, 750
Vanillylmandelic acid, 747
  urine, **347-348**
Varicella-zoster virus, HSV culture in, 455-457
Varices, 496-499, 562-564
Variola, 77, 545-546
Vascular disease
  arteriography in, 580-583
  cardiac MRI scan in, 634-636
  cerebral angiography in, 540-542
  cold stimulation test in, 735-736
  orbital radiography in, 545-546
  renal CT scan in, 636-638
Vascular lesions, EEG in, 671-673
Vascular malformations
  CT scan of spine in, 625-627
  renal angiography in, 596-598
Vascular tortuosity, fluorescein angiography in, 546-548
Vasectomy, semen analysis in, 417-420
Vasopressin-resistant diabetes insipidus, sweat test findings in, 433-435
Vasopressin. See Antidiuretic hormone.
VDRL. See Venereal Disease Research Laboratory test.
Venereal Disease Research Laboratory test, **310-311,** 747
Venous abnormalities, angiography in, 546-548
  congenital, 560-562
  ultrasonography in, 519-522
  venography in, 560-562, 598-601
Ventricular arrhythmias
  electrophysiology in, 705-707
  signal-averaged ECG in, 693-694
Verapamil, serum levels of, 750
Vertebral disorders, radiography in, 607-608
Vertebral radiography, **607-608**
Vesical diverticula, voiding cystourethrography in, 601-602
Vesical fistula, retrograde cystography in, 588-590

Vesical trabeculae, retrograde cystography in, 588-590
Vesicoureteral reflux, 80
  retrograde cystography in, 588-590
  voiding cystourethrography in, 601-602
Vestibular and cerebellar dysfunction, **722-723**
Viral disease, ANAs in, 277-279
Viral hepatitis, 31, 150-151
Viral infection, cold agglutinins in, 285-286
Virilism, 17-OHCS urine levels in, 342-343
Viruses, **290-301**
Visual acuity tests, **710-711**
Vitamin A and carotene, 80, **244-245**
Vitamin B_2, **245,** 246
Vitamin B_6 deficiency, 374-375
Vitamin B_{12}, 87-88, **246-247,** 465
Vitamin C, 80, **247-248,** 375
Vitamin D_3, 80, **248-249,** 379t
Vitamin K deficiency, 81
  capillary fragility test in, 110-111
  INR values in, 125-126
  PT time in, 114-115
Vitamins, **244-250**
  urine tests for, **374-375**
VMA. See Vanillylmandelic acid.
Voiding cystourethrography, **601-602**
Von Gierke's disease, ß-hydroxybutyrate levels in, 190
Von Willebrand's disease, 81, 110-113
VZV. See Varicella-zoster virus.

W

Waldenström's macroglobulinemia
  Bence Jones urine protein levels in, 353
  ESR levels in, 88-89
Wasting, 17-KGS urine levels in, 346
WBC count. See White blood cell count.
Weber test, 717-719
Wegener's granulomatosis, paranasal sinus radiography of, 552t
Whipple's disease
  D-xylose absorption in, 741-742
  small-bowel biopsy in, 463, 465
Whitaker test, **602-604**
White blood cell count, **102-103**
  urine, normal values in, 747
White blood cell differential, **103-107,** 746
Whooping cough, 81-82, 441-442
Wilms' tumor, 82
  gallium scanning in, 656-658
  percutaneous renal biopsy in, 485-486, 488

Wilson's disease, 82
  ceruloplasmin levels in, 175
  urine copper levels in, 380-381
  urine uric acid levels in, 360
Wolff-Parkinson-White syndrome, Holter monitoring in, 691-693
Wound culture, **447-449**
Wound infection, wound culture and, 447-449
Wryneck. See Torticollis.

XY

Xerophthalmia, vitamin A levels in, 244-245

Z

Zinc deficiency, 82, 251-252
Zinc test, **251-252**
Zinc toxicity, 251-252
Zollinger-Ellison syndrome, 234
  basal gastric secretion test in, 387-389
  gastric acid stimulation test in, 389-390